Veterinary
TREATMENTS
&
MEDICATIONS
for Horsemen

All Rights Reserved

Last printed 2001

ISBN 0-935842-01-2
Copyright ©1977 by Equine Research, Inc.
P.O. Box 8618   Tyler, Texas 75711-8618

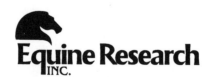

Equine Research
INC.

P.O. Box 8618   Tyler, Texas 75711-8618
(U.S. & Canada) (800) 848-0225
(Other Countries) (903) 894-9203

WRITTEN BY:

the research staff of Equine Research Publications

VETERINARY RESEARCH EDITORS:
H. Richard Adams, D.V.M., Ph.D. and
Lorraine W. Chalkley, M.S., D.V.M.

EQUINE PRACTICE EDITOR:
Terrell M. Buchanan, D.V.M.

EDITOR/PUBLISHER:
Don M. Wagoner

ACKNOWLEDGEMENT

Equine Research Publications wishes to express sincere appreciation to:

W. L. Anderson, D.V.M. (Equine Practitioner; President, A.V.M.A., 1977-1978)
S.L. Burns, D.V.M. (Equine Clinician)
W.C. McMullan, D.V.M. (Equine Clinician)
E.L. Morris, D.V.M. (Diplomate, American College of Veterinary Radiology)
N.C. Ronald, Ph.D. (Parasitologist)
M.L. Ward, D.V.M. (Equine Practitioner)

for their technical contributions and invaluable assistance in the preparation of this book.

TABLE OF CONTENTS

INTRODUCTION

VETERINARY TREATMENTS AND MEDICATIONS FOR HORSEMEN is a unique and unprecedented text designed to bridge the communication barrier between the horseman and veterinary medical science. It is a necessary guide for serious horsemen that contains numerous detailed treatment procedures and a comprehensive introduction to veterinary medications and pharmacology. Abundant photographs and illustrations, as well as an informative glossary, appendix and extensive index enhance its instructive nature. This book also comprehensively describes procedures the veterinarian may perform, enabling the horseman to understand more clearly the rationale behind the veterinarian's prescribed treatment.

VETERINARY TREATMENTS AND MEDICATIONS FOR HORSEMEN is the companion text to **THE ILLUSTRATED VETERINARY ENCYCLOPEDIA FOR HORSEMEN**. Whereas **THE ILLUSTRATED VETERINARY ENCYCLOPEDIA FOR HORSEMEN** contains detailed descriptions and explanations of various equine ailments and disorders, **VETERINARY TREATMENTS AND MEDICATIONS FOR HORSEMEN** describes the treatment procedures and techniques that are employed after the horse's dysfunction has been diagnosed.

Since a major objective of this text is to facilitate communication between the horseman and the veterinarian, medical and scientific terms are presented throughout the book in conjunction with common names. Specific topics are listed in the index in association with related subtopics in order to enable the horseman to quickly locate information on any condition and its associated treatment. Every effort has been made to provide scientifically accurate information in a format that will be of optimum usefulness to the horseman both for interesting and enjoyable reading and as a technical reference source. The single most important goal of **VETERINARY TREATMENTS AND MEDICATIONS FOR HORSEMEN** is to aid the horseman in providing his horses the very best health care possible.

DISCLAIMER

To insure the reader's understanding of some technical descriptions offered in **VETERINARY TREATMENTS AND MEDICATIONS FOR HORSEMEN**, brand names have been occasionally used as examples of particular substances or equipment. However, the use of a particular trademark or brand name is not intended to imply an endorsement of that particular product, or to suggest that similar products offered by others under different names may be inferior. Nothing contained in **VETERINARY TREATMENTS AND MEDICATIONS FOR HORSEMEN** is to be construed as a suggestion to violate any trademark laws.

Although every effort was made to present scientifically accurate and up-to-date information based on the best available and reliable sources, it should be appreciated that results of medical treatments depend upon a variety of factors (including proper diagnosis) not under the control of the publishers of this book. Therefore, Equine Research Publications assumes no responsibility for and makes no warranty with respect to results that may be obtained from the procedures described herein. Equine Research Publications shall not be liable to any person for damage resulting from reliance on any information contained in **VETERINARY TREATMENTS AND MEDICATIONS FOR HORSEMEN**, whether with respect to diagnosis, treatment procedures, drug usages and dosages, or by reason of any misstatement or inadvertent error contained herein.

Also, it must be remembered that Equine Research Publications does not manufacture, package, ship, label or sell any of the drugs or appliances which are discussed in this book. Accordingly, Equine Research Publications cannot be responsible for the results that may be obtained with products manufactured by others.

The horseman is encouraged to read and follow the directions published by the manufacturer of each product or drug which may be mentioned herein. And, if there is a conflict, the manufacturer's instructions should, of course, be followed.

I. GENERAL CARE & ROUTINE PROCEDURES

1

PHYSICAL EXAMINATION OF THE HORSE

The Importance of Good Health Records

Comprehensive and accurate records are an invaluable part of any horseman's operation. These records should be sufficiently detailed to provide any pertinent information required, and their recording should be systematic. Specialized horseowner's recordbooks or file folders are available for this purpose and should be used in a professional horse enterprise. A satisfactory substitute, however, can be made for an individual horseowner from a calendar that has space for notes under each date. For the sake of continuity and order, all relevant information should be consistently logged, and there should be a specific location where these records are kept.

It must be stressed that continuity of the record keeping system is important, for it is through such an approach that the compiled information is made easily transferable. In the event that there is a change in the operation's ownership or management, such transferable data will be greatly desired.

IDENTIFICATION RECORDS

Record keeping should begin with identification of each horse. The description of every animal should be accurate and complete enough so that each horse could be easily identified by a person unfamiliar with it. Necessarily, each description must include information on the horse's age, breed, sex, color and markings, permanent scars, etc. (refer to "Identification.") These identification records, the horse's health certificate, and other related papers can be kept with the animal's record book in a safe and convenient place.

HEALTH MAINTENANCE ENTRIES

Complete records of maintenance treatments given to each horse should be kept, since the horseowner's memory will almost never suffice for accuracy. Some of the data that should be included in the maintenance records are listed below:

1. vaccination dates, types of vaccines
2. deworming dates, anthelmintics used
3. dates of hoof trimmings, dates of shoeings, special shoes applied
4. dental treatments
5. medications and dates given; dietary changes
6. dates of illnesses and injuries

Breeding farms, of course, will require additional information on the following:

1. teasing
2. breeding dates
3. palpation
4. speculum examinations
5. stallion semen evaluations
6. foaling dates, etc.

Such records will not only serve as a reminder of when it is time to deworm, retrim, or revaccinate a horse, but, additionally, will aid the veterinarian. Suppose, for example, that a heavily parasitized horse has been dewormed with an organophosphate anthelmintic and develops an impaction from the massive number of dead worms. If the veterinarian is informed of the type of anthelmintic used, he will not administer a phenothiazine-derived tranquilizer to the animal. (Such action could cause serious side effects; refer to "Drugs and Related Topics.")

Anytime a change in a horse's appearance or behavior is noticed, a notation should be made, since such changes may indicate an impending illness. If a horse's daily routine is rearranged, or if his diet (amount of feed, time of feeding, proportions of grain to hay, feed and forages used, etc.) is adjusted, an entry recording this action should be made as well. Proper notation in these instances is important, for sometimes a difference in stable management will precipitate an ailment (colic, for example). An attending veterinarian, consequently, would need to know of such changes in order to determine the probable cause of the horse's illness.

RECORDING DISEASE AND INJURY TREATMENTS

When a veterinarian is required to examine a horse for suspected illness or injury, complete records of all disease and injury treatments should be at hand to assist the attending doctor with his diagnosis and treatment, thereby possibly saving an animal's life. There are several sound reasons for this. For instance, some medicines are antagonistic, meaning that one cancels the effect of another. If medication has been administered to a horse as part of a first aid treatment, the attending veterinarian would probably not want to administer one of the drugs antagonistic to it. Other medicines are synergistic, meaning that their combined effect is multiplied,

HEALTH AND VACCINATION RECORD

| name of horse | breed | reg. no. | color and markings |

| foaling date | owner | address |

Record information on worming in the space provided below. The type of worm medicine is important because they are selective in action.

date	veterinarian	anthelmintic

Record information on trimming and shoeing in the space provided below. Include information on corrective trimming.

date	farrier	work done

Record information on vaccinations in the space provided below. The necessity for vaccination against each disease varies from one geographical location to another. The advice of a veterinarian should be sought.

WEE/EEE   VEE

date	veterinarian

TETANUS

date	veterinarian

RHINO   INFLUENZA

date	veterinarian

OTHERS

date	veterinarian	disease

MEDICAL RECORD

Record information on each veterinary visit in the space provided below with as much information on the nature of the problem as possible.

DATE	DESCRIPTION OF ILLNESS OR PROCEDURE

Fig. 1-1   Health and vaccination record.

and, when a horse has been premedicated with certain substances, a synergistic effect may result from the combination of added drugs. Such a response could be more exaggerated and dangerous than might normally be expected. (Refer to "Drugs and Related Topics" for more information about the interaction of medications.)

Therefore, to facilitate safe treatment, medical records for every horse that has required previous treatment should always be available. These records might contain information regarding the horse's temperature, his past physical examinations and lab test results, and all medications given (brand, concentration, dosage, and time administered). The horseman, to supplement these records, must enter in each horse's health record any other first aid treatments given to an animal before the veterinarian's arrival.

As a final consideration, medical records of past treatments are particularly valuable when a veterinarian new to a horse must attend the animal, especially in an emergency. For a veterinarian to decide whether to give a horse that has suffered a puncture wound tetanus antitoxin or tetanus toxoid, he must know if the animal has been on a regular program of immunization, and how long it has been since the last toxoid injection (refer to "Vaccination Program"). Also, in treating chronic problems, a pattern of illness or lameness, etc., may become apparent when a horse's total medical record is considered, thus aiding veterinary diagnosis and treatment.

MAINTAINING OTHER RECORDS

In addition to those already mentioned, other records should be kept. Complete records are also required for insurance purposes. And finally, if the horse operation is a business, rather than a hobby, records are needed for tax purposes.

The Importance of a Good Case History

A good case history is quite helpful and often essential to a veterinarian in the differential diagnosis of equine diseases. This case history will include the following detailed and specific information:

1. the horse's age, breed, color and sex; whether castrated or intact
2. the horse's vaccination history
3. records of past illnesses and injuries
4. records of past medications
5. schedule of the horse's deworming dates
6. dental records
7. records of the horse's diet and stabling
8. records of the horse's use

9. the horse's origin and date acquired by present owner

10. information on nearby horses with similar problems

In making a diagnosis, the veterinarian will consider the horseman's major complaint, and will make a systematic, thorough physical examination of the horse to make certain that any factor contributing to the problem is not overlooked.

In his attempt to secure a good case history, a veterinarian might ask questions about things that seem unrelated, but may in fact be pertinent to an accurate diagnosis. (A careful reading of the section on "Vital Functions" will enable the horseowner to more effectively communicate with the veterinarian.) In answering these questions, it is best to be accurate, objective, and complete. There should be no exaggeration of signs or minimizing of the length of time that a horse has shown signs of illness. Non-objective information that seems to conflict with the results of a horse's physical examination will only cause confusion and perhaps give an unfavorable impression of your responsibility as a horseman.

Vital Functions

The vital parameters of temperature, pulse, respiration, mucosa color, skin pliability, urine, feces, and gut sounds are all excellent indicators of a horse's general health and physical condition. Because of this, a familiarity with these normal vital signs can help an individual determine whether or not an animal requires a veterinarian's attention, and subsequently enable him to supply the veterinarian with a more informed report on the horse's condition. (Refer to "Normal Vital Function Values of the Horse" in the Appendix for more information.)

Other than the above, it is also important to tell the veterinarian of any marked loss of appetite, depression, nasal discharge, coughing, swelling, or abnormal behavior recently shown by the horse.

TEMPERATURE

The normal temperature of an adult horse at rest is approximately 100.4°F (38°C), although it can vary from 99.5° to 101.5°F (37.5° to 38.6°C) without cause for alarm. Normally, a younger horse will have a slightly higher temperature than a more mature horse.

Internal and environmental factors both can cause increases in a horse's normal temperature. Consequently, an animal's temperature may increase when he is exercised (particularly in warm weather), excited, in pain, or suffering from an infectious disease. His temperature will also increase, to an extent, when the air temperature rises. For instance, a horse's temperature may be 101.5°F (38.6°C) in very hot weather and 99.5°F (37.5°C) in very cold weather.

An abnormal increase in the horse's body temperature (i.e. fever) is described as continuous (constant); remittent (varying, with marked increases and decreases); intermittent (marked by distinct ups and downs, the temperature returning to normal before rising again); and recurrent (marked by alternating periods of fever and normal temperature). A horse's fever is considered mild at 102°F (38.9°C), moderate at 104°F (40°C) and high at 106°F (41°C). It is possible for a horse's temperature to go higher than this in such conditions as heatstroke, tetanus, and influenza, but when it rises above 106°F (41°C) the prognosis is usually considered grave. Both abnormally high and low temperatures may indicate a health problem and should be duly reported to a veterinarian. A sub-normal temperature should not be overlooked, as it may indicate shock or impending shock. (Note: The section on "Hyperthermia" gives instructions on lowering a horse's fever in cases of heatstroke and heat exhaustion.)

TAKING THE TEMPERATURE

To precisely determine body temperature, a veterinary-type rectal thermometer is required. A veterinary model is preferable to a human thermometer because of its increased size (5 to 6 inches) and special construction which allows for its safer insertion and removal. Most types have a loop located at one end through which a string with an attached clip can be passed, making recovery of the instrument possible if it slips too far into the rectum. However, should the instrument slip inside and for some reason not be retrievable, it will probably be expelled by the horse's natural bowel movements. It is best, in this instance, to merely confine the horse rather than attempt to recover the thermometer by rectal palpation or enema.

Before using the thermometer, it should first be shaken down to a reading below 95°F (35°C) and coated with a suitable lubricant such as petroleum jelly. The horse's tail can then be raised, and the instrument gently inserted with a rotating motion until about 75% of its length is within the rectum. As the temperature is being taken, it is best to either hold the thermometer's end or clip the attached string to the horse's tail hair to prevent the thermometer from accidentally going too far into the rectum. To accurately register the horse's temperature, it should be left in place for at least two minutes.

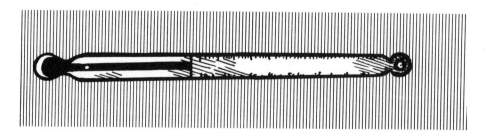

Fig. 1-2   Veterinary thermometer.

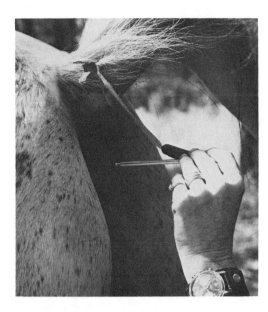

Fig. 1-3 Inserting the thermometer; note that it is clipped to the tail hairs

PULSE

A horse's pulse rate varies according to its age and sex. In the newborn foal, a pulse rate of 80-120 beats per minute is normal; in older foals, 60-80 beats per minute is counted as average; in yearlings, 40-60 beats per minute is average; and in the adult horse, a pulse rate of 28-40 beats per minute is considered normal. Mares, it should be noted, generally have a slightly faster pulse rate than do stallions or geldings.

The horse's normal pulse rate can be affected by any number of factors. The rate is increased by hot weather, exercise, excitement, fright, etc., and decreased by poor health, old age, cold weather, or exhaustion. Further-more, a severe infection accompanied by a fever will often result in a greatly increased pulse rate, ranging from 80-120 counts per minute in an adult horse. A less serious infection might also increase the pulse, perhaps at a rate of eight beats per minute for each Fahrenheit degree of fever.

The pulse throb itself results from the beating of the heart and the resultant waves of increased pressure coursing through the arteries. An even pulse rate is considered normal, and an uneven one, abnormal. An irregular pulse beat should be reported to a veterinarian, for it may be an indicator of heart disease. The pulse can be detected with the fingers (except for the thumb, which has its own pulse that could be confused with the horse's) pressed against an artery at any one of the following places:

1. the back edge of the lower jaw (the cheek), four inches below the eye; (facial artery)
2. the inner surface of the groove under the lower jaw; (external maxillary artery)

3. the inside of the foreleg; (median artery)
4. inside the left elbow, up and forward, against the chest wall; (heart)
5. behind the carpus (knee); (digital artery)
6. under the tail, close to the body; (medial coccygeal artery)

Since it is difficult for a horse to remain absolutely still for an entire minute, the pulses can be counted for thirty seconds and multiplied by two to determine the actual pulse rate per minute.

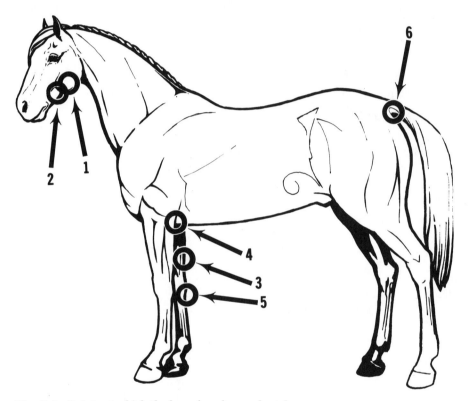

Fig. 1-4   Points at which the horse's pulse can be taken.

RESPIRATION

The frequency of respiratory movements is often checked to reveal dyspnea (difficult or abnormal breathing) and other problems. A horse normally breathes at the rate of 8 to 16 respirations per minute, but respiratory increase related to exercise, hot weather, fever, pain, stomach distension, pregnancy, and variation in age is not uncommon. At no time, however, should the respiration rate exceed the pulse rate.

The horse's respiration rate can be ascertained by watching the movements of his nostrils or flanks. When counting flank movements, it is important not to mistake individual movements of the muscles between the ribs (intercostals) for separate respiratory motion. Technically, one rise and fall of the abdomen equals one respiration count. As with the pulse, it is much easier to count these movements for thirty seconds and multiply by two, than to count for a full minute.

MUCOSA COLOR

A horse's mucosae (mucous membranes) are a good indicator of the quantity and condition of his circulating blood, and can provide clues in diagnosing conditions such as anemia, congestion, icterus (jaundice), shock and colic. As part of an examination, the mucosa of the conjunctiva, nostrils, vulva and gums can be checked for color, discharge, swelling and hemorrhage. An excellent and easy way to assess the blood circulation is to note the color of the gingiva, the horse's gums. Those of a healthy animal are pink, while a sick horse's gingiva may be fiery red, brick red, bluish-purple, or pale in color, depending on the illness (anemia, for example, causes the gingiva to appear pale). Mucosa color can also be noted just inside the lips of the vulva on the mare. The previously mentioned color code for health and sickness applies here as well.

While checking the gingiva, the horse's capillary refill time can also be determined. Capillary refill time refers to the time required for the gums to regain their original color after pressure has been applied and released. Refill time can be approximated by pressing a finger against the horse's gums, releasing it, and noting how long it takes before the color returns to the spot. A healthy horse should have a capillary refill time of one to two seconds; a prolonged refill time should be mentioned to the veterinarian.

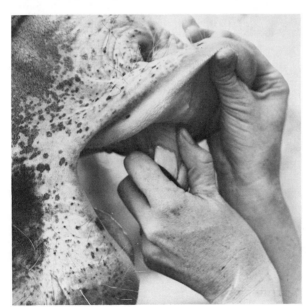

Fig. 1-5 Pressing the gums to determine capillary refill time.

SKIN PLIABILITY

A healthy horse's skin is pliable and elastic. When picked up in a fold and released, it quickly returns to its original position. If the skin "tents up" (stays in a fold) when released, a horse is moderately to severely dehydrated and requires immediate attention (refer to "Fluid and Electrolyte Therapy"). When a horse in this condition has tacky mucous membranes and decreased corneal luster (dull, slightly sunken eyes), he will already have lost four to five percent of his body water, a dangerous amount. Therefore, when "tenting" of a horse's skin or other signs of dehydration are noticed, a veterinarian should be called to begin treatment as soon as possible.

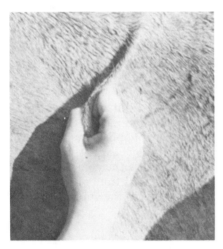

Fig. 1-6 a. Grasping the skin in a fold to check pliability.

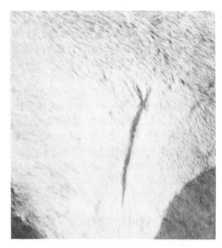

Fig. 1-6 b. "Tenting" of the skin, indicating dehydration.

URINE

A normal horse will produce from three to nine quarts of urine daily. The average is about 5.5 quarts. This urine production will decrease when water intake is reduced or when environmental temperature rises. A greatly reduced volume of urine is abnormal, however, and may mean that the animal is dehydrated.

The urine's color will vary from a deep yellow to brown, and on standing, its color may change to an even darker brown. When urine is allowed to stand, its pH changes from neutral (7) to slightly alkaline (8). Turbidity, or cloudiness, in the urine is caused by the presence of calcium carbonate crystals, which increase in concentration when the urine is retained in the bladder for a prolonged period of time. Besides these characteristics, urine will normally be somewhat viscous because of mucus and epithelial debris.

There are some abnormalities in urine production that are at once recognizable, and may, or may not be associated with serious conditions. For example, difficulty or straining in urination (strangury) may be symptomatic of muscle or nervous disorders, or of kidney disease (though the latter is quite rare). The discovery of free blood (hematuria) in the urine can mean that a urinary or genital tract infection is present. Such a sign, of course, should be conveyed to a veterinarian, since serious illness may result. A port wine-colored urine is a sign of azoturia, which also requires veterinary attention. In this condition, the pigment that is observable in the urine is myoglobin, a product of the muscle breakdown associated with azoturia.

FECES

A horse normally passes feces several times a day. Feces are usually tan or yellow to dark green and should be well-formed rather than hard or soft. In the horse, passage of loose feces or prolonged constipation should be considered a possible sign of some disorder. Constipation, for example, may lead to impaction colic, while chronic loose stool may be seen in a poor-doing horse with a malabsorption problem. Loose stools that occur in foals should receive quick attention, as a foal could become rapidly dehydrated if not promptly treated. If the feces become watery and fetid, a veterinarian should be contacted immediately.

GUT SOUNDS

Waves of muscular contractions along the horse's gut wall (peristaltic movements) produce sounds known as borborygmi. These sounds can be

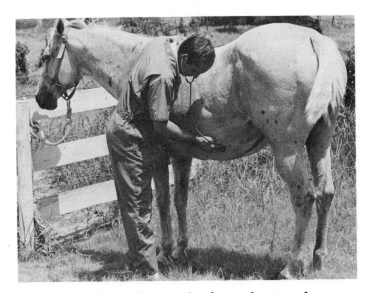

Fig. 1-7   Veterinarian listening for abnormal gut sounds.

heard by placing one's ear or a stethoscope against the horse's flank, and carefully listening. When listening for gut sounds, either excessive intestinal noises or the complete absence of sounds (gut stasis) should be noted. A total absence of borborygmi is generally considered to be the more serious of the two conditions. If normal and abnormal gut sounds are at first difficult to distinguish, good practice can be had by listening to a healthy animal and immediately comparing his gut sounds with the ones produced by a sick horse (refer to "Auscultation").

The Health and Soundness Examination

When considering a horse for purchase, many horsemen rely on a veterinarian to examine the animal for health and/or soundness. This is true even when the owner presents a veterinary certificate for the horse, as the certificate means only that the horse was sound at the time of examination. Therefore, it is conceivable that he may have developed an illness or unsoundness since that examination date. A veterinary examination conducted for insurance purposes will probably be similar to the exam for purchase, although it may vary slightly with each agency. In any case, the veterinarian conducting the examination will follow the guidelines of the particular company involved.

CRITERIA FOR DETERMINING SOUNDNESS

A sound horse should possess no physical flaws that will interfere with or prohibit its intended use. Consequently, a basic criterion for determining the soundness of any horse is the animal's intended use. Because of this, a horse suitable for a child's use may not pass a soundness examination for a stadium jumper. Soundness can furthermore be determined as either work-related or breeding-related, again depending upon the projected utilization of the animal. The difference between the two is easily demonstrated, as it is possible for a racing stallion, for instance, to fail a working soundness examination because of traumatic injury, and still be considered very desirable for breeding purposes. There are many conditions occurring in horses that constitute unsoundnesses, or that may develop into an unsoundness depending on how the horse is to be used.

CHECKING VISION

The category of vision defect includes such conditions as periodic ophthalmia, cataracts, corneal opacities, and blindness. When vision is checked, the eyes are extensively examined for these abnormalities, and the horse may be submitted to an obstacle course examination if a visual

---

Soundness Examination Date: _____

            Time: _____ AM _____ PM

Examination Requested By: _____

Address: _____ Phone No.: _____

Owner: _____ Phone No.: _____

Address: _____ Animal Location: _____

Animal name: _____ Breed: _____

Color: Chèstnut Age: 4 Sex: Filly Species: *Equine* X-Rays: _____

Markings: Star, strip, snip; RF white fetlock; LH sock;

                    Lip tattoo: None

Intended use: Pleasure/Show/Breeding

Respiratory System:	Normal	Abnormal	Rate: 16
Circulatory System:	Normal	Abnormal	Pulse Rate: 40 Temp: 99.6
Reproductive Organs:	Normal	Abnormal	

Eyes: Left Normal Abnormal

    Right Normal Abnormal

Skin: Normal Abnormal

Locomotion: Normal

  Right fore leg: Normal Abnormal

  Left fore leg: Normal Abnormal Toes in;

  Right hind leg: Normal Abnormal Thoroughpin;

  Left hind leg: Normal Abnormal Thoroughpin;

Has horse been nerved: No

Other Examinations: Reproductive: Ovaries, uterus normal on rectal;
           Cervix and vagina normal on speculum exam;

Remarks:

It is my opinion that this animal is (Sound, Serviceably sound Unsound) at the time of examination for the use intended.

Copy to: Signed: _____

Fig. 1-8 Soundness examination.

defect is suspected. If, during an obstacle course examination, a horse seems overly alert or hypersensitive to sounds, moves his ears constantly, picks his feet up high and occasionally stumbles when in motion, he is probably suffering from some visual defect, perhaps even blindness (refer to "Eye Examination").

CHECKING THE RESPIRATORY SYSTEM

Respiratory impairments that constitute unsoundnesses include roaring, heaves, chronic cough, and pharyngitis. In checking for these conditions, a horse's respiration is usually noted both before and after exercise. The animal's wind may be auscultated with a stethoscope while he is at rest, and to facilitate listening, a veterinarian will sometimes hold the horse's nostrils shut for about a minute to accentuate both lung and heart sounds. Any signs of difficult or abnormal breathing (dyspnea) may mean that the nasal and sinus cavities are obstructed, a possibility which a veterinarian will duly investigate. As part of this examination, a veterinarian may also pinch the trachea to make the horse cough. By doing this, he is able to note the presence of any possible obstruction.

CHECKING THE CIRCULATORY SYSTEM

The horse's cardiovascular system is examined before and after he is worked to detect any abnormalities that could affect performance. In this check, the heart is auscultated and mucosa color and capillary refill time are noted. A veterinarian may again hold off the horse's wind for a minute or two to increase and accentuate abnormal heart and lung sounds, and may suggest that a complete blood count (CBC) be made if the horse seems anemic.

CHECKING FOR LAMENESS

Checking for lameness is one of the most important parts of the soundness examination. Each horse, therefore, should be carefully inspected for lameness, which may be caused by the following conditions:

1. splints
2. ringbone
3. sidebones
4. curb
5. bone spavin
6. bog spavin
7. thoroughpin
8. stringhalt
9. thrush
10. cracked hoofs
11. quittor
12. bowed tendon
13. dropped sole
14. navicular disease
15. windgalls
16. laminitis

Any of these causes of lameness may be considered a disqualifying unsoundness, depending upon its severity.

In addition to this thorough inspection, a check is also made for signs of swelling, sensitivity, and damage of the hoof and leg, and for natural faulty action (which may be considered an unsoundness if it could result in future lameness). An examination of the tendons and check ligaments for any thickening that could indicate tendinitis is also made. If a horse shows scars from a neurectomy, it is probable that his future use will be limited and that he may be uninsurable. When these scars are noticed, the veterinarian in attendance should inquire as to the specific reason for the surgery.

To facilitate the detection of lameness, a horse is walked and trotted over a hard surface. The person leading the animal at this time should allow the horse a free head, since a tight grip close to the halter may conceal the head nod that is characteristic of some lamenesses, and will often make even a straight gaited horse move crookedly. Another individual may be needed to walk behind the horse and keep it moving forward as the animal is turned in small clockwise and counter-clockwise circles. (Refer to "Examination of Leg and Foot.")

CHECKING FOR DISEASE

Disease, whether respiratory, dermal, intestinal, etc., may interfere with a horse's use and render him unsound. For this reason, certain vital functions such as temperature and mucosa color are recorded to help diagnose the animal's present health (refer to "Vital Functions").

EXAMINING FOR BLEMISHES

Blemishes may be defined as somewhat superficial defects that detract from a horse's appearance, but usually do not affect his performance. The following are examples of common blemishes:

1. capped hock
2. capped elbow
3. windgalls (without arthritis)
4. scars
5. thoroughpin
6. saddle sores
7. crooked tail
8. splints (not causing lameness)
9. firing marks
10. sitfast
11. mouth deformities (including abnormalities of teeth)
12. skin conditions

Some of these blemishes can be considered unsoundnesses, depending upon their severity or upon their cause or location. For example, a defect caused by accidental injury probably will be only a blemish, whereas one resulting from poor conformation may be considered an unsoundness, since it is likely to recur and/or worsen. As part of the check for blemishes, a horse's mouth is inspected for parrot mouth, bulldog bite, missing or defective teeth, etc. (a valid recorded birthdate may be necessary to help identify a horse whose teeth are somewhat worn away by cribbing). The tongue is also inspected to locate any lacerations caused by bits or foreign objects that may interfere with the horse's use in riding. Other checks that may be made for blemishes include examinations of the horse's skin for evidence of external parasites, fungal infections, sarcoids, melanomas, etc.

CHECKING CONFORMATION

Because poor conformation may cause a horse to develop a future unsoundness, obvious flaws in conformation that predispose the horse to lameness should always be listed on the veterinary certificate. To illustrate the necessity of this practice, a sickle-hocked horse, a calf-kneed horse and a straight-pasterned horse are candidates for curbs, carpal injuries and navicular disease, respectively, and should be identified as such.

IDENTIFYING VICES

Vices that interfere with a horse's intended use may also be checked during a soundness examination. Commonly seen vices include:

1. cribbing
2. windsucking
3. weaving
4. tail-rubbing
5. stall-walking

CHECKING FOR INHERITABLE AND SEXUAL-REPRODUCTIVE DEFECTS

The examination for breeding soundness should identify sexual-reproductive disorders and inheritable defects such as poor conformation or faulty action that predispose the horse to lameness.

Typical reproductive unsoundnesses in the mare are the following:

1. windsucking conformation
2. rectovaginal fistula
3. hard, small, and fibrous ovaries
4. pyometra
5. uterine and vaginal adhesions
6. thickened cervix
7. umbilical hernia
8. scarred udder (from mastitis)
9. venereal disease

Palpation is used in the examination of horses intended for breeding. Culturing for bacteria is another diagnostic tool often used in checking barren mares for possible infections (refer to "Uterine and Cervical Cultures"). Histories of heat periods and past reproductivity are of additional value in determining the reproductive efficiency of the mare.

Typical examples of breeding unsoundnesses in the stallion include:

1. cryptorchidism (undescended testes)
2. abnormalities of the penis
3. lack of libido
4. umbilical or scrotal hernia
5. venereal disease

In the examination of the stallion, semen samples are often collected and evaluated to determine the semen volume, sperm concentration, motility, morphology and to detect infection. And, when possible, the stallion may be observed as he mounts the mare, in order to note any possible psychological problems that he may have.

Diagnostic Techniques

AUSCULTATION

Auscultation, defined as the act of listening for sounds within the body, can assist a veterinarian in determining the health of the heart, lungs, digestive tract, and other organs. When auscultation is practiced, it is most successfully done in a quiet place with a stethoscope, and most safely done on an animal that is properly restrained. The listening process itself is initiated by placing the stethoscope (or sometimes the ear) either against the horse's chest near the elbow (olecranon), or against his flank.

AUSCULTATION OF HEART SOUNDS

When correctly conducted, auscultation and the subsequent interpretation of the resulting heart sounds are quite helpful in discovering the condition of the heart. Using this technique, a veterinarian can learn if a horse has signs of arrhythmia (irregular heartbeat), valvular lesions, vascular disease, myocardial or pericardial disease, or a congenital heart condition.

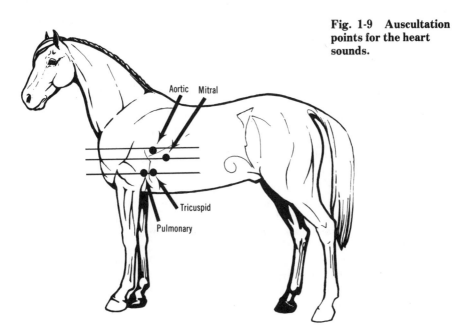

Fig. 1-9 Auscultation points for the heart sounds.

Aortic   Mitral

Tricuspid

Pulmonary

In describing heart sounds, the veterinarian may mention certain properties such as frequency, amplitude, duration, and quality. Frequency, or heart rate, refers to the number of heartbeats per unit of time (beats/minute). A fast heartbeat is described by the term tachycardia, while bradycardia is the term that refers to a slow heartbeat. The term amplitude is descriptive of the loudness of the heart sound, and duration refers to the length of the sound produced. Collectively, frequency, amplitude, and duration are all considered in describing the overall quality of the heart sound.

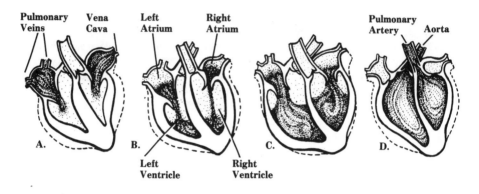

Fig. 1-10   The cardiac cycle. a. Atria are filled with blood from pulmonary veins and cranial and caudal venae cavae. b. Ventricles filling with blood from atria. c. Ventricles are nearly full as atria contract. d. Ventricles are contracting, which forces blood into aorta and pulmonary artery. [Dotted lines indicate the full capacity of the heart.]

Cardiac (heart) sounds in the horse result from four distinct causes. The first sound happens when the heart's atrioventricular valves begin to close during systole (contraction of the heart). This sound is recorded over the mitral and tricuspid areas of the thorax. The second heart sound is caused by the closing of the pulmonary and aortic valves, which occurs during the beginning of diastole (relaxation of the ventricles). In the horse, this sound is often doubled, since the two valves do not close at exactly the same time. It usually is listened for at the pulmonary and aortic areas of the thorax. Rapid filling of the ventricles with blood produces the third heart sound, which is most easily auscultated over the mitral area of the thorax. The fourth heart sound, not present in every horse, is also detected over the mitral area of the thorax. It is caused by the contraction of the atria as they force blood into the ventricles, making the muscular walls vibrate.

It should be mentioned that although heart murmurs can be linked with valvular disease (such as bacterial endocarditis), some murmurs may be innocuous in the horse. Murmurs are produced by the noisy turbulence of the blood as it rushes through the heart's valves, and can occur during either systole or diastole.

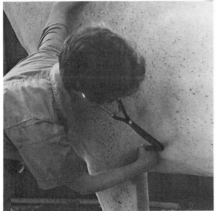

Fig. 1-11   Auscultating the heart.

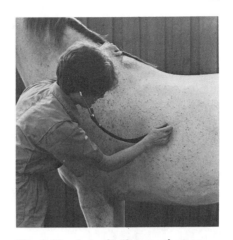

Fig. 1-12   Auscultating respiratory sounds.

AUSCULTATION OF RESPIRATORY SOUNDS

Apart from determining the condition of the heart and detecting heart-related disease, auscultation is generally used to identify respiratory ailments. For example, rhinitis, pharyngitis, and laryngitis are all conditions which will cause abnormal sounds to be heard when the larynx and trachea are auscultated. Particularly loud sounds heard over these areas may be signs of various other conditions, such as occlusion of the larynx, pharynx, or trachea. The sound of rales, in pneumonia, is recorded over the ventral half of the thorax in the disease's early stages, while it is later heard over the dorsal lung areas. A veterinarian will be able to tell if the rales are dry (no fluid is present) or moist (fluid is present) and prescribe proper treatment.

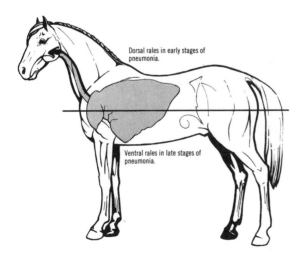

Dorsal rales in early stages of pneumonia.

Ventral rales in late stages of pneumonia.

Fig. 1-13   Areas for lung sounds in pneumonia.

AUSCULTATION OF BORBORYGMI

Borborygmi (bor"bo-rig'me) are normal gut sounds made as food, fluid, or gas passes through the gastrointestinal tract. Most of these gut sounds result from the continuous wave-like movement of the gut's muscular wall, called peristalsis, as it propels substances along the intestinal tract. These sounds may be heard with an ear or, preferably, stethoscope pressed to the horse's flank. To help determine whether the borborygmi are normal or abnormal, an inexperienced person may need to compare the gut sounds of a healthy horse with those of an unhealthy one. The normal gut sounds usually increase when a horse has diarrhea or spastic colic, and decrease when an animal has obstructive colic. Complete absence of sound, as found in gut stasis, is very abnormal and may be followed by bloating; the veterinarian should be contacted immediately.

PERCUSSION

Percussion is the striking of a body area with short, sharp blows, and is used as an aid in diagnosis. Using percussion on the horse's body surface, a veterinarian may be able to determine the condition of an underlying body part from whence the resulting sound originates. And, although it is not that widely used in veterinary medicine, there are times when even an inexperienced person may gain diagnostic information through its practice.

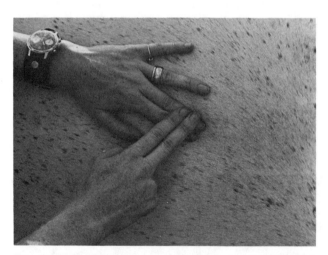

Fig. 1-14 Performing percussion; the veterinarian is tapping the body to reveal abnormalities.

One percussion technique makes use of either the fingers or an instrument called a pleximeter. This technique may be used to identify areas of lung consolidation (airless regions) in pneumonia and to define a fluid line in either the thoracic or abdominal cavity. The veterinarian may be able to ascertain such a fluid line by differentiating between percussion sounds as he produces them. The sounds produced by percussion below the fluid line will be dull, whereas percussion above the fluid line will result in more resonant sounds. This same mode of percussion is important, for it can also be combined with auscultation when necessary for diagnosis.

Diagnostically, percussion can also reveal abnormalities such as marked enlargement of the heart and hydropericardium (fluid in the sac surrounding the heart) through the dull sound emanating from the cardiac area. Other conditions that will cause dull percussion notes are large tumors and granulomatous masses. When large quantities of gas are suspected, as in acute gastric dilatation, or when there may be fluid in the peritoneal cavity, abdominal percussion can be performed to aid in diagnosis of the suspected condition.

EYE EXAMINATION

If a horseowner frequently notes the appearance of a horse's eyes, he may be able to discover signs of possibly serious conditions in time to arrange for prompt veterinary diagnosis and treatment. For example, a protruding nictitating membrane is at times caused by tetanus infection; an off-color conjunctival mucous membrane may indicate anemia, toxemia, or jaundice; and an eye that appears dull and sunken, without its normal moistness and luster, is an indication that dehydration has occurred. All of these are serious conditions.

The horse's owner or caretaker should therefore know what constitutes normal and abnormal eye appearance, and should contact a veterinarian when an ocular problem is suspected. At this time, as well as during the

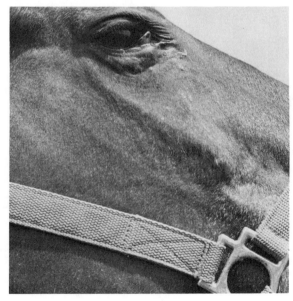

Fig. 1-15 A protruding nicti-tating membrane, which could indicate tetanus.

course of a routine soundness examination, a veterinarian will likely conduct a complete ophthalmic examination. The veterinarian will thoroughly check the eyes and note abnormalities which indicate the presence of a specific condition. Exemplary of this relationship are conjunctivitis and epiphora (tearing), often caused by nasolacrimal obstruction; and corneal edema, blepharospasm (closed eye), and photophobia, frequently caused by recurrent uveitis (moon blindness).

When an ophthalmic examination is conducted, it is the horseman's responsibility to assist the veterinarian with his diagnosis by supplying him with an accurate description of any ocular discharges, increase in stumbling or shying, or head trauma that has occurred. The veterinarian should additionally be supplied with information regarding previous treatment of the suspected problem, as some of the prior medications may have hidden lesions or worsened the condition.

PRELIMINARY EXAMINATION PROCEDURES

Before the examination can begin, the horse must be adequately restrained. Although a rope halter is often sufficient, a twitch or even tranquilization is sometimes required. As a tranquilizer, xylazine generally provides good chemical restraint for detailed ophthalmic examination, though it also reduces intraocular pressure. For the examination to be conducted properly, the horse's eyes will need to be topically anesthetized with a drug such as tetracaine or proparacaine. It may also be necessary, during the examination, to block the nerves around the eyes to prevent the horse from closing his eyelids (refer to "Nerve Block"). Lidocaine, injected into the region of the palpebral branch of the facial nerve (7th cranial), is a local anesthetic used for this purpose.

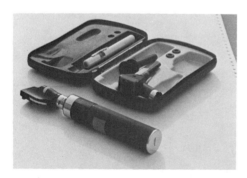

Fig. 1-16   Ophthalmoscope.

The examination is best conducted in a room that can be darkened when necessary for certain parts of the examination. Many structures of the eye, including the orbit, eyelids, adnexa, conjunctiva, cornea, anterior chamber, iris, and lens must all be inspected while the room is well-lighted. However, because sunlight causes pupillary constriction and undesirable reflections on the cornea that interfere with a veterinarian's study of the eye's interior structures, the pupillary reflexes and interior portion of the eye are all checked when the room is dark. A penlight or other bright light source such as an otoscope is commonly used to examine the cornea, anterior chamber, iris, lens and corpora nigra. An ophthalmoscope, a more sophisticated optical instrument, is used to examine deeper structures. The ophthalmoscope contains a perforated mirror and lenses in addition to a light source.

CONDUCTING THE EXAMINATION

The eye examination itself consists of three parts:

1. An evaluation of pupillary reflexes (direct and consensual light responses)
2. An inspection of the structures surrounding the eye and anterior segment of the globe itself
3. An examination of the deep vitreous and ocular fundus, visualizing the retina and optic disc

Before Dilation

In the first part of the examination, pupillary reflexes are tested to check the ability of the horse's pupils to dilate and constrict in reaction to light. While the state of the pupillary reflexes does not in itself indicate if the horse can actually see, it does reveal something about the condition of the retina, optic nerve, sphincter muscles of the iris, etc. This part of the examination is done before the horse's pupils are artificially dilated with a mydriatic, such as atropine.

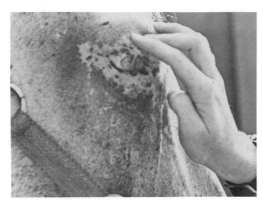

Fig. 1-17   Palpating the eyeball.

As the examination continues, the orbit is inspected to determine whether it is normal in size and shape. Any discharges that are present are noted at this point and a check made for defects of the nictitating membrane (3rd eyelid) such as inflammation, hypertrophy, protrusion, and neoplasms. Intraocular pressure is also evaluated, as a variation in it can be serious. The veterinarian conducting the examination estimates this pressure by palpating the eyeball through the upper eyelid with two fingers, thereby revealing normal pressure, increased pressure (glaucoma), or decreased pressure (hypotony).

During examination of the eyelids, any neoplasm, ectropion (out-turning), or entropion (in-turning) is noted. If the veterinarian suspects a condition such as conjunctivitis, he may collect specimens to culture before anesthetizing the eye for further examination. Then, after anesthetization, a fluorescein solution can be injected into the upper puncta of both eyes to locate any obstructions in the nasolacrimal ducts. If a duct is blocked, the injected solution will flow more slowly, revealing the obstruction. To help localize the blockage, he may then choose to inject an iodized compound into the nasolacrimal duct and x-ray it. The subsequent radiographs of the area will show an outline of the duct along with the area of the obstruction.

When the cornea of the eye is examined, the presence of small, deep blood vessels in the area reflects an inflammation of the anterior uvea. The appearance of any large, branching blood vessels, on the other hand, means superficial lesions are present. Any corneal ulcers that may be present can be detected at this point in the examination with an application of fluorescein dye, a substance that will remain in the ulcerated areas. To apply the fluorescein substance, the veterinarian may use fluorescein strips, moistened with a drop of saline solution or artificial tear solution and touched to the conjunctiva at the upper outside corner of the eye. As previously mentioned, the fluorescein will stain a corneal ulcer upon contact.

After Dilation

After dilation, the lens, vitreous, and ocular fundus are examined. It is at this time that the anterior chamber is examined for transparency, depth, and contents. The aqueous humor of the eye should be found to contain no abnormal substances such as blood, parasites, or neoplastic cells. The lens is inspected for cataracts, and may be examined with an ultraviolet light in order to discover abnormalities such as dislocation (luxation). Iris irregularities such as posterior synechia and atrophy of the corpora nigra may also be disclosed during this segment of the examination. The corpora nigra ("black bodies") are an eye structure that reduce the amount of light which enters the horse's eye. A condition such as atrophy of the corpora nigra can be indicative of recurrent uveitis, whereas extremely large corpora nigra may sufficiently interfere with a horse's vision to cause him to shy.

When the vitreous of the horse's eye is checked, it should appear as a clear gel, although some fibrinous strands may be present in an aging animal. An inspection of the ocular fundus is made to reveal pigment irregularities and to determine the condition of the retina and optic nerve. A veterinarian will use an ophthalmoscope to conduct this part of the examination.

The actual testing of a horse's vision is sometimes reserved for the obstacle course test. In conducting this test, each eye is alternately covered, and the horse is led on a long lead rope through an unfamiliar course of obstructions. If a horse is blind, he will react very sensitively to sounds, constantly move his ears, step high, and sometimes stumble.

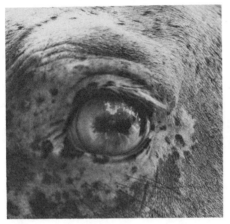

Fig. 1-18 A "glass" eye in which the internal structures are more easily visible than in a dark eye.

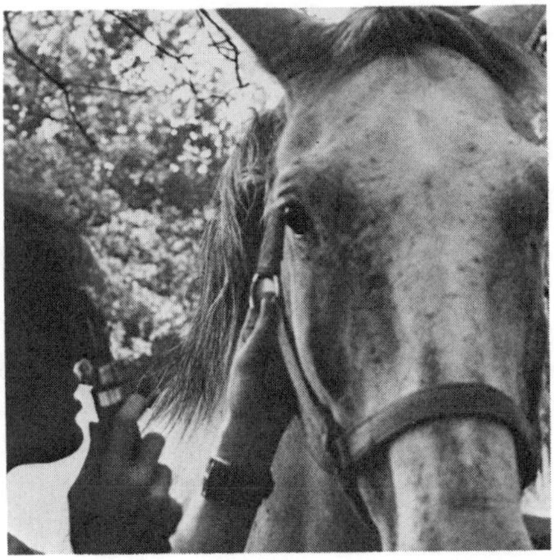

Fig. 1-19 Examining the eye with an ophthalmoscope.

EAR EXAMINATION

An ear examination is sometimes conducted by a veterinarian as a part of a horse's physical examination. This first involves visually checking for any peculiar ear positions and the general appearance of the ears. Some horses, of course, are naturally lopped-eared and carry their ears to the side. However, if a dropped ear is noticed (one that cannot be held erect), a veterinarian will examine it for a possible broken cartilage. This condition, usually affecting only one ear, may result from a horse being "eared" or from abusive use of a twitch on an ear. When it occurs, it often causes the afflicted animal to be head-shy.

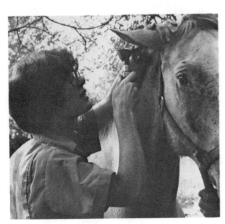

Fig. 1-20 Examining the ear with an otoscope.

The ears are additionally examined for swelling, signs of hematoma or neoplasm, notches and lacerations, and the interior surface (pinna) checked for aural plaques. When these plaques are found, they are often of little consequence, though they are permanent, and there is little or no treatment for them. Discharges in the ears caused by bacterial infections are rarely seen, but other discharges caused by dentigerous cysts (dermoid cysts, conchal fistula) are occasionally noticed. These cysts require surgical removal.

If the examination reveals that a horse is carrying his head abnormally low, Meniere's Disease (a syndrome affecting the inner ear) may be suspected. It is likely, however, that some peculiar ear positions and head-shying result, not from this condition, but from the presence of parasites such as ear ticks. The spinose ear tick and the Lone Star tick are found in the flap of the ear, and, when left untreated, can cause intense itching and rubbing which may lead to a deformed ear. Severe infestations will cause an accumulation of debris that requires removal (refer to "External Parasites" and "Application of Topical Medications").

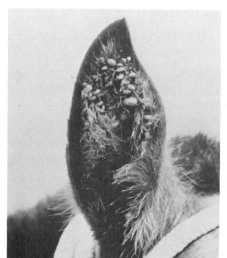 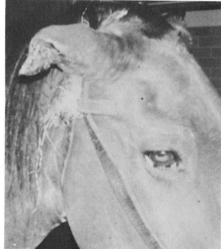

Fig. 1-21   A severe tick infestation [left] may result in permanent ear damage [right].

The only test of a horse's hearing is direct observation of his response to noise. This, however, is not quite as simple as it sounds, for horses can sense sound vibrations through the ground, hence even a deaf horse may respond to a noise.

MOUTH EXAMINATION

Examination of a horse's mouth is routinely conducted by a veterinarian as part of the general physical exam. Examination of the mouth is useful

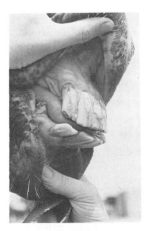

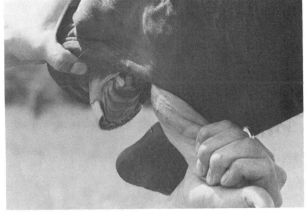

Fig. 1-22 Teeth of an aged horse; note the angle of bite.

Fig. 1-23 Holding the horse's mouth open by pulling the tongue out the side of the mouth.

for diagnosing certain conditions, and also as a means of approximating a horse's age based on teeth development (dentition), shedding, and wear. Age determination by dentition is usually quite accurate until the horse is about five years of age, but then becomes less exact. At five years, a horse has a full mouth of adult teeth and relatively little wear is detectable. Thereafter, however, grazing conditions begin to affect teeth wear, and two horses of similar age may have dissimilar mouths because of differences in grazing conditions. (Refer to the Appendix for specific information on determining age.)

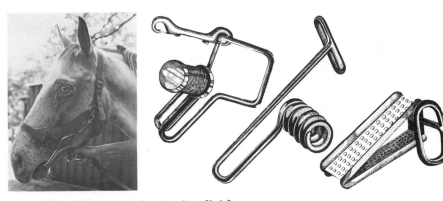

Fig. 1-24 a. Mouth speculum in place [left].
b. Various forms of mouth speculums [right].

Some signs that indicate the need for an oral examination are weight loss, pain that is related to eating or drinking, an increased amount of whole grain in the feces, bits of partially chewed food dropped from the mouth, and eating with the head tilted to one side. In young foals, milk running from the nostrils when the head is lowered often indicates the foal has a cleft palate.

The equipment used in conducting a mouth examination includes a dose syringe and bucket for rinsing the mouth, a penlight or flashlight, and an oral speculum. Should a speculum not be available, however, the examiner can keep the mouth open by holding the tongue out of the mouth and to the side. For the examination to be conducted effectively, some form of physical or chemical restraint may be necessary. (Note: xylazine, when used for chemical restraint, causes a horse to drop his head.)

CHECKING THE TEETH AND MOUTH

As part of the oral examination, a check is usually made for proper mouth conformation. Correct conformation of the teeth and bone is important to the effective grasping and chewing of food (prehension and mastication). One conformational deformity seen occasionally is overbite, or parrot mouth (brachygnathism). In parrot mouth, the lower jaw is abnormally short, causing the hard palate to be situated over the lower incisor teeth. This could result in an injury to the palate when the animal bites. Bulldog bite (prognathism) is a condition that is just the opposite, i.e., the lower jaw is unusually long in this deformity, and the upper incisors are found directly above the floor of the mouth. In both brachygnathism and prognathism, frequent floating of the teeth is required to prevent the intruding teeth from lacerating the soft tissue of the mouth.

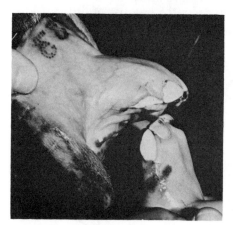 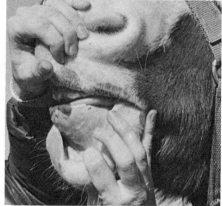

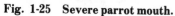

Fig. 1-25 Severe parrot mouth.   Fig. 1-26 Bulldog bite.

There are other problems involving the teeth that may be detected during the course of an oral examination. Two particularly common conditions are uneven wear of molar teeth surfaces and molar teeth with long, sharp edges. Uneven surface wear results, in part, from the natural aging process, appearing in some older horses as wave mouth, shear mouth, step mouth, etc. Long, sharp edges on teeth are the result of a physiological phenomenon. In the horse, the mandible, or lower jaw, is about 30% narrower than the upper jaw. Therefore, the outer edges of the teeth in the upper arcade and the inner edges of teeth in the lower arcade are somewhat incorrectly aligned, and are able to grow long and sharp because there are no opposing surfaces to wear against. The teeth, of course, are continual eruptors and grow throughout the animal's life. When a tooth is missing or when two opposing surfaces are incorrectly aligned, all or part of the opposing tooth/teeth will grow too long and require shortening with molar cutters or rasping with a float to prevent laceration of the soft tissues of the mouth, cheek, and tongue.

Wolf teeth (first premolars) can be extracted if they are found to interfere with bit placement in the mouth. Since spiked protrusions sometimes occur on the last molars and hooked projections can occur on the first upper cheek teeth, both upper and lower arcades must be thoroughly inspected.

A painful condition that is sometimes seen is patent infundibulum. In this condition, cement necrosis causes the affected teeth to be left with open centers, which can only be filled after any infection has been corrected. This condition is often accompanied by sinus infection and by pus drainage from the nostrils.

In some horses, extra teeth may be present; when this condition exists, the supernumerary teeth must be removed to prevent malocclusion.

Other than the teeth, the mouth itself is inspected for imbedded foreign bodies such as splinters and thorns. The tongue is checked for lacerations, and the mucous membranes are examined for color, hemorrhage, and ulcerations.

LEG AND FOOT EXAMINATION

Examination of a horse's legs and feet is very important, for it is through this systematic procedure that lamenesses and possible causes of lameness can be discovered. Moreover, the leg and foot examination serves to locate the exact site of a lameness problem and define its cause. To assure that a complete diagnosis and treatment procedure results from the examination, an accurate account of the horse's condition is necessary. It is, of course, the horseowner's duty to supply this history of the horse's current problem to the attending veterinarian. A sample history might include information relating to the following questions:

1. What signs of lameness have been noticed?
2. How sudden was the onset of the present condition?
3. Is the lameness getting progressively worse, or is it improving?
4. When was the last time the horse was ridden?
5. Does the lameness seem to improve or worsen after exercise?
6. What possible causes or contributing factors (if any) are there?
7. Has the horse had similar problems previously?
8. What activity is the horse used for?

9. What medications or other treatments have already been administered to the horse?

BASIC CHECKS FOR LAMENESS

After considering the horseman's report, a veterinarian can begin the examination to locate the lameness and define its cause. In the process, various techniques and diagnostic aids are used to administer both general and specific checks for detection of lameness. The results of these checks are then used along with a veterinarian's mental notes on the horse's history and conformation to arrive at a final diagnosis.

There are a number of conformation points that a veterinarian will consider during the course of the examination. The following constitutes a sample listing of some of these points: small feet, base-wide, base-narrow, toes out, toes in, calf knees, over at the knees, bench knees, knock knees, stifle and hock (80% of hindleg lamenesses), camped out, bow-legged, post leg (straight stifle), pastern too long or too sloped, pastern too short or too upright, sickle hock, and cow hock.

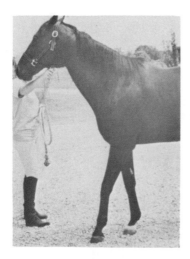

Fig. 1-27 Horse pointing the toe, an abnormal position that may indicate a condition such as navicular disease.

In the basic examination, it is usual for a horse to be observed both while at rest and while in motion. When a horse is at rest, a determination of how the animal holds his lame leg and foot can easily be made. A horse, for example, may point the toe, flex it, or turn it up, depending on the specific cause and site of his lameness problem. A veterinarian will consider this aspect, just as he will note foot shape and the condition of the horse's hoof wall, sole, frog, etc. At this time an inspection of the horse in motion is usually conducted. The animal is often trotted in clockwise and counter-clockwise circles, walked and trotted in a straight line away from the observer, backed up, and tightly turned. These maneuvers may serve to furnish relative information on such aspects as toe breakover, stride length, degree of lameness, gait variations (hard and soft surface), and foot position (in the air and at landing). Before more specific tests are begun, the foot may be palpated to discover any "hot spots" or a strong pulse, as well as to determine the pliability of the lateral cartilages, heel bulbs, and coronary band.

SPECIFIC TESTS AND USE OF DIAGNOSTIC AIDS

After the more general segment of the leg and foot examination has been concluded, specific tests can be conducted for certain kinds of lamenesses. Diagnostic aids such as hoof testers, nerve blocks, and radiography may be used to further facilitate diagnosis. In the following paragraphs, a few of the specific tests and diagnostic aids are examined more thoroughly.

Test for Upward Fixation of the Patella

In this test, a horse is turned in short circles toward the side of the affected limb to detect any catching of the patella. There may be a characteristic clicking sound when the patella momentarily catches. Also, in an attempt to lock the leg into extension, the limb may be manually forced upward and outward. The veterinarian, to perform this test, must stand directly behind the leg in question and as close as possible to the horse's body to attempt to manipulate the patella. If it does lock, the horse will be judged as being predisposed to upward fixation, and the test will be termed positive.

Test for Bone Spavin

In this test, both hindlegs are tested for the sake of comparison. This involves flexing the hock for 2 or 3 minutes, releasing it, and immediately moving the horse out at a brisk trot. Special care must be taken not to cramp the pastern while the hock is being flexed. If the lameness appears more pronounced as the horse is trotted, the test is considered positive. However, since it is possible for some normal, sound horses to show a positive reaction to this test, the veterinarian must still use his judgement to decide if the cause of lameness is actually bone spavin.

Test for Shoulder Lameness

This test involves several movements of the foreleg. First, the shoulder is deeply palpated. Then, the foreleg is lifted, brought all the way forward, and retracted as much as possible. After this, the limb is abducted (stretched or pulled away from the body). Pain or sensitivity during these movements is indicative of shoulder lameness.

Test for Stringhalt

In this test, a horse is first rested, then turned or backed up. If stringhalt is present, the lameness should be pronounced during the animal's first few steps, and hyperflexion of the hocks should be very evident.

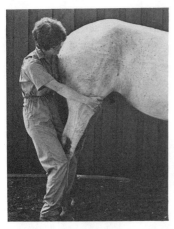

Fig. 1-28   Test for upward fixation of the patella. Attempting to lock the patella [top, left].

Fig. 1-29   Test for bone spavin. a. Flexing the hock [center left] b. Trotting the horse out [center, right].

Fig. 1-30   Test for shoulder lameness. a. Extending the leg forward [below, left] b. Abducting the leg [below, right].

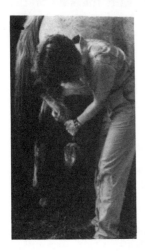

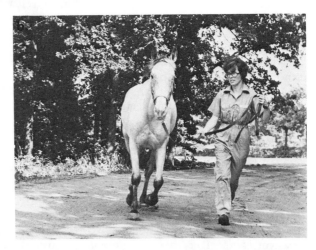

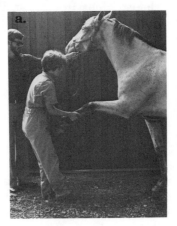

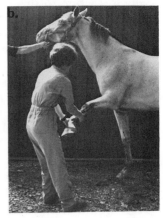

Use of the Hoof Tester

The hoof tester is a diagnostic aid used to locate lameness-causing conditions in the foot. It may be employed at any time that hand pressure is insufficient to detect specific areas of sensitivity, and its use usually facilitates a quick and accurate diagnosis of the problem. Some of the conditions that may be detected with the hoof tester include the following:

1. puncture wounds
2. laminitis
3. fracture of the third phalanx
4. sole bruises
5. gravel
6. corns
7. navicular disease
8. sidebones

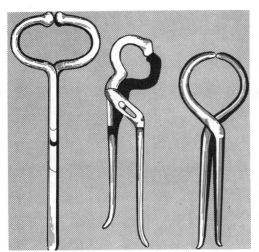

Fig. 1-31   A variety of hoof testers.

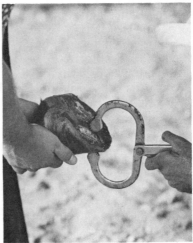

Fig. 1-32   Using the hoof tester.

Ideally, proper application of the hoof tester requires two people, one to apply pressure with the instrument and one to note the horse's reactions to the pressure. Normally a horse will flinch when the tester is applied to a painful area. However, the first compression of the tester may cause some sensitive horses to flinch, even though they are not lame. As the apparatus is applied, its jaws are opened, placed around a specific site, and closed with gradually increasing pressure to test the site's sensitivity. This procedure is applied to the heels, the quarters and toes, to nail sites (from shoes), and to the side of the frog from the opposite heel. The entire application procedure should be conducted for both sides of the foot.

Pain responses may be variously interpreted as the hoof tester is applied to the different structures of the foot. In the region of the frog, a locally sensitive area may be caused by a puncture wound. Other causes of local pain in this area are sole bruises and gravel-based infections. Pain that seems centralized in the middle of the frog could be a sign that the horse has developed navicular disease. If the animal exhibits signs of pain over the entire sole and hoof area, laminitis or an extensive infection may be present, or there may be a fractured third phalanx (coffin bone).

Sometimes, as is the case with over-trimming, a horse may flinch from pressure applied to the sole when there appears to be no reason for a painful response. If this happens, the sole should be checked to see how much it gives to pressure, as a sole that is too springy may be thin and has probably been over-trimmed. When there is pain in any area, the corresponding part of the opposite foot should be checked for comparison.

Use of Nerve Blocks

Nerve blocks are diagnostic aids used in selectively locating and pinpointing causes of lameness. Nerve blocks are effected through injection of a local anesthetic such as lidocaine into certain areas of the leg and foot to desensitize nerves in those regions. Their use can facilitate the final diagnosis of lameness, and sometimes serves as a preliminary to further diagnosis by radiography or treatment by neurectomy (refer to "Radiography" and "Neurectomy").

Nerve blocks are used only when the leg causing the lameness has been definitely identified. When used in diagnosis, nerve blocks are systematically administered, starting low on the foot and moving toward the top of the leg. In spite of their local anesthetizing effects, nerve blocks only partially desensitize joint surfaces. Joints, therefore, are most effectively blocked out by injection of the particular anesthetic into the joint itself. This is a very painstaking procedure that always requires the skill of a veterinarian and close adherence to proper sterile technique (including a surgical scrub and the same precautions that would be taken for any aseptic surgical procedure). When a nerve block is used prior to surgery, as is sometimes the case, the injection of local anesthetic will decrease the amount of general anesthetic required.

One of the more common drugs used for nerve block anesthesia is lidocaine, which is often preferred to procaine (Novocaine). Ethyl and isopropyl alcohol are two substances which are not recommended for injections as nerve blocks. Both drugs have a tendency to cause sloughing of the hoof, and both are unpredictable in their anesthetic effects, at times causing nerve blocks that last for days or weeks.

Regardless of which drug is chosen for the block, it is generally administered in the smallest quantity possible, to avoid irritation. The injection itself is given with a short, small (25 gauge) needle, after the block site has been cleansed as it would be for surgery. To insure that an injected drug has taken effect, a veterinarian may use a sterile needle to prick the area, checking the horse's sensitivity to pain. The anesthetic effect of a nerve block usually lasts for several hours.

In using nerve blocks to diagnose lameness, the foot is generally anesthetized first. Anesthetization is achieved by applying a posterior digital nerve block which desensitizes the posterior one-third of the foot. This particular block is given at a point halfway between the horse's fetlock and coronary band, and one of its major uses is as a test for suspected navicular disease.

After the posterior block takes effect, the horse is gaited (as he is after any block is given) and his action closely monitored. If there is no sign of lameness, navicular disease is a possibility.

Two additional blocks used to desensitize the foot are the sesamoid block and the palmar, or volar block. The former block is given at the point of the fetlock where the nerves cross the sesamoid bones. This block anesthetizes most of the foot without including the fetlock joint itself. The other nerve block, called a palmar or volar block, is given at a point above the fetlock joint and desensitizes the entire foot and pastern area except for a narrow V-shaped area at the front of the pastern joint.

Should any of these blocks not be successful in locating the lameness site, a veterinarian can perform what is known as a ring block. A ring block can be done above the pastern joint to anesthetize the area below the injection site including the foot. If, after the block has taken effect, the horse is gaited and found to be sound, the cause of lameness will have been isolated in this area. Similar ring blocks may be done at various locations on the leg to anesthetize the areas immediately below and to localize the specific area responsible for lameness.

As previously mentioned, a horse is gaited and examined for signs of lameness after each nerve block is given. The gaiting process, including walking, trotting, turns, and pivots, allows the veterinarian an opportunity to note the horse's movements for signs of pain. During this test, the horse is moved on a loose lead, as a tight shank could affect the animal's normal gait.

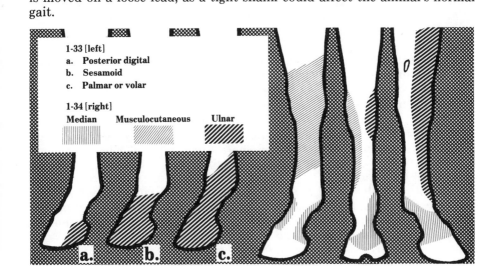

1-33 [left]
a. Posterior digital
b. Sesamoid
c. Palmar or volar

1-34 [right]
Median   Musculocutaneous   Ulnar

Fig. 1-33 & 1-34   Areas desensitized by nerve blocks.

Use of Radiography

Radiographs of the leg and foot are taken to confirm a suspected diagnosis, e.g., navicular disease, laminitis, carpal chips, etc., or to further investigate a problem area that has been identified through the use of other aids. However, a diagnostic radiograph of an area is not always an all-purpose tool. For example, although generally successful in locating a lameness-causing injury that is bone-related, radiography is not as successful in detecting injury to soft tissue. Consequently, radiographs are more useful in confirming the presence of fractures, bony lesions, or exostoses than they are in detecting sprains, strains, etc.

Radiographs are also used to reveal the stage of epiphyseal maturation in the knees of horses, by indicating the degree of closure (maturity) of the horse's knees.

REPRODUCTIVE EXAMINATION

The reproductive examination is a necessary part of the care of mares and stallions used for breeding. Although the examination is obviously different for each sex, it is generally conducted to reveal any factors that might reduce breeding efficiency in both mare and stallion. The examination thus serves to evaluate the breeding condition of both sexes.

INSPECTION OF THE MARE

The mare is normally checked for conformation, soundness, and health at purchase, with special attention paid to inheritable conditions such as umbilical hernia (detected by palpation of the naval region). At the time of purchase, any leg or foot problems that might be aggravated by the additional weight of foal-carrying should be discussed.

The mare's reproductive examination consists of several procedures, including a rectal exam of the entire reproductive tract, a vaginoscopy (speculum exam) to view the cervix and vagina, and for problem mares, a possible cervical culture and/or uterine biopsy. In addition, the endoscope may sometimes be used to visualize the interior of the reproductive tract. These tests are all conducted by a veterinarian, who may also check the mare's mammary glands for previous mastitis (rare) and scar tissue. Records of past reproductive history, heat cycles, foaling dates, and response to the teaser stallion should be very helpful to a veterinarian as he conducts the examination for each mare.

During the course of the exam, there are several abnormal conditions that may be revealed. For instance, pneumovagina is the result of a conformation fault (either tipped vulva or a lack of vulvar tone) wherein the presence of air in the vagina and/or the uterus leads to infection and infertility. Pneumovagina can be confirmed by a speculum examination, by visualizing bubbles of air on the cervix. In fact, the "windsucking" noise that is characteristic of this condition is caused by inrushing air entering the genital tract. This conformation defect is most prevalent in thin mares, old mares, and in mares with a high tail carriage. It can be surgically corrected by a Caslick's operation. A veterinarian may have to open a previously sutured vulva prior to breeding, and will always be required to open it before foaling.

Rectovaginal fistulas or perineal lacerations may also be present. When there is a communicating passageway between the rectum and vagina due to trauma of a previous foaling, the mare is rarely able to conceive. This is due to the chronic contamination and infection caused by feces in the vagina, the result of which will likely be chronic vaginitis and/or metritis. Surgical correction is often possible for these conditions; however, a year of the affected mare's reproductive life is lost.

A vaginoscopy examination is used to reveal tears in the vaginal wall or cervix, as well as inflammation and abnormal exudates that indicate infection and the need for treatment. In a normal mare, the color and size of the cervix are indicators of the stage of the estrous cycle and of optimum breeding time.

Uterine enlargement with loss of uterine tone and thickened uterine walls (from scar tissue) are other unfavorable conditions that decrease breeding efficiency. In the mare, hematoma in the broad ligament of the uterus indicates hemorrhage of one of the uterine arteries at foaling. Such a condition as this might cause one to delay breeding a particular mare. In any event, a mare with this problem would have to be closely attended during subsequent foalings, since rupture of an artery often results in fatal hemorrhage.

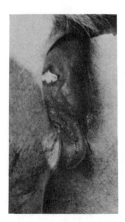 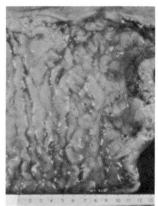

Fig. 1-35,1-36 A mare with windsucking conformation [left] in which air can be introduced into the uterus during breeding as shown by the bubbles [right].

Rectal palpation is used to check the ovaries for normal size and follicular activity. A mare that fails to cycle may have a large ovary with a granulosa cell tumor that can be surgically removed. After surgery has been performed, this type of mare may begin to cycle normally and later be able to conceive. Palpation may also reveal the absence of ovaries, which may be either a congenital defect or due to a spaying operation (surgical removal). Other infertile mares are occasionally seen to have infantile (immature) or absent uteri. Other conditions noted by the veterinarian during rectal palpation are the size and consistency (tone) of the uterus, and the length of the cervix.

It is routine practice for large breeding farms to employ veterinarians to examine their mares. By using the previously mentioned methods of rectal palpation, vaginoscopy, and a good teasing program, optimum breeding dates are thus determined. After a mare is known to be in good breeding condition, getting her in foal with a minimum number of services from the stallion becomes the immediate object. This saves the stallion and reduces infection rates in problem mares.

INSPECTION OF THE STALLION

Inheritable abnormalities in the breeding stallion are potentially more serious than in the mare, for the stallion may sire considerably more offspring during his lifetime. Therefore, inheritable abnormalities that could cause future breeding problems receive attention first. For example, umbilical and scrotal hernias and their repair are noted, if present, as well as undescended testicles. The testes and epididymis are palpated for normal size and texture, and a check is made, usually with the aid of tranquilization, of the stallion's prepuce and penis. Abnormalities that may be revealed during this procedure are edema, squamous cell carcinoma, lacerations, habronemiasis, and screwworm lesions. Any leg or foot problems which might interfere with normal breeding procedures should also be considered at this time.

A semen evaluation is required to obtain an insight into the stallion's breeding future. Although it is true that a normal semen evaluation is not always reflective of the fertility promise of a stallion, it usually does give an idea as to what an animal's future performance will be. In fact, for expensive horses and for stallions serving a large number of mares, a recorded periodic evaluation of semen is generally required before purchase.

Semen collection is accomplished by exposing the stallion to a mare in heat, then collecting the samples in an artificial vagina. If two samples are taken about one hour apart, they should be of nearly equal volumes, though the second should have about one-half the total number of sperm as the first. The most important factor to consider in evaluating a stallion's semen is the sperm concentration. However, if the semen quality is for any reason questionable, the stallion is often given a few days' rest and re-evaluated. Abnormalities that may be encountered on microscopic examination of the sample are the following:
1. low sperm count
2. decreased progressive motility (the sperm's ability to move forward)
3. abnormal morphology (shape)
4. hemospermia (red blood cells in semen)
5. a high number of leukocytes (white blood cells) in the sperm
6. dead sperm

Low concentrations of sperm and sperm with poor motility are both signs that could indicate a future of unsatisfactory breeding performance.

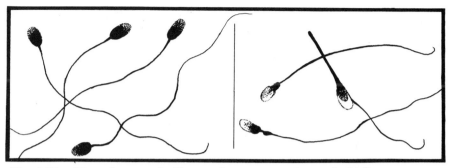

Fig. 1-37 a. Normal sperm. b. Abnormal sperm; note the crooked tails, etc.

Characteristics of Normal Stallion Semen

Volume	30-250cc
Sperm Count / ml	30-600 million
pH	6.9-7.8
White Blood Cells/cmm	fewer than 1500
Red Blood Cells/cmm	fewer than 500
Normal Morphology	minimum 65%
Live sperm	minimum 60%
Motility	minimum 40%
Longevity at room temperature	40-50% alive at 3 hrs
	10% alive at 8 hrs

SKIN EXAMINATION

A skin examination may be made by a veterinarian to evaluate the overall condition of this organ and to help disclose the state of a horse's health. Skin disease of any kind, whether fungal, bacterial, or parasitic, is always checked for in this examination; and any dermatitis, allergic reactions, saddle sores, lacerations, contusions, and hematomas are also noted if present. The skin is additionally inspected for neoplasia, particularly in older horses of grey coloration. Melanomas, which are neoplastic growths, are most frequently found on grey horses and may often be noted around the anus. Excessive patches of white, especially in the areas of the eyelids and genitals, may indicate that a horse is predisposed to other neoplastic growths such as squamous cell carcinomas. Diagnostic tools such as skin biopsy, bacterial and fungal culture and sensitivity tests, and skin scrapings may be required when a problem exists, especially if prior treatment has failed to clear up the condition.

As a part of a thorough examination, a veterinarian will look for scars that have resulted from old wounds and past operations. Scars on the edges of the ears from trimming operations, neurectomy scars on the pasterns, and firing patterns on the cannon area are characteristic blemishes that are sometimes detected. Old blemishes, such as from blistering, can often be detected by the presence of white hairs. Even though scars may have little immediate signifigance, their appearance can furnish some insight into the kind of attention and care that a horse's injuries have received in the past. A check is also made for current injuries such as rope burns and proud flesh, and an inspection conducted for abnormally hot or swollen areas.

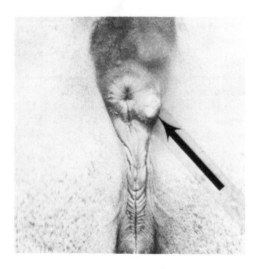

Fig. 1-38 The melanomas under the tail of this horse may be benign or malignant; if malignant, they can metastasize quickly.

An evaluation of the skin's hydration state can be made by "tenting" a skin fold (as described in the section on "Vital Functions"). A shiny, healthy looking skin and haircoat are usually indications that the animal has received proper care and attention. When a horse's skin outwardly appears this way, he may be described as showing "an overall bloom of health," a subjective, but nevertheless fairly accurate, indication of his general health and condition.

Signs of Illness

The following discussion considers certain noticeable signs that indicate the relative state of a horse's health.

CHANGES IN BEHAVIOR

A change in behavior may indicate impending illness and such changes may involve a variety of different behavioral patterns. For example, a decreased appetite, refusal to eat, and quidding (rolling the food into balls, then dropping it) are examples of abnormal behavior indicating possible illness. Other behavioral characteristics that are often associated with illness include unusual restlessness or listlessness, pawing and rolling, and biting at the flanks. Biting at the flanks is especially associated with colic in the horse. When a horse is not well, he may tire easily when exercised and show a desire to lie down at inappropriate times. Then, when he is at rest, a sick horse may adopt some unusual position, such as pointing or holding up a foot or holding his head to one side.

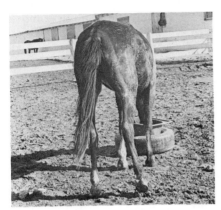 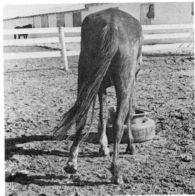

Fig. 1-39 & 1-40 **Horse shifting weight from one side to another, abnormal behavior which may be a sign of illness.**

CHANGES IN PHYSICAL APPEARANCE AND ACTIONS

Other than behavioral changes, a horse's physical appearance and actions can provide clues to his health status. For instance, a dull, staring haircoat, sunken eyes, and excessive sweating are signs which imply that a horse is not well. Excessive salivation can occur when a foreign body is lodged in the mouth, in association with esophagitis or with some central nervous system disorders. Attempts to vomit are always serious in the equine, because of the likelihood of an accompanying stomach rupture. Other unusual discharges, whether nasal, vaginal, ocular, etc., should be reported to a veterinarian, as well as any abnormal physical movement of the limbs, indicating persistent or severe lameness.

CHANGES IN VITAL FUNCTIONS

A veterinarian should be contacted when there is any distinct change in temperature, pulse, respiration, or any of the horse's other vital functions. The advice on temperature, pulse, and respiration holds true in all cases other than when the noticed change is the normal result of exercise or other exertion from which the horse soon recovers. Usually, a temperature above 103°F is considered serious and should be assumed to be a sign of illness. An increased respiratory rate, difficulty in breathing, and frequent or harsh coughs are also abnormal and should be interpreted as signs of illness.

A change in fecal color and consistency, if it cannot be correlated with a known change in diet, may indicate digestive system trouble. In this kind of illness, the feces may appear excessively hard or they may be covered with mucous. Excessive diarrhea or constipation are additional signs of digestive problems.

Other abnormalities pertaining to vital functions include straining to urinate, passing red or otherwise stained urine, loss of skin pliability, and a variance in gingiva color or increase in normal capillary refill time. (Refer to the section on "Vital Functions" for information on normal and abnormal values for these functions.)

SIGNS OF ILLNESS CHECKLIST

Behavior:
1. Change in appetite
2. Unusual eating habits
3. Restlessness: pawing, rolling, biting at flanks
4. Tiring easily
5. Unusual resting postures
6. Tail-wringing

Appearance and Actions:
1. Dull haircoat
2. Dull and/or sunken eyes
3. Excessive sweating
4. Excessive salivation
5. Vomiting
6. Unusual discharges: ocular, nasal, etc.
7. Unusual movement: lameness

Vital Functions:
1. Fever above 103°F (40.5°C)
2. Frequent cough
3. Difficult breathing
4. Change in feces
5. Difficulty in urinating
6. Colored urine
7. Changes in normal skin tone, gingiva color, capillary refill time
8. Abnormal or absent gut sounds

When the veterinarian examines the horse, he will conduct a general physical, in addition to checking the specific area of illness.

Identification

A written description of a horse is not in itself completely satisfactory as a means of medical identification. Such a description, for instance, cannot distinguish between two horses of the same age, sex, and color, and could therefore cause mistaken identity. Of course, proper identification of valuable, registered horses is always necessary to avoid serious, costly mistakes, whether unintentional or otherwise. Fortunately, accurate and positive identification is possible and can be established from records of a horse's natural and man-made markings, as well as from individual blood types and unique scars.

NATURAL MARKINGS

Natural markings such as whorls (swirls of hair) and chestnuts are much like human fingerprints; every horse has a unique set. It is possible, then, to positively identify a horse through the use of photographs of his chestnuts, taken under uniform lighting at a standard distance. Whorls are an excellent means of identification because, like chestnuts, they are permanent, unchanging, and unalterable. The location of a horse's whorls and white markings can also be marked on a diagram of the horse and used as his passport whenever the horse is shipped.

Natural white markings have pink skin underneath and are readily distinguished from fakes when the animal's hair is wetted. However, because of certain differences that exist in the definition of colors and white markings, the horse that one person refers to as sorrel may be called chestnut in another part of the country or by a different breed registry. Young grey horses are likewise variously described as roans, and it is at times difficult to distinguish between dark bay and brown animals.

HOT BRANDING

Hot branding is one of the oldest methods of identifying horses. However, it is being used less frequently now because of the pain associated with this procedure. Moreover, hot-branding prominently scars the skin and disfigures the animal. It sometimes causes a keloid to develop at the brand site, requiring surgical removal.

FREEZE BRANDING

Freeze branding is accomplished with a marking iron that is cooled to approximately -175°F (-80°C). Any attempt to alter these symbols will deface the original brand. This precaution assures the owner that the freeze brand cannot be changed for illegal identification purposes.

Before a brand is applied, the selected area is always clipped and washed with alcohol. The horse to be branded is then marked with the iron, usually on the neck under the mane. This causes the pigment-producing cells to die, leaving the site permanently marked with a white brand. If the iron is left in place for a longer period of time, the hair follicles themselves will be killed, resulting in a bald brand. This longer application time required for a bald brand may be necessary when marking a grey or white horse. Although there may be some initial local swelling at the brand site, freeze branding is quick and generally painless.

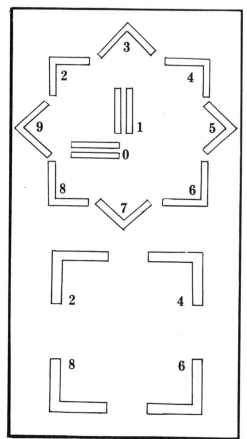

Fig. 1-41   Freeze branding symbols.

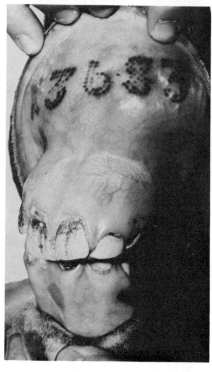

Fig. 1-42   Identification by lip tattoo.

LIP TATTOOING

Lip tattoos are commonly applied to race horses, at the track before their first race, as a means of identification. Both Quarter horses and Thoroughbreds (under the auspices of the AQHA and Jockey Club respectively) are tattooed. The tattoo usually consists of a unique letter-numeral combination. The major disadvantage of this method is that the tattoos gradually become illegible after a few years.

ELECTRICAL IMPLANTS

This is somewhat of an experimental method of identification that involves the implanting of an electrically sensitive device under a horse's skin. When examined with the proper device, this implant would give off an electrical impulse peculiar to that horse. However, because the implants conceivably could be switched, this method would not be entirely foolproof. Electrical implants are not currently being used for identification purposes.

BLOOD TYPING

Blood typing is another means of identification now in use by some horse registries. Blood types are, of course, unalterable, and because there are theoretically so many possible blood types, it is very unlikely that any two horses (other than identical twins) would have the same type.

Besides being used in identification, blood typing is also valuable when determining or verifying parentage and in discovering incompatible blood types as a prevention of neonatal isoerythrolysis (refer to "Crossmatching Blood Types").

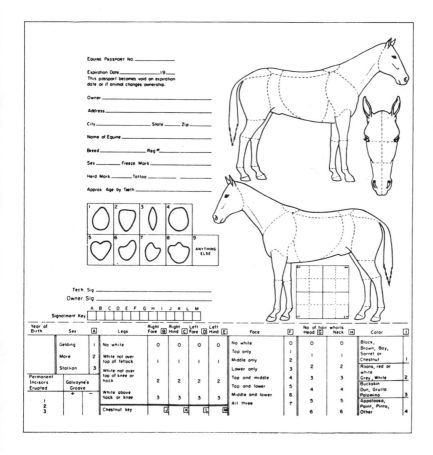

Fig. 1-43   A complete identification record form.

Equine Insurance

Many insurance companies require that the horse be examined by a veterinarian and certified to be in acceptable health before the insurance takes effect. This examination must include a check of all major internal systems and of eyesight, conformation that might cause lameness, and genitalia if the horse is used for breeding.

The horse's owner must agree to take adequate care of the animal and to acquire a veterinarian's services when the horse is sick or injured. And, if there is sickness or injury, the owner must immediately notify the company of the horse's present condition.

The insurance company must also be notified, this time by the horse's veterinarian, at any time that injury or sickness makes destruction of the animal necessary. This notification will allow the company time to send another veterinarian to verify the horse's condition. If both veterinarians and the owner agree that destruction is necessary, the insurance will pay its claim after the horse has been euthanatized. In any case of death, the veterinarian will have to carry out a post-mortem examination and complete a report for insurance records.

There are, of course, certain exclusions for which insurance companies will not assume liability, such as some types of surgery. Unless the owner has notified his company and in some instances paid an extra premium, the insured horse will have no coverage for any surgery other than an emergency, life-saving operation. Cancellation of the policy, then, would in most cases occur the day before any common surgical procedure such as castration was to be performed. (Note: It is sometimes possible for an owner to procure an extension from the insurance company regarding this matter.)

One particularly important stipulation affecting horse owners who intend to perform many minor veterinary procedures themselves is the exclusion made for procedures, such as inoculations, unless they are administered by a veterinarian. This exclusion includes preventive treatments as well as those needed because of injury or ailment. Basically, this means that much of the insured horse's care and medication must be administered by a veterinarian.

2

PREVENTATIVE HEALTH CARE

A Good Vaccination Program

Preventative medicine is a good economic measure in view of the rising costs incurred in raising and maintaining today's horse. Consequently, vaccinations are widely used for prevention of infectious diseases. The treatment of these infectious diseases is very costly today in terms of medication used, performance days lost, and possible loss of the horse itself. Therefore, a good immunization program is indeed very inexpensive insurance. The following is offered as a discussion of the basic, necessary vaccines that are currently available.

TETANUS TOXOID AND ANTITOXIN

One of the diseases that can be controlled through vaccination is tetanus, a debilitating disease caused by the introduction of a bacterium, **Clostridium tetani,** through a wound, or, in young foals, through the gastrointestinal tract. Also known as "lockjaw," tetanus is a highly dangerous disease in the horse, with a mortality rate of at least 80%. There are two different biologicals that provide protection against this condition: tetanus toxoid and tetanus antitoxin.

The toxoid, derived from tetanus toxin, takes four to eight weeks to build up an adequate level of protection. It is fairly safe, and is unlikely to cause an adverse reaction in most horses. When given to a healthy horse for the first time, the toxoid should be administered in two doses, from four to eight weeks apart, to allow the horse's immune system to develop adequate antibodies. To a pregnant mare, a tetanus toxoid injection should be given about one month before parturition so that the mare can develop a high level of antibodies. After birth, her foal will receive these antibodies through the mare's colostrum. The foal can then be given its first tetanus toxoid injection between three and twelve weeks of age. A previously immunized horse that undergoes a major surgical procedure or suffers an injury, particularly a puncture wound, should immediately receive a tetanus toxoid injection as a booster.

Immediate, temporary protection against tetanus can be provided by tetanus antitoxin, which gives only a few weeks of immunization. This injection is required when an injured horse has not been previously immunized with toxoid, when a newborn foal is not able to consume colostrum, or if the dam did not receive a tetanus toxoid injection within one month of foaling. Because the antitoxin is prepared from a donor horse's blood, it does carry the minimal risk of causing certain reactions such as hepatitis, anaphylaxis, or post-vaccination liver atrophy in the recipient horse. However, because tetanus is a fatal disease, and because the horse, among all domesticated animals is most susceptible, a horse of questionable immunization status that has been injured should definitely be given the antitoxin. A tetanus toxoid injection may be given at the same time that tetanus antitoxin is administered. The recommended practice, of course, is to administer yearly tetanus toxoid boosters to assure constant immunity.

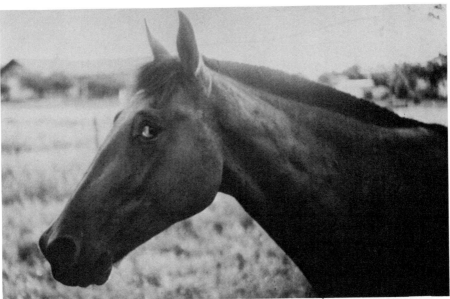

Fig. 2-1   Horse afflicted with tetanus; notice the protruding nictitating membrane.

ENCEPHALOMYELITIS VACCINES

Eastern Equine Encephalomyelitis and Western Equine Encephalomyelitis

Eastern and Western encephalomyelitis (EEE and WEE) are two potentially fatal diseases that can be prevented by proper immunization. However, the vaccine that is given for both types of "sleeping sickness" provides only a short duration of immunity and must be given annually to insure proper protection. The annual inoculation program consists of a

Fig. 2-2   BIOLOGICALS AVAILABLE FOR IMMUNIZATION

Disease	Product	Brand Name	Company	1st Vaccination	Booster	Immunity
TETANUS	Antitoxin	- - - -	[Abbott] [Ft. Dodge] [Haver-Lockhart] [Jen-Sal] [Pro-Bio] [Colorado Serum]	1500 units, S.C. 1. post-surgery 2. wound treatment 3. newborn foals	1. as indicated 2. may give toxoid at the same time	2 weeks
	Toxoid	- - - SUPER-TET TETOID UNITOX T-TOXOL	[Bio-Ceu] [Ft. Dodge] [Pro-Bio] [Colorado Serum] [Haver-Lockhart] [Affiliated] [Jen-Sal] [Cutter]	2 or 3 doses I.M. 4-8 weeks apart	1. annually 2. post-surgery 3. pregnant mare 1mo. prior to foaling	Up to several years
ENCEPHALOMYELITIS EASTERN/EEE WESTERN/WEE	Vaccine	CEPHALOVAC ENCEPHALOID I.M. ENCEPHALOMYELITIS VACCINE ENCEVAC EQUILOID MYELOVAC ENCEPHOL TC	[Jen-Sal] [Ft. Dodge] [Pro-Bio] [Haver-Lockhart] [Ft. Dodge] [Norden] [Cutter]	2 doses I.D. 1 week apart or 2 doses I.M. 2-4 weeks apart	Repeat as a two injection series annually	6-12 mo.
VENEZUELAN/VEE	Vaccine	VEE-VAC CEPHALOVAC, V, VEW	[Norden] [Jen-Sal]	1 dose S.C. or combined with EEE/WEE	Every other year	At least 2 yr.

Disease	Product	Brand Name	Company	1st Vaccination	Booster	Immunity
INFLUENZA A1/A2 STRAINS	Vaccine	EQUICINE EQUI-FLU II FLUMUNE FLUVAC FLUCINE	[Haver-Lockhart] [Jen-Sal] [Norden] [Ft. Dodge] [Cutter]	2 doses I.M. 6-12 weeks apart	1. annually 2. prior to training	6-12 mo.
RHINOPNEUMONITIS	Vaccine	PNEUMABORT RHINOMUNE	[Ft. Dodge] [Norden]	Nasal spray 1 or 2 doses I.M. 4-8 weeks apart Pregnant Mares: at 60 days and no later than the 7th month of pregnancy	Annually	4 months
STRANGLES	Strep Equi Bacterin	EQUIBAC II	[Ft. Dodge]	3 doses I.M. 1 week apart No Pregnant Mares	More than 12 Mo. after: 1. last immunization 2. natural infection	1 year
RABIES	Vaccine	ERA STRAIN	[Jen-Sal]	1 dose I.M.	Annually	Up to several years
COMBINATION: EEE/WEE INFLUENZA A1/A2 TETANUS TOXIOD	Vaccine	ENCEVAC-4	[Haver-Lockhart]	2 doses I.M. 3-4 weeks apart	1 dose I.M. annually	1 year

series of two separate injections from either of the two programs available. Either two intradermal injections are given one to two weeks apart, or a pair of intramuscular injections are given about a month apart, depending upon the vaccine used. Since Eastern and Western encephalomyelitis are spread by mosquitoes, the two-part vaccination program is best begun in late winter or early spring, before the mosquito vector is able to reach its adult stage. One manufacturer's vaccine is now approved to be used as a single annual booster, although primary immunization the first year still requires a series of two injections 3 weeks apart.

Eastern and Western encephalomyelitis vaccines are commonly found combined with tetanus toxoid in a single combination dose. It is also possible to administer a single injection that immunizes against EEE, WEE, VEE, and tetanus. Other combinations available include EEE-WEE-influenza-tetanus, and EEE-WEE-VEE.

VENEZUELAN EQUINE ENCEPHALOMYELITIS

The original vaccine for Venezuelan equine encephalomyelitis (VEE), introduced during the threat of a VEE epidemic, was thought to have a slight tendency to cause brain lesions and cerebral hemorrhages. The present vaccine does not have these problems, however, and should be given to all young horses to combat the disease. Furthermore, the United States Department of Agriculture has recently recommended that all horses receive VEE booster shots every two years. Boosters should also be given as required by shows, races, and interstate shipping regulations.

A simple plan would be to vaccinate horses of all ages during even numbered years and only weanlings during odd numbered years. Although VEE is a tropical disease and has not been a problem in the United States since 1971, it could recur at any time. Besides the specific VEE vaccine, there are several products on the market that combine protection against EEE, WEE, and VEE into a single intramuscular vaccination.

OTHER BIOLOGICALS

The biologicals mentioned thus far represent the basic ones that should be given to all horses. In addition to them, however, there are other vaccines and bacterins that the horseman may use to inoculate against other infectious diseases.

EQUINE INFLUENZA VACCINE

Equine influenza viruses account for a substantial percentage of the cough that afflicts race and show horses, commonly called "flu," or "racetrack cough." The disease causes a very high fever, and the persistent cough renders the horse useless for work for periods of from three to six weeks. Both type A1 and A2 equine influenza can be prevented by vaccination.

To successfully prevent equine influenza, those horses that travel or are under stress (as race and show horses commonly are) should be vaccinated prior to the time that they are sent to training. In general, horses may be vaccinated as sucklings, and after that age, they should receive the vaccine as weanlings, yearlings, and annually thereafter, particularly if they are under stress. In some areas it may be advisable to vaccinate twice yearly, so consult your veterinarian. Initially, two intramuscular injections are given in the hindquarters two to twelve weeks apart. Although this program is successful in immunizing against the myxovirus type A1 and type A2 equine influenza, there are other types which are not controlled by this vaccine due to dynamically changing viruses and the periodic emergence of mutant forms for which new vaccines have yet to be developed.

EQUINE RHINOPNEUMONITIS

Equine rhinopneumonitis, caused by equine herpes virus I, is responsible for a considerable number of the nasal discharges occurring in sucklings and weanlings during the autumn; moreover, up to twenty percent of the cough complexes seen in race and show horses are attributable to it. Consequently, because of the relation of this virus to "cough" in race and show horses, it is highly recommended that all horses be protected by vaccination.

Equine rhinopneumonitis is also one cause of viral abortion, which may occur in an individual infected mare or as an "abortion storm" involving most of the mares on a farm. The mare affected with rhinopneumonitis usually has a subclinical form of the disease wherein she experiences an uncomplicated abortion and gives birth to a dead or dying fetus. Most abortions occur between the eighth and eleventh month of pregnancy, and, although the aborting mare should breed back with no complications, she will have lost a year of her reproductive life. Obviously, an outbreak of rhinopneumonitis could be very costly, and should be prevented if possible.

In the past, before the development of a vaccine, planned infection was sometimes introduced into breeding herds by a live virus nasal spray to initiate a mild outbreak and provide immunization against more severe occurrences. Now, an attenuated live virus vaccine, which is given in two intramuscular injections at a four to eight week interval, is available and may be given to horses at any time after the age of three months. Some restrictions apply, however, to pregnant mares. A mare should be past her 60th day of gestation when she is first vaccinated, and should receive the second dose no later than the seventh month of pregnancy. The mare's annual booster should likewise be administered after the 60th day of any subsequent pregnancies.

STRANGLES BACTERIN

Certain biologicals may be used on a particular farm because of problems peculiar to the specific premises or herd. An example of a disease that may have to be controlled with such a biological is strangles. Strangles is a bacterial respiratory disease, caused by **Streptococcus equi** or

Streptococcus zooepidemicus. It may vary from a mild, upper respiratory disease to full-blown pneumonia and death. Strangles vaccine is really a bacterin (a suspension containing chemically killed strangles-causing bacteria) initially administered in three intramuscular injections at one week intervals. This three-shot series may cause considerable local swelling at the injection site. An annual booster shot can be given to horses that have already received the initial series, but should not be given to those horses that have had strangles, nor to those that have had their previous immunization within the last year.

The strangles bacterin occasionally causes local tissue reaction. Because of this, some veterinarians only recommend use of the bacterin where there is either an outbreak or a threatened outbreak of strangles.

SALMONELLOSIS VACCINE

Salmonellosis, an acute enteric disease, is another example of a condition that exists on some farms but not on others. When there is a problem on a specific farm, a veterinarian may treat it by administering a bacterin or a mixed infection vaccine. Autogenous bacterins, those made from bacterial cultures isolated from sick animals on a particular farm, may be required for an unusual disease problem that has developed in a certain herd.

LEPTOSPIROSIS

Although leptospirosis is a bacterial disease that is uncommon in horses, some veterinarians believe that there is a correlation between it and some cases of periodic ophthalmia (refer to "Eye Examination" and "Eye Conditions"). However, vaccination with leptospirosis products is not routinely done, though it may be recommended by some veterinarians.

RABIES VACCINE

Rabies vaccine should be considered for administration in areas where rabies is enzootic to the wildlife population. The vaccine is given as a single intramuscular injection to horses over four months of age, and a single booster is administered annually. This vaccine may also be used as a prophylactic treatment in a horse that has been exposed to rabies.

SUGGESTED FOAL VACCINATION AND DEWORMING PROGRAM

The primary goal of a foal vaccination program is to provide protection while avoiding stressing the foal. This can be aided by keeping intervals between doses at the length recommended by the vaccine manufacturer, by not administering several different products at one time, and by completing the program near weaning time.

Many variations are possible in foal vaccination programs. The following table is offered as a guideline to a vaccination and deworming program for foals.

Age	Preparation
birth	tetanus antitoxin (optional) [1] antibiotics (optional) [2]
8 weeks	deworm [3] 1st tetanus toxoid
12 weeks	2nd tetanus toxoid 1st EEE/WEE [4] [5]
16 weeks	deworm 2nd EEE/WEE 1st influenza 1st rhinopneumonitis
20 weeks	2nd influenza 2nd rhinopneumonitis
24 weeks	deworm VEE

1 For foals that nurse their dams, tetanus antitoxin is not required if the mare was given a tetanus toxoid booster two to eight weeks prior to foaling.

2 Antibiotics are required if the mare dripped a large volume of colostrum prior to foaling or if the foal is deprived of colostrum for any other reason e.g., death of the mare, neonatal isoerythrolysis, etc.

3 Acceptable foal dewormers: thiabendazole, mebendazole, piperazine, pyrantel pamoate.

4 If the intradermal EEE/WEE vaccine is used, the 2nd dose is given 1 week later, at week 13.

5 Strangles bacterin is given at weekly intervals for 3 doses beginning at about 12 weeks of age. It is generally used on premises that have a problem with the disease.

Control of Internal Parasites

The presence of internal parasites in horses is a major health problem. Nearly all horses are infested with parasites; it is only the degree of infestation that varies from one horse to another. These parasites often rob the infested horse of valuable nutrients, causing many problems. A rough haircoat, loss of weight, anemia, lethargy, diarrhea, and general poor performance may each be attributable to parasite infestation. Infestation also puts a stress on the horse, making him less resistant to bacterial and viral infections. Worst of all, the larval stages of some parasites migrate through the body's tissues, damaging the liver, lungs, circulatory system, and other specific organs and systems.

Perhaps the most insidious of the parasitic migrations is that of

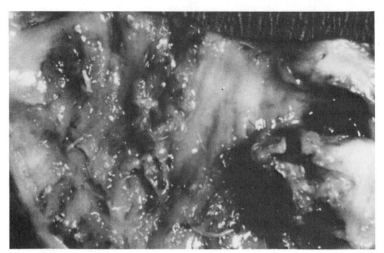

Fig. 2-3   Intestinal damage caused by large strongyles.

Strongylus vulgaris (the bloodworm). The larval stage of this parasite does extensive damage to the anterior mesenteric artery which supples blood to a large portion of the intestine. When this artery is extensively damaged, a thrombus (blood clot) will form. Small pieces of a clot, known as emboli, may break off and partially obstruct the blood flow to much of the intestinal tract. Some researchers feel that up to 90% of all colics are related to damage done by **Strongylus vulgaris.**

BASIC PARASITOLOGY

TERMINOLOGY

A brief discussion of the terminology of parasitology at this point may enable the reader to better understand the text, as well as the deworming program recommended by his veterinarian. When considering internal parasites, we are talking about the helminths (intestinal worms or worm-like parasites) and the botfly (Gastrophilus) in their various stages. The adult helminths reproduce sexually, producing ova (eggs); the larva, or juvenile, is the sexually immature form of the helminth, and the host, of course, is the animal that is parasitized. Bots (the larvae of botflies), unlike other internal parasites, are not really worms.

Helminths are classified as follows: oviparous, meaning that the undeveloped eggs pass from the worm; ovoviviparous, meaning that the eggs contain larvae when they pass from the worm; or viviparous, meaning that the worm passes active larvae, which are then passed by the equine host. The life cycle of a parasite is defined as one generation in its life, and, in the helminths, there may be several stages in the complete life cycle, separated by a period of some months.

THE PREPATENT PERIOD

The prepatent period in the life cycle of a parasite is the elapsed time between entry of the infective stage into the final host and demonstration that the parasite is present. For example, a veterinarian will be able to see parasitic eggs in the feces on microscopic examination when the prepatent period is over. Thus, the infection is said to be patent, or visible, when attempts at diagnosis can be made successfully.

DIRECT AND INDIRECT LIFE CYCLES

A direct life cycle is one in which only one host is involved. In this cycle, the parasite usually has a free-living phase; in other words, it undergoes some larval development outside the host before it becomes infective. The important worm parasites affecting horses are for the most part characterized by direct life cycles and a period of development outside of the host, which takes place in pastures and in paddocks.

In an indirect life cycle the larval development takes place in one or more animals called intermediate hosts. The intermediate host is required in this case for completion of the parasite's life cycle and development to the infective stage. When there are multiple hosts, the definitive, or final host, is the animal in which the adult reproducing stage of the parasite occurs.

DEWORMING

Deworming programs consist of the intelligent use of anthelmintics to minimize the internal parasite load in the horse. Today's anthelmintics do an excellent job of removing most of the adult worms and the botfly larvae from the infested animals. Unfortunately, however, the immature or larval stages of many parasites have already been able to do much damage by this time. A persistent parasite control program is therefore almost always necessary to at least minimize the reinfestations that inevitably occur.

In exceptional cases, it is possible to eliminate some types of worm larvae with anthelmintic treatment. For example, high doses of thiabendazole have been used as a larvacidal dose for **Strongylus vulgaris,** especially in horses subject to frequent bouts of colic and suspected of permanent parasite damage. Another anthelmintic, one of the gel types of dichlorvos introduced directly into the mouth, is being used to kill the first larval stage of the botfly, which resides in the mouth. In general, however, worm larvae are difficult to eliminate, and the best, sometimes the only treatment is preventive measures. (Refer to "The Oral Administration of Medicine" for more information on dewormers and their applications.)

FREQUENCY OF DEWORMING

Climate, concentration of horses, and results of fecal examinations all have some bearing on the frequency of deworming. For example, there will be a vast difference in the deworming requirements of a single horse on a large, arid ranch and the needs of horses on a breeding farm or in a large training operation. Deworming can usually be done less frequently when a horse is kept on dry pasture or in a dry lot situation than it can when an animal is kept on moist pasture. In addition, horses kept in a climate with sharp demarcation of seasons and cold winter weather require deworming less often than animals raised in a more temperate area.

In general, horses that are dewormed show a marked reduction in egg counts for at least 4 weeks. At 6 weeks, however, a moderate increase is noticeable, and the marked increase seen at 8 weeks indicates a need for retreatment. In climates and under high-intensity management conditions where frequent deworming is necessary, an alternating program of tubing and feed additive anthelmintics, administered every two months, is adequate. In colder or drier areas, tube deworming is probably only necessary twice yearly. Consult your local veterinarian to determine the recommended frequency of deworming in your area.

FECAL SAMPLES

A fecal sample can be taken at two month intervals for evaluation of the anthelmintic program, if the efficacy is in doubt. A persistently high egg count may be a clue to resistance to the anthelmintic. When the fecal sample is taken, the fresh sample should be stored in a sealed plastic bag and kept in a cool, dark place until it can be examined. Examination should ideally take place as soon after collection as possible, as either a time lapse or a warm environment will allow the eggs to hatch, making the exam inaccurate.

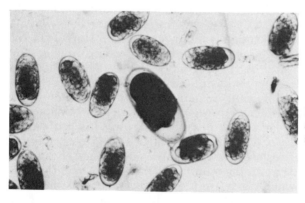

Fig. 2-4 Parasite eggs are visible in this fecal sample.

CONSIDERATIONS IN ESTABLISHING AND MAINTAINING A DEWORMING PROGRAM

SANITATION

1. Prevent fecal contamination of hay racks, feed boxes, and water sources.
2. Clean up manure daily in stalls and small paddocks.

3. Properly handle manure to be spread on pastures.
   a. compost manure before spreading
   b. use a manure spreader
4. Practice pasture rotation.
   a. let pasture rest for at least 3 months
   b. alternately graze cattle and horses on the pasture

USE OF ANTHELMINTICS

Note: The choice of an anthelmintic depends upon many factors, such as the internal parasites involved, the age of the horse, and the drug resistance of the parasites. Since each anthelmintic differs in its efficacy and recommendations, a veterinarian should be consulted before deworming.

1. Deworm all animals on the premises at one time, since parasites are a herd problem.
2. Quarantine and deworm new additions and transients before turning them out with horses already on the program.
3. Deworm at frequent intervals (6 to 12 weeks); remember, after deworming, there will be:
   a. marked reduction in eggs passed for about 4 weeks
   b. small increases in egg numbers at 6 weeks
   c. marked increases at 8 weeks
4. Alternate anthelmintics to avoid the build up of resistant worm populations.
5. Have the veterinarian conduct fecal checks at 8 week intervals to assess the efficacy of the program, if its effectiveness is in doubt.
6. Remember the following about egg counts; they can be misleading because:
   a. large strongyles, which are a more serious parasite problem, can be more difficult to remove than small strongyles; therefore, a marked decrease in eggs per gram of feces may reflect highly effective removal of small strongyles only.
   b. a single fecal sample on a single day may not be representative of the actual parasite load.
7. Calculate dose by body weight. Remember that dewormers are toxic substances and must be handled carefully.
8. Remember the routes of administration.
   a. stomach tube: preferred because the horse receives the entire calculated dose; must be done by the veterinarian.
   b. dose syringe: liquids or gels placed on the back of the tongue; effective if the horse swallows the full dose.
   c. feed additives: effective if the horse will consume the feed; can be used between tube dewormings.
9. Take necessary precautions when deworming foals, pregnant mares, heavily parasitized, or debilitated animals.
   a. use only anthelmintics safe for foals and broodmares.

   b. since deworming can stress a heavily parasitized or debilitated
      horse, it should only be done under veterinary supervision.
10. Deworm broodmares 60 days before foaling to reduce exposure of
    the foals to parasites after birth.
11. Note directions for proper product storage to preserve efficacy.

MAJOR INTERNAL PARASITES

Strongyloides (Intestinal Threadworm)

Strongyloides westeri: affects foals up to 6 months of age; the larvae
penetrate the skin, causing lesions, then move to the lungs, where they are
coughed up and swallowed; the larvae relocate in the small intestine, where
they irritate the lining, causing diarrhea; diagnosed by eggs or larvae in the
feces; they require 6 to 12 weeks to mature.

Ascarids (Roundworms)

Parascaris equorum: the most common parasite; they infest all horses,
but usually cause damage only in young foals up to one year of age and in
old, debilitated horses; they migrate from the liver to the lungs, through
the capillaries, alveoli, bronchioles, bronchi, trachea, and pharynx; they
cause diarrhea, impaction colic, lung damage (characterized by cough),
impaired growth and development, pot belly, and rough haircoat, and may
lead to a perforated or ruptured intestine; in the horse, they require 10
weeks to develop, with complete life cycle taking three months; eggs are
very resistant to adverse environment.

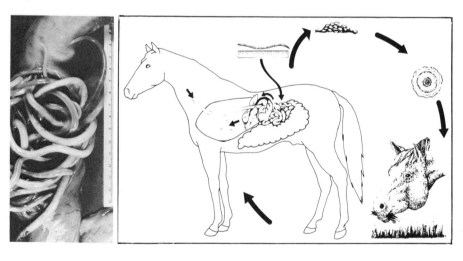

Fig. 2-5   Ascarids. Fig. 2-6   Life cycle of ascarids.

Strongyles (Bloodworms)

Strongylus vulgaris (large strongyles): most serious kind of parasite in the horse; affect all ages of horses; the eggs, laid in the large intestine, pass out through the feces; the 3rd stage infective larvae live on the underside of grass, then, when ingested, go to the cecum or large intestine where they burrow through the gut wall and migrate through the body; they damage the endothelium of blood vessels, causing a fibrin build-up and the development of a thrombus; this blockage can cause lameness, verminous colic, infarction of the gut, hemorrhagic inflammation, and death; the larvae require 6 months to mature and begin producing eggs; a routine fecal exam cannot differentiate between the eggs of large and small strongyles; fecal cultures are necessary for this.

Strongylus edentatus: has an 11 month life cycle, spends 1 month in the liver, then goes to cecum and colon.

Strongylus equinus: has a 9 month life cycle; stays in the abdominal wall for 3 to 4 months, then goes to cecum.

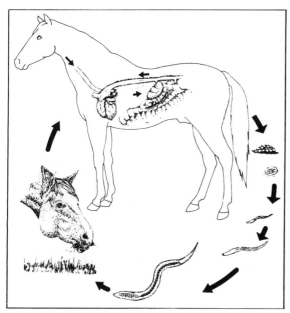

Fig. 2-7 Life cycle of large strongyles.

Tridontophorus (Small Strongyles)

Tridontophorus tenuicollis: can cause diarrhea and constipation; have a 3 week long life cycle; they migrate to the small intestine and are much less destructive than the larger strongyles.

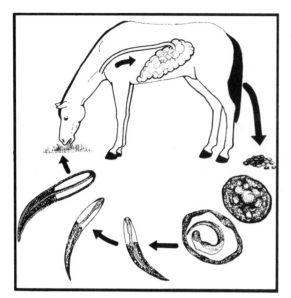

Fig. 2-8   Life cycle of small strongyles.

Habronema

Habronema muscae, Habronema majus, and Draschia megastoma: part of these worms' life cycle is spent in the common housefly; ingestion of the worm larvae can cause stomach ulcers, but the main problem is the infestation of wounds with larvae deposited by flies; larvae migrate through tissues, causing slow-to-heal "summer sores"; these larvae can also cause conjunctivitis if deposited in the eyes.

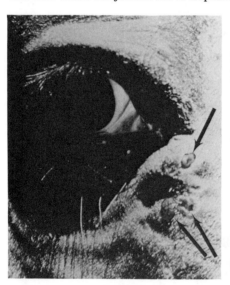
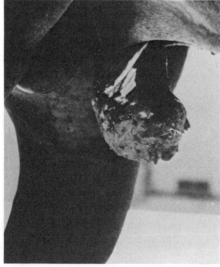

Fig. 2-9   Habronema lesions near the eye [left] and on the penis [right].

Trichostrongylus

Trichostrongylus axei: the only helminth which can affect both horses and cattle.

Gastrophilus (Bots)

Gastrophilus intestinalis(horse botfly): most common type of botfly; they affect horses of all ages; botflies lay yellow eggs on the horse's forelegs, a process which annoys the horse; when the horse licks the eggs, the larvae emerge and burrow into the mucosa of the tongue and mouth; irritation is caused by the burrowing, which may interfere with feeding, bitting, and perhaps cause cribbing; stays in the tongue for 3 to 4 weeks, then migrates to the stomach, where large numbers can hinder digestion and passage of food from the stomach; stays in the stomach for ten to twelve months; may cause anemia and stomach ulcers.

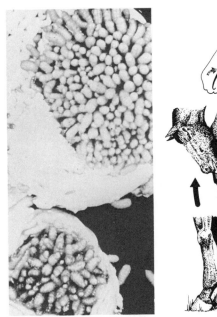

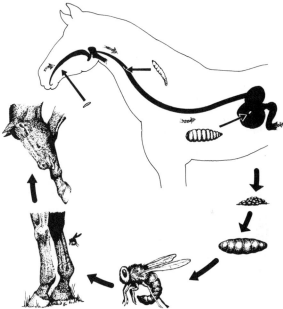

Fig. 2-10 Bots in the intestine.

Fig. 2-11 Life cycle of the bot.

Gastrophilus nasalis (throat or chin botfly): the larvae hatch from the eggs (which are laid on the throat or chin) and make their way to the oral tissues; otherwise has same cycle.

Gastrophilus haemorrhoidalis (nose botfly): the larvae burrow through the skin over the muzzle and wander into the mouth; otherwise has same cycle.

Fig. 2-12 COMPOUNDS EFFECTIVE AGAINST INTERNAL PARASITES

Anthelmintics	Ascarids	Strongylus Vulgaris	Strongylus Edentatus	Strongylus Equinus	Small Strongyles	Bots	Pinworms [adults]	Pinworms [larvae]
Cambendazole	94-99	98	98	98	94	-	-	-
Dichlorvos	99	99	85	98	90	90	99	99
Mebendazole	95-99	98-99	92	100	85-98	-	98-100	99
Phenothiazine/ Piperazine/ Carbon Disulfide	99	90	85	-	90	80	75	45
Piperazine	94	50	-	-	70	-	75	15
Piperazine/ Carbon Disulfide	99	50	-	-	90	80	75	15
Pyrantel	96-99	90-95	75-80	85-100	90	-	60-90	75
Thiabendazole	25-90	90	90	-	90	-	90	30
Thiabendazole/ Piperazine	90	90	90	-	90	-	90	30
Thiabendazole/ Trichlorfon	99	98	97	-	99	98	99	-
Trichlorfon*	90	40-90	15-40	-	80-90	90-99	90	5
Trichlorfon/ Phenothiazine/ Piperazine	95-99	40-95	15	-	60-90	90	90	-

% of Major Parasites Removed from Host

*Trichlorfon and carbon disulfide are contraindicated in pregnant mares. Check labels for other precautions involving pregnant mares, foals, and sick or debilitated animals. Dichlorvos and trichlorfon are cholinesterase inhibitors.

Oxyuridae (Pinworms)

Oxyuris equi: pinworms travel through the intestines, finally reaching the cecum and colon where they consume vegetative matter; female lays eggs on the skin surrounding the anus; these eggs cause intense itching resulting in tail-rubbing and loss of hair; pinworm life cycle is 5 months.

Anoplocephala (Tapeworms)

Anoplocephala magna and Anoplocephala perfolita: these are most commonly found in horses up to one year of age; they live in small intestine; rarely cause problems unless present in exaggerated numbers, when they can interfere with digestion or cause an obstruction.

Control of External Parasites

Flies, mosquitoes, lice, ticks, and other external parasites can transmit a number of serious equine diseases. These include piroplasmosis, equine infectious anemia, and encephalomyelitis. Such parasites are additionally very annoying to horses, and can cause nervousness and loss of condition.

FLIES

Flies are probably the most prevalent external parasite affecting the horse. Biting stable flies, horse flies, deer flies, and horn flies are all very irritating to horses. Even non-biting flies such as some house and face flies are annoying, while blow flies can severely infect wounds.

Bites of house and stable flies cause areas of edema with a small central scab. These bites are extremely painful to young horses, and may result in self-mutilation since an affected horse often will bite the swollen areas. In this case, a horse should be treated with antihistamines, tranquilizers, and an analgesic.

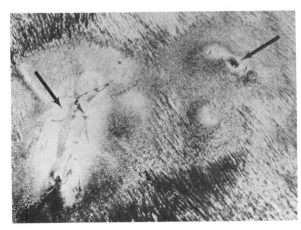

Fig. 2-13 A grub has been surgically excised as shown on the left, while a blowhole for another grub is visible on the right.

Face flies feed on the secretions from the eyes, and are very irritating to most horses. An insecticide wipe or roll-on can be applied on the horse's forehead to control these parasites.

Heel fly larvae are known as cattle grubs; these parasites burrow under the skin and make their way to the horse's back, where they may cut an airhole. A horse with grubs often cannot be ridden until the grubs are surgically removed and the wound healed. Dusts or washes are used to kill grubs that have already cut an airhole through the horse's skin.

The screwworm, a widely known blowfly larva, infects wounds on horses, often causing death. Insecticide sprays and smears are used to control blowflies. If any screwworm larvae are found on a horse, contact your county agent or veterinarian. They will be able to provide a special shipping carton, and can send the larvae to the following address:

Screwworm Eradication Program
P.O. Box 969
Mission, Texas 78572

MOSQUITOES

Mosquito bites on horses resemble the bites of house and stable flies, with the exception that they do not have a central scab. Mosquitoes can be controlled in much the same manner as can flies.

LICE AND TICKS

Lice and ticks are other serious pests that infest horses. The two species of lice that commonly affect horses are the horse sucking louse **(Haematopinus asini)** and the horse biting louse **(Bovicola equi)**. Especially problematic in winter, these parasites cause irritation and subsequent hair-rubbing. Fortunately, several species of lice and winter

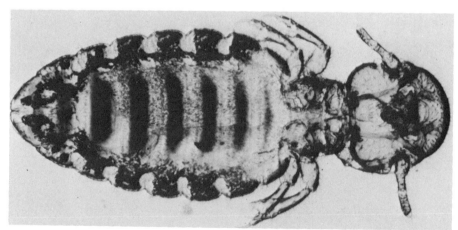

Fig. 2-14   A biting louse, greatly enlarged.

Fig. 2-15   INSECTICIDES EFFECTIVE AGAINST FLIES

Insecticide	Form	% Concentration Necessary for Control					
		CATTLE GRUB	HOUSEFLY	STABLE FLY	BLOWFLY	HORNFLY	FACE FLY
Carbaryl	spray	-	0.5	0.5	-	0.5	-
Ciodrin	spray	-	0.15-1	-	0.3	0.3	0.3
	spray	-	2	2	-	-	-
Coumaphos	spray	-	0.125	0.125	0.25	0.6	-
Dioxathion	spray	-	0.15-0.6	0.15-0.6	-	0.15	-
Dichlorvos[1]	spray	-	1	1	-	-	0.5
Malathion[2]	spray	0.5	0.5	-	0.5	-	-
	dust	-	-	-	4-5	-	-
Methoxychlor	spray	-	0.5	0.5	-	0.5	-
Ronnel	spray	-	0.25	0.25	-	0.5	-
Toxaphene	spray	-	0.5	0.5	-	-	-
Pyrethrins[3]	spray	-	0.05-0.1	0.05-0.1	-	0.05-0.1	-
Rotenone	dust	1.5	-	-	-	-	-
Lindane	spray	-	-	-	-	0.03-0.06	-

1   Dichlorvos also used as space spray for house and stable flies at 0.5-1%
2   Malathion also used as bait for house and stable flies at 0.5-2%.
3   Pyrethrins also used as space spray for house and stable flies at 0.1-0.25%

ticks can be controlled with two or three thorough applications of insecticide sprays or dusts. Some species, however, require more stringent treatment for eradication. The Lone Star tick **(Amblyomma americanum),** for instance, must be treated every two to three weeks for adequate control.

Spinose ear ticks **(Otobius megnini)** can cause head shaking, shying, cauliflower ears (from rubbing), etc., and the nymph stage of these parasites may remain in the ear for several months. Although dusting insecticide powders into the ears usually removes those ticks lodged near the surface, deeper-dwelling ticks must be removed with an oilbase insecticide mixture, such as:

    1 part 25% lindane (emulsifiable concentrate or wettable powder)
    12 parts cottonseed oil
    12 parts pure pine oil

In this mixture, the cottonseed oil is added to the pure pine oil, then mixed thoroughly with the lindane. The mixture should be applied deep in the ear with an oil can. A rubber tube over the oil can spout will protect the ear during application. The ear should be massaged after treatment, and the application repeated in 3 weeks. Below is a table of other insecticides for use against lice and ticks.

INSECTICIDES EFFECTIVE AGAINST LICE AND TICKS

Insecticide	Form	Concentration Necessary for Control	
		lice	ticks
Carbaryl	spray	0.5%	0.5%
Ciodrin	spray	0.3%	0.3%
Coumaphos	spray	0.125%	0.125%
Dioxathion	spray	0.15%	0.15%
Lindane	spray	0.03-0.06%	0.03-0.06%
Malathion	spray	0.5%	0.5%
	dust	4-5%	4-5%
Ronnel	spray	0.75%	0.75%
Toxaphene	spray	0.5%	0.5%

METHODS OF CONTROL

External parasites are best controlled through the use of stringent sanitary measures, aided by chemical control whenever necessary. Listed below are some specific sanitary control measures.

1. Clean manure daily from stalls and pens in stables.
2. Remove manure at weekly intervals from paddocks and pastures.
3. If manure is spread on pastures, spread it thinly with a manure spreader so that fly eggs will be killed by drying. Pastures may also be harrowed to break up manure piles and destroy fly breeding sites.
4. If manure is to be composted, place it in a fly-proof container for 2 to 4 weeks to kill all fly eggs; then spread as fertilizer on pasture.
5. Pick up and compost dog droppings, leaves, grass clippings, wet litter, and decomposing meat, fruit, and vegetables.
6. Use electric fly and mosquito traps with baits such as corn syrup to improve efficiency.
7. Distribute fly predators throughout the stable area. (Fly predators are small flies, harmless to horses, whose larvae feed on the eggs of stable flies).

The following is a list of suggestions for chemical control.

1. Apply residual sprays to surfaces where flies light.
2. Use space sprays applied as fogs or mists in stalls, alleyways, and other enclosed areas.
3. Apply larvicides to breeding grounds such as manure piles, compost piles, and garbage cans.
4. Apply sprays and sponged-on products directly to the animals. Proper dilution and application are necessary if toxicity and skin reaction are to be avoided.

PRECAUTIONS TO OBSERVE WHEN USING INSECTICIDES:

1. Use only insecticides approved and recommended for use on horses; those intended for other classes of livestock may prove injurious to horses.
2. Follow label directions carefully; use the insecticide in the manner and concentration which the manufacturer recommends.
3. Exercise particular caution when applying insecticides to debilitated or stressed horses; these animals are much more susceptible to the toxic effect of the product.
4. Avoid contaminating feed and water supplies.
5. Place baits where children and animals cannot get to them; replenish at weekly intervals.
6. Store insecticides out of the way in a safe place.
7. Know the toxicity signs of insecticide poisoning.

Fig 2-16   COMMON EXTERNAL PARASITES

External Parasites	Pathology	Breeding Areas	Methods of Control
stable fly horse fly deer fly horn fly mosquitoes	bite bite bite bite bite	moist, decaying matter standing water	insecticide sprays fly predators
face fly	irritates carries pinkeye	fresh manure	insecticide smears/ treated halters
house fly	nuisance	horse manure	sprays, baits
screwworm	maggots destroy live flesh	wounds	sprays, smears
botfly	non-biting internal parasite	eggs laid on legs, pupate in manure	oral anthelmintics
lice	suck blood feed on skin debris	eggs attached to hair	dipping, sprays, dusts
spinose ear ticks	severe irritation	eggs laid in protected areas	dusts/powders
hard ticks	biting, spread piroplasmosis	eggs laid in protected places	dips, sprays, dusts
mites	mange		dips, sprays

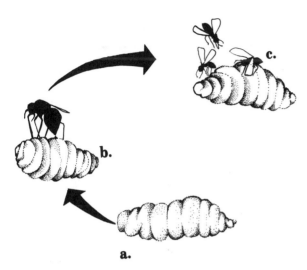

Fig. 2-17 Life cycle of fly predators. a. Egg case of house or stable fly. b. Fly predator laying eggs in the house or stable fly egg case. c. Young fly predators hatch.

Nutrition

Adequate nutrition is necessary for establishment and maintenance of good equine health. Nutritionally related diseases like colic, laminitis, heaves, and azoturia are often related to improper feeding practices. When a horse is well-fed, he is much more resistant to disease and is apt to recover from sickness more quickly than is an underweight, unthrifty horse. A horse's body requirements of energy, fat, minerals, vitamins, and water must be met or exceeded by his diet for him to be in good, healthy condition. Good nutrition, however, although always desirable, is not always simply attained. Of course, complete information on equine nutrition can only be found in a book specializing in such; however, the following covers the general aspects of nutrition.

For the most part, nutritional requirements vary according to a horse's age, weight, and required labor. For example, a young, lactating mare requires more and higher quality feed than does a mature, idle gelding. Recommendations made by the National Research Council can be used as guidelines to tailor each horse's ration to his individual needs. These recommendations can be found in FEEDING TO WIN, a book specifically concerned with equine nutrition.

The following tables can be used to determine the approximate number of kilocalories a horse requires at different levels of work, as well as provide a guide to the amount of feed, expressed as a percentage of the horse's weight, that should be fed daily.

FEED AND ENERGY REQUIREMENTS

Amount of Feed Required

Age of Animal	% of Body Weight
nursing foal	3½ to 4%
weanling	2½ to 3%
lactating mare	3 to 3½%
mature	2 to 2½%

Work	Definition	Kcalories Required per Hour
light	slow jog, lope	2000
medium	fast jog	6000
heavy	gallop, jumping	11000
severe	polo, speed work	19000

PROTEIN SUPPLEMENTATION

In addition to basic feeds that provide roughage and energy, horses may sometimes require supplemental protein from some high quality protein source. The essential amino acids that proteins are made from must be contained in the diet, because the horse's system cannot manufacture them. Moreover, each of the essential amino acids must be present in sufficient quantity so that there is no limitation of the body's ability to produce proteins.

When selecting any protein supplement, protein quality should always be considered as important as the percent of protein contained in the supplement. Quality of protein refers to the balance of amino acids. A high quality protein contains the essential amino acids in the correct proportions and ratios to facilitate the body's protein synthesis.

The following table shows the approximate protein requirements, expressed as percentages of the horse's total ration, required by horses at various stages of life.

Classification	% Protein Required
3-6 month foal	18 to 22%
weanling	15 to 18%
yearling	12 to 14%
2 year-old	12 to 14%
lactating mare	12 to 14%
show & performance horse	12 to 14%
mature horse	10 to 12%

VITAMIN AND MINERAL SUPPLEMENTS

Depending on the roughage/concentrate mixture fed, horses may need supplements of vitamins and minerals. Regardless of the vitamin/mineral supplement used, only one such supplement, used at its recommended level, should be fed to a horse. Horses which do develop vitamin/mineral deficiencies or toxicities are often the recipients of multiple vitamin/mineral supplements from well-meaning owners who think that if one is good, several will be better.

Some of the minerals considered most important to equine nutrition are calcium, phosphorus, and magnesium. The balance between calcium and phosphorus must be correct to avoid signs of mineral toxicity or deficiency. Included in the table below is information regarding the correct calcium to phosphorus ratio for horses of various ages.

Calcium to Phosphorus Ratios Ca:P			
AGE OF HORSE	MIN. RATIO	OPTIMUM RATIO	MAX. RATIO
nursing foal	1 to 1	1.2 to 1	1.5 to 1
weanling	1 to 1	1.5 to 1	2 to 1
yearling	1 to 1	1.7 to 1	3 to 1
mature	1 to 1	1.4 to 1	5 to 1

A vitamin B complex injectable or 3 tbsp/day of brewer's yeast may be used in the ration of a sick or debilitated horse, as well as in the ration of a performance horse, to stimulate appetite.

Supplements high in vitamin D should not be overfed to any horse. This is because vitamin D is rarely deficient in the horse, due to the fact that the average animal receives an adequate amount from sunlight and/or sun-cured hay. This caution also results from the fact that an excessive amount of vitamin D can cause signs of toxicity such as calcification in the heart.

FEEDING SUGGESTIONS

Because of their relatively small stomach capacites (two to four gallons), it is best to feed horses at least two or, preferably, three small meals per day instead of one large one. It is also recommended that horses be fed on a regular schedule, since they learn to anticipate feeding time (even when on pasture) and can be upset by an erratic feeding timetable. Feeding should be done, however, at times other than just before or after exercise to avoid digestive upsets. The feed that is used should be free of debris, mold, and dust, which are contributing factors in problems of colic and heaves. Ample quantities of good quality hay or pasture should also be provided. Where hay is included as part of the diet, it should, ideally, be provided prior to the feeding of the grain ration. (For more detailed information on feeding management, refer to the text FEEDING TO WIN.)

Horses should also be provided free access to clean, fresh water and to some salt. A container of loose salt in a location where it is protected from the elements is preferable to a salt block. All water and feed should be offered from clean equipment, rather than from the ground, to safeguard the animals' health. This means that all troughs, buckets, feeders, etc., must be regularly inspected and cleaned when necessary. Ground feeding, which leads to ingestion of dirt and an increased parasite load, is not recommended.

When possible, it is suggested that horses be fed separately. This practice helps prevent fighting among the animals and assures that each horse receives his individually correct ration of feed.

FEEDING BY WEIGHT

The term "correct ration" refers more nearly to the true weight measurement of a feedstuff than to its volume measure. Weight and volume are often confused at feeding time because of the common practice of feeding from one-pound cans and similar-sized containers. A one-pound coffee can, of course, generally holds one pound of coffee, but may hold more or less than a pound of feed grains or supplements. This is because grains and other feeds of varying densities may differ greatly in weight per volume measure. The one-pound coffee can, for instance, will hold a much greater weight of corn than of oats. Thus, using such a can or similar container as a weight measure for all grains is not recommended. Of course, this means that quart measures and arbitrary weight measures such as coffee cans should be used only after their contents have been weighed.

A device for measuring true weight, a simple baby scale for instance, should prove a helpful and valuable addition to the feed room when fixing rations and changing from one feedstuff to another. In the event that rations are switched, they should be changed gradually to prevent colicking the horse or putting him off his feed.

FEEDSTUFF	Approximate Pounds/Quart
oats	1.0
heavy northern oats	1.2
cracked corn	1.7
molasses	0.8
wheat bran	0.8
sweet feed	1.0
calf manna	1.7

Two factors which can positively or negatively affect nutrition are an animal's parasite load and the condition of his teeth. For this reason, adequate dental care, particularly in regard to floating the teeth, and a proper deworming program are essential (refer to "Control of Internal Parasites" and "Floating the Teeth"). It might be noted here that a horse that is free of parasites and on a diet of adequate protein will likely have a shiny haircoat. The luster of the haircoat can generally be brightened by feeding a source of the polyunsaturated fatty acids linoleic, linolenic, and arachidonic. Corn oil is a good source of linoleic acid, but there are also commercially available products that contain these fatty acids. Such supplements as linseed meal and linseed oil are not as satisfactory as corn oil for conditioning the haircoat, although they may be used for this purpose. Boiled linseed oil certainly should never be fed to a horse, as it is treated for use in paints and is extremely poisonous.

Weight gains in horses of different ages and conditions may vary, but a nursing foal that receives adequate nutrients should gain approximately two and one-half pounds per day. A thin horse in need of extra weight can safely be fed enough to effect a gain of two pounds per day, and, in the case of a dehydrated animal, weight gains of up to four pounds per day may be expected.

DIET-DEFICIENT BEHAVIOR

When a horse does suffer from a dietary deficiency, the result may be an abnormal or depraved diet. Coprophagy (the eating of feces), for example, is sometimes the result of a mineral deficiency in the diet, and any unusual behavior in the form of eating feces, eating tree bark, chewing on fences, etc., can be interpreted as a possible diet-related phenomenon. Admittedly, these conditions may also result from boredom, particularly if a horse is kept stalled and fed a pelleted ration; their occurrence, however, should prompt an investigation of the animal's ration just the same. To ensure a properly fed horse, consult those publications, such as FEEDING TO WIN, that deal specifically with equine nutrition.

Grooming

Proper grooming makes a substantial contribution to the good health and physical condition of a horse. Grooming helps tone up the circulation as well as remove external parasites and improve overall appearance. At the same time, and perhaps most importantly, regular grooming provides the horseowner with an excellent means of discovering abnormal skin conditions, lacerations, abrasions, and swellings that might otherwise go unnoticed.

ROUTINE GROOMING PROCEDURES

BRUSHING THE COAT

A daily grooming program that includes a thorough brushing can do more toward making a horse's coat gleam and giving it a healthy appearance than can any supplemental coat conditioning product. More importantly, however, daily brushing makes a horse feel better by removing dirt and other debris and also allows an individual a chance to closely inspect the skin for any abnormal conditions, etc. Daily brushing is therefore recommended.

REMOVING BOTFLY EGGS

During botfly season, the yellow bot eggs should be removed from a horse's coat before they can be ingested and damage the stomach. These eggs are usually found on the front legs (particularly below the knees) and

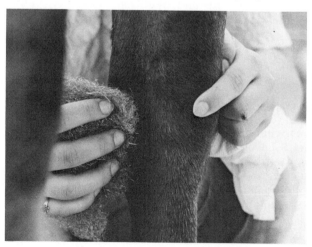

Fig. 2-18 Removing bot fly eggs with a steel wool pad.

on the chest. The eggs can be removed by either scraping the hair carefully with a razor blade, a sharp pocket knife, a serrated bot-removing knife, a bot block, a steel wool pad, or sandpaper, or by application of a commercial preparation designed to loosen the adhesive. The application of warm water will cause the larvae to emerge from the eggs; however, recent reports show that animals treated with weekly hot water baths were as heavily infested as pastured horses that were not bathed, so this is not really an effective way to control bots. However, those that were dewormed every other month with a boticide had healthy stomachs.

CLEANING THE EYES, EARS, NOSE, AND DOCK

As a part of thorough grooming, a damp cloth should be used to wipe clean the eyes, nostrils, and ears. Also, the area under the tail and around the anus should be wiped clean of debris that could cause skin irritation and infection if neglected. The udder of the mare and sheath of the stallion or gelding also require attention periodically.

CARE OF THE HORSE AFTER RIDING

When a hot, lathered horse is brought in from a day's hard riding, he should not be immediately unsaddled and turned out. This practice invites digestive disorders and laminitis, and may cause a horse to develop a sore back. Do not quickly unsaddle the horse; rather, first loosen the girth (cinch) and allow the horse a small amount of cool (not cold) water. Too much water can cause a horse to colic or founder, so the amount given is important. The saddle should not be removed until the horse has had a chance to cool off for approximately fifteen minutes to avoid too-rapid dilation of blood vessels in the back.

While cooling out, a horse should also be kept moving at a slow pace, to help prevent colic, laminitis, or chilling. This can be accomplished by either hand-walking a horse or by putting him on a hotwalker. A horse's water intake should also be restricted when cooling out, as another possible preventive for colic or laminitis. Small amounts should be given at about three to five minute intervals until the horse is completely cooled out and no longer thirsty.

SPECIALIZED GROOMING PROCEDURES
CLEANING THE SHEATH

Cleaning the sheath of a stallion or gelding is an area of grooming that should not be neglected. The sheath, over a period of time, can collect secretions and dead skin cells which together are called smegma. Sometimes an unclean sheath causes irritation, which in turn causes a horse to rub his tail. Occasionally, smegma even accumulates in a mass above the opening of the urethra. The resulting "bean" may become large enough to interfere with urination if not removed. In addition, in locales where they are prevalent, screwworm larvae are often attracted to dirty sheaths, where they may cause serious wounds and infection.

Most horses, therefore, should have their sheaths cleaned at least every six months. Those animals, however, with lightly-pigmented genital areas, such as Pintos, tend to accumulate smegma more quickly and should be cleaned more often.

The horse needs to be restrained so that he is not able to move around while his sheath is being cleaned. Having an assistant hold the head, and putting the horse next to a fence or wall is preferable to having the horse tied, and may be sufficient restraint with a horse accustomed to this procedure. Of course, caution should be observed when cleaning a horse unaccustomed to this treatment.

Cleaning, itself, is a relatively simple matter that requires only a bucket of warm water, some cotton, and a mild soap, such as Ivory. First, the cotton is soaked in the warm water, then soap is applied to it. The soapy cotton is then applied to the sheath to clean the penis, after which the area above the urethra can be checked by hand for smegma accumulation. When one piece of cotton is dirty, another clean one should be used. A very thorough rinsing with as much water as is necessary should follow the soapy cleaning. If a horse is very relaxed, a hose can be used to rinse the area.

CLEANING THE BREEDING STALLION

A breeding stallion needs to be washed both before and after breeding a mare. Before breeding, the stallion's penis should be cleansed with warm water and disposable cotton after he has had an erection. For the sake of cleanliness, disposable gloves should be worn by the individual performing this task. Also, the cotton used for washing should be disposed of as it is used; it should not be put back into the clean water. Washing not only cleanses the penis, it also serves to stimulate the stallion just before he is bred. After breeding, the penis should be gently rinsed with an antiseptic such as a weak solution of tamed iodine.

CLEANING THE MARE

Occasionally, a smegma-like substance collects between the teats on a mare's udder. This substance can be very irritating and cause the mare to rub her tail. Consequently, it is a good idea to check this area periodically for cleanliness.

Hoof Care

IMPORTANCE OF CLEAN STABLING

Proper hoof care begins with preventive measures, and good stable management is essential for prevention and treatment of hoof ailments. Horses should not have to stand in dirty bedding or in stalls with muddy floors, because both conditions predispose horses to thrush and canker.

Stalls should therefore be cleaned daily and floors occasionally disinfected with lime, after stripping of all bedding, to reduce odors. (Care should be taken not to lime the stalls too often, however, as too much lime will irritate a horse's mucous membranes.) Additionally, any dips or hollows in stall floors need to be filled and leveled to prevent horses from injuring themselves when lying down or straining their legs while standing.

CLEANING THE HOOFS

Hoofs should be cleaned daily with a hoof pick, and trimmed or reshod every four to six weeks (refer to "Maintenance Trimming and Shoeing"). When picking up a horse's feet, face the rear, lean into the animal, and pick up the foot as the horse's weight shifts. Holding the lifted foot and leg as close as possible to the horse's body will help his balance and reduce struggling.

After becoming accustomed to having his hoofs picked up, a horse will learn to lift his feet readily at a pinch of the tendon behind the fetlock.

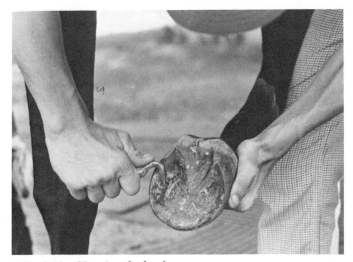

Fig. 2-19   Cleaning the hoof.

MAINTAINING MOISTURE IN THE HOOF

Moisture, of course, is necessary for a hoof to maintain its springy action. It is this spring-like action of the bars of the hoof that allows the hoof wall to expand laterally when weight is placed on the structure. The preferred way to preserve moisture in the hoofs is to stand or walk the horse in water or mud frequently. If this is not possible, application of a hoof conditioner can help preserve proper hoof moisture, especially on horses housed in dry stalls. These animals often develop quarter cracks because their dry bedding actually pulls moisture from their hoofs.

Hoof conditioners help maintain the integrity of the hoof wall by increasing its flexibility, thus reducing the chance of cracking and splitting, and improving brittle hoofs.

A hoof conditioner should be applied to the hoof wall and coronary band when necessary to prevent dryness. It should never be applied to the sole of the foot.

Hoof conditioners, though useful, do not stimulate hoof growth. To encourage hoof growth, a horse should be kept nutritionally sound and his coronet area frequently massaged. This massage will increase blood circulation, possibly accelerating production of new hoof wall.

It is possible for a hoof to contain too much water; when this happens, elasticity is lost and there is a tendency for the hoof wall to overspread when weight is placed on the hoof. In this case, the hoof wall may eventually separate from underlying tissues. This could be a problem if a horse is kept on damp, muddy ground for an extended period of time.

SOAKING THE HOOF

Contracted heels and brittle feet are examples of two hoof conditions that can definitely benefit from daily soaking in water to replenish hoof moisture. Additionally, if infection is present in the hoof, as it is in cases of thrush, quarter cracks, gravel, puncture wounds, canker, and subsolar abscesses, a supersaturated solution of magnesium sulfate (epsom salts) can be effectively used. Drying agents such as formalin and Kopertox may be used on the sole as well. Depending on the condition, iodine, antibiotic powders, or chlorine bleach may also be beneficial in the sole area.

PACKING THE HOOF

Clay packs can be used in a horse's hoofs to keep his feet soft and moist or to prevent the accumulation of manure and the resulting possibility of thrush. When applying a clay pack, just enough water should be added to

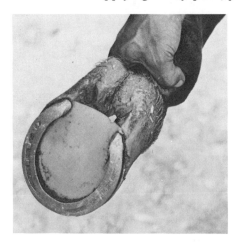

Fig. 2-20 Horse shod with a leather pad for protection of the sole.

the clay to facilitate working it into the hoof; too much water will allow it to fall out easily. A handful of coarse salt can be added during the packing procedure to help retain moisture and soothe the foot. The clay should be packed into the hoof with a paddle, which can be used to smooth over its surface. Once the hoofs have been packed, a piece of heavy brown paper can be applied to the bottom of each hoof to help keep the clay from falling out.

Other packs may need to be bandaged into place to keep them from falling out. Such bandaging not only keeps the packing material in, it also keeps dirt and debris out of an injured foot. For this purpose, a leather pad with a pine tar and oakum pack can be used in conjunction with any special shoe required. On a bruised sole, a silicone rubber pad or one of tire retread rubber may be tried instead of leather. Leather hoof pads, as palliative treatment, can also be used on horses with navicular disease to help reduce hoof concussion. This is of some importance, as further treatment for navicular disease includes walking exercise to increase circulation.

APPLYING A POULTICE TO A HOOF

A poultice is used as a drawing agent or to create moist, local heat and provide counterirritation. When used, a poultice can be retained either in a horse boot or in an innertube sleeve that has been slipped over a leg and folded at the bottom. Another way to keep a poultice on the sole of a hoof is to use an Easyboot.

Poultices are sometimes used as palliative treatment for navicular disease. Examples of some poultices and their ingredients are: magnesium sulfate; aluminum silicate; boric acid paste; kaolin, glycerine, water and aconite; zinc oxide glycerine, gelatin and water (Unna's paste). (Refer to "Bandaging" for more information.)

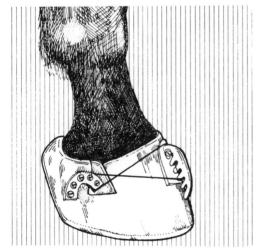

Fig. 2-21   An Easyboot.

TRIMMING AND SHOEING

Horses do not always need to be shod. However, when they need extra traction, when their use causes excessive wear on their feet, or when they have incorrect gaits, they should be shod. The object of shoeing a horse is to protect and decrease the wear of the hoof wall. To an extent, however, shoeing interferes with the natural movement of a horse's foot. Because of this, the underlying theory of shoeing is to add shoes of such design and weight that they help the horse do his best with the least amount of unnatural interference. Most trimming and shoeing requires a farrier (or a farrier's expertise).

When trimming and shoeing are necessary, they should be done every four to six weeks on most horses (some horses may be able to go 8 weeks). Performance horses, however, involved in more strenuous activity, may require attention more often. The purpose of trimming is to level the foot and make the foot axis as normal as possible. The axis is a straight line that passes through the center of the pastern and continues through the hoof to the sole. A normal angle (viewed from the side) is about 45-50° in front and 50-55° in back, and can be measured with a foot protractor. It is important to remember that each horse has a normal axis of his own; trimming, therefore, does not aim at the creation of a "perfect foot."

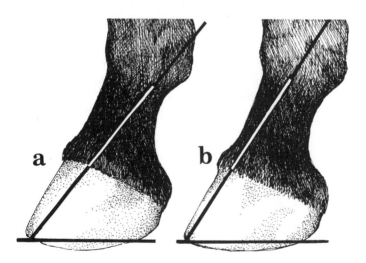

Fig. 2-22 Ideal foot and pastern angle. a. Front foot is 45-47°. b. Hind foot is 50-55°.

In general, a horse performs best if he is trimmed and shod according to his own angle of hoof and toe conformation, keeping hoof and pastern axis unbroken, in other words, as an individual. Before trimming, each horse should be viewed in motion and at rest to establish which foot angle is best suited to him.

After the angle is decided, the hoof should be cleaned with a hoof pick, and the loose, dead areas of the frog and sole scraped away with a hoof knife. Cleaning the areas between the angles of the bars helps prevent accumulation of dirt and debris which can result in the formation of corns. After cleaning, the hoof wall should be trimmed to about the level of the frog, but never past the sole, then leveled and smoothed with a rasp. Since the sole is concave, the wall should be trimmed closer at the toe than at the heel. If a horse is to be left unshod, about one-quarter inch more of hoof wall should be left than if he is to be shod. The hoof wall can then be beveled to prevent splitting.

The shoe itself should conform to the shape of the hoof wall, with its branches extending about one-sixteenth inch beyond the wall at the heel and quarter to allow for expansion. At the heel, the shoe should normally be from one-sixteenth inch to one-quarter inch longer than the hoof.

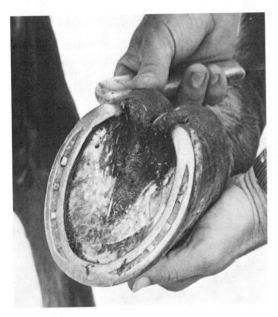

Fig. 2-23 **Improperly shod hoof; notice that the lateral heels are not supported by the shoe.**

The shoes a horse wears should be specifically adapted to the work he does. On pleasure horses, for instance, regular plate shoes are preferable to shoes with heel caulks or toe grabs. These special devices, designed for added speed and traction, are found on many racing shoes. Neither heel caulks nor toe grabs are meant to be used on horses that must make quick turns, i.e., barrel racers and cutting horses (refer to "Corrective Shoeing and Trimming").

Shoes may be reset once or twice, though they should not be reset if the toe has worn thin. Shoes that are not particularly worn, but have enlarged nail holes, should not be reset either. Borium is sometimes added to shoes to make them wear longer.

REMOVING A SHOE

It is sometimes necessary to remove a shoe without the aid of a farrier in order to promptly and adequately treat a foot injury or to take off a shoe that has become loose. For example, in cases of close nail, pricked sole, bruised sole, and corns, a horse's shoe must be removed from the affected foot. Required tools for this procedure include a pair of pulling pincers and a clinch or rasp.

The first step in removing a shoe is to cut or rasp off the clinched nail ends. After this has been done, the foot should be lifted, held between the knees, and the hoof supported in one hand to prevent the foot from turning and damaging the fetlock joint. It is suggested that the shoe be loosened a little at a time, starting with one heel and moving toward the toe. Both heels should be loosened in a like manner, and the loosening procedure continued back and forth up the sides of the shoe towards the toe. If the nails loosen from the shoe, they should be removed one at a time; if they remain seated in the nail creases, they will come out with the shoe. To actually pull the shoe off once it has been sufficiently loosened, each heel of the shoe should be grasped in turn with the pulling pincers and pulled with a short, hard pull towards the toe and middle of the foot. The shoe should then be lifted off carefully, without twisting the pincers. After removal, it is important to make sure that all pieces of nail are out of the hoof wall.

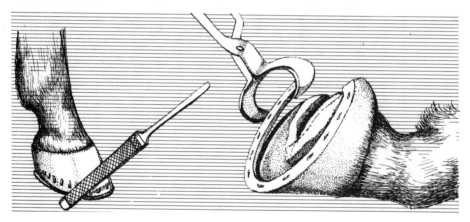

Fig. 2-24 Removing a shoe.

Vices

Horses are occasionally afflicted with vices (bad habits) that are annoying both to other horses as well as to their owners. Many of these vices result from the boredom of being constantly stalled, and often disappear when a horse is allowed to run out on pasture. This is especially true when an animal is turned out before the habit becomes too ingrained.

If the horse must be kept stalled, a hanging object to play with (such as a tetherball) is often successful in curing a boredom-caused vice. In addition, more frequent attention, grooming, and exercise is psychologically better for the horse.

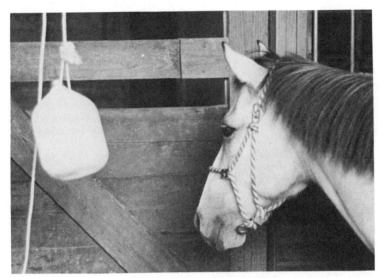

Fig. 2-25   A hanging object in the stall, such as a tetherball or a plastic bottle filled with pebbles, will often help distract a bored horse.

This section will discuss only those bad habits that are considered to constitute a health hazard to the horse as well as an irritation to the owner. If suggested treatments for any of the following vices are not successful, the afflicted animal should probably be quickly separated from other horses. This action is necessary because bad habits will often be imitated by surrounding horses. Each of the following vices may be serious enough to be considered an unsoundness by some people, and should be prevented if at all possible.

CRIBBING AND WINDSUCKING

The terms cribbing and windsucking are often used interchangeably to mean either wood-chewing and/or the swallowing of air. For the purposes of this discussion, cribbing will be defined as wood-chewing, and windsucking as aerophagia.

CRIBBING

Cribbing, which is the act of chewing wood, is a relatively common vice. Cribbing horses usually chew the wood of their stall doors, fencing, trees, etc., often inhaling air through the mouth (and eventually becoming windsuckers) in the process. Cribbing often results from boredom, but may be caused, at least in some horses, by a dietary deficiency. Should this be the case, one-half cup of apple cider vinegar added to the horse's daily ration and some free-choice monosodium phosphate may be beneficial.

However, if cribbing continues, the number of wood surfaces that are available for the animal to chew should be reduced. Such a reduction can be effected either by removing some objects, by coating everything with a distasteful substance, or by capping all wood surfaces with metal. Several commercial preparations are available on the market for coating wood surfaces, most of which have a base of creosote or red peppers.

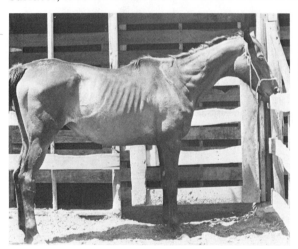

Fig. 2-26 A windsucker; notice the poor condition of this horse.

WINDSUCKING

Windsucking, or aerophagia, is the act of grabbing a firm object with the teeth and inhaling air through the mouth. Cribbing is often a part of this problem, although, occasionally, a veteran windsucker can indulge in this vice without even grasping an object. Because this condition impairs digestion, many horses that windsuck are very thin and pass foul-smelling gas. Horses with the vice of either cribbing or windsucking often develop a peculiar wear pattern on the labial surface of the incisor teeth, that can be used to identify the horse as a windsucker.

A metal-reinforced leather collar may be effective in the prevention of aerophagia when placed around the throatlatch. These collars are available with spikes or a single metal piece that digs into the horse as he tenses his neck for windsucking. The collar must be adjusted tightly enough to prevent the horse from cording his neck muscles, but not so snugly as to interfere with his breathing. The advantage of such a collar is that it does not deter the horse from eating or drinking, as tying him in cross-ties does. Since a horse must be able to create a vacuum in order to windsuck, the use of a fluted bit may provide a method of prevention.

Windsucking is a vice that might be cured by turning the horse out to pasture and giving him a vacation for an extended period of time. This is most successful if the horse is not a windsucker of long habit.

The most radical method of curing windsucking is surgical intervention. The surgery entails the incision of the muscles inserting on the hyoid bone, thereby restricting the horse's ability to swallow air. Although there is a danger of physical disfigurement, the operation is fairly successful. Experiments with electric shock-based corrective methods have recently been successful, and may hold some promise in treating windsucking.

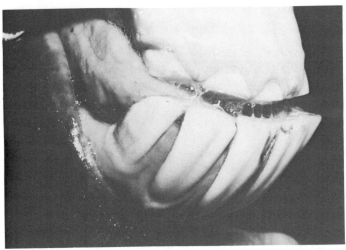

Fig. 2-27 Teeth of a cribber or windsucker; upper incisors are almost completely worn away.

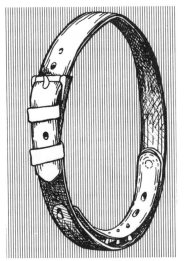 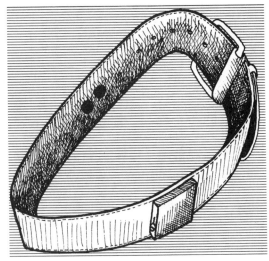

Fig. 2-28 Windsucking collars; a spiked collar [left] and an electrical collar [right].

WEAVING

Weaving, the shifting of the horse's weight from one lateral pair of legs to the other, is another undesirable vice that can cause a horse to lose condition and energy. Moreover, this vice may cause the tendons of the forelegs to weaken.

For distraction and entertainment, a tether ball, or a plastic bottle filled with pebbles or grain, can be suspended from the barn rafters as a toy for the horse to play with. This may relieve some stall-related boredom and solve a weaving problem. A goat may also help alleviate the problem by providing companionship.

Since many horses weave with their heads over a stall door, closing the door's upper half (Dutch door) will often solve the problem. If the door is just a half-door, burlap strips or even tin cans hung over the opening with strings may dissuade the horse from putting his head through.

MASTURBATION

Masturbation is a vice that may cause poor performance and, in breeding stallions, may result in lower fertility. It is usually described as a solitary habit; that is, it usually is done by a horse at night, or when the animal is alone. Masturbation is less frequently seen in stallions that are housed where they can see other horses.

Sometimes, an accumulation of smegma in the prepuce may cause irritation and encourage masturbation. To help eliminate this accumulation, the sheaths of both stallions and geldings should be regularly cleaned as part of the grooming routine (refer to "Cleaning the Sheath" under "Grooming").

In addition to these precautions, there are some physical devices available for controlling masturbation. Examples of specific devices are the plastic stallion ring made to fit on the penis about an inch above the glans, and the corrosive-resistant metal stallion cage which fits around the glans. Both of these devices are fitted to the size of the relaxed penis and prevent an erection. Any apparatus used should first be disinfected, and must be removed from time to time (once a week) to check for possible irritation.

Masturbation in stallions can almost always be stopped, and the previously affected horses quickly returned to good breeding condition.

PAWING, KICKING, AND STALL-WALKING

A horse that constantly paws in his stall is capable of making deep holes in a dirt or clay floor. This is more serious than may be immediately evident, for an uneven stall floor is very hard on a horse's legs.

Kicking in the stall can result in scarred hind legs and capped hocks. Sometimes this behavior can be controlled simply by putting a different horse in an adjacent stall, or by stalling the kicker where he cannot see other horses. Both kicking and pawing can frequently be controlled by fastening chains (about 14 inches long) to the horse's legs with padded leather straps, either above the knees or hocks (depending upon whether the horse paws or kicks). When the horse attempts to paw or kick, he will hit himself with the chains and soon stop.

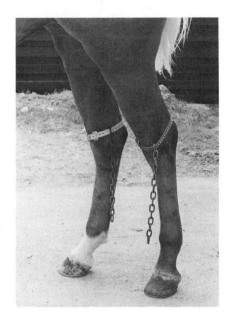

Fig. 2-29 Chains are an effective restraint to prevent kicking or pawing; ideally, the straps should be padded to prevent chafing.

A stall-walker needs as much quiet as possible, and, if necessary, may have to be kept in cross-ties. As with a weaver, a tether ball or other hanging object in the stall will often give the stall-walker something to play with and occupy his time. Stall-walking is one of the most serious vices.

BOLTING THE FOOD

Bolting food is, of course, dangerous. Any horse that bolts his food, besides endangering his nutrition, also risks the possibility of choking. Placing large, smooth stones in the horse's feeder may help to eliminate this vice. ♞

3

RESTRAINT OF THE HORSE

Physical Restraints

Nearly all horsemen are familiar with restraints such as halters, twitches, and hobbles, and realize their value in controlling horses for medical treatment and convalescence, as well as for grooming. However, the very fact that restraints are such useful and valuable means of control necessitates discussing a few of the commonly used types in some detail.

REASONS FOR RESTRAINT

Restraints are most often necessary to physically control an injured horse before beginning treatment, to facilitate the treatment itself, to prevent further harm to the animal, and to prevent injury to the handler. Popular restraints like hobbles help immobilize a horse, while such well-known physical restraints as twitches and war bridles help control an animal by causing him pain if he continues to struggle. While these methods of restraint quiet most horses, there are those animals that will panic when restraints are applied. Abrupt or indecisive movements by the handler can be misinterpreted by a horse and further excite him; therefore, a direct approach and application of the restraint is suggested. It is important, then, to apply the restraint calmly, carefully, and confidently, preferably in an area such as a large stall or shed where the horse can do little damage if he continues to resist.

INITIAL EVALUATION

Initially, a careful evaluation of a horse's temperament and size, the kind of work to be done, the necessary location and duration of the restraint, and the handler's ability will aid in making a knowledgeable choice of the mildest restraint that will provide humane control. There will, however, be times when physical restraints must be used with other methods to obtain the desired control (in a few cases, no matter how much care is taken or what methods of restraint are attempted, some horses cannot be controlled unless sedated). Consequently, chemical restraints such as sedatives or tranquilizers may be necessary, or in special instances, general anesthesia may be required (refer to "Chemical Restraints").

THE TWITCH

The twitch is a basic restraint that is preferred because it is a mild and humane control. Commercially, the basic twitch often consists of a 36-48 inch handle with a rope or chain loop on one end. A twitch with a chain loop is a better choice, as a chain is less likely to cut off circulation or abrade the lip than is a rope loop. Other types, such as the tong twitch, are becoming more popular and are discussed later.

Since a horse will swing away from a twitch, the person applying it should stand in front and to the same side as the person treating the animal. This positioning will allow an alert handler the leverage required to quickly turn the horse away from the person administering treatment, if necessary. This is normal procedure, but it may have to be amended somewhat when a horse is "tubed." In tubing, either mechanical interference would occur between the two individuals or else one of them would be forced to stand directly in front of the horse in the animal's strike zone. In this instance, the operator usually picks the side he prefers and the handler works from the opposite side. The twitch can then be readily applied when the operator is ready to proceed.

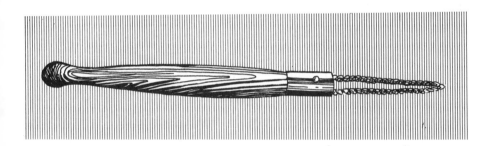

Fig. 3-1 Chain twitch.

The principle of the twitch is that its application causes pressure on the sensitive nerves of the lips, and the resulting discomfort diverts the horse's attention from the procedure/treatment being performed. The necessary firmness with which the twitch is applied will vary from horse to horse. While a twitch must always be twisted at least enough to prevent slipping, it will have to be applied more tightly on some horses to obtain the desired control.

Caution and judgement are required here, for excessive pressure or application time can result in a cut lip. Moreover, as mentioned previously, a twitch distracts a horse's attention by compressing the nerves in the upper lip and causing pain. If applied to this area for too long a period of time, a twitch would cut off circulation, the lip would become numb, and the desired diversionary effect would be lost. Pressure should therefore be alternated, so that circulation and sensitivity in the lip are maintained.

APPLICATION

A simple twitch can be applied from either side of the horse. To apply a standard rope or chain twitch from the left side, take these steps:

1. Grasp the twitch handle firmly at mid-shaft with the hand.
2. Loop the chain or rope around the middle three fingers of the left hand. This will prevent the chain from slipping around the wrist of the handler.
3. Grasp the animal's upper lip with the left hand and slide the chain or rope around the lip while folding the lip. (If applied to an ear, a twitch may break the conchal cartilage that supports the ear, or injure a muscle or nerve. The result would be a blemished horse.)
4. While holding the folded lip with the left hand, rotate the handle clockwise so that the chain tends to climb up the face rather than down and off the lip.
5. With both hands, hold the lead shank and twitch handle simultaneously, near the end of the handle.
6. If the procedure is prolonged, occasionally rotate the twitch back and forth on its long axis to keep the animal distracted. Tapping on the handle of the twitch after it is applied will often work to distract the horse's attention, should this become necessary.

Remember that all restraints should be applied for as short an interval as possible. Since there are a few horses that will not tolerate a twitch, it may sometimes be best to choose another method. In these cases, for example, a chemical restraint such as a tranquilizer may be required. Other horses are easy to handle once the twitch is in place; however, they may require a momentary distraction while it is being applied. For these animals, grasping a roll of skin over the scapula or holding an ear (refer to "Body Restraints") will often suffice. Once the horse is distracted and the twitch is in place, it should always be held firmly enough to prevent the horse from flailing it about.

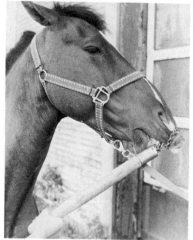

Fig. 3-2 Chain twitch in place; notice that the chain is not in contact with the inner lip surfaces.

OTHER TWITCHES

TONG TWITCH

There are several other types of twitches that are useful as restraints. A nose-clamp, or tong twitch, is a popular type of restraint that can be attached to the halter, if necessary, thereby removing the need for an assistant to hold it. It is a nutcracker-shaped clamp with an attached nylon cord which is wrapped around the twitch to hold it closed. A snap at the cord's end is fastened to the halter, keeping the nose-clamp in place. Like the standard twitch, the tong twitch should be applied to the folded upper lip, which should be massaged after removal of the clamp to help restore circulation.

ENGLISH TWITCH

Another restraint, the humane or English twitch, consists of a metal screw clamp that is applied to the upper lip. While this twitch doesn't require an assistant to hold it, it does require more time to put on and remove, a disadvantage which could cause problems in dealing with an uncooperative animal. A humane twitch is rather awkward to apply and therefore not as satisfactory as one of the other types.

ONE-MAN TWITCH

A more complex restraint, the one-man twitch is so named because its application only requires one person. It consists of a metal bar, 10 inches long, with a metal ring at each end, one ring twice the diameter of the

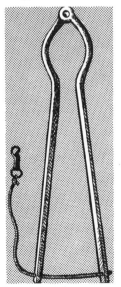 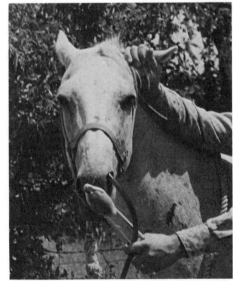

Fig. 3-3 a. Tong twitch.   b. A tong twitch can be applied for restraint during minor procedures, such as deworming. Holding the ear can be used as additional restraint.

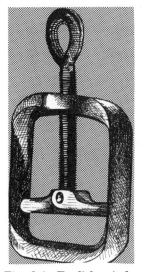

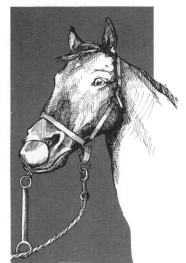

Fig. 3-4   English twitch.   **Fig. 3-5   One-man twitch in place; notice that if the horse pulls back, the halter will take the shock before the lip.**

other. In applying it, a loop of nylon cord is brought through the smaller ring and placed around the horse's upper lip. After tightening the loop by twisting the bar, the halter rope is passed through the larger ring and tied to a solid object. If the horse becomes frightened and pulls back, the halter absorbs the strain instead of the twitch, thus reducing the chance of injury to the animal's lip.

RING TWITCH

A ring twitch consists of a metal ring with an attached loop of rope. The loop is placed around the horse's upper lip and the ring turned to increase

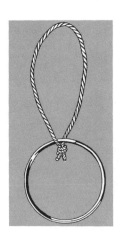

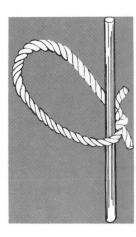

Fig. 3-6   Ring twitch [left].

Fig. 3-7   Simple rope twitch [right].

pressure. Some ring twitches have metal snaps that fasten on the horse's halter so an assistant is not needed to hold them. A simple twitch can be made from a piece of rope (tied in a loop) and a stick, which is put through the loop and twisted, somewhat like a tourniquet, to apply pressure on the horse's lip.

THE WAR BRIDLE

Horses that fight a twitch, or are vicious, can sometimes be controlled by the use of a war bridle. Basically, a war bridle is a more stringent restraint that applies pressure on the poll, the gingiva (gums), the jaw, or on a combination of these. The war bridle tends to be harsher in action than a twitch, and might not be as good a choice for restraint with most horses. War bridles are also used as training devices, and may have greater value as such; their occasional value in restraint is usually as a control method to be used in conjunction with a twitch.

CHAIN-TYPE WAR BRIDLE

One type of war bridle consists of a leather halter with a chain shank. The chain is attached to the right-hand cheek ring on the halter, and can be used in a variety of ways. It can be passed through the mouth, over the muzzle, under the jaw, or over the upper gingiva, and then run through the left cheek ring. (This restraint is particularly useful for controlling a stallion.) Since the chain under the jaw may cause the horse to rear, care should be exercised in its application; the same care must be taken when the gingiva are involved to insure they are not injured by excessive pressure. As an additional safety precaution, a horse should never be tied using this restraint.

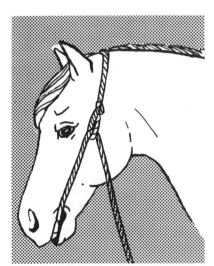

Fig. 3-8   Yankee war bridle.

NERVE BRIDLE

The other major type of war bridle is called a rope gag, or nerve bridle. This gag, made from rope approximately the size of sash cord, should always be used with a halter and a lead rope, and must not be used to tie a horse. Nerve bridles are particularly useful in controlling a rearing horse, since the poll pressure forces the animal down.

Yankee War Bridle

One type of nerve bridle is the Yankee war bridle, which causes diversionary pain. In forming it, a small loop is tied in one end of a 10 foot piece of five-sixteenth inch or three-eighth inch rope, and the other end passed through this eye to form a loop 3 feet in diameter. This loop should be placed over the horse's face, across the poll, down the sides of the face, and over the upper gingiva. When the free end of the rope is pulled, pressure on the poll and gums causes the animal pain.

Magner's Modified War Bridle

Another of the many variations of this type of restraint is Magner's modified war bridle, which applies pressure on both the poll and the gingiva. This restraint is applied by placing a non-slip noose around the lower jaw, then passing the other end of the rope up the right side of the head and over the poll. The rope is bent behind and below the left ear and held, while the free end of the cord is passed down the right side of the horse's head, under the upper lip, and over the gingiva. The rope is then brought up the left side of the head, through the loop at the ear, and down underneath the noose around the jaw.

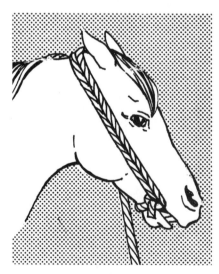 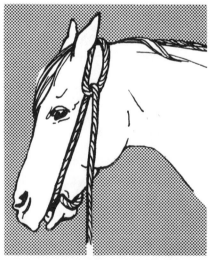

Fig. 3-9 a. Magner's modified war bridle [right view].

Fig. 3-9 b. Magner's modified war bridle [left view].

TYING A HORSE

When tying a horse, particularly when restraining an injured horse, the most appropriate equipment should be used. A fractious or distressed horse can break leather halters, lightweight nylon leads and halters, and lightweight tie-rope snaps, perhaps injuring or re-injuring himself in the process. And, since breakage, in part, depends not only on the quality of material used in the rope and halter, but on the snap construction as well, only equipment with heavy-duty hardware should be used.

Although very strong nylon leads and halters are good, some of the better ones available are made of cotton rope. Nylon rope, although strong, is harder to handle than cotton rope and is more likely to cause rope burns on the hands of the person holding the horse, should the animal jerk the rope (one reason the rope should never be looped around a hand). Cotton ropes, especially round ones (as opposed to those of flat webbing), are also better able to hold knots and thus are better used in tying than are nylon ones.

Regardless of what equipment is used, it is imperative that a horse be tied to solid, stationary objects such as fence posts set well into the ground or, ideally, into concrete. As another general precaution, a horse should be tied at least as high as his head to reduce the chance of neck injuries. When properly tied, it should be virtually impossible for a horse to catch a leg over his lead rope.

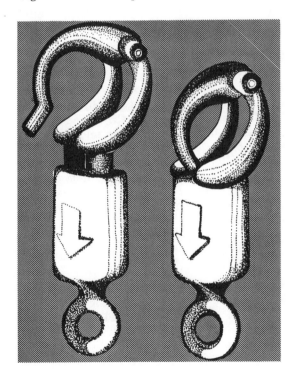

Fig. 3-10 A quick-release snap; a sharp pull downward will release the snap immediately, even if the horse is pulling hard.

COMMONLY USED KNOTS AND METHODS OF TYING

Cotton Neck-Rope

Should a horse continue to pull on his lead rope, he can be tied with a cotton neck-rope. This rope should be about 10 feet long, with a heavy snap on one end and a heavy metal ring approximately 18 inches from the snap. This rope is placed around the horse's neck, as close to the poll as possible, and the snap fastened to the ring. The free end of the neck rope is then tied to the same object as the lead. It should be tied shorter, though, so that the neck rope will receive the initial strain if the horse decides to pull back again.

Quick-Release Knot

A certain knowledge of knot tying and the uses of various knots is very helpful for purposes of restraint because different knots lend themselves to specific uses. For example, to avoid injury, a quick-release knot is a good one to use when tying and restraining a horse. This knot can be quickly undone even when a horse is pulling back. The quick-release knot can be made by putting the lead rope around a stationary object, making a large loop with one end, and then pulling a smaller loop made with the free end through the first one. The second loop is then pulled tight to complete the knot. If the horse succeeds in loosening this knot, the tail of the rope can be threaded through the first loop to prevent untying. (See accompanying illustrations.)

Bowline Knot Used With Burlap Sack

Another humane way to tie a horse by the neck involves the placement of a folded burlap bag around the horse's neck, directly behind the poll. The ends of the bag are tied together with rope, and secured by a non-slip bowline knot. This knot is tied by first making a loop in the left end of the rope and passing the right end through the loop, down and over the opposite side of the loop. This end is then continued under the left hand strand and back up through the loop. The bowline is a good knot to use because it doesn't slip, it will not draw tight, and it is easily untied. It is much preferred to the slipknot, which is not a good knot to tie a horse with because of the risk of injury. If the horse was to panic, the slipknot would tighten like a noose, possibly causing strangulation or serious injury.

Tying the Tail

Sometimes a horse's tail may need to be tied to discourage kicking or to move it out of the way during a rectal examination. In tying the tail, a rope is placed over the tail, just past the dock, and the remaining part of the tail folded up over the rope. The left end of the rope is then folded under the tail, and brought up to the right hand side where it is doubled (made into a bight). The bight is carried over the folded tail and brought through the

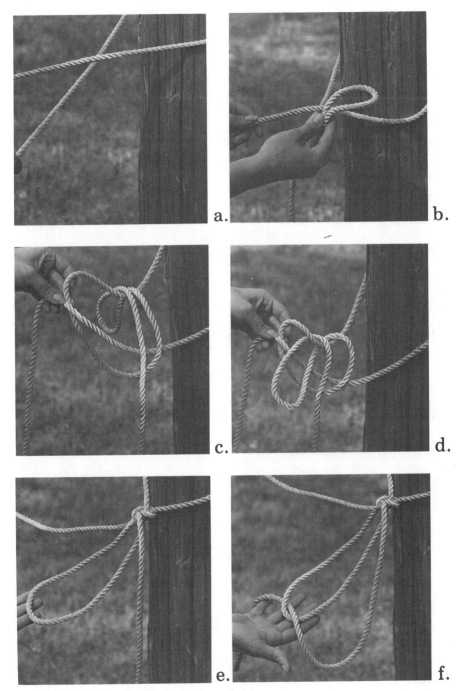

Fig. 3-11 Steps in tying a quick-release knot.

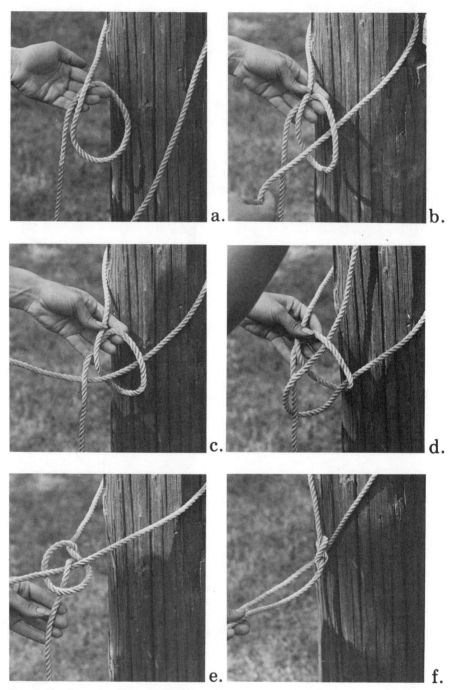

Fig. 3-12   Steps in tying a bowline knot.

loop around the tail, then pulled tight to finish the tie. The tail is then held to the side by the rope. A tail rope is always held by hand, never tied to a stationary object.

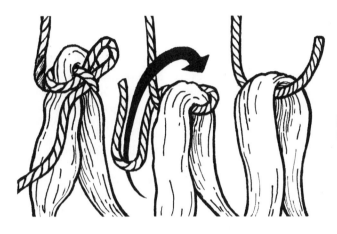

Fig. 3-13 Steps in tying the tail.

Tying a Foreleg

It sometimes becomes necessary to restrain one or more of a horse's legs to prevent moving or kicking. When restraining a foreleg, a person should choose the one on the same side of the horse as he is working, since lifting that limb will normally keep the horse from kicking with the hindleg on that side.

There are several ways to control a foreleg, the simplest of which is to have an assistant hold the leg up in a bent position. The leg can also be held by a kneestrap buckled around the cannon and forearm of the flexed limb. This method, however, is not recommended because of the difficulty of unbuckling the kneestrap. If a horse restrained in this manner became very excited, he might harm himself before the strap could be undone. A similar restraint for a foreleg can be fashioned from an old stirrup leather of an English saddle. When the horse's leg is bent at the knee, the leather strap is put around the bent leg and one end drawn through the metal ring at the other end. It can then be drawn tight and tied with a half hitch.

Still another method of foreleg restraint uses a rope with a quick-release knot, which requires the aid of an assistant. (Note: Any time a rope is used on the leg, it should be a soft cotton one. If other types are used, abrasions can be prevented with hobbles or bandages used around the limb, at the point of contact with the rope.) In applying this restraint, one end of the rope is tied around the pastern, and the other end is brought up over the horse's withers. The assistant standing on the side opposite the roped foreleg can then hold the limb up with the rope after the foot has been lifted.

A similar method of foreleg restraint allows the handler to stand in front of the horse instead of at his side. The procedure for tying is the same except that the rope is continued over the withers and around the animal's chest to the side it is tied on. It is taken under the rope over the withers, then pulled to the front by the handler. The person holding the rope can easily release it if the horse becomes excited.

Tying a Hindleg/Use of a Sideline

In order to prevent kicking, to distract a horse during a rectal examination, or to allow for the performance of a minor operation, a hindleg can be restrained through the use of a sideline. One variation of the sideline is made by forming a non-slip loop with a bowline knot in one end of a 15-20 foot piece of soft cotton rope. This loop must be large enough to be placed loosely around the horse's neck. When the loop is in place, the rope is passed backwards, between the hindlegs, and around the pastern of the leg to be restrained. By bringing the rope forward and passing it through the neck loop, the foot can be brought to and held in any position by pulling the free end of the rope. A rope burn can be avoided by using a hobble, hobble strap, or bandage around the pastern of the leg. If a hobble strap is used, the rope is passed first through the inside D-ring, then through the outside D-ring.

A second method again uses 15-20 feet of rope. In this method, one end is fastened to a hobble around the pastern of the leg to be restrained. Next, the free end is brought forward between the forelegs and continued up along the opposite side of the neck from the leg (example: left hindleg, right side of neck). The rope is returned to the same side as the restrained leg, and just back of the withers it is brought down and around the part of rope between the hobble and forelegs. This procedure will form an adjustable half hitch over the shoulders.

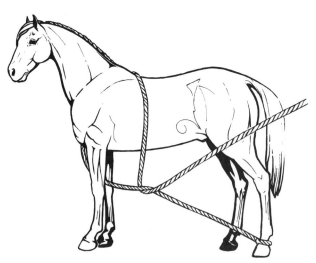

Fig. 3-14 Sideline restraint.

HOBBLES

Hobbles are restraints of soft cotton rope, woven rope, or leather used around a horse's legs to help immobilize him. They can be used as restraints to help prevent a horse from kicking, striking, and rearing. Hobbles usually consist of strong strips of material wrapped around the pasterns of either the forelegs or hindlegs, and tied or buckled on. There are, however, numerous variations, some of which are designed to fit around only one leg and attach to a rope which connects every other leg. One other variation, a hock hobble, is different from others in that it fits the hock area of the leg instead of the pastern. Generally, a woven or leather hobble is superior to a piece of rope used as one, since the rope is more abrasive and can come off more easily if the horse moves about. Although they often provide a useful method of restraint, it is possible for a horse to move with hobbles on; they are not, therefore, ideal as a single method of immobilizing a horse. It is important to remember that since a horse will often struggle when hobbled for the first time, it is best to select a soft location for him to stand in case he throws himself.

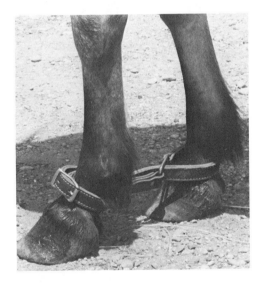

Fig. 3-15   Leather hobbles in place.

BREEDING HOBBLES

Breeding hobbles are one kind that has somewhat specialized uses. They are very helpful in any situation where the hindlegs must be restrained, particularly in assisting breeding, rectal palpation, and vaginal examinations. Although commercial breeding hobbles are available, a satisfactory set can be made from a long (40 foot) piece of soft cotton rope. A double rope collar is first formed by doubling the rope, forming a loop, and placing it around the horse's withers and chest where it is secured with a bowline knot. The knot should at this point rest low and comfortably on the animal's chest. The doubled rope ends are then taken down between the horse's forelegs and passed back to the rear legs. Here, one strand is passed around each hindleg above the hock from outside to inside, carried over itself, then passed back around the leg below the hock from inside to outside. This forms a double half hitch around each hock. The remainder of the rope can then be tied with a slipknot at the hock; pulled forward and tied at the collar; pulled forward and held; or taken forward, passed under the collar, pulled backward and held.

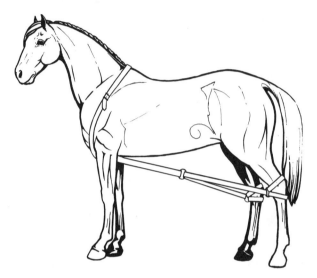

Fig. 3-16   Breeding hobbles in place.

It is important that the hobbles are properly adjusted to remove any slack, and that they can be quickly removed if necessary. If the breeding hobbles are adjustable, they may be moved from the hock to the pastern area. Attaching them at the hock is safer for the mare, though not as safe for the stallion, as he could get tangled in the ropes more easily when they are higher. Consequently, the ropes may be dropped from hock to pastern just before the stallion mounts the mare. A form of hindleg restraint known as Scotch hobbles is really more of a sideline, and is discussed under "Use of a Sideline."

FOUR-WAY OR FIGURE-X HOBBLES

Four-way, or figure-X hobbles, often provide an effective control. Four-way hobbles consist of an X-shaped chain fastened at each of its 4 ends to each of the horse's legs. Because a horse hobbled in this way cannot easily move, he may relax and cease to struggle more quickly than he otherwise would. In some cases, however, the use of four-way hobbles can actually agitate the animal into a state of panic. Therefore, their use is normally restricted to situations of absolute necessity (and any horse so hobbled should be on a soft surface).

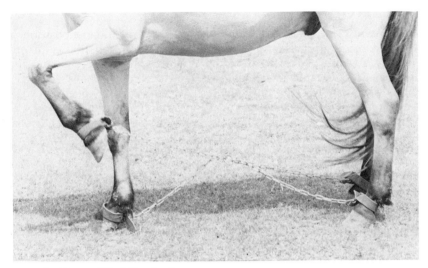

Fig. 3-17   Figure-X hobbles in place.

ENGLISH AND CALIFORNIA HOBBLES

These hobbles are also specialized types. English hobbles are comprised of four leather straps that buckle around the pasterns. Each strap has a metal D-ring through which a chain (anchored to one strap) is passed, thereby immobilizing the legs. California hobbles are similar, except that they attach, via double ended snaps, to a large steel ring instead of a chain. English and California hobbles can be employed as a means of restraining the legs of an already anesthetized horse.

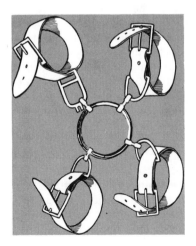

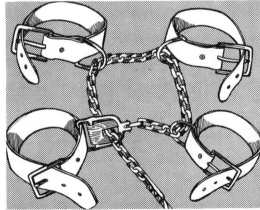

Fig. 3-18   California hobbles.   Fig. 3-19   English hobbles.

CASTING

A horse will rarely need to be forcibly held in a recumbent position, and thorough consideration should always be given to the possibility of injury before any attempt at casting is made. When casting is necessary (usually for treatment by a veterinarian), great care is vital in moving the horse onto his side. Choosing a soft, smooth place for him to go down and avoiding tight ropes and strained positions which can cause nerve injuries are also important considerations. Ideally, anyone attempting to cast a horse should have previously witnessed this casting procedure as performed by a knowledgeable, skilled person.

THE CASTING HARNESS

The casting harness operates on one of two principles; it either flexes the hindlegs and sets the horse down before putting him on his side, or it pulls all four legs from under him at once. The former method is much safer, as it reduces the likelihood of damaging the horse's knees, head, or spine. There are various kinds of casting harnesses, but all have a band of leather, webbing, or another material that goes over the horse's withers, and similar straps that fit around the girth and pectoral (chest) areas. These straps form a kind of harness that in turn is attached to the rear legs by long ropes. The ends of these ropes are held by those persons assisting in casting the horse.

CASTING A PONY

It is not necessary to use a casting harness when casting a pony or small horse (under 12-13 hands). Instead, a person should stand at the animal's side, lean over its back and grasp the halter. Then, while pulling the head around slightly with one hand, he should grasp the tail with the other hand. The tail should be passed forward between the pony's hindlegs to the flank on the opposite side from the person. The halter and tail are then pulled upward and backward toward the handler, who uses his knees as a fulcrum to upset the pony and bring it to the ground. (The actual skin of the flank should never be used as a handhold in casting foals or ponies, as this skin is easily damaged.) Once down, the pony can usually be held there by someone holding its head while another person holds the tail between the pony's legs.

STOCKS

When a horse must be almost completely controlled or immobilized for breeding, applying medication, or cleaning purposes, he can be put into stocks. Such doctoring stocks, designed to protect the handler from kicking or striking, can be constructed with either pipe or stout lumber. Approximate measurements for construction are 30 inches wide by 6 ½ - 7 feet long. Two to four inch steel pipe can be used, and constructed to a height of 7 feet if necessary. Removable wooden panels can also be added to form solid sides.

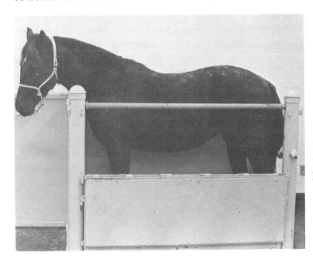

Fig. 3-20 Safe stocks with removable side panels.

BODY RESTRAINTS

SKIN ROLL

It is frequently possible to dispense with using objects to restrain a horse, and simply use his own body to prevent movement. To discourage striking during minor procedures, the skin over the scapula can be grabbed with both hands and rolled forward into the neck. This skin roll can also be tried on the horse's head, where the skin is rolled from the poll to ear. A skin roll can be especially effective in momentarily restraining a horse while a twitch is being applied. Both of these methods usually work for only very short periods of time.

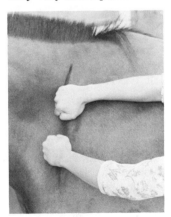

Fig. 3-21 Rolling the skin over the scapula.

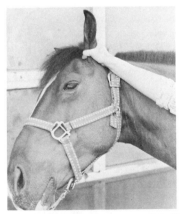

Fig. 3-22 The first step of holding an ear is to grasp it firmly at the base.

HOLDING AN EAR

If neither of the skin rolls succeed, it is sometimes possible to restrain a horse by holding his ear. The person attempting to restrain a horse in this way should slowly move his hand up the horse's neck and reach for the ear, which is then pulled down and forward by grasping it at its center base. After it is released, the ear should be gently rubbed to help restore circulation. If the ear is pulled or twisted too hard, or held too strongly, the possible result may be a broken ear or a head-shy horse.

FOAL RESTRAINTS

TAILING

One type of restraint especially effective with small horses, ponies, and foals, is tailing. In tailing, the halter is grasped in one hand while the tail is held firmly near its base by the other hand, and turned forward over the animal's back. Care should be taken because, if done abusively, tailing can result in pain, bone distortion, coccygeal fractures, or paralysis. Consequently, the use of tailing as a method of restraint is not a recommended procedure for the novice.

CRADLING

Anyone desiring to restrain a foal should initially try to do so in the safest manner possible, which is cradling the foal in one's arms. The halter should not be held even if the foal is halterbroken, as his neck is easily injured at this age. Instead, one arm should be placed firmly around the foal's neck where it joins the chest, and the other arm put around his rump just above the hocks. The arm shouldn't be put under the chest, since it would then put pressure on the rib cage and possibly displace or fracture a rib. If the foal is too large for this, he may be tailed instead, keeping the precautions mentioned above in mind. One other method of restraint which may be tried is putting the foal between your body and a wall to keep him from moving.

SPECIAL RESTRAINTS

RESTRAINTS TO PREVENT BANDAGE CHEWING

Occasionally, circumstances require specific kinds of restraints. At times, for instance, special devices may be necessary to restrain a horse from reaching his legs or sufficiently moving his head to chew his bandages. A horse that chews bandages, besides destroying them, can pull the bandage and possibly bow a tendon or grossly mutilate a wound; restraint, therefore, is very important. Numerous ways to accomplish this exist, most of which work by in some way restricting the animal's movement. An exception, however, is the application of red pepper or creolin to the dressings. Commercial preparations designed to prevent wood chewing also work, but great care should be taken to apply the preparation only to the bandage. The reason for this caution is that many commercial preparations contain phenol (carbolic acid) or similar irritating substances. If applied to the skin, they will cause chemical burns. The use of these products will discourage most horses from bandage chewing; unfortunately, they also will stain the bandages. The following restraints are also effective in preventing self-mutilation after a horse has been fired, sutured, or injured.

Muzzle

A muzzle can be tried expressly to prevent a horse from chewing his bandages. It should be constructed with sufficient openings to allow the horse to breathe easily and to drink. The muzzle, of course, will have to be removed for feeding, at which time the horse should be watched and stopped from any attempts at chewing the bandage.

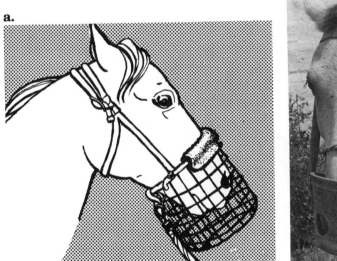
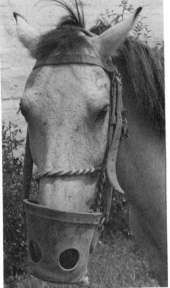

Fig. 3-23   Both of these restraints will prevent bandage-chewing & self-mutilation. a. Wire muzzle. b. Leather muzzle in place .

Neck Cradle, Bib, and Sidestick

A neck cradle is another kind of special restraint that will prevent the horse from bandage chewing. It is a wooden collar that extends down from the throatlatch, and prohibits the horse from bending his neck far enough to reach his legs (though it does permit him to walk around in the stall). If the neck cradle keeps a horse from reaching down to his feed, either the feed will have to be raised to him or the neck cradle will have to be removed at feeding time to allow the horse to eat. If the horse learns to circumvent the cradle by holding his leg up to chew the bandages, a leather or plastic bib can be attached underneath the neck cradle or directly to the halter. When a hindleg has been injured and bandaged, a side stick running from the halter to a full girth or surcingle will often hinder movement just enough to protect the leg.

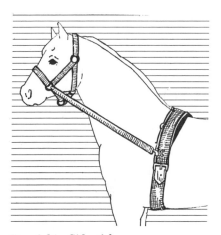

Fig. 3-24   Sidestick.

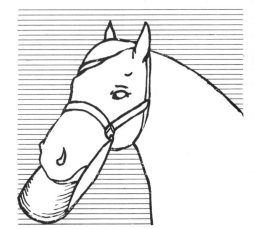

Fig. 3-25   Leather bib.

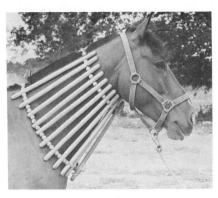

Fig. 3-26   Neck cradle.

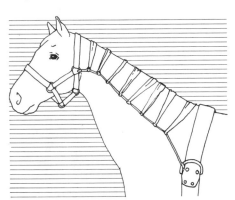

Fig. 3-27   Overcheck.

Overcheck

For a horse that needs more restraint than the previous examples, the following may be tried. Two one-quarter inch cords can be run up each side of the horse's neck from the halter to a surcingle or full girth. These cords are taped or fastened together at six inch intervals, causing the horse to be unable to flex his neck far enough to disturb his bandages. As a result, the animal will not be able to lie down, though he will be able to move about in his stall. (An overcheck from a harness will serve this same purpose.)

Swivel Tie

If a horse still succeeds in chewing his bandages, an overhead swivel tie can be used. The overhead swivel consists of a rope dropped from a beam and attached to the noseband of the halter with a swivel snap. It is important not to hook the snap onto the halter crownpiece, because the horse might slip it over the back of his head. When restrained in this fashion, a horse is prevented from lying down, but is permitted some movement around the stall. A rope tied to the ceiling of the stall and fastened to the horse's lead with a metal slip ring will serve in a like manner, while permitting the horse considerable freedom of movement.

The Cross-Tie

If all else fails, a horse may have to be cross-tied to prevent his bandage chewing. As a means of restraint, cross-tying is also used to keep a horse from biting, from bothering a wound, or to restrain while bandaging, grooming, or a like activity is being performed. A cross-tie can be simply constructed by hooking two leads into opposite cheek rings of a halter, then tying these leads up just snugly enough to prohibit the horse from lowering his head too much. The leads can be tied to heavy-duty screw eyes set in the wall, or to posts. The leads should be fastened to the wall or the posts at a minimum height of just above the horse's head. (Note: A cross-tie used when shipping a horse should be tied lower than this to prevent injury). When cross-tied, a horse will be prevented from moving his head excessively and from lying down. Though the leads should be slack enough to allow the horse some movement, they must not be so slack that he is able to reach his bandages.

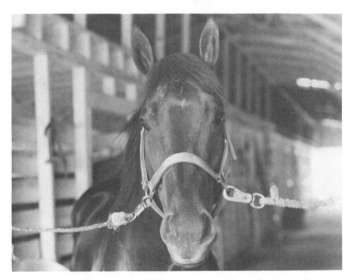

Fig. 3-28 A horse in cross-ties; notice that the cross-ties
are as high as the horse's head.

OTHER SPECIAL RESTRAINTS

The Body Sling

A body sling is a device used to support part of a weak animal's weight, or to help raise a weakened horse to a standing position. The sling is best indicated when a horse is willing or able to support at least some of his own weight.

Though infrequently used, a sling is invaluable because there is usually no suitable substitute. Good body slings are sturdily made and are easily adjustable. They normally consist of a breast collar, a wide belly strap, a hindquarter strap, fastening chains, and a hoist which is to be firmly anchored in the ceiling. When a horse is standing in a sling, there should be about 1 inch of space (or the width of a hand) between the abdominal strap and the horse's belly so that the animal's breathing is not impaired. Any horse restrained in a sling should be allowed easy access to food and water.

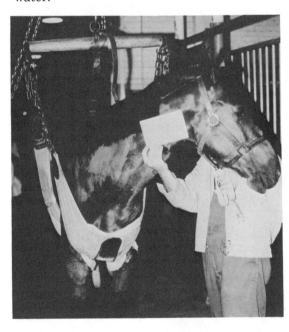

Fig. 3-29 A horse in sling; unfortunately, few horses will tolerate a sling.

The Blindfold

A blindfold is a means of providing quick protection and restraint for a cast horse. It can also be tried as a means of quieting and persuading a balky horse to move. An emergency blindfold can be made by simply placing a jacket over the horse's eyes and tying the sleeves around the animal's neck. A blindfold, however, should never be relied on as the sole means of restraining a sick horse, for it will sometimes unnecessarily stimulate a sick animal.

Chemical Restraining Agents

The use of only physical force to overpower and restrain a struggling animal for treatment is rarely necessary today because of the availability of useful chemical restraints such as tranquilizers and sedatives. So common has the use of tranquilizers become, that promazine and acepromazine are now familiar drugs to many horsemen. In addition, sedatives, painkillers, and short-acting general anesthetics may now be given outside of the veterinary hospital to enable a veterinarian to perform short surgical procedures, such as castrations, on ambulatory calls. (Refer to "Drugs and Related Topics" for an in-depth discussion of the pharmacological agents mentioned below.)

TRANQUILIZERS

Tranquilizers are in widespread use in equine medicine. (They also have been abused by unscrupulous individuals as an aid in the sale of unsuitable horses.) Tranquilizers are most often used when it is desirable to control the movement of a horse or when surgical procedures are to be carried out under local anesthesia. Common examples of indications of tranquilizer use are: simple examinations, laceration repair, pregnancy diagnosis, hair clipping, shipping, and as a preanesthetic agent. The advantages of tranquilizers are that:
1. they can be injected, or certain ones can be given in the feed
2. horses can usually be allowed to continue to eat and drink prior to, and immediately after, tranquilization
3. the effects of tranquilizers are often longer-lasting than the effects of some sedatives.

As premedication for general anesthesia, tranquilizers have the following advantages:
1. induction is easier
2. the anesthetic dose required is reduced
3. the recovery is smoother

The disadvantage is that recovery time is also lengthened.

It is essential that a horse not be excited prior to administering a tranquilizer since an excited horse may respond adversely. Therefore, a tranquilizing drug is best given while an animal is undisturbed before removal from his stall. Silence and a lack of commotion are required after the tranquilizer is administered, and a horse should not be moved until after the drug takes effect. The dosage for each horse is calculated according to body weight.

Phenothiazine derivatives such as acepromazine maleate and promazine hydrochloride are commonly used tranquilizers in horses. The phenothiazine tranquilizers may potentiate the effects of organophosphates and should therefore not be given to animals that have recently been exposed to these compounds (e.g., a horse that was dewormed with dichlorvos or trichlorphon). Although phenothiazines are usually safe, death can be caused if the drug is accidentally injected in the carotid artery instead of the jugular vein. Neither tranquilizers nor sedatives should be relied upon too heavily in restraining a nervous or aggressive horse.

SEDATIVES

Sedatives are drugs used to quiet a horse. They may be used prior to a standing operation, one in which nerve blocks or local or epidural (above spinal cord) anesthesia is required. Sedatives are also useful for procedures involving momentary pain such as injecting the carpal joint.

Xylazine (Rompum) is a sedative with analgesic properties useful as a preanesthetic agent. It works well for routine examinations and minor surgical and dental procedures. However, it is best used for procedures that require dropping the horse's head, since that is one of the effects of xylazine.

Pentazocine (Talwin) is a non-narcotic used today for sedation and control of abdominal pain. It is especially helpful in those cases of colic that sometimes terminate fatally due to fear and the resulting shock associated with abdominal pain.

Chloral hydrate, usually administered with magnesium sulfate, may be used as a sedative. This solution is given intravenously "to effect," and should be stopped before the horse becomes unsteady and goes down.

LOCAL ANESTHETICS

The local anesthetic most commonly used in horses is lidocaine, with procaine being second in popularity. The most frequent uses of lidocaine and procaine are for subcutaneous infiltration around lesions requiring minor surgery (biopsy and small tumor removal) and for suturing lacerations.

GENERAL ANESTHETICS AND MUSCLE RELAXANTS

Glyceryl Guaiacolate (guaifenesin) with a small amount of thiobarbituate is sometimes given to a horse that has been premedicated with a tranquilizer. It provides good restraint and light general anesthesia for 15 to 30 minutes, and, as respiration is not markedly depressed, there is usually a wide margin of safety. A disadvantage of this drug is that a relatively large volume must be given intravenously. Commonly used solutions require one ml/lb or one liter/1000 pound horse.

4

THE HORSEOWNER'S
TREATMENTS AND TECHNIQUES

Equine First Aid Kit

Certain medical supply items should be kept readily available by the horseowner since, in case of serious emergencies, time should not be wasted in searching for first aid supplies. Such items should be kept together in a convenient place and periodically checked to make sure that the contents are in usable condition.

Most of the following items can be purchased at a feed store, tack shop, drugstore, or through a veterinarian.

BANDAGING SUPPLIES

1. a box of 3 inch square gauze pads
2. a non-stick (Telfa) pad for protecting wounds
3. a roll of conforming gauze (Kling)
4. two or four 4 inch wide elastic bandages (Ace), adhesive elastic (Elastikon), or doubleknit bandages made from fabric scraps
5. a 2 inch wide roll of adhesive tape
6. a one pound roll of cotton, or sanitary pads (for larger wounds or pressure bandages)
7. padding: sheet cotton, quilted pads, disposable diapers, etc.
8. a roll of black electrician's tape (to hold ice packs and poultices on the leg)
9. cotton swabs (Q-tips)

ANTISEPTICS AND DISINFECTANTS

1. a mild surgical soap (Betadine, Septadine, pHisoHex)
2. hydrogen peroxide
3. disinfectant (70% isopropyl alcohol, Nolvasan)
4. tamed iodine solution

MEDICINES

1. nitrofurazone salve (or other non-irritating tissue-soluble ointment)

116

2. nitrofurazone powder or spray
3. antibiotic eye ointment
4. a mild liniment
5. epsom salts
6. a caustic powder with copper sulfate or calcium hydroxide (for use on old wounds with proud flesh)
7. sodium bicarbonate
8. physiological saline solution (1 tsp. salt to 1 pint sterile water

EQUIPMENT AND INSTRUMENTS

1. bandage scissors
2. a veterinary rectal thermometer
3. a sharp knife
4. a bucket
5. twenty feet of cotton rope
6. a twitch
7. hemostat or tweezers
8. hoof nippers (to pull shoe)
9. a sponge
10. clippers

MISCELLANEOUS

1. petroleum jelly (for mild abrasions, and to protect the skin below draining wounds)
2. fly repellent

Basic Care of a Sick Horse

STABLE REQUIREMENTS

A sick horse should have complete rest during and immediately after an illness. Indeed, for many illnesses, adequate rest is one of the more important areas of treatment. Every precaution should therefore be taken to allow a sick horse as much rest as possible during an illness.

In part, this can be accomplished by taking care to see that a horse is properly stalled. A sick horse should be put in a clean, roomy, well-bedded stall that is free of draft and dampness. As bedding material for stalls, good quality wood shavings are preferable to straw. Shavings are warmer and softer, and may encourage a horse to lie down and rest.

Many sick horses seem to prefer resting in quiet, darkened stalls, somewhat removed from other animals. Horses that are suffering from an eye disorder, like photophobia, or from a nervous disorder, like tetanus, can benefit especially from this kind of stalling. Of course, a segregated stalling arrangement is always necessary when a horse has a communicable disease.

QUARANTINE STALLING

A horse with a contagious disease should be kept separated from other animals. The degree of quarantine necessary for an animal depends on the disease involved and the methods by which it is transmitted. For instance, equine infectious anemia and encephalitis are transmitted by insects, and horses with these or similar diseases, require a type of quarantine, such as screened stalls, that will prevent insect contact. Other conditions, such as strangles, which are commonly spread by nasal discharges, and influenza and rhinopneumonitis, which are spread in the air, require different stalling arrangements for effective quarantine.

An excellent facility for quarantining a sick horse is a detached, separately ventilated stall located away from other stalling. Ideally, the stall should have a small, adjacent entry room in which grooming tools, veterinary instruments, coveralls, rubber boots, etc., can be kept.

Such a stalling arrangement, although ideally suited for effective quarantine, is not always feasible. Its basic concepts, however, when slightly modified become much more practical and remain effective. In such a plan, the quarantine stall should have an outside entrance and face away from other stalls. A pair of coveralls and rubber boots reserved for wearing in the stall should be provided, in addition to a disinfectant foot bath kept just outside the stall door and changed daily. If special clothes are impractical, one must be especially careful not to contact the sick horse with any article of everyday clothing. Of course, a disinfectant soap should be used before handling other animals.

A helpful suggestion for caring for a quarantined horse is to arrange all handling schedules so that the sick horse is treated after all healthy horses have been attended.

After a term of illness, the stall in which the sick horse was kept should be thoroughly disinfected before it is used again. Disinfection can be accomplished by following these four steps:

1. completely remove all bedding
2. lime the stall floor
3. spray disinfect the walls
4. clean and disinfect feed troughs and water buckets

Of course, the feed troughs and water buckets should be disinfected during the illness as well as afterwards.

FEEDING THE SICK HORSE

It is normally recommended that an unhealthy horse be fed small portions of feed at frequent intervals, and that any food not eaten be removed within a few hours. If a sick animal is unenthusiastic about eating, he can often be enticed to eat by the addition of slight quantities of bran mash, chopped carrots or apples, molasses, honey, grass, or alfalfa added to his ration. Or, hand-feeding may be tried, as a sick horse will sometimes eat or even take medicine from his owner/rider's hand when he would not otherwise eat.

To make eating a little easier, any hay that is to be fed should be dampened slightly to reduce irritating dust. Vick's Vaporub applied in the nostrils will also help prevent dust irritation and mask the telltale scent of some medicines as well.

Fresh water should be made available at all times and changed frequently. If unpalatable medicines given in the water tend to decrease an animal's water consumption, they should be administered in another manner or discontinued. If necessary, a little salt may be sprinkled on a sick animal's ration to increase water consumption and make the feed taste better. A sick horse becomes dehydrated easily, so maintaining water consumption is very important.

CARE DURING COLD AND WARM WEATHER

During cold weather, every attempt should be made to keep a sick horse warm. Besides being blanketed, a horse can also have his legs loosely bandaged for protection against the cold. And, if the weather warrants it, a heat lamp may even be placed in the horse's stall.

In hot weather, there are two objectives. One is to keep a sick animal cool. Electric fans may be used for this purpose, but they should have protective screens over their blades, and should be installed in a safe place out of all animals' reach. The second objective is to protect the horse from insects which, especially at this time, can be extremely annoying. Such protection can best be effected with insect repellents, insecticides, and flysheets.

OTHER CARE

An ailing horse should not be annoyed by unnecessary grooming; therefore, a simple, daily sponging of the eye areas, nostrils, and dock should be conducted in lieu of more elaborate procedures. Other than this, a hand-rubbing should be sufficient.

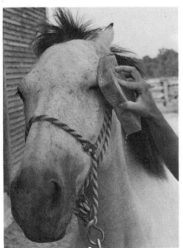

Fig. 4-1 Sponging the eyes, nostrils and dock of a sick horse is a satisfactory substitute for grooming.

If a horse has a fever, he can be given aspirin, either in his feed or as an electuary, a drug made into a palatable paste with honey or syrup (refer to "Oral Administration of Medicine"). For detailed care of specific ailments, refer to sections covering those problems elsewhere in this book.

Cleansing and Treating Wounds

There are six basic types of wounds; abrasions, contusions, incisions, lacerations, punctures, and burns. Abrasions are superficial scrapes or friction burns that may scab as they heal; contusions are bruises and swellings that have no external drainage; incisions are cuts which have clean edges and often heal with little scarring; lacerations are cuts with jagged tears and uneven edges; and punctures are wounds that are deeper than they are wide. The medical management of burns is specifically discussed under "Burns."

Although wound treatment varies according to the type and age of the wound, best treatment results occur when the injured horse is in good general health. Regardless of the kind of wound, tetanus antitoxin or a tetanus toxoid booster is always recommended for an injured horse as a precautionary measure.

FIRST INTENTION AND GRANULATION HEALING

Wounds can heal in one of two ways: by first intention or by granulation healing. First intention, also known as primary intention, means that the edges of a cut heal together with a minimum of infection and scar or fibrous tissue formation. This kind of healing is the desired goal in the management of surgical incisions and wounds.

However, if the initial wound involves considerable tissue loss, if harsh antiseptics are used, or if infection occurs, an injury will heal by granulation. Healing by granulation involves the proliferation of red vascular tissue, which bleeds easily, within the wound. This tissue grows from the inside out. With granulation healing, there occurs a greater amount of fibrous tissue and a wider, more prominent scar than with first intention healing. Fortunately, a scar left by granulation healing contracts, and in time may be only about 10 to 15% of its original size.

Occasionally, a granulating wound will appear to cease healing. Should this happen, the veterinarian may hasten development of new granulation tissue by the application of an irritant such as scarlet oil. Alternatively, hydrotherapy, also used on veterinary advice, can be employed to stimulate the growth of granulation tissue. Any treatment, however, to stimulate the growth of granulation tissue should be discontinued when the granulation tissue reaches the level of the surrounding skin. This must be done because new epithelial cells that are formed to bridge the gap during skin repair only proliferate horizontally on a flat granulation bed, and are not able to proliferate and cover elevated granulation tissue. Extended growth beyond the skin level may result in the formation of proud flesh.

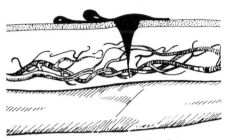

Fig. 4-2   The process of healing.
a. Trauma breaks the skin and bleeding starts.

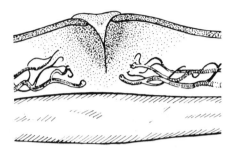

b. Exudates enter the injured area from the blood vessels, causing swelling which helps stop the bleeding.

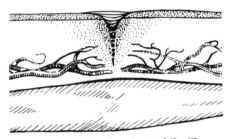

c. A scab begins forming, while fibrous adhesions develop between the wound edges.

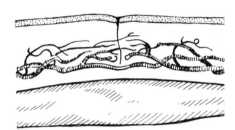

d. The fibrous adhesions form a scar which eventually contracts the area. The scar tissue has a poorer blood supply and less strength than normal tissue.

EVALUATION OF WOUNDS

There are several important considerations that preface the treatment of a wound. With severe injuries, the prevention or treatment of shock is vitally important and should always be begun before wound therapy commences (refer to "Shock"). Otherwise, basic considerations that influence wound treatment include:

1. adequate drainage of the site
2. increasing circulation to promote healing
3. preventing and retarding infection
4. avoiding or, at least, minimizing damage to surrounding tissue
5. allowing for an adequate air supply

INITIAL TREATMENT OF WOUNDS

If hemorrhage occurs, the first step in wound treatment obviously is to control bleeding. Although the bloodstream of a typical 1000 lb horse can contain over 11 gallons of blood, circulatory shock can occur if excessive bleeding continues unabated. A severed artery, characterized by spurting, bright red blood, should be treated with a pressure bandage until a veterinarian arrives. If blood seepage occurs, a clean pressure bandage should be applied evenly over the wound and left in place, even though it becomes bloodsoaked, until bleeding has completely stopped. Removing the bandage too soon will destroy the forming blood clot and allow bleeding to recur.

If a bandage is not available to stop the bleeding, a piece of clothing may suffice. A warm, moist teabag may also be tried as a hemostatic agent. In some outdoor emergencies, applications of cold water, snow, or ice will decrease minor bleeding by constricting the blood vessels, but may contaminate the injury. Commercial "blood stoppers" containing hemostatic ingredients such as tannic acid and alum can be purchased, but they probably should not be used except for very minor injuries, since the introduction of any foreign material into a wound may interfere with later wound treatment. After bleeding has been stopped, a wound should be cleansed, preferably with a weak saline solution, though water or mild soap and water can be substituted.

The combination of salt and water in the ratio of 1 teaspoon salt to 1 pint sterile/boiled water is known as physiological saline solution, and is a good rinsing solution for cleansing fresh wounds. Another acceptable rinsing solution for older wounds can be made from salt, citrate of soda, and boiled or sterile water, as directed below:

1. mix 4 parts salt with one part citrate of soda
2. add 1 tablespoon of this mixture to each pint of boiled water

If there is a lot of secretion from a wound, the above solution should be applied to clean bandage material and applied to the wound with gauze, then left in place for 24 to 48 hours. When the bandage is removed, all extraneous material, including scabs, should come off on the bandage, leaving the wound clean.

Antiseptics are used in treating wounds, however, they should not be used to rinse fresh injuries. Although antiseptics kill bacteria, their effectiveness is reduced when they are contaminated by organic matter, such as blood. Moreover, antiseptics, particularly ones that contain acetone or alcohol, interfere with normal healing and many invariably kill tissue at the edges of wounds. This increases the amount of fibrous tissue and results in a larger wound, slower healing, and a more prominent scar once healing does take place.

Antiseptics do have real value in wound treatment, but their value is as a disinfectant rather than a cleansing agent. When antiseptics are applied directly to wounds, they only slow healing and at times interfere with further treatment. As a point of fact, a veterinarian may refrain from suturing a wound that has been treated with antiseptics. These wounds, which might have healed by first intention, are then forced to heal by granulation.

ABRASIONS

Most mild abrasions may be treated by simple cleansing. A more serious abrasion should be carefully managed and probably wrapped with a pressure bandage to prevent the formation of proud flesh, a frequent complication. Products that contain petroleum jelly or lanolin may also be of some help in treating more serious abrasions.

CONTUSIONS

A contusion may be treated immediately after its occurrence by application of ice or cold packs. Once tissue reaction to the injury has developed, however, a contusion is allowed to eventually be reabsorbed by the horse. If a hematoma has formed, a veterinarian may be required to establish drainage about one to two weeks after formation of the blood clot (refer to "Hematomas").

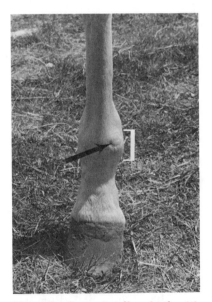 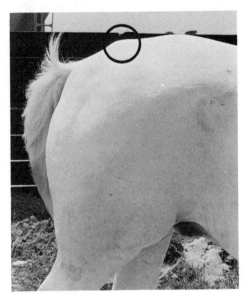

Fig. 4-3 Contusion [bracket] with an abrasion [arrow].

Fig. 4-4 Hematoma [encircled area].

INCISIONS

Small incisions that are not deep should be cleansed initially, preferably with saline solution, to prevent contamination and infection. Shallow incisions on the lower legs may then be bandaged for additional protection. Deep incisions that are uninfected can usually be sutured, unless they occur on the lower legs where the skin is tight and there is much movement. Incisions that are successfully sutured often heal with little scarring, particularly when they are well protected (refer to "Suturing").

LACERATIONS

Lacerations, whether large or small, should generally be cleaned, and treated with a non-irritating dressing such as nitrofurazone ointment or a comparable product. For deep lacerations, antibiotics may be required to prevent infection. Additionally, large lacerations often require a period of surveillance during which they must be cleaned and kept free of flies and other irritants. Lacerations on the legs and hoofs should usually be bandaged after initial treatment. After this, an ointment containing a combination of antibiotics and enzymes may be used in treatment.

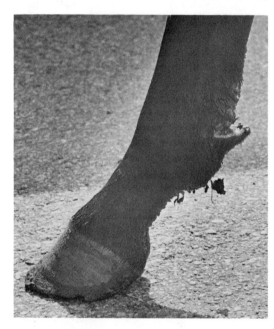

Fig. 4-5   A laceration which will require debridement before treatment.

PUNCTURES

One of the more serious types of wounds is a puncture wound. This type of injury is deeper than it is wide, and consequently is hard to cleanse. Thus, a wound of this type is often a prime site of infection. Puncture wounds may be classified in three ways:

1. as penetrating wounds, which go into a body cavity
2. as perforating wounds, which go into a body cavity and back out again
3. as stabbing wounds, which go only into deep tissue

Because puncture wounds cannot be completely reached by air (due to their characteristic shape), they are often susceptible to infections of tetanus, a disease caused by germs active only in anaerobic (airless) conditions. Although signs of this disease may not appear for up to three weeks after a wound has healed, it is vital that a toxoid or antitoxin injection be given within 24 to 48 hours after an injury occurs. The booster of tetanus antitoxin or toxoid, depending on past immunization, is immediately necessary, for the toxoid or antitoxin will have no effect after the signs of tetanus have appeared.

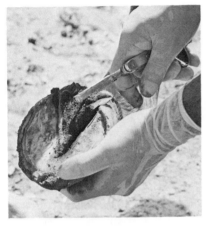

Fig. 4-6   Puncture wound of the frog.

a. The veterinarian is paring down the frog to establish drainage [left].

b. Cleaning the wound with an antiseptic such as iodine [below left].

c. Flushing an antiseptic solution deep into the wound [below right].

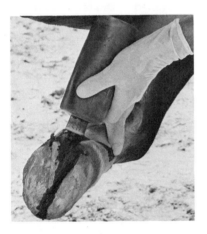

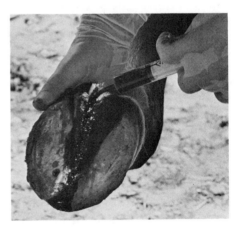

Punctures of the Hoof

Most puncture wounds that occur in the hoof are the result of nail injuries. If a nail is found in the hoof, it should be carefully pulled out and its site of entry noted. If the nail has dislodged and the location of the hole is not known, hoof testers can be used to detect the sore area in the foot. Once the entry site has been located, the sole should be pared with a hoof knife until the hole is reached, and an opening for drainage made from the bottom of the hole, widening as it extends toward the surface of the sole. If infection is suspected, the foot should be soaked in either hot, antiseptic solutions or in warm water with magnesium sulfate (epsom salts) added.

The hole can then be packed with iodine-soaked cotton, which should be changed daily for several days. If swelling and inflammation do not subside, an operation to drain the abscess will often be required. Usually, after this operation, a horse may be shod with a shoe having an attached steel plate or rubber pads which can be periodically removed for examining the injured area.

Punctures of the Leg

Puncture wounds on the leg frequently swell because of the effect of gravity. To prevent or reduce edematous swelling, a puncture wound can be soaked in a magnesium sulfate (epsom salts) solution, or covered with an anti-inflammatory paste, and wrapped with gauze and elastic bandages. Antibiotics may be administered both systemically and locally.

EYE WOUNDS

Anytime an eye has been injured, a veterinarian should be called at once. However, if a foreign body is lodged in the eye's conjunctiva, it should be removed immediately only if removal can be done without causing further damage; if possible, discuss removal of the object with the veterinarian before attempting this procedure. A Q-tip, moistened with sterile water or sterile saline solution, or a dab of eye ointment can be used to remove some objects. To reduce injury-related pain, the eye can be covered or the animal put in a darkened stall. If there are no racing blinkers or goggles available for covering an eye, a piece of innertube can be glued over the eye with a non-toxic glue. The piece of rubber used for a patch should be circular and approximately 4 ½ inches in diameter. There are commercial eye patches made specifically for cattle with pinkeye that can also be used.

If no veterinary assistance is immediately available, the following preparation can be used temporarily to soothe an eye and wash out any foreign material:

  1 heaping teaspoon of baking soda
  1 heaping teaspoon of borax
  1 heaping teaspoon of table salt

These ingredients should be dissolved in a quart of boiled water and a tablespoon of glycerine added. Commercial eye washes, such as Murine or Visine, may also be used to rinse out the eye. Other compounds such as castor oil will also help relieve the pain of an eye injury, but no compound containing cortisone should be used without specific instructions from a veterinarian.

MOUTH WOUNDS

If the mouth is damaged, it should be checked for debris which, if present, should be promptly removed. If a wound is not serious, a strong saline solution can be used to rinse the mouth out several times daily. Swabbing mouth lesions with a mild antiseptic solution such as boric acid or hydrogen peroxide should also be helpful. Besides this, the injured horse should be kept on a soft or liquid ration to avoid any further irritation. If an injury is severe, a horse should not be allowed to eat until professional help arrives, in order to keep the wound as clean as possible. Severe tongue wounds, often caused by misuse of bits, can be sutured to facilitate correct healing.

TREATING INFECTED WOUNDS

If a wound is not treated within several hours of its occurrence, it is considered to be infected and treated as such. The eventual result of an infection depends on the injury's location, the infectious microorganisms present, and the treatment supplied; notwithstanding this, an infected wound is usually allowed to heal from the inside out to prevent abscess formation.

When infection occurs, it is most often necessary for the veterinarian to treat the horse systemically and locally with antibiotics. Foreign matter lodged in wounds may be removed by flushing with one of the solutions previously mentioned. If this proves unsuccessful, a sterile gauze soaked in warm saline solution can be used to lift the debris away. If contaminants are deeply lodged and tissue excessively damaged, the veterinarian may elect to surgically remove the contaminated tissue. To keep hair out of the injury, the surrounding hair should either be shaved and carefully brushed away or coated frequently with petroleum jelly. Petroleum jelly can also be applied to the skin beneath a wound for protection against irritating wound exudate.

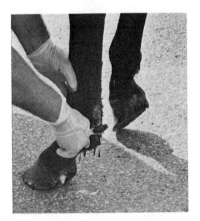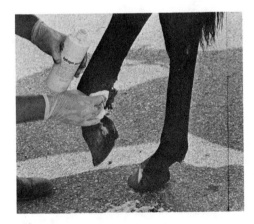

Fig. 4-7 Veterinarian debriding a laceration.

TREATMENT OF SCABS

Scabs are formed from wound secretions, as healing and contracting of tissues take place underneath. If a scab is loose and seeping, infection may be present, and the scab should be removed to prevent healing retardation.

If an area will not scab, it is possible to form one by painting the injury with an irritant such as formalin or iodine for several days until a scab appears. This treatment should be used only on mild abrasions; if there is any doubt about whether an injury should have a scab, consult a veterinarian.

WOUND SUTURING

Not all wounds should be sutured. Ideally, a wound suitable for suturing should be a clean, incised cut, containing no crushed tissue or foreign bodies. "Selection" of wounds, however, is impossible, and "clean" wounds are not always encountered. Early treatment is always beneficial, though, and best results are obtained when suturing is conducted as soon after the wound occurs as is feasible. If suturing is delayed, infection will likely develop, leading to abscess formation and possible dehiscence and reopening of the wound.

In suturing, which is of course a veterinary procedure, all devitalized tissue in the wound area is cut away leaving as much healthy skin as possible. The wound edges are then brought into apposition and sutured.

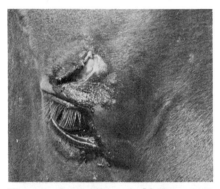
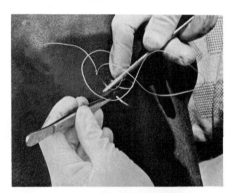

Fig. 4-8 a. Laceration suitable for suturing.   b. Suturing wound edges together.

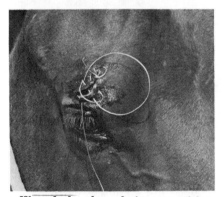
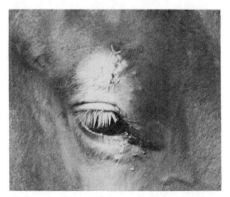

c. Wound edges brought into apposition.   d. Sutured wound dusted with antibiotic.

Because of inadequate drainage, a sutured wound normally has more swelling than an unsutured one, therefore a small portion of the cut may be left open to promote drainage. For large, complex wounds, drain tubes may be sewn in and left for 3 to 10 days. After suturing, a wound is frequently bandaged for protection, and antibiotic therapy, continued for several days, is often necessary (refer to "Suturing").

Wound Dehiscence

Wound dehiscence (de-his'ens) is defined as the separation of layers of a surgical wound. Dehiscence may be partial and superficial, or it may be serious enough to cause total disruption of the sutured area. (Sutured areas are sometimes severely damaged during recovery from general anesthesia.) When dehiscence occurs, a wound that would normally heal by first intention healing is forced to heal by granulation, unless devitalized tissue is cut away and resuturing is attempted.

Excessive movement that stresses the suture line is one cause of dehiscence. Immobilization, therefore, is a preventative in some cases; for instance, when a lightweight cast can be used to immobilize a lower limb. Direct interference with sutures is also disruptive. If such interference is the result of a horse chewing on his sutures, physical restraint in the form of a neck cradle, bib, or sidestick will likely be required (refer to "Restraints").

CONTROLLING PROUD FLESH (EXCESS GRANULATION TISSUE)

Sometimes, granulation tissue grows uncontrollably and "proud flesh" results. This is especially prevalent in wounds below the knee and hock. Proud flesh is usually brought about by the use of excessively strong antiseptics or by continual movement of the injury which retards complete healing. To help prevent the formation of proud flesh, antiseptics should not be applied to a fresh wound, and a wound should be bandaged snugly after treatment, particularly if on or below the knee.

If extraneous granulation tissue has already formed, it can be removed by the veterinarian by careful application of escharotics, which cauterize the excess tissue. Powdered copper sulfate, commonly called "bluestone," can be dusted over a wound for this purpose, and the wound tightly bandaged afterward. After 48 hours, when the bandage is taken off, a thin layer of granulation tissue will be removed. In some cases, a stronger escharotic such as hydrochloric acid/sulfuric acid paste may be used. However, before this type of paste is applied, the hair and skin surrounding the wound should be protected with a coat of petroleum jelly. After treatment, the wound should be bandaged snugly with a dry dressing. Although escharotics do remove proud flesh, they also damage new epithelial tissue and can cause severe scarring if misused. Thus, treatment with escharotics is recommended only as a veterinary procedure. Large areas of proud flesh are usually best treated through surgical removal, cryosurgery, and skin transplants.

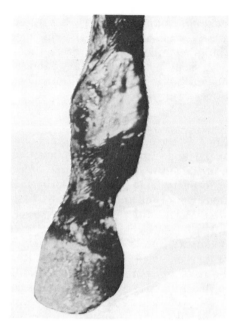

Fig. 4-9 Neglect or improper treatment of a wound, particularly one below the knee or hock, can result in proud flesh.

THE USE OF CASTS IN WOUND THERAPY

A cast can be helpful in the treatment of wounds because it effectively immobilizes an injury, thus reducing the chances of wound dehiscence and proud flesh formation. Casts are especially effective in treatment of deep wounds of the fetlock, pastern, and coronary band regions.

SUGGESTIONS FOR TREATING WOUNDS

WHAT TO DO

1. Try to control bleeding with direct pressure or with a hemostatic agent.
2. Clean the wound with saline solution or with mild soap and water.
3. When a wound must be sutured, try to immobilize it and see that it is attended to promptly. If there is any question about the severity of the wound or the need for suturing, call the veterinarian.
4. When instructed by the veterinarian, use antibacterial drugs to prevent infection.
5. When necessary, bandage a wound until it has sufficiently healed and can be uncovered.
6. Immunize against tetanus.

WHAT NOT TO DO

1. Do not wash wounds frequently.
2. Do not apply medicine to a wound to be sutured.

3. Do not apply astringents or caustics to wounds other than surface scratches.
4. Do not apply salve to a deep, open wound.
5. Do not use strong antiseptics.
6. Do not allow excessive movement.

Bandaging

BASIC USE OF BANDAGES

At one time or another, the proper care of a horse will almost certainly require a knowledge of bandages and their practical applications. Bandages are frequently used for the following reasons:
1. to protect wounds from contamination and insects
2. to keep wound dressings, hot and cold packs, poultices, and other substances in contact with the affected area
3. to immobilize an area so that tissue repair is not disrupted by excessive motion of the injured area
4. to reduce and control soft tissue swelling
5. to stop excessive hemorrhage
6. to provide temporary support for a fracture
7. to support strains and sprains
8. to add support to a limb and prevent injury due to trauma during shipping and training
9. to control injury and contamination at breeding and foaling
10. to support a sound leg that is stressed when the opposite leg is injured and cannot bear much weight

To accomplish these purposes, there are a variety of bandages available, and diverse methods of application. The following bandages are some of the most often used:
1. wound bandage
2. quittor or poultice bandage
3. temporary cast bandage
4. "Thomas Jones" splint for fractures
5. pressure bandage
6. standing and shipping bandages
7. shipping boots, splint boots, etc.
8. support bandage
9. exercise bandage
10. running bandages used in competition
11. rundown bandages and speed patches
12. fetlock, knee, and hock bandages
13. spider web or many-tailed bandage
14. tail wrap bandage
15. anti-inflammatory bandage
16. sweat bandage

17. warmth bandage
18. cold water bandage
19. hot water bandage
20. ice bandage

BASIC MATERIALS

A variety of materials is used for the various types of bandages. Gauze bandages, however, are probably the most common type and are ideal for use on wounds that require good air flow. Conforming gauze, like regular gauze, permits air to reach a wound, but stretches just enough to conform easily to the shape of the area being bandaged and is far easier to work with, especially in the 3 inch wide size. Flannel and knits are other popular materials used for bandaging. Cotton knit bandages, called "derbies" or track wraps, are 4 inches wide and 8 to 12 feet long. Elastic or Ace-type bandages are also widely used for support. Both of these bandage materials may be washed and reused. Other materials available include adhesive elastic bandages and non-adhesive crepe. They have the advantages of conforming well to the limbs and staying in place, but they cannot be reused. Cotton adhesive tape is often used on some types of bandages to keep the end of the bandage in place.

There are several materials that are acceptable as padding for bandages. Cotton is commonly preferred. Sheet cotton, no-chafe hospital pads, quilted cotton pads, and disposable diapers are some of the materials that can be used for padding. Even sanitary pads may sometimes be of use as extra padding. Additionally, combination dressing (combine roll) made of rolled cotton with a gauze outer casing is good for padding because it holds up well under a bandage. However, when any material is used as padding, it should be applied thickly enough to be of value. When padding is applied, it should protrude beneath the wrapped portion of the bandage about an inch at the top and bottom to prevent the bandage from interfering with circulation. Stockinette, which is often used under cast bandages, can also be employed to help keep dressings in contact with a wound.

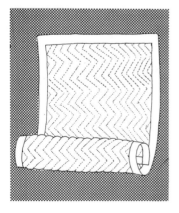

Fig. 4-10 A quilted cotton pad suitable for use under a bandage.

GENERAL PRECAUTIONS

Before any bandage is applied, dirt and other possible irritants should be removed from the haircoat by a gentle rubbing in the direction of the hair's growth. Wounds should be gently flushed with plain water or saline solution. This will prevent contaminating particles from being wrapped over and irritating the area. The tightness of the applied bandage should vary according to its purpose and location on the horse's body. However, pressure necrosis could be an inadvertent result if a bandage is too tightly applied. If a bandage is required to protect a wound, it should not be left on for more than 24 hours at a time, unless so directed by a veterinarian, so that any changes in the condition of the injury can be noted soon after they occur. In addition, a bandage protecting a wound should be kept dry and removed if it becomes wet.

Remember:

1. Use ample sheet cotton or quilted leg pads to allow for even pressure on the legs without cutting off circulation.
2. Apply leg wraps and gauze smoothly and without wrinkling, with the cotton and bandage wrapped in the same direction; wrinkles can cause soreness and tendinitis.
3. Understand and follow the instructions for any medication applied under the bandage.
4. Tie the bandage strings on the lateral surface of the leg, not the front or back where they could cause undue pressure, especially on tendons.
5. An animal chewing at a bandage, or swelling below a bandage, are indications for veterinary advice and probable removal and replacement of the bandage.

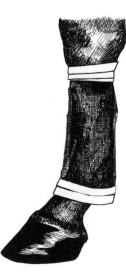

Fig. 4-11 Taping a piece of screen over a wound will protect it from insects.

WOUND BANDAGES

When bandaging a dressing in place on a wound, it is important to remember that excessive snugness can restrict circulation and retard healing. The bandage, therefore, should be just tight enough to keep the dressing in place on the wound.

When it is necessary to leave a wound open to the beneficial effects of fresh air, yet protect it from flies and other insects, a piece of nylon or plastic window screen can be taped over an injury. The screen will prevent insects from lighting, yet will allow medication to be applied through the mesh.

LEG BANDAGES

LEG INJURIES

Two of the best bandages for use on leg injuries, particularly injuries of the upper leg or knee, are adhesive elastic wrap and non-adhesive, clinging crepe. While these types of bandages cannot be reused, they fit more closely without injuring the leg, and stay in place better than most reusable bandages.

Track wraps and other non-adhesive bandages can be fastened with safety pins. or with Velcro strips, or their strings can be tied in a bow around the leg. As previously mentioned, to prevent binding a tendon when using strings, the knot must be tied at the lateral side of the leg instead of in the back or front. If safety pins are used for fastening, they should be large, strong ones that will not accidentally open. For greater security, two safety pins should be fastened in an X-shape on the lateral side of the leg and covered over with a piece of adhesive tape to keep them from opening. When the bandage is taped in place, the tape should be wrapped diagonally, rather than in circles, for circular layers form an unyielding band around the leg.

On a young foal, a bandage can often be held in position by placing the injured limb into one leg of a pair of support-type pantyhose, and tying the other leg around the foal's neck to hold the hose up.

A minor injury of the lower leg should first be cleansed and treated with an ointment such as nitrofurazone before it is covered with a non-stick gauze pad. At least two layers of sterile sheet cotton or another type of padding should be wrapped evenly around the leg to assure proper circulation, and a bandage started ½ inch from the bottom of the padding and wrapped up the leg to within ½ inch of the top of the padding and back down again. Each turn of the bandage should cover about ⅓ of the width of the preceding strip, and the wraps should be parallel to each other to even out the pressure. The bandage should be pulled snug from the front of the leg towards the rear so that pressure is not directed against a tendon.

Bandaging the Knee, Hock, and Fetlock

With some leg injuries, the greatest problem is that of keeping the bandage in its proper position. The hock is a difficult area to bandage correctly, and any bandage there could cause the skin to slough over the Achilles tendon. On the hock, it is usually a good idea to use an adhesive or elastic bandage, either of which will readily stay in place. Bandaging of the hock may be done in a figure-eight pattern, using the flexor (anterior) surface of the hock joint as a crossover point (see the accompanying illustrations on figure-eight bandaging). For a capped hock, adhesive or elastic bandages should be used over sheet cotton padding (no gauze is necessary) and wrapped in a similar manner.

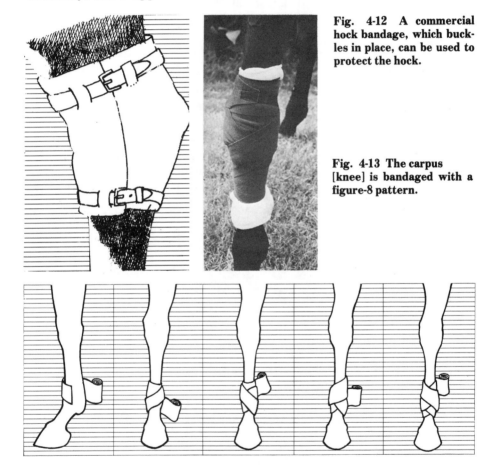

Fig. 4-12 A commercial hock bandage, which buckles in place, can be used to protect the hock.

Fig. 4-13 The carpus [knee] is bandaged with a figure-8 pattern.

Fig. 4-14 A support bandage can be successfully applied to the fetlock by following these steps.

Bandaging the carpus (knee) may also be accomplished with the figure-eight pattern using the flexor (posterior) surface as the crossover points.

To bandage the fetlock for support, a criss-cross pattern is generally used, employing either adhesive or non-adhesive elastic bandages (see the accompanying figure).

Sometimes, in order to keep a bandage in place over the knee or hock, it may be necessary to apply a standing bandage over the lower leg to provide support for the bandage above. A standing bandage is simply a track wrap rolled evenly over padding. When applied to the lower leg, this bandage forms a shelf-like base on which the knee or hock bandage can rest. To test the standing bandage for correct application and even pressure, insert two fingers between the top and bottom of the bandage and the horse's leg. There should be no pinching at any point on the leg.

a.   **b.**

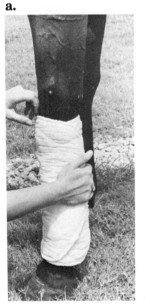 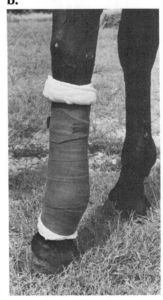

Fig. 4-15 Standing bandage. a. Wrapping the padding evenly around the leg. b. Finished bandage; note the padding left uncovered at the top and bottom.

Spider Web or Many-Tailed Bandage

A spider web or many-tailed bandage is used in areas of extensive motion and/or areas that require support. It is fashioned so that its ends can be tied together over the flexing surface to secure the bandage and permit free movement. This bandage is cut from a rectangle of muslin as indicated in the accompanying illustrations, and is placed over the wound dressing and cotton padding. The knots used to tie the bandage in place are tied on the flexing surface of the limb to allow for motion. If the bandage is applied to the knee or hock, a standing bandage below will help prevent the spider web bandage from slipping down the leg. (Refer to the illustrations for specifics on making and applying the spider web bandage.)

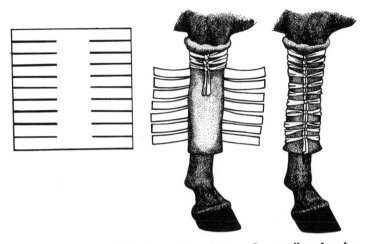

Fig. 4-16 Spider web bandage; the numerous knots allow freedom of movement.

A very large version of this bandage can be used for abdominal support. In such a case, the tie ends of the bandage must be well-padded with cotton to prevent pressure sores.

Temporary Cast Bandage

Commercially available, plaster impregnated bandages are available for use as temporary casts; some are packaged wet, while others are to be wetted before application to the leg. These bandages are semi-firm and are designed to give added support when a light cast effect is desired. They are not intended to replace an actual cast, and should only be used in emergency situations, or at the advice of a veterinarian.

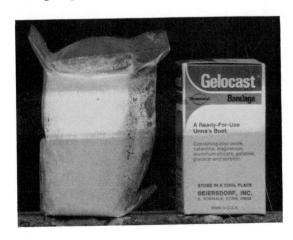

Fig. 4-17 A commercial plaster-impregnated tempo-rary light cast.

If the temporary cast bandage used is packaged moist, it must be applied immediately after its removal from the package and allowed to dry on the leg. One of these may be applied over cotton padding as a support for an acute injury and to retard swelling.

"Thomas Jones" Emergency Splint for a Fracture

A fractured leg should be immobilized immediately to prevent further injury. The best way to quickly immobilize a broken limb is to apply a pillow splint, which is known as a "Thomas Jones" bandage. This bandage forms a soft cast which will help support the horse's leg until a veterinarian arrives.

A large bed pillow, several elastic or adhesive bandages, and a strong stick are needed to fashion this splint. If there is an open wound, as there might be with a compound fracture, the wound should be bandaged with gauze, cotton, and an elastic bandage (as described previously) before the pillow splint is applied.

When placed on the fractured leg, the pillow should be wrapped lengthwise around the leg and held in position by a tight wrapping of the elastic or adhesive bandage. It is not likely that even a very tight wrapping would injure the horse, for the pillow should provide ample padding. If the front leg is involved, the wrapping should move upward first, finishing just above the knee. Then, a second wrapping should be applied down the pillow and back up. After this, boards or sticks may be placed on either side of the leg and secured by additional wrapping with elastic or adhesive bandages. (For more information on the "Thomas Jones" bandage, refer to "Casts.")

Pressure Bandages

Pressure bandages are typically used for the following conditions:
1. prevention of proud flesh
2. support of tendons and ligaments
3. prevention of leg swelling (stocking up) in cases of fresh cuts and abrasions
4. to hold a pack in place on a punctured sole
5. to stop blood flow
6. to prevent edema under new suture lines

When a pressure bandage is applied to stop blood flow, sterile gauze is placed against the wound and the leg wrapped with sheet cotton or cotton quilting, then covered with track wrap or an elastic bandage. Blood seepage through the bandage is normal in cases of extensive wounds, and should not cause great alarm if arterial bleeding has been stopped. (Arterial bleeding can be recognized by its bright red, pulsating flow.)

Adhesive elastic tape wrapped snugly over padding and gauze dressings makes a very effective pressure bandage for most conditions, such as the prevention of proud flesh. The pressure bandage should be applied evenly beginning at the coronary band, and extending up the area requiring treatment. A pressure bandage must be applied in an exceptionally careful manner to avoid binding the leg, since excessively tight bandages can cause skin sloughs because of restricted circulation. A cast bandage, mentioned earlier, may also be used as a pressure bandage.

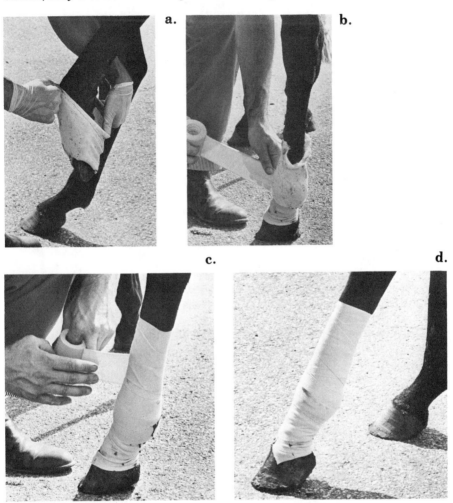

a.   **b.**

c.   **d.**

Fig. 4-18 **Pressure bandage.** **a. Pulling a stockinette over the injury.** **b. Rolling gauze evenly over the dressing to hold it in place.** **c. Adhesive elastic wrap is applied.** **d. Completed pressure bandage.**

Poultice Bandage

To limit infectious or noninfectious inflamed swellings, it is sometimes useful to bandage a poultice to a wound. This is especially true when treating a puncture wound. This bandage will tend to draw out heat and infection as well as relieve pain. Strained fetlock joints, banged knees or hocks, and sole bruises and punctures may be treated this way.

To be fully beneficial, poultices should be bandaged in place for 12 to 48 hours and remoistened at regular intervals. This much time is necessary because the purpose of a poultice is to supply moist heat, and the purpose is defeated if the poultice is removed too soon or allowed to dry.

Quittor Bandage

This bandage is known as a quittor bandage from the fact that quittor is one of the conditions in which this bandage may be employed in treatment. Quittor bandages are also used to draw out heat and relieve pain in cases of sole abscess, sole bruises, and gravel. To bandage a poultice in place on the hoof, the following procedure should be used:

1. Place the poultice mixture in the middle of a piece of waxed paper or plastic wrap.
2. Fold the paper up around the foot and cover it with a 12 inch by 12 inch combine pad.
3. Hold the combine pad in place over the paper by wrapping 3 inch gauze around the foot several times, from the coronary band and pastern to the toe, until the hoof is completely covered.
4. Use adhesive tape to hold the gauze in place.

The bandage must be protected from excessive wear in one of the following ways:

1. Place the bandaged foot on a burlap sack, fold the sack up around the foot, and tape the sack in place with a standing bandage
2. Use a burlap bag protector, cut as shown in the accompanying illustration, to cover the hoof.
3. Wrap the entire bandaged foot with an adhesive elastic bandage

This same bandage, minus the poultice mixture, may be used to protect sole or coronary band injuries.

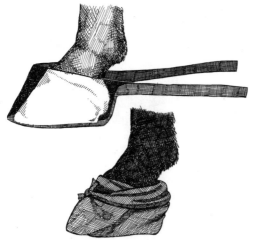

Fig. 4-19 Quittor bandage.
a. A burlap sack can be cut in the shape shown.

b. Bandage in place.

Unna's Paste Poultice

One popular anti-inflammatory poultice is Unna's paste, which is used in treating sprains and strains. It consists of the following ingredients:

5.3 ounces each of zinc oxide and gelatin
5.6 ounces each of water and glycerine

Unna's paste is made by mixing the solid ingredients together, then combining them with the liquids and stirring and heating all ingredients together in a double boiler. The mixture is ready to be used when it attains the consistency of thick paint.

Apply Unna's paste liberally to both the area to be bandaged and to a roll of 2 inch wide conforming gauze, which ensures that the layers of bandage will adhere to each other. The bandage should be wrapped directly onto the injured area, and the horse kept away from dust and bedding for about twenty minutes to allow the paste time to set. This bandage will dry to the consistency of foam rubber and should require nothing other than its own adhesiveness to stay in place. If necessary, this bandage can remain on the leg for a couple of days before removal.

Sweat Bandage

Old swellings that are not warm to the touch may possibly be removed by the application of a sweat bandage, which works by increasing circulation to the covered area. To apply a sweat bandage, a layer of plastic wrap is wrapped directly on to the horse's leg underneath an exercise bandage. Before using a chemical counterirritant under this bandage to increase the effect, consult your veterinarian. This is because some counterirritants may cause sloughing of the hair or skin when applied under a bandage. The leg should be washed with mild soap and water and dried after removing a sweat bandage.

Cold Water Bandage

A cold water bandage is used to cool a hot or strained leg and to minimize or reduce soft tissue swelling in an affected leg. Before the bandage is applied, hydrotherapy with cold running water can be employed for 15 minutes to 1 hour.

A cold water bandage is basically a support bandage made from a track wrap and a quilted cotton pad that has been soaked in a bucket of ice water and applied while wet. Both the track wrap and quilted cotton pad should be thoroughly wetted and applied as described under "Support Bandage"; they should not be wrung out.

Because a cold water bandage may shrink and injure a tendon, it is never allowed to completely dry out. Elastic bandages should never be used for cold water bandages because of the danger of shrinking. Rewet the bandage as it warms and dries until the length of time of application recommended by the veterinarian has elapsed. Then remove the cold water bandage and thoroughly towel dry the leg.

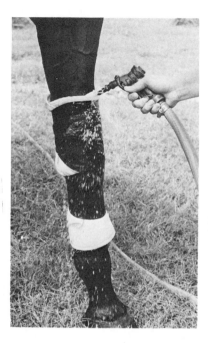

Fig. 4-20 A cold water bandage should be wetted frequently to prevent shrinking, which may constrict circulation and put pressure on tendons.

Hot Water Bandage

A hot water bandage can be applied to facilitate abscess maturation. Either flannel bandages or a quilted cotton pad soaked in a hot epsom salt (magnesium sulfate) solution can be used for this purpose, or an anti-inflammatory ichthammol dressing can be applied under the bandage as a drawing agent. After soaking the flannel or quilted pad in hot water, wring it out and apply it to the leg under a dry track wrap. For best results, this bandage should be frequently redone, in order to apply continuous heat to the injured area for the prescribed length of time. Then the bandage is removed and the leg towel-dried.

Ice Bandage

Immediately following a traumatic injury to a leg, the application of cooling gels, ice packs, and ice bandages may be very beneficial to prevent excessive soft tissue swelling. Maximum benefits are obtained if ice is applied to the injured area within the first hour after the occurrence of trauma.

Instant cold compresses packaged in plastic bags are commercially available to keep on hand for emergency situations; when activated, they cool to a temperature of approximately 20°F.

An ice bandage can be made by first wrapping the leg with a track wrap. Then a plastic bag (such as a heavy duty trash can liner) is filled with ice and secured around the leg with electrician's tape. The ice is replenished as required for the desired length of cooling time.

a.

b.

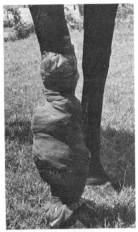
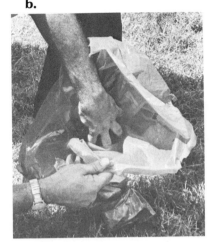

Fig. 4-21 Ice bandage. a. A plastic bag can be filled with ice. b. The bag is then taped in place.

LEG PROTECTION

Standing and Shipping Bandages

Standing or shipping bandages are used for protection of the legs, knees, coronary band, and heels during shipping, or to support a bandage applied to the upper half of the leg.

For shipping purposes, three to five layers of padding are used for additional protection, applied from the lower part of the knee to below the coronary band and heels. Then, a double length track wrap is used to wrap the leg, starting at the lower quarter of the knee about an inch from the top edge of the padding. The bandage should be applied evenly, with the wraps parallel to each other. When the bandage reaches the fetlock joint, use criss-cross wraps to allow for movement, then wrap down over the coronary band and heels. The bandage is continued in the same manner back up the leg and secured with ties, safety pins, or Velcro as described previously.

Standing bandages usually have only one or two layers of padding and are discussed under "Bandaging the Knee, Hock, and Fetlock."

Commercial shipping boots can also be used for additional leg protection during shipping. These boots provide support for the legs and help prevent the circulation in the limbs from becoming sluggish from long periods of van confinement. It is also helpful to cushion the van or trailer floor with rubber mats for even greater protection.

Support Bandage

Many kinds of bandaging materials are suitable for providing support to a horse's leg. Track wraps, rubberized elastic, non-elastic cloth, and Army surplus field bandages are all appropriate. Two to three sheets of padding are needed for a support bandage, and should be wrapped from the coronary band to the knee as the bandage is applied. The support bandage should be wrapped smoothly over the padding from near the padding's lower border and back up to just below the padding's top edge. To help the padding stay unwrinkled, wrap the bandage in the same direction as the padding. Overlap the turns of the roll bandage about two-thirds of the width of the material to provide extra support.

If done correctly, one should be able to insert two fingers easily between the horse's leg and the support bandage (although the fetlock may be safely wrapped a little more snugly than this).

When finally in place, this bandage may be fastened with tie strings, safety pins, or Velcro tape. The tie strings, of course, should be on the lateral side of the limb, away from the tendons. This basic technique of support bandaging is suitable for bandaging sprained ligaments, bowed tendons, carpitis, bog spavins, or various other injuries requiring support. It may be used after workouts and to prevent stocking-up while in the stall.

Exercise Bandage

Exercise bandages are applied to support the tendons of the lower leg during strenuous activity such as racing or training. Either a track wrap or an elastic bandage is used over a single layer of padding for this bandage.

A layer of padding is applied to the leg, extending from the bottom of the knee to the top of the fetlock joint. Next, the track wrap or Ace-type bandage is wrapped evenly over the padding, starting one-half inch below the top edge of the padding, just below the knee. Overlap the turns of the bandage about two-thirds the width of the material, and try to keep the turns parallel to the ground. To avoid excessive pressure when using an Ace-type bandage, do not pull the bandage at all when applying, but just wrap it without using tension. Continue wrapping the exercise bandage down to the fetlock to within one-half inch of the bottom edge of the padding. Then, finish the bandage by wrapping back up the leg to just below the knee again.

An exercise bandage should be fastened with two sturdy safety pins pinned in the shape of a figure X, with adhesive tape applied over the pins to help hold them in place. The tape should completely encircle the leg, while taking care to not bind the limb. Tie strings cannot be depended on to keep an exercise bandage in place during strenuous activity.

To check the bandage for correct application, insert one finger between the bandage and the horse's leg at both top and bottom. The bandage should not pinch, and pressure should be even around the leg. After the activity for which the exercise bandage was necessary has been completed, the bandage should be removed immediately.

Running Bandages

Running bandages are applied for the duration of competition only. They are usually 4 inch wide elastic or latex bandages applied without padding to the front legs from the coronary band to just below the carpus. Their purpose is to support tendons, and they are removed immediately following the event. Improper application and uneven pressure could contribute to a bowed tendon.

Rundown Bandages and Speed Patches

A rundown bandage is normally worn only during competition to protect the back surfaces of the horse's fetlocks from contacting the ground. The fetlock may be covered with orthopedic felt, which is then wrapped with an adhesive elastic tape, or a rundown patch may be applied to the fetlock, which is then covered with either an adhesive or clinging, non-adhesive elastic tape.

Speed patches are small circles of self-sticking plastic material which are generally applied to the back of the fetlock for use as rundown patches. In addition, they may be applied to any point of interference on the inside of the legs for a horse with a "speed cutting" problem.

TRUNK BANDAGES

Although most of the bandaging done on a horse is performed on the legs, larger body areas that are less frequently injured do require bandaging at times. An elastic girdle-type bandage made from adhesive elastic tape is one that can be used around the abdomen for broken ribs and abdominal puncture wounds. Because of its tendency to slip, it is usually held in place with a breastplate and crupper. Chest injuries are bandaged with a pressure bandage wrapped around the chest, which is also held in place with a breastplate and crupper. Many injuries to the chest and ribs will require a veterinarian's assistance to be correctly bandaged. In cases requiring abdominal support, a large spider web bandage may be effective.

EYE BANDAGES

An eye that has been injured may have to be bandaged to prevent contamination with foreign matter, help reduce pain, and protect the eye from light. Racing goggles that have had one of their lenses taped over make an effective bandage, or commercially available eye patches, such as those used on cattle, may be used. The eyelid itself can also act as a bandage if the eyelids are sutured together by a veterinarian (refer to "Tarsorrhapy"). Additionally, a piece of stockinette pulled over the head will make an effective eye bandage. Holes cut in the stockinette for the ears will keep the bandage in place. A dressing can be placed under the stockinette, over the wound, and adhesive tape used to secure the stockinette to the horse's face and neck.

TAIL WRAP BANDAGE

When a horse is being shipped, its tail can be bandaged for protection from rubbing. If the tail is not wrapped, considerable loss of hair (especially near the dock) may result from rubbing against the trailer door during transit. The best bandages are disposable gauze, track wraps, or elastic bandages. Disposable materials in a 3 inch width are preferred.

Although the bandage needs to be wrapped tightly enough to stay in place, one should remember that tail bandages are worn for a considerable length of time during shipping, and a too-tight bandage will cause hair loss through lack of circulation. If circulation to the tail is restricted, the tail may slough and suffer permanent damage or, at the very least, the hair will take a long time to grow back.

If the bandage is to be worn for an extended period of time, turning a few hairs back between layers of the bandage while wrapping will help prevent slippage. The tail bandage is begun at the base of the tail and continues down to the last tail vertebrae.

Tail bandages are also applied to prevent contamination and injuries during procedures involving the reproductive tract, such as breeding, culturing, speculum examination, uterine infusions, uterine biopsies, suturing the vulva, and foaling. During breeding and at foaling, a mare's tail should be bandaged for sanitary purposes, and to avoid having the stallion or mare cut by the tail hairs.

A breeding bandage is made from a material such as cotton gauze, and is started by wrapping around the base of the tail near the dock. It should be given an extra turn or two at the dock to help keep it in place, and then wrapped the length of the dock, overlapping each turn about one-third of the bandage's width, or about 1 inch. A foaling bandage is usually wrapped on after the tail has been braided into a three strand length and doubled back on itself. The tail should be wrapped just snugly enough so that the bandaging does not loosen.

Plain gauze may be wetted before applying it as a short term tail wrap. However, although dampening the gauze will allow it to conform to the tail, it should not be left in place for an extended period of time, since pressure damage could result from shrinkage.

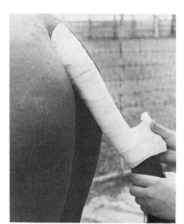

Fig. 4-22   Conforming gauze makes an acceptable tail bandage.

Application of Topical Medications

APPLYING ANTISEPTICS AND ANTIBIOTICS

Antiseptics and antibiotics are two of the most widely used topical medications. Antiseptics are drugs that inhibit the growth and development of microorganisms without necessarily destroying them. However, antiseptics can adversely affect the healing process and should therefore not be used on any injury more serious than a slight abrasion. Antiseptics and skin disinfectants are often used on skin and hair surrounding a wound, to help control wound contamination.

Control of superficial bacterial infection is often assisted by the local application of antibiotic ointments or powders. In spite of this, antibiotic ointments should not be used in an open, deep wound, as they will collect dirt and debris. Additionally, some antibiotics are inactivated by the presence of pus and necrotic debris. Certainly, a thorough cleansing should precede the application of topical medication. Corticosteroid medications should not be applied to an injury unless under veterinary supervision. They are sometimes useful in wound management at later stages of wound healing when used in conjunction with antibiotics.

Wooden tongue depressors may be conveniently used to apply topical medication to wounds or to gauze that is used on wounds. Throw-away depressors should be used for application of medications; they should not be returned to the reservoir of medicine after having once been applied to a wound.

Caustic powders are intended for the control of proud flesh but are often over-applied or used at the wrong stages of healing. Furthermore, their use in treating excess granulation tissue is often superseded by surgical excision and pressure bandaging. Like corticosteroids, caustic powders should be applied only under the direction of a veterinarian.

APPLYING FLUSHING SOLUTIONS

A safe topical medication that can be used to flush out body wounds is sterile saline solution (described in the section on "Cleansing and Treating Wounds"). On fresh wounds, it should be used in lieu of hydrogen peroxide solutions which can irritate an injury by destroying living cells. However, hydrogen peroxide and furacin solutions may be safely used to rinse out old, infected wounds. Only those substances that are soluble in tissue fluids (water-based) should be used to dress wounds.

For applying a solution, a syringe without the needle makes a very good flushing instrument. Ear bulbs and plastic squeeze bottles with nozzles can also be used for applying flushing solutions.

Boric acid solution, saline solution, and clean water are the only substances other than specific ophthalmic medications that should be used to flush the eyes. Unused eye ointments remaining from previous eye treatments should not be used without a veterinarian's approval. Ointments and drops containing corticosteroids may destroy a horse's vision if used when corneal ulcers or lacerations are present. However, corticosteroids may be safely prescribed in later stages of healing.

APPLYING LINIMENTS AND BRACES

Liniments, tighteners, and braces are all rubefacient drugs that produce redness and mild heat by increasing circulation. These substances are often given the credit for reducing edema when, in reality, it is probably the massage used to apply the rubefacient that actually lessens the swelling (refer to "Massage").

A liniment is a mixture of rubefacient drugs that is used to create superficial heat. Soreness or edema may appear after a liniment has been massaged into the skin, therefore, exercise at this time is contraindicated.

A tightener is a preparation used to "tighten" the skin around a joint capsule or tendon by aiding in the removal of edema. The massage used to apply a tightener also aids in reducing edema, thus making the tendons and suspensory ligament more easily felt. Largely, though, it is the tightener that is responsible for the apparent positive effects.

A brace is a mixture of rubefacient drugs that is normally used on the legs after exercise. It is massaged into the skin before the horse's legs are bandaged.

A blister is a much stronger rubefacient than a liniment or brace, used to increase inflammation and hasten healing by converting a chronic inflammation to an acute condition. A blister should be used cautiously, for it causes loss of hair and sloughing of the upper skin layers in the region of application. A horse that has been blistered will require an extended period of rest; it is probably this rest period that is the most important and effective part of treatment. Blistering is an older form of treatment that is no longer used as much as in the past.

Leg paints are another strong type of rubefacient preparation frequently used in conjunction with therapeutic cautery (firing). A daily application of a leg paint is usually required for an extended period of time after firing to increase the counterirritant effect of therapeutic cautery. Like blistering, the use of leg paints has decreased in recent years.

Liniments, tighteners, braces, etc., generally must be applied at least one or two times daily to be effective. Bandaging a horse's legs after application of any of these substances will increase the rubefacient effect, but it can also irritate the skin. It should be remembered that these drugs work superficially if used correctly, and do not penetrate to structures beneath the skin. (For more information on counterirritant drugs, refer to "Drugs and Related Topics.")

APPLYING INSECTICIDES AND REPELLENTS

Insecticides are available as powders, sprays, gels, wipes, and ointments.

Powders may be dusted onto a horse and into the ears (the latter application is to rid the horse of spinose ear ticks). The powdery dust of these insecticides can be very irritating to the lungs and eyes of animals and people alike; consequently, when using a powder, one should try to avoid raising a "cloud" of powdery dust.

If an aerosol insecticide is to be used for the first time, a horse should be familiarized with the spray can and its hissing noise before application is attempted. Making a hissing sound before and during spraying the aerosol will often cause a horse to relax enough so that the repellent may be sprayed directly onto his body. The spray, of course, should be kept away from the eyes at all times. There are horses that particularly object to aerosols, especially to aerosols being used around their ears. When treating a skittish horse, an insecticide can be sprayed onto a soft cloth and wiped on the animal's face and ears.

Insecticides are also available in non-aerosol spray bottles. They have the advantages of being, on the average, much easier to use on a horse and more economical than aerosols. Insecticides can also be purchased in concentrates which must be diluted before they can be wiped or sprayed. Concentrates are generally the most economical form. Insecticide wipes and gels are also available in forms to be smeared on the horse with rub rags or applicator mitts.

PRECAUTIONS AND SUGGESTIONS REGARDING APPLICATION OF INSECTICIDES

Insecticides and insect repellents should be kept out of wounds. Only insecticides specifically recommended by the manufacturer for fly and insect protection around wounds should even be used near wounds. Also, for safest application, an insecticide/repellent should be used only around the edges of the wound and not within the injury's margins. Areas of thin skin and the areas around the eyes must always be treated carefully to avoid irritation. The manufacturer's instructions should always be followed.

CHECKLIST FOR APPLICATION OF TOPICAL MEDICATIONS

1. Wash a wound with either clean water or, preferably, sterile saline solution.
2. Do not use hydrogen peroxide to clean fresh wounds; it is irritating to living tissue. (It may be safely used on older, infected wounds.)
3. Do not use topical antiseptics on any wound more severe than a mild abrasion.
4. Do not use ointments or salves in open, deep wounds.
5. Wash the eyes out with clean water, mild boric acid solution, or sterile saline solution.
6. Remember that liniments, tighteners, and braces do not help a horse as much as the massage and rest that accompany their use.

7. Apply insecticides according to label directions, keeping them out of the eyes and wounds.

Injections

Parenteral administration of drugs refers to administration by routes other than the alimentary canal. As a method of administering medication (i.e., drugs), parenteral administration has several advantages over oral and topical applications. Drugs given parenterally act more rapidly, may have a longer duration of action, and are more efficiently utilized than when given orally or topically. In addition, parenteral administration is sometimes required because certain drugs are not absorbed from the gastrointestinal tract, some are destroyed in the alimentary canal, and other medications cause gastric irritation.

The possible disadvantages of parenteral drug administration are that:

1. it is more expensive
2. it may cause local irritation
3. a sterile approach is necessary
4. the chance of systemic reaction is increased, particularly with intravenous injections

When giving an injection, the individual should have some previous experience and have learned the basic technique from a veterinarian. Furthermore, the hazards and possible consequences of parenteral drug administration should always be considered, and drugs should be administered by the horseman only after consultation with a veterinarian. This is particularly true with intravenous injections.

ROUTES OF PARENTERAL ADMINISTRATION

The following types of injections represent important routes of parenteral drug administration in horses:

1. Subcutaneous (just below the skin)
2. Intradermal (between the layers of the skin)
3. Intramuscular (in the muscle)
4. Intravenous (in the vein)
5. Subconjunctival (beneath the conjunctiva)
6. Intra-articular (into a joint space)
7. Epidural (into the epidural space of the spinal cord, usually between the first and second coccygeal vertebrae)
8. Intrathecal (into the spinal fluid)

The route of administration is a determining factor in how quickly a drug acts, how long its action lasts, and the amount of drug that is required. In general, the intravenous route provides more rapid action than the intramuscular; the intramuscular route provides more rapid action than the subcutaneous; and the intradermal route provides the slowest absorption rate.

The absorption rate of medication is determined to a large extent by the amount of blood supply to the tissues in which the drug is deposited; the smaller the blood supply, the more slowly the substance is absorbed. A substance that is slowly absorbed generally has a more prolonged effect than one that is absorbed quickly.

NECESSARY EQUIPMENT FOR GIVING INJECTIONS

The equipment necessary for giving injections consists of a sterile syringe and hypodermic needle. Disposable plastic syringes are usually adequate; they are sterile, inexpensive, and safe, that is, they won't break like glass syringes. Disposable syringes of a 3 cc size are particularly well suited to the administration of vaccines. Other sizes that are quite useful are the 6 cc and 12 cc syringes, as many drugs are given to horses in amounts between 5 cc's and 12 cc's. Syringes of 20 cc. sizes are useful for some drugs that are given in larger doses, including certain antibiotics.

Disposable syringes and needles should be thrown away after each injection, and should not be used on different animals because of the risk of spreading infection. Unclean needles have been implicated in the spread of equine infectious anemia from horse to horse. If glass syringes are used, they can be appropriately sterilized in boiling water for about 15 minutes and used again for other injections. Autoclaving, however, is preferred to boiling as a means of sterilization and should be used when possible.

THE NEED FOR RESTRAINT

Since some horses may kick or move suddenly when given an injection, it is best to have another person restrain the animal. It may even become necessary to use a twitch, particularly if several injections are to be given. If so, the horse should be hand-held and twitched rather than tied to a stationary object. Naturally, a skilled person will be better able to give injections without eliciting violent reactions.

PREPARATION FOR AN INJECTION

The first and most important step in preparing for an injection is a thorough reading and understanding of the instructions on the bottle of medicine. Instructions normally contain information on refrigeration (necessary and important for some vaccines, antibiotics, etc., which deteriorate if not refrigerated), as well as information regarding the route of administration and the medicine's expiration date. Drugs that have exceeded their expiration dates should be discarded.

After closely reading the directions for the medicine, the injection can be given in the following manner:

1. Fill the syringe with an amount of air equal to the amount of injectable to be used (e.g., use 10 cc of air for 10 cc of drug).
2. Inject the air into the bottle of drug through the cleansed rubber seal. Caution: Injecting air hastens the deterioration of certain injectables, such as some vitamin complexes, and is not recommended when the remainder of the drug will be stored for future use.
3. With the needle inserted into the vial, hold the vial upside down or at a steep angle, making sure that the end of the needle is not in an air pocket.
4. Slowly pull the plunger back until it is a little above the mark for the amount of drug needed; for example, withdraw 11 cc of substance if 10 cc is required.
5. With the needle still in the vial, hold the syringe and vial upside down and give the syringe a few gentle taps on the side to dislodge air bubbles that may be present.
6. Finally, push the plunger down just enough to expel air and the extra medicine in the syringe and pull the syringe and needle straight out.

If a medicine has been kept refrigerated, it is best warmed to body temperature before it is injected. This can be done by holding the filled syringe in one's hand until the correct temperature is reached.

Although alcohol is effective in removing oil and dirt from the hair, it is a weak disinfectant and requires several minutes to kill bacteria. Thus, there is little immediate bactericidal effect of alcohol when it is applied to the skin of a horse as a preparation for an injection. If an effort is made to clean the skin, it is more beneficial to use a pHisoHex-type cleanser or iodine cleanser. Shaving the injection site is unnecessary and is not recommended.

SUBCUTANEOUS INJECTIONS

A subcutaneous (SC) injection is given when slow absorption of a drug into the bloodstream is required. An appropriate site for a subcutaneous injection is in an area where the skin is loose, such as the middle of the side of the neck. For a subcutaneous injection, a small diameter needle of about 18 or 20 gauge should be used. The small diameter prevents too large a hole from being made in the horse's sensitive skin. The needle's length should be approximately five-eighths inch to one inch.

To give the injection, the skin should be lifted and the needle inserted at a direct angle into one end of the fold. Raising a fold reduces the horse's reaction to the needle and prevents injecting the medication intradermally (i.e., between the layers of the skin).

To insure that a muscle mass isn't penetrated, the needle should be backed up slightly and held under the skin with the thumb and fingers

a.

b.

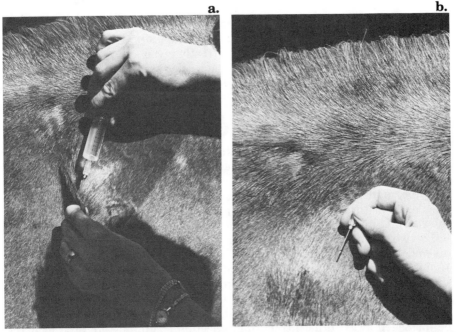

Fig. 4-23 Subcutaneous injection. a. The needle is inserted beneath the fold of skin. b. Completed injection leaves a small lump beneath the skin.

a.

b.

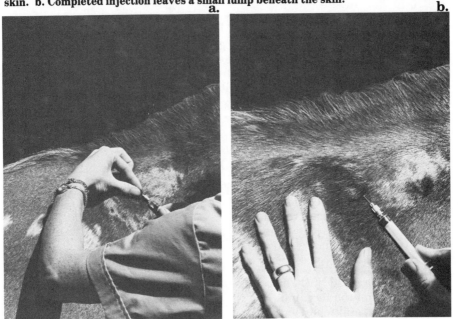

Fig. 4-24 Intradermal injection. a. Injection made into a small pinch of skin. b. Completed injection leaves a bleb beneath the skin.

while the injection is made. Moving the needle from side to side under the skin (called fanning) or massaging the injection site will cause additional trauma, and is not recommended. A correctly given subcutaneous injection will temporarily leave a small lump just under the surface of the skin. If this lump is not present, the injection given may have been a shallow intramuscular injection which will have dispersed the drug into the tissues.

INTRADERMAL INJECTIONS

Injections between layers of the skin are sometimes used to administer encephalomyelitis vaccines or antigens in allergy testing. This type of injection should be given in an area which will not be chafed by tack, for example, under the mane or between the front legs. A 22 to 25 gauge needle, from three-eighths to five-eighths inch in length, is useful for an intradermal injection.

To give an intradermal injection, a small fold of skin should be pinched up and the needle slipped into the fold at a very oblique angle (about 160°). Pinching the skin reduces the pain of the injection. The medicine should be slowly injected; if it flows too easily, the injection being made is in subcutaneous tissue instead of in intradermal tissue. A correctly given intradermal injection will leave a hard bleb (small, raised area) that cannot be massaged away. If an intradermal injection is administered too near the skin's surface, the drug may cause sloughing of the skin.

INTRAMUSCULAR INJECTIONS

An intramuscular injection (IM) is given when more rapid drug action is desired. The needle used for this type of injection should be either 18 or 20 gauge, and the length is determined by the size of muscle at the site of injection. Needles of one and one-half inch length are convenient to use. The length of the needle must allow it to penetrate the skin, enter the muscle, and remain there during the injection. Too short a needle could result in a subcutaneous injection.

AREAS OF ADMINISTRATION

Sites at which intramuscular injections are commonly given are:
1. the lateral muscles of the neck
2. the biceps femoris muscle
3. the semimembranosus muscle
4. the semitendinosus muscle

Less frequent sites are:
1. the long head of the triceps muscle, near the shoulder and above the elbow on the forelimb
2. the pectoral (chest) area
3. the gluteal region (rump)

The most common of these areas of injection is the lateral muscles of the neck. This is also the safest place for drug administration for the person giving the injection. In this region, there may sometimes be a local reaction such as a knot, caused by swelling of muscle tissue. Performance horses are often injected in the neck, since an inflammation here would least affect their ability. Even then, the neck may be somewhat stiff. If local swelling or stiffness causes concern, the injection can be given in the biceps femoris muscle mass of the hindquarters. When an injection is given in the biceps femoris area, the horse should be approached from the side to reduce the chances of being kicked, and the injection should be given below the tuber ischium (point of buttock).

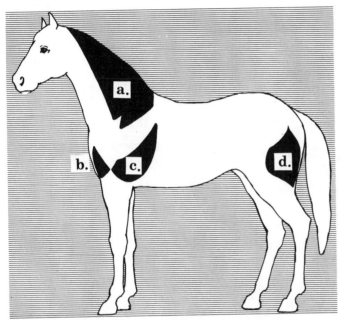

Fig 4-25 Shaded areas indicate locations suitable for intramuscular injections. a. Lateral neck muscles. b. Pectoral muscles. c. Triceps muscles. d. The lower portion of the biceps femoris, semimembranosus, and semitendinosus muscles.

An injection should not be given in the triceps area if the horse is to be saddled or harnessed within the next few weeks, for injections in this area can be irritated by the presence of tack. Injections may be easily given in the pectoral area, though drug administration here may also cause side effects. This area may swell greatly and abscess, causing a horse discomfort when he moves. In comparison, the muscle mass in the gluteal region is covered with thick skin, and swelling here is seldom seen. However, if an abscess develops from an injection into the gluteal muscles, it may spread into the pelvic area and will heal with difficulty due to poor drainage, a serious consequence. For this reason, the gluteal area is not recommended for injections.

Regardless of the injection site chosen, an intramuscular injection should always be made into the belly (center) of a muscle, away from any nerves, blood vessels, or bones. Injecting a substance into a nerve could cause the nerve's deterioration and, perhaps, eventual paralysis of the innervated area.

GIVING AN INTRAMUSCULAR INJECTION

To distract a horse and to minimize his response to the injection, the skin surrounding the injection site should be lightly patted before the needle is inserted. A good, relatively easy way to give an injection, especially for beginners, is to insert the needle alone and attach the syringe when the animal has calmed down. First, the needle should be disconnected from the syringe and held between the thumb and index fingers. Then, the horse should be thumped a few times with the side of the hand, and the needle driven in on the final thump. During this procedure, there should be no pause or any other incongruous action that would indicate when the needle is to be inserted. The syringe should then be inserted and the injection completed.

a.
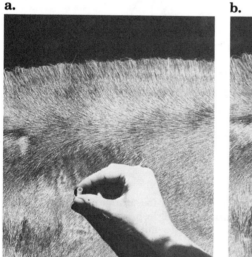

b.
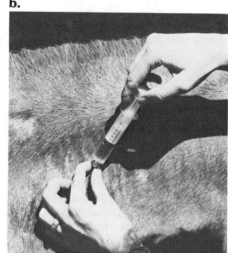

Fig. 4-26 Intramuscular injection into the neck.   a. The needle is quickly inserted with a thrust.   b. The plunger is pulled back slightly to determine whether the needle is in a blood vessel.

Before depressing the plunger of the syringe to give the drug, it should be pulled out very slightly to see if any blood is aspirated. If blood is present, the needle is in a blood vessel and the injection procedure must be repeated in a different site. When the drug is administered, no more than 12 to 15 cc of substance should be deposited at any one injection site. Therefore, if 20 cc of medication is required, the dose should be split and given as two separate 10 cc injections.

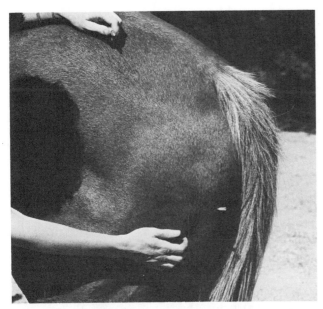

Fig. 4-27 **Intramuscular injection into the rump. The needle has been inserted below the point of the buttocks. The syringe is attached to the needle and the injection completed.**

INTRAVENOUS INJECTIONS

Intravenous (IV) injections should only be administered upon advice from a veterinarian; given incorrectly, they can easily be fatal. Also, infection can be introduced while inserting the needle into the jugular vein, and too rapid an injection of some substances may cause serious toxic effects. In addition, if the horse suffers an anaphylactic reaction to the medication, the veterinarian may be able to save the horse if only a small amount of the drug has been given and emergency drugs are available. Therefore, label directions on drugs should be implicitly obeyed, and no substance should be injected intravenously if the directions recommend administration by another route. Drugs to be given intravenously should not be mixed, because mixing could cause formation of a precipitate, or cause toxic chemical or biological effects. Nor should cloudy solutions be injected intravenously; the fact that a drug is cloudy usually indicates that it is in some way defective.

An intravenous injection is usually given in the jugular vein in the upper two-thirds of the neck. In the lower one-third of the neck, this vein is covered by muscle. The injection is often given in the right jugular vein to avoid inflammation of the esophagus that may result from the administration of an irritating substance, such as a broad-spectrum antibiotic. Irritation to the tissue around the injection site from such a drug may cause inflammation and sloughing of the skin. The esophagus is on the left side of about 90% of all horses, and non-irritating medications may be injected into the jugular vein on this side. It is possible to permanently damage the jugular vein during an intravenous injection by causing enough inflammation and irritation (phlebitis) that the vein becomes blocked. One occluded jugular vein is considered a blemish and two are considered a serious unsoundness. Giving an intravenous injection with the smallest needle practical (one of 16 to 18 gauge, one and one-half to two inches in length) should help minimize damage.

An intravenous injection is given in the following manner:

1. First, block the jugular vein by pressing the thumb against the vein between the intended injection site and the heart. This causes blood to back up and distend the vein.
2. Then, holding the needle firmly, push the needle quickly through the skin into the distended vein and thread it through the lumen of the vein until blood is flowing freely through the needle. The needle may be directed either towards the head or the tail of the horse, as explained further below.

If blood does not flow when the needle has been inserted, one of the following has happened:

1. The needle has not been inserted deeply enough.
2. The needle has gone above or below the vein.
3. The needle has passed all the way through the vein.
4. The needle is dull and has been blocked by skin.
5. Blood has clotted in the needle.
6. The bevel of the needle is resting against the wall of the vein.

If any of the above is suspected, the needle should be withdrawn one-quarter inch. Then, if blood still does not flow, the needle must be removed and the procedure repeated. Blood from a vein is dark red and will drip from the needle. If the blood is bright red and spurts from the needle, the carotid artery has been entered instead of the jugular vein. An accidental injection into the carotid artery can result in extreme, uncontrollable excitement and death. Thus, it is very important to correctly establish the needle's position in the jugular vein before the intravenous injection is made.

The needle can be directed either cephalad (toward the head) or caudad (toward the tail). When the needle is directed toward the head, drug dispersion is more even and irritation is reduced; with the needle directed toward the tail, medication is prevented from seeping out around the injection site. After proper needle placement, the syringe should be attached to the needle, a small amount of blood should be aspirated into the barrel of the syringe to recheck needle placement, and the injection made.

The needle should be closely observed during the course of the injection to insure that it does not pass through the vein, which could result in an accidental perivascular (into the tissues surrounding the blood vessel) injection, and subsequent inflammation and sloughing of the skin and tissue. If perivascular injection occurs, isotonic sodium chloride (saline) solution should immediately be injected into the site through the same needle. Five times as much saline solution as drug should be given to help counteract any inflammation. A corticosteroid solution is often injected around the site of a perivascular injection to reduce the inflammatory response, and procaine may be used to lessen the pain.

For the administration of larger amounts of medications (over 60 cc), a piece of intravenous tubing is attached to the hub of the needle in place of the syringe. The other end of this tube is fastened to the drug vial, and gravity forces the medication into the jugular vein.

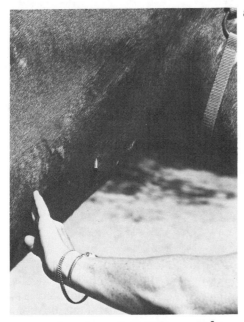

a.

Fig. 4-28 Intravenous injection.
a. The jugular vein is held off to facilitate insertion of the needle. In this
case, the needle has been directed
towards the head. b. Blood is aspirated to ensure that the needle is in
the jugular vein. c. Completing the
injection.

b.

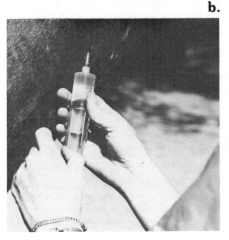

c.

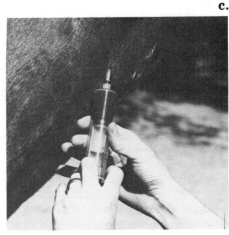

a.   **b.**

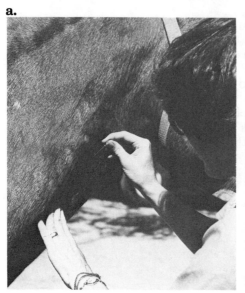
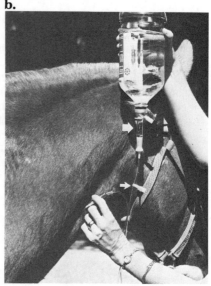

Fig. 4-29 Intravenous injection using an i.v. set for large fluid volumes. a. The needle is inserted in the jugular vein. b. The i.v. set is attached. Fluid flow is regulated by gravity [the higher the bottle, the faster the flow] and by the screw clamp [small arrow]. The rate of fluid flow is noted by observing the drip chamber [large arrow].

THE INDWELLING INTRAVENOUS CATHETER

Irritating medications that must be administered repeatedly or over an extended period of time should be given through an indwelling intravenous catheter set. To reduce the trauma that would result from multiple needle insertions, the catheter may remain in place for 3 or 4 days of repeated use, according to the need for fluids and the scheduled doses of medication. The set includes a piece of narrow plastic tubing (catheter), which is passed through a needle into the vein. A syringe with a blunt needle is then used to inject the substance into the catheter, or the catheter can be connected to a vial for gravity flow of the drug solution. Because too rapid a flow of medication can cause shock or cardiac arrest, drugs administered intravenously should be slowly dripped into the bloodstream. The veterinarian will flush the catheter with sterile saline solution and heparin after each injection to prevent a blood clot from forming in the catheter while it is still in place in the jugular vein.

An intravenous set is also employed in the administration of large amounts of liquids. Like a regular intravenous injection, injection through an intravenous set is best done by an experienced person, and should be used by the horseman only upon advice from a veterinarian.

A horse will occasionally become frightened by an intravenous outfit, and the eye on the side of the injection may have to be covered before the injection can be given. After it is used, the intravenous equipment should be rinsed with boiled water. Before it is to be reused, the equipment should be autoclaved or boiled.

NOTE: The following injection procedures should be done only by a veterinarian, as they are complicated procedures and require special skill for correct application.

THE SUBCONJUNCTIVAL INJECTION

With certain eye conditions, the veterinarian may choose to inject small amounts of corticosteroids and/or antibiotics beneath the conjunctiva. A short, small gauge needle (25 gauge) is used to deposit the medication. This route of administration prolongs the drug's action in the eye area compared to that of topical drops and ointments applied directly to the eye's surface.

THE INTRA-ARTICULAR INJECTION

An intra-articular injection is used to administer an anti-inflammatory agent and/or antibiotics directly into a joint space. This type of injection is used to relieve the pain of some kinds of arthritis, bursitis, and synovitis. It is also used to remove a sample of synovial fluid from a joint space for examination, and to relieve pressure in the joint space. When joint fluid samples are taken, they are cultured for the presence of bacteria and antibiotic sensitivity tests are performed. In addition, the intra-articular injection technique is used for saline lavage or flushing a joint (refer to "Infectious Arthritis").

The intra-articular injection of corticosteroids is particularly common, for it allows greater drug concentration in the joint capsule than systemic administration of corticosteroids. However, improper injections into a joint capsule can result in bone demineralization and retarded healing.

Sterile technique is, of course, used in preparing the site of an intra-articular injection, and the veterinarian may use a sterile syringe with a 20 gauge needle to slowly remove a portion of the synovial fluid prior to injection of the chosen drugs.

After receiving an intra-articular injection of a corticosteroid, the horse must be rested for one to six months to allow time for natural healing. If joint surgery becomes necessary, a two months' observation period between the time of injection and the operation is necessary to note the development of possible complications.

THE EPIDURAL INJECTION

This technique is used for standing surgery on the horse in the areas of the rectum and vulva, and in delivering foals in cases of dystocia. In the equine, an epidural injection of four or five milliliters of local anesthetic (e.g., 2% solution of xylocaine) is given between the first two coccygeal (tail) vertebrae. As this area becomes numb, care is required to ensure that the horse does not become unsteady and lose its footing.

THE INTRATHECAL INJECTION

The intrathecal injection is a seldom used technique reserved for collection of cerebral spinal fluid, tetanus therapy, and special radiographic techniques. The areas of injection include the region between the first two neck vertebrae (the atlas and axis), and the lumbosacral region of the vertebral column. This route of administration is used cautiously, with care taken to avoid damage to the spinal cord, and prefaced with the same careful preparation required for major surgery.

Oral Administration of Medicine

For many horsemen, the oral route of administration of drugs is frequently easier and more convenient to use than are other methods such as injections. When medicine is given orally, a horse should be in his stall or in another familiar place where he is likely to remain calm.

DRENCHING

Drenching, the peroral (through the mouth) administration of liquid medicine, is a fairly convenient method for the horseman to use. Still, there are cautions which must be observed. An oily, bland liquid with little taste, such as mineral oil, should normally not be given as a drench. This is because such a liquid does not stimulate swallowing and it might accidentally pass into the trachea where it could cause foreign body pneumonia. Additionally, horses suffering from any of the following conditions should not be drenched:

purpura hemorrhagica	semicomatose state
pharyngitis	encephalitis
forage poisoning	strangles
pharyngeal paralysis	botulism

Medicine applied as a drench will reach therapeutic levels more quickly and accurately if the animal has not eaten prior to the drug's administration.

GIVING THE DRENCH

The person giving the drug to a horse should stand at a level where the horse's head is within easy reach. Because the front of the horse's head should be horizontal, the head must be held up, either by an assistant or with a rope attached to the halter's noseband and put over a beam or rafter. If tied, the head should not be tied to a stationary object; instead, it should be fastened so that it can be rapidly released if necessary.

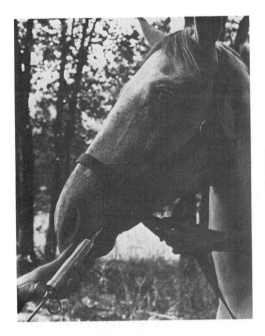

Fig. 4-30 A dose syringe can be inserted into the interdental space to administer an oral medication.

The head should not be held above the horizontal. This would interfere with the animal's ability to swallow the medicine and perhaps cause the liquid to enter the trachea instead of the esophagus.

Because some of the medication is often lost by dribbling from the mouth, small amounts should be diluted so that a minor fluid loss is not critical. The solution should be put into a dose syringe or into a plastic or strong glass bottle with a long, smooth neck. The syringe or bottle should then be placed into the space in front of the first cheek tooth, and the drench slowly poured down the horse's throat. The horse should be allowed to swallow after every few ounces of medicine have been given; otherwise, he might inhale the liquid (especially if the liquid is being given too quickly and the horse's head is above a horizontal plane). If the horse coughs or begins to choke, his head should be immediately lowered. The drenching should then be discontinued and a veterinarian consulted.

ELECTUARIES

A good way to administer anthelmintics, tranquilizers, and electrolytes is to put the medicine into a more palatable form called an electuary. This can be done by mixing the drug with corn syrup, honey, molasses, or with sugar if the medication is a liquid. The electuary can then be rubbed on the horse's teeth and tongue, where it is usually quickly dissolved and swallowed with the saliva.

PASTE ANTHELMINTICS

Some deworming compounds distributed as pastes or gels are designed for application with a plastic syringe. These anthelmintics are very convenient to give and, since the medicine adheres to the horse's mouth, there is little spillage or loss of medication. Moreover, some of these compounds are effective against early larval stages of botflies when administered directly into the mouth.

Because these anthelmintic doses are calculated according to a horse's weight, it becomes necessary to know the true weight or have at least a close approximation. Weight may be estimated with the weight tapes that are available from some feed companies. The syringe should be inserted between the teeth at the interdental space, then passed to the back of the tongue and the plunger depressed to administer the correct dose.

ANTHELMINTICS AS FEED ADDITIVES

Many anthelmintics are given orally as feed additives. Although some compounds are more palatable than others, no additive by itself is very delicious (regardless of advertising claims to the contrary). Consequently, the additives should always be mixed with a small amount of feed to encourage consumption. The taste of the more unpalatable anthelmintics may be successfully disguised by adding a package of fruit flavored gelatin dessert to the feed for two or three days, then adding the gelatin and anthelmintic at the same time.

Since some horses are skilled at sifting out grain and leaving a pile of dewormer powder at the bottom of their feed tubs, it is recommended that a powder anthelmintic be mixed with a little water and sprinkled over the ration. The use of a feed with a high molasses content will also help bind the dewormer powder to the feed and keep it from sifting through.

DEWORMING BY STOMACH TUBE

Using a stomach tube is the most accurate way to administer anthelmintics. The stomach tube guarantees that 100% of the medication will reach the horse's stomach and is therefore the most certain way of administering a calculated dose of dewormer. Administration of anthelmintics through a stomach tube is a serious procedure requiring skillful technique and should only be attempted by a veterinarian (refer to "Stomach Tubing").

CAPSULES AND BOLUSES

For most adult horses, capsules or boluses can be given either by hand or with a balling gun. Excessively large capsules should not be given to ponies or foals, as they may lodge in the esophagus, causing complications such as choke, esophagitis, and even death.

A bolus to be given by hand should first be soaked in mineral oil or

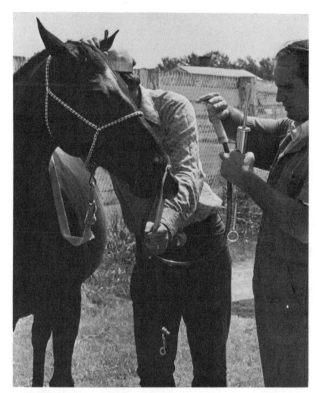

Fig. 4-31 The veterinarian is using a stomach tube to administer an anthelmintic.

glycerine for a few minutes to soften it. Then, the horse's tongue should be pulled out of the way to one side between the upper and lower cheek teeth and the bolus placed far back on the tongue. The tongue must then be released and the mouth held closed. The head should be kept in a normal position to facilitate swallowing. Standing at the horse's left side will enable one to see the movement of the bolus down the esophagus; this movement will occur in the jugular groove on the left side of the horse's neck. If the bolus stops, a massage-like push will often start it moving down again. After the capsule has been swallowed, a horse should be allowed to drink some water, and when more than one capsule has been administered, a horse should be given a couple of ounces of water as a drench. This should be done even if the capsules have previously been lubricated.

When a balling gun is used, the tongue is held in the same manner and the pill discharged onto its base. If too dry a bolus is used, however, or if a balling gun is placed too far back in the mouth, the horse may gag on the medicine and spit it out. At no time should a balling gun be jammed roughly into the mouth.

Should a capsule become lodged in the esophagus, a veterinarian should be called. The horseman should not attempt to treat this condition by giving water to loosen the bolus; water may only worsen the condition by causing the bolus to swell. Furthermore, because of pressure necrosis and contact with the irritating capsule, the area where the bolus is lodged may be quite fragile and susceptible to injury.

Upon arrival, the veterinarian may decide to pass a stomach tube, administer a small amount of mineral oil, and try to gently push the bolus the rest of the way down to the stomach. This is not a procedure for the horseman. It requires no small amount of skill and, even then, foreign body pneumonia and death are associated risks. This procedure should only be attempted by a veterinarian.

Feeding the Critically Ill Horse

LOSS OF APPETITE IN THE SICK HORSE

A depressed appetite can be caused by an illness, a change in surroundings, or by a change in feed. When there is a change in environment or feed, a horse will usually return to normal eating habits after a period of adjustment. A lack of appetite from illness is a much more serious problem, since a horse's tissue requirements increase even though his appetite decreases. Starvation, whatever the cause, inhibits the body's defense and healing capabilities (refer to "Emaciation").

ENCOURAGING A SICK HORSE TO EAT

If a horse is picking at his feed or just slightly "off his feed," he can often be encouraged to eat and drink if his food and water is made more palatable. The addition of molasses or corn syrup sweetens and improves the flavor of water and feed, and may make it more appetizing to a sick horse. Salt can also be used, as it improves the flavor of feed and makes a horse thirsty. It can be easily added to grain, or can be placed in small pinches inside the lips.

PLANNING A SPECIAL DIET

When an illness is debilitating or prolonged, a special diet should be planned to aid the horse's recovery. Any change in diet should be done gradually to prevent diarrhea or digestive upsets. When changing the concentrated food ration, never increase or decrease grain more than two pounds a day. The factors in making up a special diet are palatability to encourage eating, high protein content to facilitate healing, moderate fiber content for digestibility, and supplementation of vitamins to increase appetite.

To encourage the horse to eat, the diet should be as appetizing as possible. Some horses have difficulty picking up or swallowing grain, but are able to pick up and swallow a wet mash. Molasses and apple slices may be added along with hot water to make the mash more appealing. Alfalfa hay is more tempting to most horses and it is also higher in protein and lower in fiber than timothy hay. The intake of one and one-half to two pounds of alfalfa per 100 pounds of body weight meets the protein requirement and energy needs of an unstressed horse. A sick horse will have higher tissue requirements, and feeding alfalfa free choice is usually recommended. Alfalfa is lower in fiber and can cause diarrhea if the horse is not accustomed to it, so it should be introduced gradually into the diet over approximately a five day period.

It is important to keep a high protein content in the diet to insure the ill horse is getting a high level of nitrogen. When available in sufficient quantities, nitrogen may aid in wound healing, improve the horse's defense system, and prevent muscle wasting. If necessary, the protein content can be increased by substituting a commercial pelleted feed for grain or grain mashes. There are several pelleted feeds on the market that are both high in protein and highly digestible.

A sick horse should have only a moderate amount of fiber in its feed, since the fiber content of the diet affects the digestibility of nutrients. Too high a fiber content will interfere with the digestion and absorption of essential nutrients, however, some fiber is needed for fecal ball formation. Bran is relatively indigestible and should only be fed when a laxative effect is desired.

The last consideration when planning a special diet is the addition of vitamins. In older horses it is not necessary to supplement with fat soluble vitamins since these are stored in the body. However, a sick foal may need supplements with vitamin A since the stores are small at birth and may be used up rapidly during an illness. A horse also usually receives all the B vitamins it requires either directly from feed or by synthesizing them in the intestines from precursor ingested from feed. The B-complex vitamins may be utilized during an illness, and may contribute to a decrease in appetite. Therefore, vitamin B complex injections may be effective in increasing appetite. The response to such injections should be seen in 24 to 48 hours if therapy is successful.

FORCE-FEEDING

A serious problem occurs when a horse is so ill that he completely refuses to eat. By not eating, the animal impairs his recovery ability and causes fluid and electrolyte imbalances. When this happens, an attempt must be made to forcibly feed the horse to ensure that he receives an adequate supply of nutrients. This can be done by use of a stomach tube, by feeding through the rectum, or by intravenous solutions.

Though it has a few disadvantages, the stomach tube is usually the most effective and preferred means of force-feeding a horse. The main advantage of using a stomach tube is that it can be used over an extended period of time, however, it can cause pressure lesions on the epiglottis when left in place too long. A stomach tube cannot be used in some diseases, such as tetanus, where passing the tube is not feasible.

Feeding by stomach tube should be attempted only by or under supervision of a veterinarian. In cases where lesions are present in the esophagus or pharynx, and the affected horse will not eat, a stomach tube may be passed once and left in place for several days. This procedure will supply basic nutrients (administered by a stomach pump), yet will also allow the lesions time to heal. After the stomach tube is first passed, it is wrapped with tape where it passes from the nostril and is then sutured to the nostril by a veterinarian. The protruding end is then taped to the halter to secure it out of the way. When the tube is thus placed, further irritation or excitement and stress that would be caused by repeated tube passings is no longer a problem. With this arrangement, it becomes possible to feed a horse on a daily basis without a veterinarian's assistance.

The veterinarian will prescribe a ration for tubing, based on the horse's condition and the nature of the disease. For a diet where some fiber is desired, a complete pelleted ration can be soaked in warm water and made into a gruel. This should take from twenty minutes to an hour, depending on the consistency of the pellets, and should be done carefully to avoid fermentation which can be caused by excessive soaking. A brass marine bilge pump can be used to slowly force the suspension into the horse's stomach. Particles up to one-eighth inch in diameter can be passed with this type of pump. A funnel can also be used to get the feed into the stomach tube and the gruel will flow by gravity rather than by pumping. Since approximately five gallons is the maximum amount that a horse's stomach can comfortably hold, a forced feeding should be half this volume or less, to prevent painful stomach distension. For the maximum benefit, the horse should be fed small amounts frequently.

The following ration, administered through a funnel and tube, will provide a maintenance diet for a 1000 pound horse receiving no exercise.

3 lbs wheat flour	2 ¼ lbs soybean flour
1 ½ lbs alfalfa leaf meal	⅓ lb dry nonfat milk
3 tablespoons corn oil	1 ¼ pints molasses

One-half of this ration in two and a half gallons of water should be given to the horse twice daily. After a few days of this diet, the feces may become loose and green due to a lack of roughage.

In some cases, the veterinarian may recommend a diet with little or no fiber. Such a diet usually consists of an electrolyte mixture, an energy source, and a protein source mixed with water. The electrolyte mixture provides maintenance mineral requirements and may include:

sodium chloride	potassium phosphate
sodium bicarbonate	calcium chloride
potassium chloride	magnesium oxide

Dehydrated cottage cheese (90% digestible in the horse) can be added as a protein source, and glycerol, sucrose, dextrose, or emulsified fat can be added as an energy source. This mixture should be combined with water and should be fed three times a day to maintain a 1000 pound horse. While this diet does not meet energy requirements, it does meet protein and mineral requirements, and a horse can be kept on this ration for two weeks without an electrolyte imbalance or appreciable muscle wasting.

When tube feeding is used for more than several days, it is essential that hydration, blood glucose, and B.U.N. are regularly checked. It may also be helpful to monitor the packed cell volume (PCV) and total protein (TP) (refer to "Hematology").

FEEDING THROUGH THE RECTUM

If an illness makes passing a stomach tube impossible, a gravity flow system can be used to introduce nutrients through the rectum. It should be mentioned, however, that this method of feeding is extremely uncommon, and doses that are given must be limited to two or three quarts of such feeds as milk, starch, flour, eggs, saline solution and glucose. Inflammatory reactions in the mucous membrane of the rectum restrict this manner of administration of nutrients to a maximum period of seven to ten days. This method of administration should be attempted only under veterinary supervision.

INTRAVENOUS FEEDING

Fluids, electrolytes, glucose, and amino acids can be given intravenously, but their administration will not provide a sufficient level of nutrition to maintain life over an extended period of time. Still, intravenous feeding may be the method of choice to enable a horse to survive a crisis (refer to "Fluid and Electrolyte Therapy").

Treating Common Hoof Ailments

Some frequently encountered hoof ailments can be profitably treated by the horseowner. They include thrush, puncture wounds, abscesses, corns, gravel, seedy toe, and canker. For information about other specific hoof ailments that may cause lameness, refer to the "Lameness" chapter.

TREATING THRUSH

Thrush involves disintegration of the frog, clefts, and sole of the hoof, and is characterized by a black discharge and offensive odor. Some of the causes of thrush are unclean stabling conditions, insufficient foot expansion, failure to properly clean the hoof, and lack of frog pressure, all of which allow infection to develop.

When a horse is treated for thrush, he should first be stabled on a clean, dry surface, and his feet thoroughly cleaned with disinfectant. The affected parts of the frog should then be trimmed away and the hoof treated twice daily with one of the various thrush treatments, many of which contain a form of iodine. A suitable thrush dressing may be made by mixing one part formalin with three parts water.

For mild cases of thrush, drying solutions like Kopertox and a dilute formalin solution can be directly applied to the sole of the hoof. Other astringent medications that may be used include chlorine bleach, calomel, anti-inflammatory packs, and cotton soaked in a 10-15% sulfapyridine solution and packed into the affected area. Later, corrective shoes with bars may be used to provide adequate frog pressure. If thrush affects the sensitive structures of the foot, tetanus antitoxin or toxoid should be given.

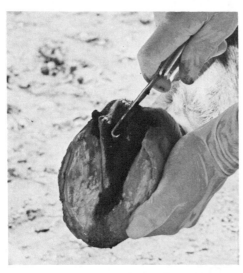

Fig. 4-32 The veterinarian is paring the frog to provide drainage at the puncture site.

TREATING PUNCTURES

Puncture wounds of the sole are fairly common injuries, most often caused by nails and barbed wire. However, a puncture can also result from improper shoeing when a farrier drives a nail either too close to, or into the sensitive hoof tissues. (This may be an unavoidable occurrence if the hoof wall is especially thin.) Treatment of a puncture wound should begin with location of the site of injury. If the wound is not evident, hoof testers can be used to reveal its location. The object must then be removed from the sole in order for the wound to drain and swelling to subside. The sole is usually pared out in the area of the puncture to facilitate drainage, after which strong tincture of iodine or a solution of one part phenol and two parts formalin can be used to dry the wound. The foot may also be treated by soaking in a hot antiseptic solution or epsom salts. Puncture wounds in cases of pricked sole and close nail may be beneficially treated with a two or three day application of a poultice such as an epsom salts poultice. The foot should be covered with a bandage during the treatment, and a shoe and full pad of leather or rubber used afterward. A pack of pine tar and oakum can also be applied to a puncture wound under a full leather pad and corrective shoe. Tetanus immunization should be provided in treating any puncture wound.

TREATING SOLE ABSCESSES

Acute abscesses of the sole of the foot can be treated with hot compresses, then opened (by a veterinarian) when they are mature. After an abscess has been opened, its contents should be drained and the cavity flushed with an antiseptic such as iodine. The sore hoof may benefit from soaking in a mild epsom salts solution. The hoof should be bandaged after treatment; this therapy is repeated daily until the discharge from the wound ceases, after which time it can be treated as an ordinary wound.

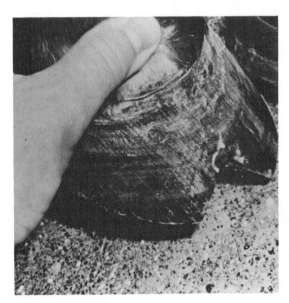

Fig. 4-33 A sole abscess which breaks out at the coronary band is called gravel. The hoof wall has been notched to relieve pressure.

TREATING CORNS

Corns are bruises of the sole usually seen in the area of the angle of the bars. When corns are present, they likely are the results of improper shoeing, or shoes that were left on too long, or of continued work over a hard surface. To treat corns, the shoes should be removed and the discolored sole area pared by a veterinarian. If the corns are suppurative (pus-forming), the pus should be drained (by a veterinarian, whenever possible). Then, a poultice should be applied for 48 to 72 hours, bandaged in place with a quittor bandage, and changed every twelve hours (refer to "Bandaging"). A soaking treatment in a warm epsom salts solution may also be beneficial. After treatment, the horse should be reshod with an appropriate type of corrective shoe (refer to "Corrective Shoeing and Trimming"). A pad may be required if an abscess was present. Because corns may be considered to be types of puncture wounds, immunization for tetanus should be provided.

TREATING GRAVEL

Gravel is an infection that usually enters the bottom of the hoof at the junction of the hoof wall and sole. It then breaks out at the coronary band and causes a severe lameness. In treating this condition, any accumulated pus should be drained (by a veterinarian when possible) and the foot soaked in epsom salts and flushed with iodine. Until drainage stops, the hoof should be bandaged with a quittor bandage or suitable substitute, and shoes with full pads used to keep dirt out of the wound. In severe cases, the veterinarian may be required to perform surgery.

TREATING SEEDY TOE

The separation of the hoof wall from the sole at the toe is known as seedy toe; it is a common sequela to road founder. In the case of this kind of infection, the diseased part of the hoof should be hollowed out before the hoof is treated. Melted wax or pitch can be poured into the resulting crevice, or it can be packed with gauze soaked in a 7% iodine solution. If a horse with seedy toe is to be reshod, the shoe should be one that will not bear on the affected portion of hoof wall (refer to "Corrective Shoeing and Trimming").

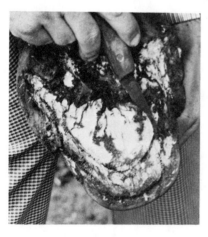

Fig. 4-34 Seedy toe, the separation of the hoof wall from the sole at the toe, may result from laminitis.

TREATING CANKER

Canker is a chronic, hypertrophic (overgrowing), moist ailment of the hoof characterized by a fetid odor. The corium (a tissue layer underneath the sole) will be swollen and exude a thick, white discharge. This disease usually affects the hind feet and may involve the frog, sole, and walls, or the entire foot. It seems to occur most often when the feet have been neglected. Before treatment for canker is begun, the diseased tissue must be removed by a veterinarian. An antibiotic such as aureomycin powder is then dusted on prior to bandaging an antiseptic pack on the hoof with a quittor bandage. Other agents that are useful in canker treatment include topical zinc sulfate and penicillin in parenteral and topical applications. A solution used in treatment is as follows:

1 oz. $CuSO_4$
1 oz. $ZnSO_4$
1 oz. lead acetate
16 oz. water

Canker is precipitated by filthy stabling which allows the feet to become infected. But canker and thrush differ in the following points:

CANKER	THRUSH
1. thick, white exudate from corium	1. black, necrotic exudate from frog
2. overgrowth of corium	2. disintegration of frog
3. bleeds easily	3. deeper than normal sulci (the grooves on either side of the frog)

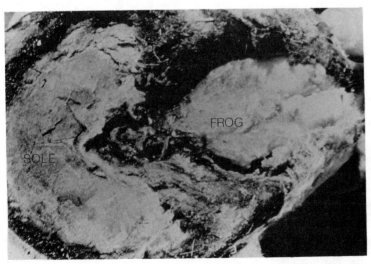

Fig. 4-35 **A severe case of canker; note the exudate from the corium.**

Massage

Massage is defined as the rubbing or kneading of parts of the body for therapeutic purposes. It may be helpful in treating many conditions, including sprains, splints, swelling from saddle sores, simple bruises, and general muscle soreness. Massage also aids lymph circulation which speeds removal of waste products, and stimulates superficial blood vessels which increases the flow of blood and nutrients to the massaged area. Finally, massage helps in freeing scar tissue adhesions between the skin and underlying tissues, though it must be repeated several times daily to be most effective. Generally, massage should be done more than once a day, and, if any real benefit is to be derived, each treatment should contain at least five minutes of rubbing.

THE MASSAGE TECHNIQUE

Technique in massage is very important. However, the technique of hand and finger movement, once mastered, may be used on different parts of the horse's body. In massage, the hands should basically be moved lightly and flexibly over the horse's body in the direction that the hair grows. Large muscular regions of the body should be massaged with the palms of the hands, while small, bony areas should be massaged with the fingers.

As an example of this, the hands should be cupped around a leg and moved slowly and smoothly down it. The thumbs should then be used to apply the massage in a rotating movement between the tendons. In this movement, the greatest pressure should be exerted on the part of the stroke directed toward the heart. When massaging the leg, this circular motion can be continued down the leg and used on the coronary band.

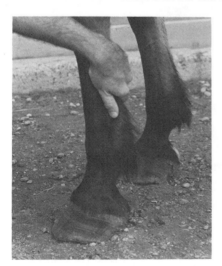

Fig. 4-36 Massaging the legs with special attention to the tendon areas.

If frequent massage begins to irritate the horse's skin, lanolin, petroleum jelly, or a liniment can be used as a protecting agent. Otherwise, no special medicinal liniments should be needed, as it is the massage itself that reduces swelling and relieves pain.

USING PETRISSAGE

If the area to be massaged has a loose skin covering (e.g., the area over the neck), the technique of petrissage can be used. It consists of gently lifting the skin from the underlying muscle, stretching it slightly while moving the fingers along it, then dropping the fold. This is best done rapidly by lifting up sections of skin one after another for a few seconds each. Although petrissage helps tone up the skin and increase dermal blood circulation, it will not reduce edema or swelling in deep muscle masses.

Hydrotherapy

Hydrotherapy is the application of water, often under pressure, for exercise and therapy. Because of its hydrothermal and hydrokinetic effects (i.e., water temperature and movement), hydrotherapy is often beneficial in the treatment of leg injuries.

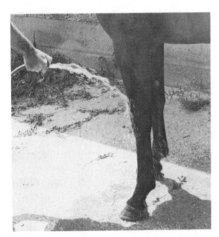

Fig. 4-37 Spraying cold water on an acute injury is a convenient method of applying hydrotherapy.

WATER MASSAGE AND WOUND HEALING

The simplest way to achieve the benefits of hydrotherapy is to hose the horse's legs with water. The jet of water will massage and cool swollen and sore legs and muscle masses, and the pulsating flow will wash debris out of any wounds present and have some toning effect as well. Water also stimulates the healing process by encouraging the growth of granulation tissue to fill in large, gaping wounds. For this reason, however, water should not be used excessively on wounds in which granulation tissue has already reached skin level, or proud flesh may result.

PRINCIPLES AND APPLICATIONS OF HEAT AND COLD

COLD

Applications of cold exert definite therapeutic effects in treating and reducing the acute inflammation and associated pain that occur early in the course of many conditions. Cold therapy may be used successfully in treating injuries affecting muscles, tendons, ligaments, joints, and in treating some wounds, though it should not be used on open wounds. The success of cold applications in treating any injury is dependent on the elapsed time between the injury's occurrence and the subsequent treatment; only during the initial 12 to 24 hour period (and preferably during the first few hours) is cold therapy actually beneficial.

Cold causes vasoconstriction (constriction of blood vessels) which limits edema and tissue swelling; excessive cold, however, can cause reflex vasodilation (expansion of blood vessels) and further swelling. Therefore, cold applications should be limited to periods of 20 to 40 minutes, separated by at least 30 minutes to one hour.

Applying Cold

Commercial ice boots are perhaps the ideal means of applying cold to a horse's leg. When in place on the leg, an ice boot resembles a canvas bag surrounding the lower portion of the limb. In lieu of commercial products, it is possible to fashion a facsimile of an ice boot by cutting across an innertube to make a long sleeve, binding the sleeve at the bottom, and filling it with ice. To keep this sleeve on the leg, a neckstrap can likewise be cut from the innertube.

To limit swelling from acute, noninfectious inflammation and to shorten the recovery time from such an injury, cold may be applied to a leg as an ice pack or cold water bandage, or a horse can stand in a tub of ice. Cold packs may also be used on a seeping wound to assist in reducing bleeding. A water hose can be used to spray cold water on a swollen leg, and, for certain conditions such as laminitis, a horse can stand in a tub of cold water. If not in a stable area, standing the horse in a cold stream or pond will give beneficial results.

HEAT

Heat, in contrast to cold, should not be applied until one or two days after an injury occurs, after the original inflammation and swelling have subsided. Heat causes vasodilation (i.e., expansion of blood vessels) and increases circulation to an area. Heat also increases the metabolism and oxygen supply, raises the local temperature, and increases blood vessel permeability. Application of heat is beneficial when used to bring abscesses to a "head" or to treat muscle soreness.

Applying Heat

Heat may be radiant, conductive, or conversive in nature. Radiant heat originates from a radiating heat source such as an infrared light; conductive heat is supplied by a heat source, such as a hot water bandage, that contacts the body and transfers heat to it; and conversive heat results from tissue resistance to diathermy or ultrasound (refer to "Deep Heat Therapy"). Hot water can be used in turbulator boots or a whirlpool bath for hydrotherapy.

SWIMMING

Swimming is an excellent form of hydrotherapy. For example, lameness that is associated with weight bearing (i.e., sole bruises and laminitis) can be aided by allowing swimming exercise during convalescence. Conditions such as myositis and muscle atrophy also respond more quickly to swimming than to some other forms of therapy.

Although the ocean is suitable for swimming horses, as is common in coastal regions, some modern facilities offer pools especially designed for horses. However, before deciding to swim a horse in one of these pools, the pool should be checked to see that it is at least 8 feet deep, and that it is spacious enough for maneuvering, especially near the entrance to the water. Large pools are best for swimming horses, and any pool used should be at least 25 feet in diameter. The horse is usually led down a ramp into the pool wearing either a halter or a bowline over the neck and attached to a leading pole. A tail rope, and sometimes two lead ropes, should be used on inexperienced swimmers.

a.
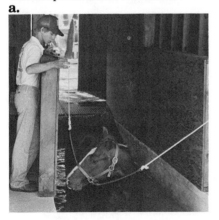

b.
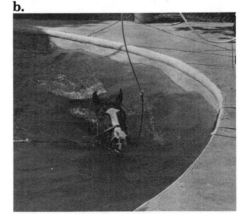

Fig. 4-38 Swimming. a. The horse is slowly lead down an incline into the pool. b. The horse is lead around the pool.

In beginning hydrotherapy, it is best to choose a moderate swimming program that at first allows one to four minutes per day and gradually increase the time to a maximum of 15 minutes daily. The chlorine level of the chosen pool should be checked before swimming commences, as improper concentrations may cause dermatitis or conjunctivitis.

Of course, a horse may be exercised in a lake, either in the area of a floating dock or behind a boat. In some cases, an innertube placed around the neck or a styrofoam float around the girth may be required for added buoyancy. Ideally, the water temperature should be about 70°F (21.1°C).

WHIRLPOOL BATHS

The whirlpool bath offers another type of hydrotherapy. In a whirlpool stall, the horse stands chest-deep in water that is agitated and treated with chemicals to help relieve soreness and aches. There are also portable whirlpool units that consist of a set of turbulator boots which fit over the legs and provide a jet-propelled water massage to the limbs.

Insect Stings and Bites

Most bites from flies, gnats, and other common insects cause only minor itching and skin irritation. With minor problems, removal of the cause of irritation will generally allow the lesions to heal and disappear within a few days or weeks. Overall, prevention of stings and bites by protection from offending insects with insecticides is probably the best form of treatment.

Allergy to certain insects may cause a permanent skin change in some horses, as in hypersensitivity to the bite of sandflies. These insects are also the intermediate hosts for a nematode, **Onchocerca cervicalis**; the microfilaria of this parasite cause skin problems such as depigmentation, ventral midline dermatitis, a strong itching sensation, and scaling of the skin at the withers, chest, and neck. Additionally, infected house and stable flies carry Habronema larvae that contaminate wounds, sheaths, and eye areas, causing habronemiasis or "summer sores."

Insects are also vectors for certain viral diseases; e.g., tabanid flies are the vector for equine infectious anemia, and mosquitoes are vectors for EEE and WEE. In addition, the mechanical trauma caused to the skin by biting insects may make the horse more susceptible to a fungal or bacterial infection.

TREATMENT

Severe insect bites and stings often cause reactions with signs similar to snakebite and should be actively treated. The injured areas should be rinsed with a weak ammonia solution or treated with a poultice of sodium bicarbonate, then a cold or ice pack applied to limit or reduce swelling. Application time should be limited to 2 or 3 hours, and the pack should be removed for a few minutes every 20 minutes.

If severe dyspnea results (perhaps from a sting on the nose), a veterinarian should be contacted to administer epinephrine and/or antihistamines, or to perhaps perform a tracheostomy to alleviate the breathing difficulty. Antihistamines are very effective if given within a short time of the onset of the allergic reaction. Corticosteroids are also given, if necessary, for their anti-inflammatory action and to combat shock. If epinephrine is not quickly given to a horse suffering an anaphylactic reaction to multiple bites/stings, death could rapidly ensue. Fortunately, swarming attacks of insects and acute reactions to individual bites and stings are not common occurrences.

To help reduce swellings associated with minor bites and stings, an oral antihistamine, such as Antiphrine granules, can be given in the feed.

Snakebite

The severity of any poisonous snakebite depends on the amount of venom the snake injects, the size of the injured horse, his general condition, the location of the bite, and the time lapse before treatment is begun. The injection of an antivenom, if given early enough, can be an important life-saving measure in cases of bites from poisonous snakes. This is especially true if the bite is on the head or neck.

Since the venom circulates through and is absorbed more quickly by the system of an active warm body, all physical activity should be kept to a minimum. The animal should be kept as quiet and still as possible until the veterinarian arrives. If the horse is exposed on a hot day, it should be slowly walked to a nearby cooler area (tree-shade, barn) if possible.

TREATMENT

Treatment of poisonous snakebites is a somewhat controversial subject in medicine, and several different types of procedures have been both advocated and discounted. Even the use of a tourniquet is sometimes questioned since, if used in an unskilled manner, it can compound the problem by producing pressure necrosis. The use of incisions in or near the bite punctures in conjunction with suction of the area has been particularly challenged by many medical authorities and this procedure is now infrequently used.

The use of antivenom is the best primary treatment currently recognized and it should be implemented as quickly as possible by both local and systemic administration. In any case, the veterinarian should be immediately contacted since the management of venomous snake bites should always be considered a veterinary-only procedure.

Depending upon the location of the bite, severity of tissue reaction, and approxmiated time lapse since its occurrence, several different procedures may be used by the veterinarian, as outlined below.

If the bite is discovered immediately after occurrence (within 15 minutes), the veterinarian may decide to make shallow one-quarter inch incisions in the wound parallel to the blood supply and attempt to remove venom with a suction cup. It is no longer recommended that poison be orally sucked from a wound by an individual, as it could be absorbed into the system. Some veterinarians recommend making a longitudinal incision (vertical with the affected limb) to open the wound.

If the bite is on a limb, a tourniquet may be applied about 2 inches above the bite to retard lymph circulation. It should remain in place for no longer than 2 to 3 hours total and may be released every 20 minutes for a few minutes. However, the continued periodic release of the tourniquet has been challenged as producing a "pumping-like" action that may increase venom dissemination. All of the factors will be considered by the veterinarian in the management of each particular bite wound.

Ice or cold water packs can be placed on the wound to reduce circulation, but they should not remain in place for more than a maximum of 2 to 3 hours total time, with the ice removed every 15 to 20 minutes for a few minutes, because cold may increase the extent of tissue necrosis that occurs at the site of most bites.

When the bite is on the head, particularly on the animal's nose, and there is rapid local tissue swelling, the greatest immediate problem will be difficulty in breathing. In an emergency, breathing can be facilitated by inserting a 4 inch piece of garden hose into each nostril. This will hold the nostrils open and allow the horse to breathe more easily. A burlap feed bag soaked in water and placed over the animal's head can also be used as a cold pack to reduce swelling. However, if the horse's breathing remains labored, a tracheostomy may have to be performed by the veterinarian. This operation introduces a tube into the trachea, through which the horse will be able to breathe more easily.

If the local tissue reaction to a snakebite is severe (as is usually the case), anti-inflammatory hormones such as cortisone or ACTH may be beneficial. These drugs will help reduce swelling and may decrease the tissue necrosis and sloughing that usually follow a bite. Antibiotics should be administered and continued for several days to a week or more, depending on the severity of the bite or abscess development at the site. A snakebite is, of course, a contaminated puncture wound and, if not treated as such, abscess formation due to infection, tissue necrosis due to cytotoxins, and sloughing of skin and muscle in the area are likely to occur.

As a precautionary measure, tetanus toxoid or tetanus antitoxin should be given according to the program that the horse is on, since a snakebite is an exceptionally contaminated puncture wound. Should dehydration and shock occur, the horse will also need fluids (administered intravenously or via stomach tube by the veterinarian) to combat shock as well as to furnish nutrients. ♞

5

EQUINE OBSTETRICS AND PEDIATRICS

Care of the Mare During Gestation

Proper prenatal care of the mare is very necessary to ensure the birth of a normal, healthy foal. In this section, some of the special nutrition, exercise, and management requirements for pregnant mares are discussed.

NUTRITION

Nutritional requirements for pregnant and non-pregnant mares are approximately the same until the last three to four months of pregnancy. For the most part, good pasture with an adequate mineral supply and other supplementation as needed are satisfactory until the last third of pregnancy, when the mare's energy and protein requirements increase. It is a mistake to allow a mare to gain too much weight, as excess fat may make foaling much more difficult and cause the foal to be small and weak. (For complete information on nutrient requirements of pregnant mares, refer to the text FEEDING TO WIN.)

EXERCISE

Especially when pregnant, a mare needs exercise to keep muscles properly toned. During pregnancy, a mare can be allowed to graze in a large pasture with a simple covered shed for shelter. Most mares will be more content at this time if pastured with other pregnant mares and separated from young horses and geldings that often are too physical in their actions. It is also safe (besides being good exercise) to ride a pregnant mare moderately for one hour a day until about one week before the expected foaling date. Well-conditioned mares may be ridden longer and even shown if necessary early in the pregnancy.

HEALTH CARE

Internal parasites should be controlled during pregnancy, just as during other times in life. There are several anthelmintics that are safe to use on pregnant mares. The last deworming should be scheduled from 30 to 60 days prior to foaling so that the foal can be born into a relatively parasite-free environment. Because of the potential for producing developmental anomalies in the early gestation period, anthelmintics probably should not be administered during the first few months after breeding.

The administration of a tetanus toxoid booster to the mare about one month before the foaling date will raise the level of tetanus antibodies in her colostrum and make a tetanus antitoxin injection at birth unnecessary for the foal. The mare's basic booster vaccination program should be begun between foaling and the next breeding.

Drugs such as trichlorfon, or corticosteroids and most other hormonal substances, should not be administered during pregnancy because they may cause abortion. Anestrus mares are often given prostaglandins, but these substances may cause abortion in mares already in foal, and a careful check for pregnancy should precede their administration. Teratogenic drugs (e.g., corticosteroids, certain hormones), which result in abnormalities of fetal development are most harmful during the first trimester of gestation.

If a mare has received a Caslick's operation (suturing of the vulva), an episiotomy will have to be performed by the veterinarian one to two weeks before the expected foaling date. Otherwise, the vulva may be severely lacerated during parturition.

ABORTION

The expulsion of the fetus before 300 days of gestation, at which time the fetus cannot survive because of immaturity, is termed an abortion. A variety of causes such as infection, conception of twins, fetal abnormalities, and nutritional deficiencies can precipitate an abortion. Death of the fetus may result in its rejection from the uterus, or the fetus may be forced out (while still alive) by hormonal imbalances or detachment of the placenta.

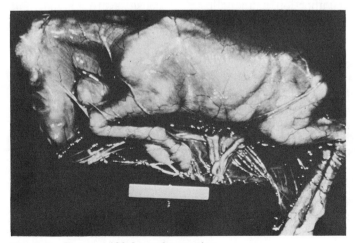

Fig. 5-1   Fetus at 180 days of gestation.

If a mare aborts before the 37th day of pregnancy, she will soon cycle again and can be rebred. However, if a mare aborts between the 37th and 120th days (approximately), the presence of a persistent corpus luteum will prevent her from showing signs of estrus. Because of this, several months are lost before the mare is discovered to not be in foal. If the mare is found to be open during this interval, and is not showing signs of heat, hormone therapy will cause the corpus luteum to regress so that she will come back into heat and can be rebred.

VIRAL CAUSES

Viral infection is a leading cause of abortion, and viral arteritis and viral rhinopneumonitis are the two major abortion-causing viruses. Once these viruses have been contracted, there is no satisfactory treatment other than allowing the horse adequate rest and providing antibiotics (when necessary) to prevent secondary bacterial infection. Vaccines against arteritis and rhinopneumonitis are available and can be used in breeding herds where viral abortion is a problem. Rhinopneumonitis is also known as equine herpes virus I and was once introduced into breeding herds in controlled situations to provide immunity. This practice, now illegal in some states and foreign countries, has been outdated by the development of a modified live virus vaccine that is much safer.

BACTERIAL CAUSES

Bacterial abortions are most commonly caused by 1. **Salmonella abortus equi,** 2. **Streptococcus genitalium,** 3. **Escherichia coli,** and 4. **Staphylococci.** Mares that abort from salmonellosis usually shed the bacteria quickly and can be successfully rebred if not suffering from metritis or cervicitis. A cervical culture should be done to ensure that the mare is free from infection (refer to "Cervical and Uterine Cultures"). Besides precipitating abortion, salmonellosis can cause severe diarrhea and anemia which are often difficult to treat. Breeding animals should therefore receive a killed bacterin to help prevent the spread of this infection. This bacterin is given annually, in three doses in the autumn. It takes time, however, for the immunity to develop and, in the event of an outbreak, vaccinated mares may still abort if they have not developed sufficient immunity.

Streptococcus genitalium can cause abortion before the fourth or fifth month of pregnancy. An infected mare often has difficulty in settling, aborts again, or delivers a weak foal. Antibiotic therapy in the form of a uterine infusion is used in the treatment of this disease.

FUNGAL CAUSES

Abortions between the seventh and tenth months of gestation may be caused by a mycotic (fungal) infection. There is little to be done after such an abortion, except to culture the mare before rebreeding to determine whether she is still infected.

NUTRITIONAL CAUSES

Nutritional deficiencies rarely cause an abortion since it is unlikely that the mare's level of nutrition will fall so low that she will abort. However, an improperly nourished mare will rapidly lose condition during pregnancy due to the nutritional demands of the fetus. In addition, deficiencies of vitamins A and D, calcium, and phosphorus (and other necessary nutrients) can cause defects in the newborn foal. Therefore, proper nutrition, particularly during the last third of gestation, is very important.

HORMONAL CAUSES

Mares that are free from infection and well-fed, and yet still consistently abort from one and one-half to eight months of pregnancy, may not produce enough progesterone to maintain the fetus. In an attempt to remedy the cause of this type of abortion, the veterinarian may administer progesterone.

TWINNING

The conception of twins is another condition that can result in abortion. This occurs because one of the twins usually dies of an insufficient blood supply and the mare expels both fetuses. Since it is unlikely that a mare will carry a twin pregnancy to full term, the veterinarian may induce abortion so that the mare may be rebred as soon as possible. If an abortion is performed, the veterinarian may also administer a uterine infusion of saline solution and antibiotics to help prevent infection. The mare will probably require six to eight months before she will become pregnant again.

Causes of Abortion

Non-Infective causes:
1. twinning
2. hormonal dysfunction
3. nutritional failure
4. twisted umbilical cord
5. trauma (kicks, etc.)
6. hereditary
    sex-linked factors
    lethal genes
7. iatrogenic
    (caused by medications)
8. pregnancy in the uterine body
9. abnormal fetus

Infective causes:
1. Bacterial
    Salmonella abortus equi
    Streptococcus genitalium
    Escherichia coli
    Staphylococci
2. Viral rhinopneumonitis
3. Mycotic (fungal)
    Aspergillus
    Mucor

DRUG-INDUCED ABORTION

An abortion can be accidentally induced by the improper administration of cathartics and steroids, anthelmintics, and other drugs. Examples of substances that may cause abortion are some organophosphate dewormers. Drugs should not be administered to pregnant mares without the veterinarian's knowledge and approval, and label recommendations and contraindications should always be heeded.

Mare and Foal Care at Parturition

PRENATAL CARE

A considerable amount of time and money is required to produce a quality foal. Thus, in addition to humane reasons, it is vital that the mare and her foal be provided with proper care at parturition in order to protect the financial investment.

Beginning about one month before her due date, the mare should be watched closely for signs of impending parturition, and an appropriate foaling area should be selected soon afterward. A clean, uncrowded pasture with no standing water or rough underbrush is suitable (except in wet or cold weather), as is a clean, dry stall (ideally, at least 12 feet by 16 feet). The stall should be thoroughly disinfected and its floor covered with a deep layer of clean bedding (ideally, straw should be used) to reduce the risks of navel ill, joint ill, etc.

SIGNS OF IMPENDING PARTURITION

Approximately two to four weeks before foaling, the mammary glands will begin to increase in size and the mare's udder will feel cool and flacid. A week to ten days prior to foaling, a depression will appear on either side of the tailhead, as the sacrosciatic ligaments relax. The mare will tend to carry her tail a little higher than usual when she walks, the vulva will double or triple in size, and the muscles in the hindquarters will relax.

Other signs of approaching parturition resemble an attack of colic. The mare may appear restless and go off by herself, gently kick at her abdomen and turn her head to look at her flanks, have frequent, small bowel movements, sweat, and grab mouthfuls of grass only to drop them again. This stage usually lasts from one to four hours.

As parturition approaches, the mare's udder will be warm and tight in the evenings. This condition is known as "making bag" and is caused by the mammary glands filling with colostrum, some of which will form golden drops at the ends of the teats. This "waxing" usually occurs 12 to 36 hours before foaling, though some mares drip milk for several days before foaling.

PREPARATION FOR FOALING

A few necessary items should be assembled in preparation for foaling.

These items include hot water, disinfectant, mild soap (Ivory soap is satisfactory), clean buckets, tail bandages (three-inch gauze), enema syringe with soft rubber hose, clean turkish towelling, iodine, and a small glass or other container. The mare's udder, vulva, and surrounding area should be gently washed with soap and water, and her tail wrapped and tied (refer to "Bandaging").

BIRTH OF THE FOAL

This stage involves the dilation of the cervix and contraction of the uterine muscles. As this occurs, the chorioallantoic sac (water bag) is pushed through the opening and ruptures, releasing two to five gallons of the fluid in which the foal has been suspended. This should proceed rapidly, lasting no longer than 10 to 30 minutes before the foal's appearance. As the mare's abdominal muscles contract, the next stage commences, and the foal begins to be expelled. Since the foal cannot remain alive in the birth canal for more than half an hour, the veterinarian should be contacted if the foal's appearance is delayed. To reduce labor contractions while waiting for the veterinarian, the mare should be walked about. Pinching or pressing down on the withers is also sometimes effective in minimizing the contractions by distracting the mare.

If the birth proceeds normally, the foal's forefeet should appear first, heels down, with one foot perhaps slightly in front of the other and the head between them. The mare will experience the greatest difficulty in passing the foal's shoulders, since that is the widest part of its body. If the mare appears to be straining but not progressing in expelling the foal, aid can be rendered in the following manner:

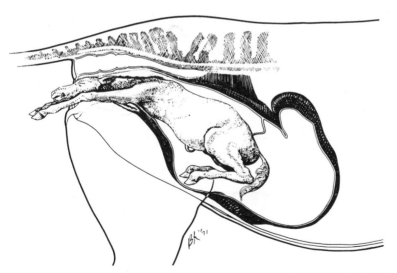

Fig. 5-2   In a normal birth, the foal is presented with the forelimbs, head, and neck fully extended.

When the mare is lying down, as is usually the case, firmly grasp the foal's forelegs and apply pressure, pulling out when the mare pushes. Keep the foal close to the ground.

Once the foal's hips are past the pelvis, direct all force down and out along the foal's natural body lines, keeping the foal close to the ground.

For standing mares, firmly grasp the foal's forelegs and pull up and out when the mare pushes.

As the foal's hips pass the pelvis, all force should again be directed out and down along the body lines; pull in an arc towards the mare's hocks.

Although a mare will ordinarily lie down, nervous or young mares sometimes deliver their foals while standing. When standing, a mare must be watched to ensure that she does not bang her foal against a wall. One should be prepared, also, to catch the foal as it is born, and ease its fall to the ground.

DYSTOCIA

Dystocia is the abnormal presentation and difficult delivery of the foal at birth, often due to uterine torsion. When dystocia is evident, the horseman should not attempt to reposition the foal except in cases of emergency since critical damage to both mare and foal can easily occur in this situation.

Instead, veterinary assistance should be obtained immediately if dystocia is suspected. Examples of abnormal positions are:

1. one or both forelegs back
2. rear presentation, hindlegs coming first
3. breech birth
4. upside down

When the foal is being presented upside down, the frogs of the forefeet will first be visible. To rotate the foal, the mare should be encouraged to stand, walk a few steps, and lie down again. This procedure may have to be repeated more than once, but it is usually successful. If the foal's forelegs are already out, the veterinarian can sometimes rotate the foal by twisting the forelegs.

In a situation where only one foreleg appears, the veterinarian assists by lubricating his hands with warm water and glycerine, inserting a hand into the vagina to find the foot, and bringing it gently through the vaginal opening. A foot caught back and pressing upwards can tear the partition between the rectum and vagina and cause a rectovaginal fistula. This injury is correctable only by major surgery and should be prevented by moving the foot in the manner just described. The same technique is also used if both front legs are bent back, that is, one leg is brought forward at a time.

If the bottoms of the hoofs appear, it is possible to determine whether they are front or hind feet by running a hand up the leg to the next joint. Obviously, the presence of a knee (the 2nd joint bends in the same direction as the fetlock) indicates a foreleg, and a hock (the 2nd joint bends in the opposite direction from the fetlock) indicates a hindleg. In a case where a foal is presented hindfeet first, or backwards, birth must proceed rapidly to ensure the safe delivery of the foal. Otherwise, the umbilical cord will be strangulated and the foal's oxygenated blood supply cut off. (The resulting carbon dioxide buildup in the foal's brain would stimulate the foal to begin breathing, which it would be unable to do while still inside the mare). At this point, the only way to save the foal is to forcefully pull with the mare's contractions; in fact, this is one situation in which it is advisable to pull even if the mare is not straining.

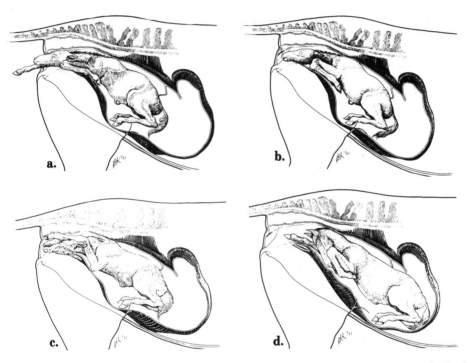

Fig. 5-3 Examples of abnormal birth presentations. a. One foreleg back. b. Both forelegs back. c. Both forelegs crossed over the foal's head. d. Head and one foreleg unextended.

When the foal's front feet appear alone, the veterinarian may insert a hand into the vagina to check the position of the foal's head. Then, the foal's chest can be controlled with one hand while the head is brought around to the birth canal with the other hand. The veterinarian may grip the foal's head by placing a thumb and forefinger in the orbits and nostrils.

It is possible for the forelegs, hindlegs, and head to be presented simultaneously, with the foal in either a frontward or backward position. In either situation, the foal's body will act as a stopper and obstruct its further passage along the birth canal. To correct this position, it will be necessary for the veterinarian to push the foal's body, head, and trailing pair of legs back in the mare to create a normal, elongated posture. The mare should be kept from straining as much as possible.

When the foal's mane can be felt but not the head, the head is probably between the front legs. As with other types of dystocia, the veterinarian should be called immediately, as a Caesarean section may be necessary. While awaiting his arrival, the mare's contractions may be reduced by walking her about.

One of the most serious abnormal presentations of a foal is breech birth. This is the term applied to a foal positioned in the uterus in an upright posture with tail towards the vagina and legs flexed. In this instance, the hindlegs must be individually brought back by the veterinarian and stretched out to permit the foal to be delivered. The foal must be held back in the uterus as much as possible while his legs are being moved to prevent them from being jammed against the pelvis when the mare contracts. The umbilical cord will be obstructed and the foal will drown in fetal fluids if rapid delivery is not accomplished.

It is important to stress that excessive force may permanently damage a mare, and should not be used to correct any abnormal foaling position. No more force than a man can normally pull (unaided) should be used.

a.   **b.**

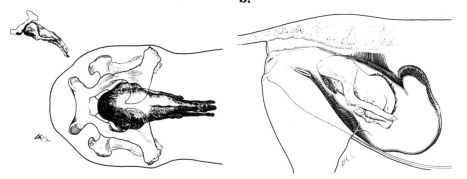

Fig. 5-4 Breech birth presentation. a. Top and side views. b. With head and knees flexed.

When Does Foaling Require a Veterinarian's Assistance?

Any of the following conditions indicate the need for veterinary assistance in order to preserve the life and health of the mare or foal.

1. when hard labor is non-productive and exceeds 20 minutes
2. during dystocia or abnormal foal presentation
3. when the foal and/or mare fail to rise within 45 minutes to 1 hour after birth
4. when the foal fails to nurse within first 2 hours of life
5. when the mare refuses or threatens the foal
6. when blood flows from the mare's vulva or the navel stump of the foal
7. when the placenta is retained for more than 2 to 3 hours

8. when the placenta is not passed intact
9. when the mare or foal is weak or depressed
10. when the foal does not have a bowel movement within six hours or is seen straining and arching the back

VETERINARY ASSISTANCE AT BIRTHS

Depending upon the type and duration of dystocia, the veterinarian may elect to perform mutation, forced extraction, Caesarean section, or embryotomy. If the foal is alive, one of the first three methods is used.

Mutation is the procedure of changing the foal's position in the uterus. Version, rotation, repulsion, and extension are all maneuvers that the veterinarian may use during this process. In performing mutation, the veterinarian will first give a local anesthetic block (epidural) to control the mare's contractions. Then, one-half to one gallon of heavy mineral oil may be infused into the uterus to take the place of fetal fluids. This oil lubricates the foal and the birth canal and relaxes the uterus. Repulsion refers to the act of pushing the foal back into the uterus; a necessary maneuver before any attempt can be made to straighten the foal's limb. Version defines the change in direction of the foal in reference to the mare, accomplished by repelling one end of the foal's body while pulling on the other end.

Forced extraction refers to the application of pressure to assist delivery. Traction is usually easier to apply when the mare is standing or when her hindquarters are elevated. The veterinarian may use his hands, obstetrical chains, or a fetal extractor. Forced extraction requires skill, for excessive traction can result in paralysis or death of the foal, rupture and bruising of the mare's pelvis and birth canal, and extensive injury of the mare's urinary bladder and urethra.

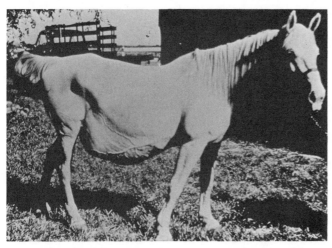

Fig. 5-5 Pregnant mare with a ruptured prepubic tendon, a condition that necessitates a Caesarean section.

In an embryotomy, the veterinarian dissects the foal to reduce its size and facilitate removal from the mare. Obviously, an embryotomy is only performed when the foal is already dead or so incorrectly situated in the mare that it must be sacrificed to save her life. This procedure may also be necessary if the foal is a fetal monster with severe developmental anomalies.

Caesarean sections are ideally performed in the early stages of labor, and in a veterinary hospital where the mare can be closely observed. The operation must be performed in aseptic surroundings, and it is important that the veterinarian is called before the mare has had a great deal of trouble. During this procedure, the mare is first tranquilized and anesthetized before a ventral midline incision is made. This incision allows more room for the delivery of the foal than one through the flank, but it cannot be performed on a mare with abdominal edema. The veterinarian will carefully incise the uterus over the location of the hindlegs to avoid accidentally cutting the foal. The foal's legs are then grasped with dry towels and the foal removed from the uterus. The umbilical cord is left intact for several minutes to permit all of the placental blood to reach the foal. Finally, the cord is broken, and the foal treated while the mare is sutured.

Under some circumstances, the veterinarian may decide that labor should be induced in the mare, although this is not often recommended. This may be required in cases of uterine atony (lack of tone and forceful contractions) and has the advantages of facilitated placenta expulsion and prevention of dystocia. However, labor should not be induced in a mare already suffering from dystocia. The ecbolic drugs commonly given to mares to induce labor are oxytocin, pituitary extract, and pituitrin. An injection is usually administered after the cervix has dilated and the foal is then normally born within 30 minutes. The mare can be successfully bred back if all other aspects of delivery are normal.

POSTNATAL CARE

After delivery, the mare and foal should be allowed to rest quietly for 10 to 15 minutes. If necessary, the membranes should be removed from the foal's nostrils to facilitate breathing. Raising the foal's head or gently shaking it will help drain excess fluid quickly, and wiping fluids from the mouth and nostrils will also ease congestion.

It is vital that the umbilical cord not be prematurely cut, broken or tied. Approximately 25 to 35% of the foal's blood supply circulates through the placenta, and premature breakage of the cord will result in a loss of one to two pints of blood. The cord will usually break at a natural constriction, after which it should be sealed by soaking in a small container of iodine. This will prevent disease and infection-carrying organisms from entering the stump. It should be noted that the blood vessels in the cord are more elastic than its outer covering, and will retract farther into the body, carrying bacteria and germs with them if sanitation is inadequate. Lack of sanitary measures at this time is the primary cause of joint and navel ill.

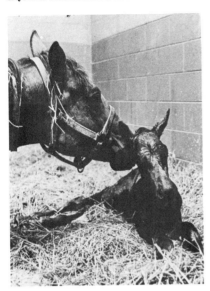

Fig. 5-6   Mare with her newborn foal.

The mare should be allowed to lick the foal unless the weather is cold or the mare is especially tired, in which circumstance the foal should be dried with a Turkish towel. The foal should be permitted to stand by itself and not be helped up. Nursing may begin from 15 minutes to 2 hours after birth, but if the foal has difficulty finding the udder, it should be guided in the right direction. Occasionally, a mare, usually a maiden mare, will refuse to let her foal nurse. But, although a twitch or sedatives are sometimes necessary, she will usually relax when she finds that nursing alleviates the pain of her swollen udder. Sedatives or other CNS depressants should be used carefully since the mare may inadvertently injure the foal if her "survival instinct" is dulled by tranquilization! If the foal is too weak to stand and nurse, some of the colostrum may be milked from the mare and given to the foal in a sterile nipple-topped bottle.

It is important that the foal receive colostrum soon after birth, for it contains antibodies that can only be absorbed during the first 24 hours of life. Ideally the colostrum should be provided within 6 hours of birth, as the foal's ability to absorb antibodies begins decreasing as early as 6 hours. Without these antibodies, the foal would be extremely susceptible to disease. When milk has been dripping from the mare's teats for several days prior to foaling, she has probably already lost her colostrum, and more will have to be obtained. Large breeding farms and veterinarians often keep a supply of extra colostrum frozen for just such emergencies.

Before using the colostrum from another mare, however, it must be checked against the blood type of the foal to prevent neonatal isoerythrolysis. When a mare is suspected of having antibodies against the blood type of her foal, the foal must be muzzled for 36 hours until he can no longer absorb the antibodies and the mare is no longer producing colostrum. This will require, if possible, the feeding of at least a pint of frozen colostrum.

The veterinarian may administer the colostrum through a stomach tube.

Any foal that does not receive colostrum will need extra protection against infection, which can be provided in the form of a five-day series of vitamin and antibiotic shots. The foal's mucous membranes of the eye and mouth should be checked daily during the first week of life for signs of jaundice. Often, an injection of penicillin-streptomycin is considered a routine veterinary practice for newborn foals.

If the mare was not given a tetanus toxoid injection one month prior to foaling, or if the foal did not receive colostrum, the foal should be given a tetanus antitoxin injection. The mare should also receive a tetanus antitoxin injection, unless on a regular immunization program, because vaginal lacerations, no matter how small, can become infected.

EXPULSION OF THE PLACENTA

The final stage of labor involves expulsion of the afterbirth. The placenta may be passed with one strong contraction immediately after the foal's birth, but it is not unusual for expulsion to require 30 to 40 minutes. When the mare stands, the membranes should be tied up in a knot with a piece of sterile gauze so they are not stepped on. A maiden mare may also shy at the afterbirth swinging at her heels and kick at it, perhaps injuring the foal. Tying up the membranes prevents this and allows their weight to naturally clean out the uterus. The afterbirth should not be pulled, as part of it may tear off and remain in the uterus, or the uterus may itself be accidentally torn. Once the placenta has been delivered, it should be spread out and checked for correct shape (it should resemble a pair of trousers with closed ends). A mare that has not passed the afterbirth within three to four hours is considered to have a retained placenta, and laminitis, colic, or septicemia may develop unless the mare is treated.

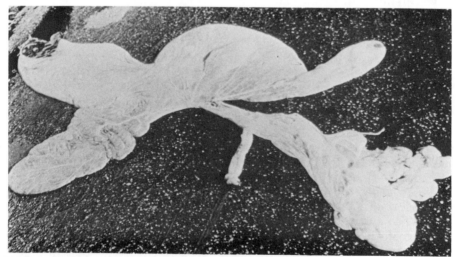

Fig. 5-7   The placenta is spread out to be checked for completeness.

Retained Placenta

A retained placenta requires veterinary treatment. The veterinarian will often check to see if there is a large amount of the afterbirth lodged in the vagina, and if necessary, may gently pull this part out. This will help to naturally cleanse the mare by asserting pressure on the portion retained in the uterus. Many veterinarians also give drugs that cause contractions of the uterus (i.e., oxytocic or ecbolic drugs) such as oxytocin or ergotamine, and antibiotics such as penicillin-streptomycin or tetracycline, as well as antihistamines. The veterinarian may use gentle traction to encourage the membrane's expulsion, but stronger force is not used because of the danger of tearing and uterine prolapse.

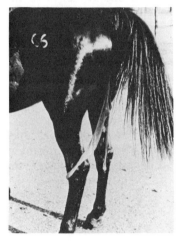

Fig. 5-8   Mare with retained placenta.

PROLAPSED UTERUS

A prolapse is an extremely serious condition that occurs when the uterus protrudes from the vulva. It may result in death from loss of blood within a few minutes. To correct prolapse, the veterinarian must sedate the mare, replace the uterus, and suture the vulva tightly. The mare will require broad-spectrum antibiotics and perhaps steroids, antihistamines, and fluids during her recovery.

POSTPARTUM COLIC

Contractions of the empty uterus may cause the mare to exhibit signs of colic from 15 minutes to several hours following parturition. The mare may act much as she did before foaling, looking at her flanks, kicking her belly, etc. Because extreme pain of this nature could cause the mare to unintentionally injure her foal, she should be closely watched at this time and kept on her feet until the pain passes. A sedative, carefully controlled, may alleviate some of her distress.

To prevent impaction of the mare's colon, the veterinarian may give one gallon of light mineral oil through a stomach tube on the morning after foaling. If the mare's feces remain dry or scarce, another gallon of mineral oil may be given two or three days later. Reducing the mare's grain intake for the first couple of days subsequent to foaling is suggested, as is deworming a heavily parasitized mare after about 5 days.

RESUTURING THE MARE

If an episiotomy has been performed, the veterinarian will perform a Caslick's operation and resuture the mare if necessary. When there is a large amount of bruised tissue at the edges of the vulva, as there often is on maiden mares foaling for the first time, the veterinarian will have to wait several days for healing to occur before suturing the area. If the mare suffered a rectovaginal fistula during foaling, several operations (over an extended period of time) will be necessary to restore her to breeding soundness.

UTERINE ARTERY RUPTURE

Rupture of the middle uterine artery is a rare complication seen most often in older foaling mares. The primary sign of this condition is the mare going into shock shortly after foaling. Since the mare may suddenly collapse and die, the foal should be removed from her side. Treatment involves keeping the mare standing, the administration of sedatives and clotting agents, and therapy for shock. Associated internal bleeding may correct itself because of the formation of internal hematomas; in this case, the mare may survive.

Caring for an Orphan Foal

If a source of colostrum is available, the orphaned foal should receive the colostrum within a maximum of 24 hours of birth (within six hours is preferable). A schedule of preventive antibiotic treatment should be quickly prepared if the orphaned foal does not receive the colostrum, else the foal will be deficient in passive antibodies and therefore less resistant to early infection.

There are several ways to raise a foal that has been orphaned by its mother's death or abandonment. Ideally, another mare may be provided to nurse the foal. Or, if this is not possible, a nanny goat may serve as a substitute, or a formula/milk replacer may be bottle-fed to the foal. A formula or milk substitute is required during the period of transition, even when a nurse animal is to be used.

FORMULA FEEDING

Unmodified cow's milk is higher in fat content and much lower in protein and sugar content than is mare's milk, and is, therefore, an unsuitable substitute. Moreover, feeding cow's milk can cause a foal to develop diarrhea, enteritis, and dehydration. Commercial milk replacers such as Foal Lac (Borden) can be used satisfactorily for formula feeding, or one of the following formulas based on cow's milk, lime water, and sugar may be given.

Formula A: 1 pint low-fat (1-2%) cow's milk
4 ounces lime water
1 teaspoon sugar

Formula B: 1 can evaporated cow's milk
1 can water
4 tablespoons lime water
1 tablespoon sugar or corn syrup

Formula C: 1 pint low-fat cow's milk
2 ½ ounces water
2 ½ ounces lime water
2 teaspoons sugar

Formula D: 20 ounces cow's milk
12 ounces lime water
2 ounces sugar

The lime water contained in these formulas is a solution of unslaked lime (calcium hydroxide) in water at the rate of 1 part lime to 700 parts water. When being prepared, this mixture should be allowed to stand for 12 hours, then the clear upper fluid, or lime water, poured off. Bottled lime water should be available at large drugstores.

All utensils and pans used in preparation of formulas must be sterile, for orphan foals are very susceptible to infection and scours. The amount of formula prepared should not exceed the amount required for a single feeding (about 1 pint per feeding during the first week) because of the possibility of bacterial growth. The milk should be heated to about 85-95°F (30-35°C) before feeding.

FEEDING PROCEDURE

When colostrum is available soon after birth, the veterinarian may administer it through a stomach tube if the foal is weak. For normal feedings, the foal should be fed from a nipple bottle and allowed to regulate its own milk intake. If the foal appears not to be consuming enough milk, the number of daily feedings should be increased. A lamb nipple approximates the size and shape of a mare's nipple and should be used on a nursing bottle for feeding. Soft drink bottles, though convenient and inexpensive, can break and cause injuries.

The foal should have an automatic suckling reflex and learn to drink from the bottle quickly. If it does not quickly adapt, the foal may be taught to drink from a pail in the following manner:

1. Pour milk into a bucket and dip two or three fingers into it. Fingers should be clean.
2. Encourage the foal to lick and suckle your fingers by placing them in his mouth.
3. Repeat this several times in succession, each time bringing the fingers down closer to the pail of milk.
4. Gradually lower your hand into the bucket of milk as the foal sucks on your fingers. The foal should soon begin to drink directly from the bucket.

FEEDING SCHEDULE

A regular feeding schedule for a foal should be adopted, and, during the first week, the feedings should be conducted approximately once each hour. Feeding may require some diligence, for the foal will not be able to drink very much formula at a feeding, but failure to provide nourishment at consistent intervals will cause the foal to be unthrifty and pot-bellied.

By the second week, a foal may be fed every 3 hours and the daily ration of milk increased to 6 quarts. If it is not possible to feed a foal regularly throughout the night, the schedule should be altered so that the foal receives more frequent feedings during the day, beginning early in the morning and continuing to late in the evening. Even with this schedule, an effort should be made to feed at least once during the night.

During the third and fourth weeks, the foal's ration may be increased to 7 to 9 quarts daily, given in feedings 4 hours apart. By this time, the foal can be started on milk pellets and the liquid formula decreased. After the first month has passed, a creep feeding program may be instituted. Just before weaning, the intervals between liquid feedings can be lengthened to 6 hours.

A foal on creep feed should eat about one pound of feed per day for each month of his age (for example, two pounds for a two month-old foal) and still receive his milk replacer pellets. If the foal does well, the milk replacer pellets may be decreased during the fourth or fifth month as the creep feed intake increases. After the foal is completely off the milk replacer pellets, it may be put with other weaned foals and treated as a normal weanling.

In cases where the foal must be fed a formula diet, a goat or small proven gentle pony should be provided, if possible, for companionship. An orphan foal will be more independent if he is around other animals and will learn to eat solid foods much more quickly if he has an example to imitate.

THE NURSE MARE

As mentioned at the beginning of this section, the best way to care for an orphan foal is to provide it with a nurse mare. When a mare is to be used, she should be stalled near the orphan foal in surroundings similar to her accustomed ones, put on high quality feed and supplements, and allowed to rest for awhile. If the mare is to feed an orphan foal as well as her own, she must be especially well-fed.

At this time, the mare is persuaded to accept the foal and allow it to nurse. Normally, but not always, a mare will allow nursing to commence within the first three days. Some mares even accept orphan foals immediately. However, there are mares that may resist attempts at nursing for several days. Therefore, because this inaction may constitute a serious problem, two methods of introduction are detailed below that will often help ensure ready acceptance.

1. Collect some of the mare's manure and urine and apply it to the foal, particularly to the flank and tail areas; this helps transfer the mare's distinct smell to the foal.
2. If the mare's own foal has died, it can be skinned and the skin placed on the orphan foal. This may cause the mare to accept the foal as her own, but it is certainly an unpleasant task for the horseman.

The foal should be introduced to the mare at a time when the mare's udder is full and uncomfortable, and the foal a little hungry and eager. The mare should be restrained by a person at her halter, with another individual near her left flank (the side from which the foal should approach), as a third person leads the foal to her. Before nursing is attempted, the mare should be allowed to smell and become acquainted with the foal. If the mare resists the foal's nursing attempt, chemical or physical restraint may be necessary. At all times, however, work should be conducted as quietly as possible to avoid disturbing the mare and foal.

Most mares will permit nursing for a few minutes to relieve the uncomfortable pressure in their udders. It is important that the foal nurse for these few minutes, as the mare's milk will cause him to smell more like her own foal. After nursing, the mare and foal should be returned to adjacent stalls and left by themselves until time for the procedure to be repeated. The introductory nursing procedure should be repeated every few hours until the mare accepts the foal's nursing calmly.

Caution remains necessary even after the mare appears to have accepted the foal. It is best to keep mare and foal separated and to watch them at nursing times to ensure that the mare doesn't attempt to harm the foal. When the mare begins following the foal, calling to it, and otherwise treating it as though it were her own, it should be safe to leave them together.

THE NURSE NANNY GOAT

When a nurse mare is not obtainable, a lactating nanny goat may be acquired as a satisfactory substitute. A nanny goat usually will accept a foal readily, call to it, and even stand on a hay bale or other raised object to make nursing easier. Of course, the foal should be started on a creep feeding program as soon as possible.

Weaning

A foal may be weaned after it is approximately five months old and well-established on a creep feed diet. Some farms, however, now wean foals as early as 3 months while other establishments prefer to wait until 6 or 7 months. Although some authorities recommend a sudden, permanent separation for the mare and foal, many individuals prefer a gradual and less traumatic separation. For instance, when there are several mare and foal pairs to be weaned, the mares may be removed one at a time from the group until the foals are completely alone. If the foal was kept alone with the mare, a gentle (proven safe with foals) gelding or barren mare should be provided as a companion, to ease the initial strain of weaning when the mare and foal are separated.

The mare's grain ration should be decreased several days prior to weaning to slow her milk production, and, during the first week of weaning, she should be kept off grain and fed hay or good pasture grass. The mare and her foal should be kept apart for a few weeks to ensure that the mare completely dries up. Because the mare's full udder may be very uncomfortable for 5 to 7 days, she may be given a bran mash with aspirin and her udder milked out the first night of separation if she appears to be in pain. Rub a mild hand lotion on the udder if it seems congested and dry; if the udder is especially warm, congested, and painful, cold packs can be applied to alleviate some of the pain. During this period, one should watch for signs of mastitis. A veterinarian should be consulted.

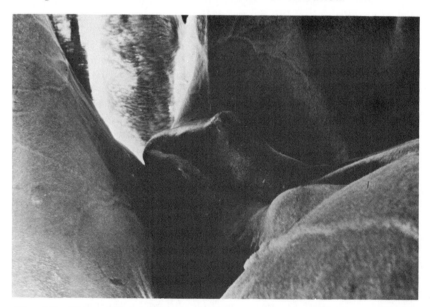

Fig. 5-9   Mare with mastitis; this condition is characterized by a hot, swollen udder and requires antibiotic therapy.

Foal Diseases and Disorders

COLIC IN NEWBORN FOALS

In foals, colic occurring within the first 48 hours of life is caused chiefly by constipation due to meconium retention. Early colic, however, is also a sign associated with more serious conditions such as atresia coli and ruptured bladder.

MECONIUM RETENTION

Newborn foals are often constipated at birth or shortly thereafter because of the collection and hardening of the fecal mass formed before birth. This condition, known as meconium retention, derives its name from the fecal mass itself, called the meconium. An affected foal may appear normal at parturition and may even eliminate a scanty amount of normal appearing feces, but at about three hours of age, the foal will begin to strain, hunch its back, swish its tail, and move as if to urinate.

Many cases of meconium retention are mild enough to be routinely treated by the horseman. Most cases of meconium retention can be prevented by routine administration of an enema to the foal shortly after birth. The enema should be given after the foal has had a chance to nurse and move about (refer to "Enemas"). If signs of constipation continue, various mixtures of milk of magnesia, mineral oil, and castor oil given orally are also helpful in encouraging meconium elimination.

A persistent constipation can be very serious and should be treated by a veterinarian. If a foal does not respond to the above treatments, the veterinarian may administer small amounts of neostigmine (at 12 hour intervals) to stimulate intestinal movement and give a sedative or analgesic such as meperidine to lessen pain. The veterinarian may eventually have to remove the fecal mass manually, though this requires great care to avoid perforating the rectum.

ATRESIA COLI AND ATRESIA ANI

Atresia coli is a congenital abnormality in which a section of the foal's intestinal tract is missing. Characteristic signs of this condition include colic and bloat occurring about 12 hours after birth. These signs may appear even though the foal seems to be nursing normally. Another indication that the foal has atresia coli is the return of clear fluid after a routine enema has been given. This, of course, is caused by the empty rectum, which, in atresia coli, ends in a blind pocket. Because surgical correction of this abnormality is impractical, atresia coli is fatal.

A related condition is atresia ani, in which the external opening of the anus is missing. Signs of this condition are similar to those of meconium retention and colic. This birth defect is surgically correctable.

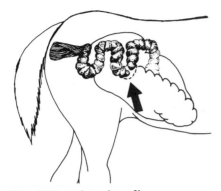
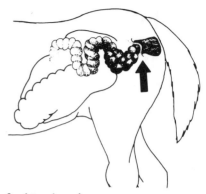

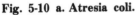

Fig. 5-10 a. Atresia coli.   **b. Atresia ani.**

RUPTURED BLADDER

Ruptured bladder is an abnormality that most often affects male foals. At birth, it produces colicky signs, abdominal distention (bloat), and causes the foal to attempt to urinate frequently with unsuccessful results. The foal's temperature may remain normal during this time, though he will lose interest in nursing. As uremic poisoning develops, the foal's breath will become sweet-smelling.

To confirm diagnosis of ruptured bladder, the veterinarian will perform an abdominal paracentesis to drain the urine. Early surgical correction followed by administration of antibiotics and fluids may allow the foal to survive.

FOAL HEAT DIARRHEA

Foal heat diarrhea is a common condition associated with the mare's first heat period which usually occurs between four and twenty days postpartum (after birth). Although the cause remains undetermined, it is not believed to be hormonal in nature. Instead, foal heat diarrhea may be caused by ingestion of lochia, the vaginal discharge excreted during the first week or two after parturiton. Lochia is a thick material which gravitates down to and sticks on the mare's teats. The foal of a mare with metritis may also develop scours.

Another cause of foal heat diarrhea is a disrupted feeding schedule. For example, if the mare is bred at her foal heat, the foal will not be able to nurse at its accustomed time and may develop diarrhea. In addition, foals are particularly susceptible to infectious enteritis during the foal heat, especially if they are in a concentrated group of horses.

In small foals, milk overload may cause diarrhea. When out on pasture and unconfined, mares escape constant nursing from their foals and the problem does not occur. Treatment of this diarrhea consists of the oral administration of two to four ounces of milk of magnesia and the application of petrolatum to the area below the anus to help prevent hair loss, dermatitis, and fly infection. Washing the hindquarters and tail with a mild soap, to remove fecal debris, will help prevent hair loss and chafing and is recommended in treating any diarrhea.

Foal heat diarrhea ordinarily disappears spontaneously, yet persistent diarrhea can quickly dehydrate a young foal and antibiotics and antidiarrheals may be prescribed by the veterinarian. A foal with severe diarrhea and dehydration will also require fluid and electrolyte therapy. Washing the mare's udder and keeping the foal's rump clean will aid recovery.

Strongyloides westeri has been incriminated as a likely cause of foal heat diarrhea. It is an intestinal parasite that can cause a severe diarrhea accompanied by a secondary infection in the damaged intestinal wall. The larvae of this parasite may be passed in the mare's milk or the parasites may penetrate the foal's skin when it beds down in contaminated areas, especially in small paddocks. If untreated, cases may increase in severity and require fluid therapy. Treatment of this diarrhea must be persistent to be effective. Administration of a mixture of thiabendazole or related dewormer and antibiotic powder, followed two days later by a kaolin-pectin mixture, should be beneficial. In cases resistant to therapy, a drug that reduces intestinal hypermotility may be required. If possible, the affected foals should be isolated from healthy ones.

PATENT URACHUS

The urachus is a fetal structure that communicates with the urinary bladder. It is contained in the umbilical cord which usually closes off when the foal is born. Improper closure, however, causes urine to drip from the umbilical stump whenever the foal strains to urinate. The dripping urine keeps the umbilical stump wet and dirty and causes the area to be prone to infection.

Patent urachus usually clears up within several days, but cauterizing the stump daily with silver nitrate or strong tincture of iodine will hasten the process. The umbilical cord should be kept clean and dry and treated with a topical antibiotic until the seepage stops. Another treatment for patent urachus is surgical correction. Regardless of the treatment used, the foal will require systemic antibiotics, as such foals are very susceptible to navel ill and joint infection.

HERNIAS

An umbilical hernia should not cause undue concern if it is small and the abdominal contents can be easily pushed back into the body cavity. Such hernias usually heal spontaneously within a year. However, when a hernia seems slow in closing, a surgical procedure will complete closure. Colic noted in conjunction with a hernia may indicate a strangulated hernia which requires veterinary treatment. A strangulated hernia must be surgically corrected before the strangulated piece of intestine develops necrosis and gangrene, resulting in death.

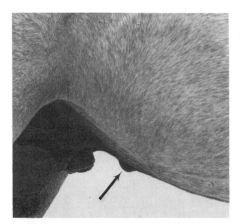

Fig. 5-11 Foal with an umbilical hernia.

CONVULSIVE SYNDROME

When the foal is a barker, dummy, or wanderer, he must be kept quiet to prevent injury. Usually, the foal that survives the barker stage of this convulsive syndrome will also survive the dummy and wanderer stages. This nervous disorder is caused by cerebral hypoxia, often due to premature breakage of the umbilical cord which deprives the foal of a portion of its blood supply. Since the stricken foal will not attempt to nurse and must be forcibly fed if he is to recover, the veterinarian will administer colostrum through a stomach tube.

NEONATAL ISOERYTHROLYSIS (HEMOLYTIC DISEASE)

Hemolytic disease is a severe anemia, affecting newborn foals, caused by the destruction of a foal's red blood cells by maternal antibodies present in the colostrum. Either through a non cross-matched blood transfusion, through a vaccine containing horse erythrocytes, or because some of the foal's red blood cells have reached the mare's circulation, the mare develops antibodies against the foal's blood type. These antibodies are concentrated in the colostrum and, when the foal nurses and absorbs them, attack the foal's erythrocytes, causing severe anemia. Thus a foal that was healthy at birth becomes jaundiced and easily exhausted as a result of lack of red blood cells. Signs of neonatal isoerythrolysis include an overall weakness, increased heart and respiratory rates, and pale, then yellow mucous membranes. Unless therapy is initiated immediately, the affected foal will die within five days.

After the veterinarian has diagnosed neonatal isoerythrolysis, he will separate the foal from its dam to prevent the ingestion of any more colostrum. The veterinarian may then give the foal a blood transfusion from a healthy donor horse while removing some of the foal's blood. The sire of the foal is always a compatible donor. If another horse is used, however, the blood must be cross-matched with that of the foal. In this way, the foal receives a new supply of red blood cells and many of the maternal antibodies are removed. The foal may require up to six quarts of blood given in this manner.

The veterinarian will probably administer antibiotics and vitamins to the foal as supportive therapy. It should be safe by 36 to 48 hours after birth to allow the foal to nurse from its mother; by this time, the foal will have lost its ability to absorb maternal antibodies through its intestinal tract.

PREVENTION OF HEMOLYTIC DISEASE

When a mare is suspected of being isoimmunized against her foal, the veterinarian can test her blood serum against some of the stallion's erythrocytes during the last month of pregnancy, or erythrocytes from the umbilical cord can be cross-matched with the mare's blood serum at parturition (refer to "Cross-Matching"). Agglutination (clumping of red blood cells) is a sign of isoimmunization and, when it occurs, the foal should be taken from its dam immediately after birth. The colostrum can then be milked from the mare and the foal returned to its mother in 36 to 48 hours. Because colostrum provides necessary antibodies, the foal should receive colostrum from another mare if it is available. Large breeding farms and some veterinarians keep supplies of frozen colostrum. When it is not available, the foal will need frequent antibiotic injections to guard against infection. While the foal is separated from its mother, it should be fed formula to supply nutrients, as discussed in "Care of the Orphan Foal."

FOAL PNEUMONIA

Young foals may develop pneumonia as a secondary complication of rhinopneumonitis, influenza, adenovirus, and other respiratory infections. In addition, a foal with immunodeficiency disease may contract pneumonia. Between the ages of one and three months, foals often suffer pneumonia as a result of **Corynebacterium equi** infection. Signs of pneumonia include difficulty in breathing, elevated respiration rate, a cough and nasal discharge, fever between 102° and 106°F (39-41°C), and loss of appetite.

The veterinarian may perform a tracheal aspiration to definitely identify the infectious organism involved and may use auscultation and percussion during additional diagnosis. Auscultation in the early stages of pneumonia will reveal moist rales, while dry rales become apparent later. After the first 12 to 24 hours of illness, there will be a dull response to percussion.

Pneumonia requires large amounts of antibiotics administered parenterally during the illness, and for several days after all signs of the disease are gone. The foal may need oxygen therapy and perhaps corticosteroids if shock is suspected. Misting or nebulizing the foal with antibiotic solutions and bronchodilators may help alleviate respiratory distress and combat infection.

Good supportive therapy, in the form of fluids, electrolytes, vitamins, etc., is recommended, as is warm, dry housing and adequate nursing care.

At least two or three weeks are necessary for complete recovery from pneumonia.

SEPTICEMIA AND VIREMIA IN FOALS

A foal may become infected due to a lack of colostrum and develop septicemia or viremia. This condition can be caused by one of the following infectious organisms:

1. Escherichia coli
2. Actinobacillus equuli (Shigella)
3. Salmonella abortus equi
4. Streptococcus pyogenes
5. Salmonella typhimurium
6. Pseudomonas aeruginosa
7. Corynebacterium equi
8. Viruses

A foal with septicemia or viremia will have diarrhea and become dehydrated. The white blood cell count and the level of blood will increase as well. The foal's temperature will be increased over 102°F (38.8°C), and it may become lame if joint infections are present. The eyes of affected foals may have a grey-green appearance, caused by leukocytes (white blood cells) in the ocular fluid. It is possible for a foal to become infected either before or after birth. Foals infected in the uterus are often born weak and may die within 12 hours. Depending on the causative organism, the foal may be a "dummy" with poor coordination and electrolyte imbalances. The veterinarian will be able to isolate the infectious organism from the foal's tissues or fluids for a definitive diagnosis.

The treatment of septicemia or viremia requires large doses of antibiotics, administered parenterally two or three times daily for at least several days after all signs of illness are gone. The foal will also require supportive therapy such as blood transfusions, vitamins, electrolytes, and corticosteroids. Unfortunately, many foals that recover from septicemia or viremia, and appear to be normal, have eroded articular cartilages which only become apparent when the horse begins training.

JOINT ILL

Actinobacillosis, also known as shigellosis or joint ill, is an acute, infectious disease that occurs suddenly and with great intensity, with frequent localization in the foal's joints and tendon sheaths, particularly in the hock and carpus. It is usually seen at birth or within the first two weeks of life, and 40% of all deaths from this condition occur within the first three days. The causative agent is a normal inhabitant of the gastrointestinal tract. While it is possible that a foal could be infected in the uterus, the organism probably enters through the umbilical cord or is ingested at birth or soon thereafter. The infection is generalized in the blood stream and localizes in the brain, kidney, liver, joints, and tendon sheaths. If the foal survives over a day or two, pus formation, abscesses, and joint lesions will be observed, and the intestinal tract will be very inflamed. Joint ill is diagnosed through a blood culture. The prognosis is poor, with death occurring in acute cases in two or three days and chronic cases lingering for as long as two and three months.

Preventive measures include providing a clean place for the mare to foal, dipping the navel of the newborn in iodine at birth, and giving antibiotics to the foal soon after birth. Treatment consists of early use of antibiotics (such as chloramphenicol, gentamicin, and streptomycin), antidiarrheals, fluids, electrolytes, nutrients through forced feeding, and blood transfusions from the dam to supply antibodies. The infected joints can also be drained and infused with antibiotics.

If the foal survives joint ill, it may be permanently lame, especially if there has been serious involvement of the joints. Such a horse will always be of the type known as a "poor doer."

SLEEPY FOAL DISEASE

Sleepy foal disease, resulting from an in utero infection, causes the foal to be unable to nurse at birth, and a veterinarian should be consulted if this condition is suspected. The mare's colostrum will have to be milked into a bottle and fed to the foal to provide sufficient antibody protection. An injection of antibiotics, such as penicillin-streptomycin, should be given and repeated every six hours until the foal recovers.

IMMUNODEFICIENCY DISEASE IN FOALS

The immune system protects the body against infectious diseases. It accomplishes this either through antibodies or through the activity of certain cells. Occasionally, however, a foal will have a deficient immune system and be less resistant to disease.

Immunodeficiency disease may be caused by:

1. a lack of maternal antibodies, either through
   a. a failure of the foal to receive colustrum at birth, or
   b. an inability of the foal to absorb the maternal antibodies
2. an incomplete immune system
3. an inhibited immune system

COLOSTRUM DEFICIENCY

A foal that cannot nurse at birth is deprived of the mare's vital colostrum and inherent antibodies. Thus, a foal that is incapable of producing any antibodies of his own for several months will be very susceptible to infectious disease. The foal that has been deprived of colostrum requires antibiotic therapy for one to two weeks after birth to ward off infection.

PRIMARY IMMUNODEFICIENCY

A foal with primary immunodeficiency disease suffers from an incompletely developed immune system. The cause of this is an inherited defect called combined immunodeficiency disease (CID). Affected foals cannot produce antibodies, due to a lack of T or B lymphocytes, and cell-mediated immunity fails to develop. Cell-mediated immunity refers to the ability of certain cells to either inactivate or kill bacteria and viruses, reject foreign matter, and destroy tumors. Combined immunodeficiency disease is believed to be a recessive trait in which the carrier parents appear normal.

The foal with CID has 1000 or fewer lymphocytes/cmm of blood as compared to 4000 lymphocytes/cmm for a normal, healthy foal. If the foal has from 1000 to 1500 lymphocytes/cmm, it has lowered disease resistance, but may survive with good nursing care.

The foal usually becomes ill with an adenovirus, causing an upper respiratory disease sometime between 10 and 35 days of age. Signs include poor general condition, weakness, depression, and fever. In addition, the foal will have a discharge from the eyes and nose, a cough and an increased respiration rate due to secondary bacterial infection. Some afflicted foals also develop diarrhea and/or oral ulcers. The foal eventually weakens and dies. Although adenoviral disease is the major cause of death, the foal will occasionally succumb to another ailment. Primary immunodeficiency is always fatal, and most foals with CID die within 2 to 12 weeks after birth.

SECONDARY IMMUNODEFICIENCY

Secondary immunodeficiency disease is caused by an inhibited immune system that is incapable of protecting the horse because of some stress. Conditions that may result in this disease include equine infectious anemia, malnutrition, chronic diarrhea, drugs such as corticosteroids, or any chronic, debilitating illness. Because of the weakened defenses, the horse becomes very susceptible to parasites, bacteria, and viruses. Unlike the primary type, secondary immunodeficiency can affect mature horses.

TICK PARALYSIS

Tick paralysis, a rare condition caused by engorged ticks, can cause paralysis in suckling foals. Treatment consists of removal of the parasites, after which recovery should occur in six to twelve hours. Supportive therapy, antibiotics, and B complex vitamins may speed recovery.

ANGULAR DEFORMITIES OF THE LIMBS

KNOCK-KNEES

Congenital deformities in foals most often affect the forelegs, causing them to be either both curved in the same direction (from cramping in the uterus) or to be curved inward (knock-knees). The latter condition often corrects itself spontaneously within a few days after birth. If the condition does not improve, however, the veterinarian may either apply a plaster cast to the affected limb or limbs for a period of ten to fourteen days to help straighten the deformity, or recommend a few weeks of stall rest with no exercise.

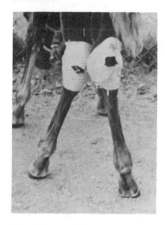

Fig. 5-12   Foal with an angular deformity.

If this problem continues, the veterinarian may surgically insert staples into the epiphyseal plate from the convex side of the leg to inhibit growth on that side and allow the opposite side's growth to catch up. On a foal with knock-knees, insertion is performed on the inner, or medial, side of the leg. Since this procedure requires several weeks to be fully effective, the staples must be inserted quite some time before the epiphyseal plates close and the bone ceases to grow in length. The fetlock should be stapled before six months of age and the carpus and hock before fifteen months, preferably as early as possible (refer to "Stapling the Epiphysis").

CONTRACTED TENDONS

Another congenital limb deformity is contracted tendons, which, if severe, results in "knuckling over." In treating mild cases, the veterinarian may choose to apply splints to the foal's legs to straighten the limbs.

In more severe cases, the veterinarian may apply a plaster cast or perform surgery. Surgical repair of contracted tendons is known as a tenotomy and involves cutting and lengthening the superficial and, possibly, the deep flexor tendons. After a tenotomy, a cast is required for stabilization.

Since contracted tendons may be the result of a deficiency of calcium, phosphorus, or vitamin A in the pregnant mare's diet, her ration should be analyzed for proper nutrients. If the condition is found to be nutrition-related, it will recur (even after surgery) unless the foal's ration is supplemented. A foal is occasionally born so severely deformed that euthanasia is recommended.

Contracted tendons occurring at a later age are said to be acquired, and are usually caused either by a nutritional deficiency or an injury. (Refer to "Contracted Tendons" under "Lamenesses.")

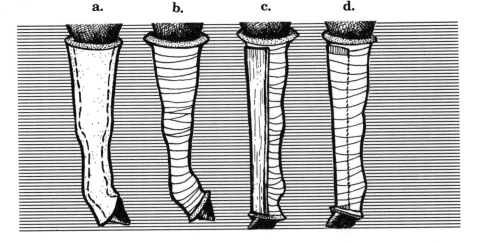

a.   **b.**   **c.**   **d.**

Fig. 5-13   Applying a splint to contracted tendons.
a.   Cotton padding.   b.   Gauze bandage wrap.
c.   Splint. d.   Additional tight wrap with more bandage material.

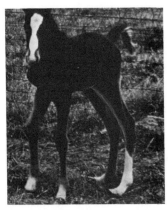

Fig. 5-14   Foal with a slightly contracted tendon of the right forefoot; this foal also has weak flexor tendons of the hindlegs.

WEAK FLEXOR TENDONS

Occasionally, a foal will be born with weak flexor tendons (down in the pasterns) which may allow the fetlocks to hit the ground. Usually, this condition improves spontaneously within a few days. If necessary, a bandage may be applied to protect the fetlock surfaces. When the condition persists, the veterinarian may apply a trailer shoe to support the foot. (Refer to "Weak Flexor Tendons in the Foal" under "Lamenesses.")

EPIPHYSITIS

Inflammation of the epiphyseal plate occurring in horses one to two years old is discussed under "Lamenesses." A nutritional form of this disease occurs in highly conditioned young horses that are overfed. In other words, they carry too much weight for their stage of development and the growing skeletal system is adversely affected. In addition, oversupplementation of minerals may cause a calcium/phosphorus imbalance that results in nutritional hypoparathyroidism, in which the foal develops epiphysitis. A foal may also develop this condition if suffering from malnutrition due to a low-protein ration.

PARASITE PROBLEMS IN FOALS

Early control of parasites is vital if a foal is to grow to its genetic potential. Parasites that are not controlled will stunt the foal's growth and cause a potbellied, rough-coated appearance. Foals infested with **Strongyloides westeri** may require deworming as early as nine days of age. Otherwise, all foals should be on a regular deworming program by six to eight weeks of age. (For specific information about parasites and recommended deworming schedules, refer to "Control of Internal Parasites.")

COPROPHAGY IN FOALS

Coprophagy in foals may be innocuous, since most foals eat some of their mothers' droppings, and this causes no apparent change in a foal's appearance. Coprophagy may result from a feeding problem such as an inadequate milk supply or a vitamin/mineral deficiency, and indicate a need for supplementation. Regardless of the cause or apparent seriousness, two major problems can result from this practice.

A foal that ingests many parasite ova (eggs) will become infested. If so, it will exhibit characteristic signs of parasitism; colic, rough haircoat, potbelly, etc., and probably will be a "poor doer." The other problem often associated with coprophagy is the appearance of a transitory diarrhea. The diarrhea may be treated with symptomatic therapy and removal of droppings in the foal's environment. A small dose of kaolin and pectin given in combination with an intestinal antibiotic and mild foal dewormer such as thiabendazole or piperazine is a possible treatment. In some cases, a veterinarian may use a stallion catheter as a stomach tube to administer medications.

WHITE MUSCLE DISEASE

White muscle disease, or nutritional myopathy, occurs in newborn foals and in those up to seven months of age raised on selenium deficient pastures and is quite common in New Zealand. Subclinical cases of the disease are thought to occur in the United States. Signs of white muscle disease include lethargy and a stilted, stiff gait. When muscle damage is extensive, the affected foal will go down and usually die unless treatment can be given immediately after the onset of clinical signs. Therapy involves two or more injections of selenium and vitamin E given a week apart.

In areas where nutritional myopathy is known to occur, preventive measures should be taken. Vitamin E and selenium should be administered to the pregnant mare approximately one month before her expected foaling date. The foal should also be given an injection of both substances at birth and later at monthly intervals.

ABNORMALITIES OF DEVELOPMENT OBSERVED IN YOUNG FOALS

The incidence of developmental problems in newborn foals is between 2 and 4%. Following is a list of some of the more common developmental abnormalities:

CONDITION	SIGNS	TREATMENT
Cleft palate	regurgitation of milk	euthanasia is usually recommended
Heart defects	auscultation murmurs and fainting	no treatment
Hernia: scrotal or umbilical	defect in abdominal floor, intestines may be felt just beneath skin	surgery
Hydrocephalus	dome-shaped skull, CNS signs	no treatment
Hyperflexion of limbs	contracted tendons, knuckling over	splints, casts, surgery
Hypoflexion of limbs	down in the pastern, lack of tone in muscles and ligaments	bandage support, splints, casts, good nursing
Microphthalmia	small, undeveloped eyes	no treatment
Parrot mouth	undershot lower jaw (overshot lower jaw also occurs)	no treatment
Patent urachus	umbilical cord stem wet with urine	cautery, antibiotics surgery
Ruptured bladder	colic, straining 2 to 3 days after birth	surgery

II. EQUINE AILMENTS

6

LAMENESS

General Conditions Affecting the Musculo-Skeletal System

This section deals generally with the causes and treatments of lameness, and does not cover the specifics of treatment procedures. For example, under "Arthritis," therapeutic cautery, casting, and radiation therapy are all mentioned treatments. Since each of these topics is discussed fully elsewhere in the book, few specifics are given here to avoid repetition. And, rather than repeatedly refer the reader to these topics, the reader should refer to the index for the sections that offer detailed information on the treatments mentioned.

The following is a sample list of treatment procedures that are recommended in the text. The reader may find more specific information on each of these treatments by referring to the index.

Ankylosing a Joint
Bandaging
Casting
Cleansing and Treating Wounds
Corrective Shoeing and Trimming
Cryosurgery
Drugs and Related Topics

Flushing a Joint
Use of Hoof Testers
Hydrotherapy
Massage
Neurectomy
Radiation Therapy
Radiography
Therapeutic Cautery

ARTHRITIS

Although arthritis can be defined simply as an inflammation of a joint, it is actually a complicated condition that can involve the bones, articular cartilages, joint capsule, and associated ligaments of a joint or joints. Primary arthritis results from direct trauma such as penetration of a foreign body into a joint or a physical blow to the joint. Secondary arthritis, as its name indicates, is secondary to other problems and can be caused by:

1. poor conformation that predisposes a horse to joint trauma
2. bone disease
3. localization of a systemic infection in a joint

Acute arthritis is characterized by a rapidly developing, severe joint inflammation. Acute arthritis can eventually dissipate, leaving a healthy joint, or it can develop into a chronic condition. Chronic arthritis is defined as a slowly developing, low-grade joint inflammation that usually results in some degree of permanent damage.

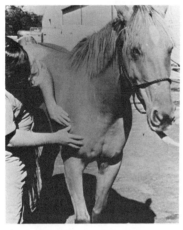

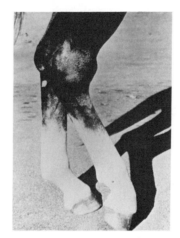

Fig. 6-1 Deep palpation of the shoulder joint of a horse with arthritis.

Fig. 6-2 Arthritic pastern joint.

SEROUS ARTHRITIS

Serous arthritis is usually caused by trauma, and is characterized by excessive accumulation of serous fluid in the joint space. This condition often occurs in poorly conformed horses. The synovial membrane is inflamed, but the bony structures of the joint appear normal in radiographs. Serous arthritis can either be acute in onset or recur periodically on a chronic basis.

Treatment: Supportive treatment for the acute phase of serous arthritis is directed toward relief of pain and consists of sedatives and local anesthesia. Usually, at least two weeks of absolute rest, in either a plaster cast or heavy bandaging, is required. The veterniarian may inject a corticosteroid, or a mixture of corticosteroids and DMSO, into the joint to reduce the acute inflammatory response. After the initial two week rest period, hot epsom salt packs and liniments can be used to help return mobility to the joint. The joint should then be bandaged for another four to six weeks. The veterinarian may administer a systemic anti-inflammatory agent, such as phenylbutazone or a corticosteroid, during the course of treatment. Chronic serous arthritis may be treated with intra-articular injections of corticosteroids, as well as by local heat, liniments, and closely controlled exercise. In the treatment of fetlock and carpal joint arthritis, intra-articular injections of sodium hyaluronate have been used. The veterinarian may also employ radiation therapy, ultrasound, diathermy, or therapeutic cautery. The horse will require from one to six months rest to recuperate.

OSTEOARTHRITIS

Osteoarthritis is a severe type of arthritis characterized by deterioration of the articular cartilage, damage to the joint surfaces, and bony involvement. This condition is most frequently seen in older horses and is commonly associated with chronic joint problems. In working horses, this type of arthritis often results from the trauma associated with continued use of a horse suffering from serous arthritis. This is particularly true if excessive corticosteroid injections are used to provide temporary relief from serous arthritis without allowing an adequate rest period for healing. As with serous arthritis, a poorly conformed horse is predisposed to osteoarthritis; however, this condition can also be simply a consequence of old age and the gradual wearing of the joint cartilage which results in cartilage and bone degeneration.

Treatment: Surgical fusion of the affected joint, called arthrodesis, may be used to reduce the pain of osteoarthritis. In addition, the veterinarian may inject corticosteroids intra-articularly (within the joint). However, since chronically affected joints may exhibit increased susceptibility to infection, an intra-articular injection could cause an infection. In fact, careful precaution is always exercised by the veterinarian to ensure that any joint is entered only under aseptic conditions.

INFECTIOUS ARTHRITIS

Infectious organisms entering the joint through a wound, or via the blood or lymph systems can cause an infection that results in a distended joint capsule which feels hot to the touch. This infection destroys the joint cartilages and underlying bone and causes new bone growth which results in ankylosis or osteoarthritis.

Treatment: The first step in treating infectious arthritis involves culturing a joint-fluid sample in order to identify the infectious organism. The veterinarian will aspirate the joint space before injecting an antibiotic into the space. Prior to injecting the antibiotic, the veterinarian may thoroughly flush the joint using a saline lavage. This technique effectively washes a number of infectious organisms from the joint space. The joint is then bandaged and systemic antibiotic therapy is maintained for ten to fourteen days (at least five days after all signs of infection are gone). In some cases, the veterinarian may choose to flush the joint and surgically install drains. If the joint has been opened, it will require a plaster cast or bandaging until healed.

The best response to therapy is seen when treatment is started within a few hours of the introduction of the infective organism, or before the infection becomes "fullblown."

ANKYLOSING ARTHRITIS

Ankylosing arthritis is characterized initially by severe degeneration and ulceration of the articular cartilages, accompanied by erosion and flattening of the underlying bone. These severe degenerative processes result in new bone growth across and occluding the joint space until that area is eventually obliterated. This type of arthritis may be the end result of osteoarthritis, infectious arthritis, or a severe injury, such as a fracture or puncture wound. Radiography of the joint will reveal that the joint space has been replaced by bony growth.

Treatment: Possibly the only treatment for ankylosing arthritis is to hasten the fusion of the joint, which will restrict movement and reduce pain. The prognosis largely depends on which joint is affected. If successful, the therapy may make the horse sound for breeding, but it is unlikely that the animal will ever return to working soundness.

BURSITIS

Another general cause of lameness that can affect several different areas of the body is bursitis, an inflammation of a bursa. Bursitis may be a very mild inflammation of the synovial membrane, or it may be severe enough to include suppuration (formation of pus) with abscess formation. True bursitis is the inflammation of naturally present bursa, whereas acquired bursitis involves the development of a false bursa. Acquired bursitis usually results from trauma, such as in hygroma of the carpus.

Treatment: Treatment of all types of bursitis includes the prevention of repeated trauma to the injured area. The veterinarian may aspirate (remove by suction) the fluid from the bursa and inject corticosteroids locally into both the bursa and the surrounding tissue. A pressure bandage should be applied in order to protect the area from further injury. If this treatment is not successful, the veterinarian may surgically remove the bursal sac.

MYOSITIS

Myositis is defined as inflammation of muscle, and includes such conditions as azoturia and "tying up." These ailments are thought to have basically similar etiologies (causes), which are related to metabolic malfunction associated with electrolyte imbalances and cellular energy metabolism. Contributing factors include weather, temperament, diet, extent of exercise, and level of fitness of the horse. A ration excessively rich in carbohydrates, combined with a vitamin E and/or selenium deficiency, may precipitate myositis. In some cases, the diet is also sometimes found to be deficient in calcium, sodium, and the B-complex vitamins.

AZOTURIA

Paralytic myoglobinuria, more commonly known as azoturia, occurs most often in horses that are normally exercised heavily and well fed, then rested for a few days while still being fed a high energy ration. Soon after renewal of exercise after the rest period, the horse begins to exhibit muscle tremors and hesitates to move. If the horse is forced to continue working, the symptoms worsen and the animal may go down. The horse will sweat heavily, and may pass dark, coffee-colored urine (the color results from myoglobin released by the breakdown of affected muscle tissue). The femoral, gluteal, and iliopsoas muscles become hard, swollen and painful.

Treatment: Because continued exercise will increase muscle damage, the horse should not be moved after diagnosis of this condition. Since the affected muscles will become inflamed, application of cold packs to the hindquarters may help reduce the swelling if applied soon after myositis becomes apparent. The application of heat in the form of moist, hot blankets (suggested in past years) will only serve to increase circulation in the affected muscles and increase swelling

The veterinarian may administer a muscle relaxant and anti-inflammatory drugs, such as phenylbutazone, for pain. One of the most common treatments, which has also been successfully used prophylactically, is the injection of a vitamin E/selenium mixture. This combination is effective in aiding the removal of the by-products of anaerobic metabolism. Recently, the drug naproxen has been shown to have a protective effect against the muscle damage that accompanies this condition when given in the feed ration for about a week to ten days after an attack of azoturia. Additionally, the administration of lactated Ringer's solution, calcium gluconate, and the B-complex vitamins are often used in the treatment of this condition. Because the affected horse may occasionally have difficulty in urinating, a diuretic may sometimes be administered or a catheter may be passed. During recovery from azoturia, the horse's grain ration should be eliminated and the animal should be allowed only a gradual return to full ration and exercise. High-quality hay, especially alfalfa hay (which is rich in calcium) should be the initial diet. As the grain ration is increased, it should not exceed more than one-half pound/100 pounds of body weight. Limestone salt, and Lite salt (KCl,NaCl) are added to the diet to correct the electrolyte imbalance. Lite salt may be given at the rate of one tablespoon per day.

TYING UP

Since "tying up" is usually considered a mild version of azoturia, treatment for the two conditions is almost identical. Some veterinarians, however, do recommend mild exercise if the horse is willing to move. Otherwise, the horse should receive the same therapy as for azoturia.

PREVENTION OF MYOSITIS

Myositis may be prevented if careful attention is given to the horse's diet and exercise regime. A well-conditioned horse accustomed to considerable exercise on a regular basis should not suddenly be deprived of exercise, stalled, and fed a high-energy grain ration. This is particularly important if he has suffered an attack of azoturia or tying up in the past. During periods of forced inactivity, the horse's grain should be reduced and his hay ration increased. As a preventive measure for a horse that has demonstrated a susceptibility to myositis attacks, a vitamin E/selenium combination may be injected once a week for a month, then once every other week for two months, and, finally, once a month for three months.

FRACTURES

Fractures are usually due to trauma, but can be precipitated by heredity (small, weak bones), poor conformation, poor nutrition (vitamin/mineral deficiency or imbalance), and age. When a bone fractures, the surrounding soft tissue is injured and the bone's blood supply is reduced. In addition, infection may be introduced through a resulting wound when a compound fracture occurs.

CONSIDERATIONS IN LONG BONE FRACTURE REPAIR

Several factors are considered when the veterinarian evaluates a fracture and decides on treatment and prognosis. The first aspect to be considered is the type of fracture that has occurred. Simple, compound, and comminuted are terms that describe the relative degrees of severity. A simple fracture is one that does not break the skin; a compound fracture includes an open wound at the fracture site; and a fracture that is comminuted is one that involves crushed or fragmented bone.

Fractures may also be classified as complete or incomplete. If early diagnosis of an incomplete fracture is not made, and the fractured part is not rested and protected, complete separation of the bone fragments may occur in a few days. Fractures may be transverse, oblique, longitudinal, or spiral in direction, according to the forces of bending, shearing, or twisting that the bone was subjected to at the time of injury. The direction of the fracture line can influence the chances of successful repair. For example, a spiral fracture has a poor prognosis.

The fracture's location is also a determining factor in the healing process. The straight conformation of the forelegs lends itself well to immobilization in case of injury, and fractures there are thus more easily treated than in the hindlegs. Also, fractures below the carpus or hock heal more readily than injuries above these joints.

Another factor to be considered is the injury's estimated healing time. Since the immobilization device may be retained for a limited period (about 10-12 weeks), healing within this time period must be possible for the fracture to be considered repairable.

Age must be considered in the injury's prognosis, for immature horses heal more quickly than mature animals due to superior callus formation.

Additionally, foals are naturally inclined to lie down more than older horses and therefore are not as likely to unduly stress an injured leg.

Other factors that affect the chances of recovery are the horse's disposition and the animal's intended use. Disposition is important because successful recovery depends in part on the patient's calmness and stability. The horse's intended use will indicate the required perfection of fracture repair. In other words, a horse may recover to breeding soundness but not to working soundness.

Treatment: When a fracture is suspected, the limb should be immediately immobilized and veterinary assistance acquired. While the veterinarian is en route, the injury can be effectively immobilized by the application of a pillow splint (refer to "Bandaging"). Immediate treatment is important, for a simple fracture may be quickly converted to an irreparable compound fracture if the limb is not immobilized promptly.

More permanent treatment of fractures consists of reduction and immobilization of the bone, accomplished through the use of external or internal fixation devices. The term external is applied to splints, casts, slings, and close confinement, while internal denotes pins, screws, and compression plates.

The injured horse will also require supportive therapy and tetanus immunization. If the fracture is compound, the accompanying wound will require treatment and there will be a greater danger of osteomyelitis or bone infection.

One very real problem in limb fractures of the equine is that, within 7 to 10 days after the initial fracture repair, the opposite limb may break down. Unless the opposite leg is also protected by support bandaging, muscle and tendon fatigue may occur as well as joint problems and secondary laminitis.

CONSIDERATIONS IN CHIP FRACTURE REPAIR

Overextension of a limb can result in bone chips occurring on the first phalanx, carpus, or tibial tarsus. Lameness from a chip fracture is often most pronounced at the trot, and four or five radiographic views are frequently necessary for an accurate diagnosis. Surgical removal of the bone fragments is probably the best treatment. However, if the joint has been injected with a corticosteroid, an eight week delay will be necessary before surgery can be performed, otherwise, possible reaction to the corticosteroid, such as increased susceptibility to infection can occur.

LUXATIONS AND SUBLUXATIONS

A luxation is a complete dislocation of a joint whereas subluxation involves partial displacement of a joint. Continuous or intermittent lameness is usually present. Any joint can be involved, but the most common luxation seen in horses is that of the patella or stifle joint. A subluxation sometimes encountered in jumping horses is subluxation of the sacroiliac joint or "Hunter's bumps."

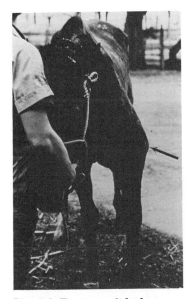 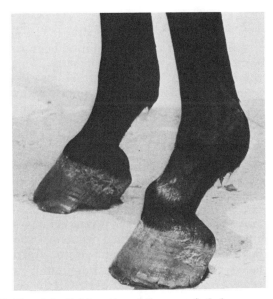

Fig. 6-3 Fracture of the humerus.   Fig. 6-4   Subluxation of the second phalanx.

a.   **b.**

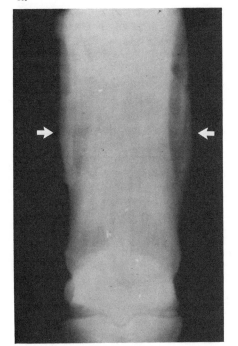 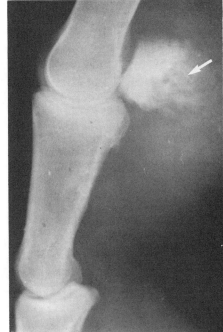

Fig. 6-5   Osteomyelitis [bone infection] involving a) third metacarpal [cannon bone] and b) proximal sesamoids.

OSTEOMYELITIS

Inflammation and infection of bone caused by pus-producing microorganisms are known as osteomyelitis. This infection can result from either comminuted or compound fractures. If the fractured ends of the bone puncture the skin, there is an open pathway for the entrance of infectious organisms. Osteomyelitis is an exceptionally serious, often fatal condition. The infection is characterized by chronic drainage from the wound and delayed healing of the fractured bone.

Treatment: The veterinarian will completely debride the wound caused by a compound fracture, set the fracture, and apply a cast for eight days to two weeks. If the injury is not healing normally by first intention at the end of that time, the veterinarian may apply a cast with a window over the wound. This cast will allow daily flushing of the injury with antibiotics and enzymes to encourage the formation of granulation tissue.

In cases of comminuted fractures where a separated piece of necrotic bone is the source of drainage, the fragment must be surgically removed before the wound will heal. Parenterally administered antibiotics, given for several weeks, are also necessary in the treatment of osteomyelitis.

MYOPATHY

Fibrotic and/or ossifying myopathy may result from old muscle injuries, particularly with the hindquarters. Fibrotic adhesions, caused by the healing of torn muscles that resulted from sliding stops, etc., can form between the semitendinosus, semimembranosus, and biceps femoris muscles of the hindlimbs. These lesions, which may ossify (i.e., have calcium deposited in the tissue as bone-like material), limit the action of the muscles and thus affect the horse's gait.

Treatment: The veterinarian will surgically remove a portion of the semitendinosus tendon at the stifle joint, separate the fibrous adhesions, and cut away any bony cover over the semitendinosus muscle. The horse will require three days to one week to show the full effect of the surgery. Although almost all horses show improvement following treatment, some may still exhibit signs of myopathy.

WOBBLER SYNDROME

Wobbler syndrome is a lack of coordination that first affects the hindlimbs and later gradually affects the forelimbs. Necropsy of a horse with wobbler syndrome will often reveal vertebrae lesions that are thought to cause incoordination. An inherited tendency to develop these lesions, an excessively high protein diet in early age, or an injury are all suspected causes of wobbler syndrome. The affected horse will usually be healthy except in its coordination and will often stay at a certain level of disability. Although some horses do learn to compensate for the loss of nervous control of their limbs, a wobbler is not safe to ride and may fall easily, particularly when tired.

Treatment: There is no definite, known treatment for wobbler syndrome. Injection of corticosteroids may have a temporary beneficial effect, but even that effect ceases when the medication is stopped. Supplemental feeding of vitamins and minerals is sometimes recommended. Basically, there is no effective treatment for this condition and the prognosis is poor.

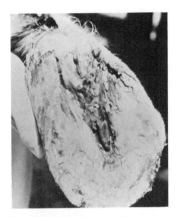

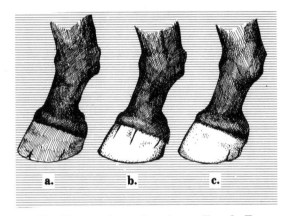

Fig. 6-6 Contracted heels with canker.

Fig. 6-7 Types of sandcracks. a. Toe. b. From the coronary band. c. Quarter.

Foot

The more common hoof conditions (i.e., corns, bruised sole, thrush, canker, gravel, seedy toe, and puncture wounds) are discussed in the section on "Treating Common Hoof Ailments," as they can often be treated by the horseman. Other causes of foot lameness are discussed in this section.

CONTRACTED HEELS

Narrowing of the heels and frog due to a lack of frog pressure is a condition known as contracted heels. The front feet are affected with this ailment more often than the hindfeet.

Improper shoeing and trimming or cutting away of the bars can cause the heel to contract. The frog eventually will atrophy, leading to loss of shock absorption and to lameness. The veterinarian will diagnose this condition by the extremely narrow appearance of the heels.

Treatment: The treatment for contracted heels requires corrective shoeing to provide frog pressure (refer to "Corrective Shoeing and Trimming").

SAND CRACKS

Cracks in the hoof wall, whether originating from the bearing surface of the hoof or from the coronary band, are known as sand cracks. Either the front or hind feet may develop cracks. Depending upon their location, sand cracks are termed toe, quarter, or heel cracks.

Cracks beginning at the bearing surface of the hoof wall are usually due to excessive hoof growth and can best be prevented by proper trimming of the feet. An injury to the coronary band can result in a sand crack starting from the coronet and extending downward. If the crack reaches sensitive tissues of the foot, the horse will become lame.

Treatment: A crack originating at the bearing surface of the hoof is first cleaned, then the bearing surface at the crack is raised to prevent the horse's weight from spreading the crack further. If necessary, the veterinarian may use acrylic to repair the defect.

A sand crack originating at the coronet is also cleaned and then repaired with acrylic. Depending upon the severity of damage to the coronary band, the hoof may grow out permanently defective (refer to "Acrylic Hoof Repair").

KERATOMA

A keratoma is a rare, benign tumor of the hoof wall that causes pressure on the laminae, thereby causing pain and lameness. The tumor may even eventually change the shape of the foot.

The veterinarian will locate the keratoma through the use of percussion, hoof testers, and radiographs.

Treatment: A keratoma must be surgically removed and the foot bandaged after the operation. Occasionally, the defect will be filled in with acrylic while the foot is healing. The foot may be shod after the horse regains soundness.

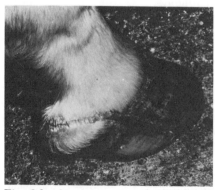

Fig. 6-8 An injury to the coronary band can result in a permanent hoof defect.

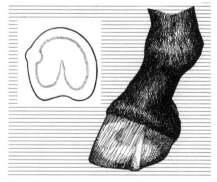

Fig. 6-9 A keratoma presses on the sensitive laminae [inset].

LAMINITIS

Acute laminitis is a medical emergency, in which the sensitive laminae of the foot become inflamed and possibly suffer permanent damage. Treatment must begin early (within 16 hours) if irreversible damage is to be prevented. This condition is characterized by the following signs:

1. heat and pain at the coronary band
2. pounding digital pulse
3. congestion (accumulation) of blood in the laminae
4. a peculiar stance in which the horse attempts to get as much weight as possible off the affected feet

Laminitis may be precipitated by any of the following situations:

1. ingestion of excessive amounts of grain (grain founder)
2. ingestion of lush pasture (grass founder)
3. ingestion of excessive amounts of cold water (water founder)
4. allergic reaction to proteins in highly concentrated feeds
5. retained placenta at parturition (postparturient founder)
6. overuse on hard surfaces (road founder)
7. standing for long periods during transport
8. obesity

These situations result in the development of organic toxins, hormonal imbalances, bacterial endotoxins, or concussion, any of which can lead to laminitis.

MECHANISM OF LAMINITIS

In laminitis, there is a great release of histamine into the circulating blood. In addition, vascular changes occur, including a severe decrease in the arterial blood supply to the terminal arch of the foot. If left untreated, acute laminitis may become chronic and can lead to severe alterations in the foot (e.g., rotation of the third phalanx and subsequent penetration through the sole of the foot). These changes are often irreversible.

ACUTE LAMINITIS

Acute laminitis is characterized by the typical "founder stance," in which all four feet are forward of the normal position, the head is low, and the back is arched. The horse may lie down (especially if all four feet are affected), and may lie flat on one side. In addition, the horse will have great difficulty in getting up and down. Other signs of acute laminitis include local heat and pain at the coronary band, increased digital pulse, muscle tremors, and sweating. The horse will also show a marked increase in heart rate, a rapid, shallow respiration, and have an expression of great anxiety. The entire foot will be tender when examined with hoof testers.

If left untreated, the third phalanx (coffin bone) may rotate and even drop through the sole of the foot. Eventually, the hoof may slough, if the wall and the sensitive laminae separate at the coronary band.

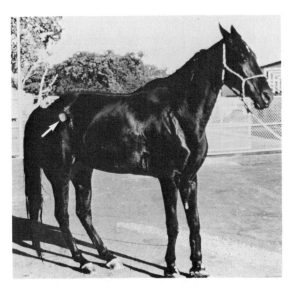

Fig. 6-10   Typical "founder stance"; note the forward position of the feet. The injury [arrow] was caused by the horse lying down to relieve pain.

CHRONIC LAMINITIS

In chronic laminitis, the third phalanx rotates, and may protrude through the sole of the foot. The hoof will grow very rapidly, especially at the heel, resulting in long, dished feet with many horizontal ridges. In very severe cases, bulging will occur at the coronary band at the front of the hoof, and growth of the hoof will occur at the heels only. This is due to alteration of the blood supply to the foot, and the prognosis is poor in such cases. In addition, the hoof wall tends to separate from the surrounding structures, and seedy toe may develop. Such an animal has clumsy gaits and may be subject to repeated attacks of laminitis. In any event, radiographs are of value to determine the degree of rotation of the third phalanx, the type of trimming required, the probability of sole penetration, and the prognosis.

GENERAL TREATMENT

In cases of laminitis, veterinary assistance should be secured immediately. Since laminitis is a true medical emergency, time is of the essence, and immediate treatment often determines whether an acute case will recover or degenerate to the chronic form.

Probably 90% of all cases of laminitis are precipitated by grain overload. Mild purgatives in mineral oil should be given in the early stages of the condition to remove any toxic ingesta. If the horse is shod, the shoes should be removed. Periodically soaking the feet in ice water may bring

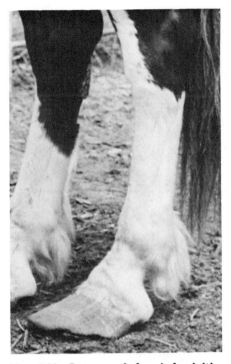

Fig. 6-11 In cases of chronic laminitis, the hoofs assume a "dished" appearance.

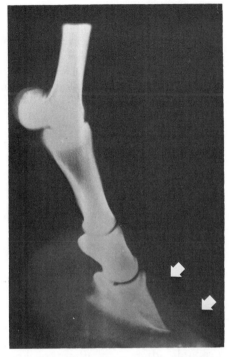

Fig. 6-12 In chronic laminitis, the third phalanx [coffin bone] may rotate away from the hoof wall. Note that the third phalanx is no longer parallel to the hoof wall [arrows].

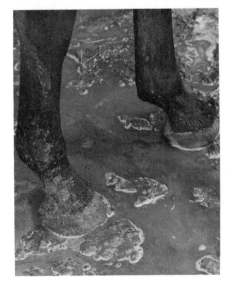

Fig. 6-13 Standing the horse on a soft surface, such as mud, is sometimes recommended as general treatment for laminitis.

some relief when the first signs of laminitis appear.

If begun within 24 hours, several injections of antihistamines are beneficial. Analgesics, such as phenylbutazone, are used to help relieve pain and inflammation. Diuretics are occasionally used to reduce edema. Short periods of forced exercise at frequent intervals have also been found to be of value, as exercise will increase the blood flow through the foot. To aid in walking, rubber or foam padding material may be secured to the sole of the foot with electrician's tape, however, casting the hoof may prove more satisfactory. If the affected horse is still reluctant to move, it may be necessary to perform a nerve block to relieve the pain enough that the animal can be walked.

Specific treatment for laminitis will depend on the suspected cause and the particular horse involved. In all cases, grain should be removed from the diet and parenteral antibiotics should be administered. The veterinarian may prescribe the addition of methionine and Lite salt to the horse's ration. Lite salt, added to correct the potassium deficiency, may be given at the rate of two tablespoons a day. In chronic laminitis, corrective shoeing will aid in restoring the normal angle of the third phalanx.

Grain Founder

Regardless of whether or not signs of laminitis have appeared, therapy for grain founder should begin as soon as it can be substantiated that the horse has eaten an excessive amount of grain. The veterinarian will probably administer mineral oil and cathartics in order to increase passage of the grain through and out of the digestive system. The horse will also be given antihistamines and antibiotics. Walking will increase the venous blood flow from the feet and is therefore beneficial. If the horse hesitates to move, the veterinarian can inject a local anesthetic into the volar nerves to reduce pain. For maximum benefit, the horse should be exercised for one hour three times daily. Grain will be removed from the diet and a high-quality hay substituted.

Soaking the horse's feet in hot water (in some cases, alternating with ice water) will increase blood circulation and remove edema and toxic products. The use of ice water is somewhat controversial, but has been used when laminitis was recognized early in the onset of the condition. The administration of antihistamines and phenylbutazone will also reduce inflammation. In addition, the horse may require fluid and electrolyte therapy.

Forced exercise, standing the horse on a soft surface, such as sand, and lowering the horse's heels will all help prevent rotation of the third phalanx.

Postparturient Founder

In treatment, the retained placental membranes must be removed from the uterus by the veterinarian, after which the uterus can be treated with antibiotics. The attending veterinarian may choose to administer a drug that increases constriction of the uterus in an effort to increase expulsion of placental membranes. The mare should receive antibiotics parenterally (either intravenously or intramuscularly) for three to five days. In addition, antihistamines and phenylbutazone may be administered. Forced exercise should also be helpful since it stimulates the venous blood flow of the foot.

Grass Founder

The horse that founders on lush pasture will be given a purgative and an antihistamine, along with an anti-inflammatory agent (such as phenylbutazone). Other treatments include hot packs for the feet and forced exercise. The horse's diet should be restricted to a low-protein ration, such as dry grass hay, for at least 72 hours. The typical horse that grass founders usually needs to lose some weight, and will often be found to be hypothyroid.

Water Founder

Treatment for laminitis caused by a too-rapid intake of large amounts of water (particularly after strenuous exercise)is similar to treatment for grass founder. The veterinarian will probably give the horse a purgative, antihistamines, and phenylbutazone. Soaking the horse's feet immediately in ice water (warm water may be used later), followed by forced exercise, will help reduce edema and increase circulation.

Road Founder

Laminitis can also result from excessive concussion over hard surfaces. In such a case, the horse should be rested from work over hard surfaces. Both soaking the feet in hot water and packing them in ice have been suggested as treatments for road founder. Forced exercise and a veterinarian's attention are also necessary for the best prognosis.

Other Types of Laminitis

If a horse suffers a severe injury in one leg (for example, a cannon bone fracture of a foreleg), the extra weight placed on the opposite good leg will often cause laminitis to occur in the good foot. This is especially true in stalled horses that are completely without exercise. To help prevent this occurrence, the horse should be allowed exercise, if possible, to aid blood circulation in the hoof. Additionally, a support bandage will help provide extra support to the good leg, thus reducing the chance of laminitis. Unfortunately, if the horse should founder in one front foot while the opposite foreleg is recovering from an injury, euthanasia is often the only alternative.

SIDEBONES

Ossification of the collateral cartilages of the foot (particularly the forefeet) is known as sidebones. This condition slowly and naturally occurs in older horses, but it may be hastened by concussion or by poor conformation. A base-narrow horse will more often develop lateral sidebones, while a base-wide horse will more frequently have medial sidebones. Improper shoeing that increases concussion may precipitate this condition. Another possible cause of sidebones is a wire cut that damages the collateral cartilage.

Sidebones are infrequently a cause of lameness, unless severe inflammation characterized by local heat and pain is present. Pressure exerted on this area may cause the horse to flinch and the quarters to bulge at the coronet, and radiography of the horse's foot will reveal the ossification of the cartilages. Occasionally, a sidebone will appear to fracture due to multiple centers of ossification.

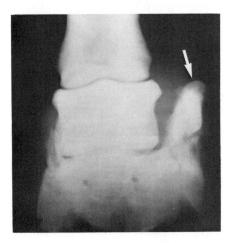

Fig. 6-14 A severe case of sidebones.

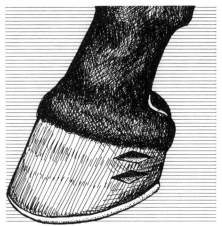

Fig. 6-15 Grooving the quarters may relieve the pain of sidebones.

Treatment: If lameness is actually caused by the sidebones, grooving the quarters will allow the horse's foot to expand and relieve the pain of ossification. Corrective shoeing for this condition is sometimes necessary.

If the horse is persistently lame, and the veterinarian believes that the cause is sidebones, a posterior digital neurectomy may be performed. Small proximal chips from fractured sidebones can be surgically removed and the damaged area pressure bandaged for two weeks. Large proximal fragments, however, are not removed; instead, the horse's foot is immobilized until the fracture heals. Afterwards, the horse will need to be rested until the inflammation has subsided.

Therapeutic cautery and blistering, although used as treatment for this condition in the past, appear to be of no real benefit.

QUITTOR

Quittor is a chronic, purulent inflammation affecting the collateral cartilages of the foot. It usually occurs in the forelegs and is characterized by cartilage necrosis and sinus drainage tracts through the coronary band. Quittor may be caused by direct trauma that results in a subcoronary abscess, or by a wire cut or bruise that interferes with blood circulation to the cartilage. A puncture wound through the sole and interfering are two other causes of quittor.

The affected area of the coronary band will be swollen, hot, and painful, and one or more drainage tracts will be present. Sidebones appear and a permanent swelling may develop. Eventually, the horse's foot may become deformed.

Treatment: In the early stages, quittor may be treated by daily escharotic injections into the draining tracts. An enzyme solution or ointment may be administered to help remove the necrotic cartilage. After treatment, the hoof is bandaged.

Chronic cases of quittor may necessitate surgical removal of the necrotic tissue followed by postoperative application of a topical antibiotic and bandaging. The veterinarian may recommend the use of a poultice to increase circulation to the area.

NAVICULAR DISEASE

Navicular disease is an inflammatory condition affecting the surfaces of the navicular bone and the deep flexor tendon in the navicular bursa (i.e., the bursal space between these two structures). The tendon surface gradually deteriorates and the tendon adheres to the navicular bone, thus mechanically limiting the horse's stride. In advanced cases of navicular disease, the suspensory ligament of the navicular bone calcifies, and the horse may develop arthritis of the coffin joint. Demineralization of the navicular bone itself is often the most prominent sign, and is revealed by radiographic examination. Although navicular disease can affect the hind feet, it is almost always seen in the forefeet.

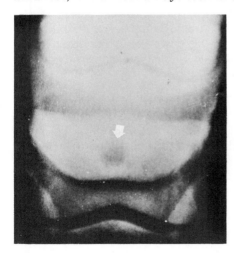

Fig. 6-16 Demineralization of the navicular bone.

Too high or too low heels (as a result of poor conformation or improper trimming), concussion from work on very hard surfaces, and upright pasterns all can precipitate navicular disease. A tendency towards this condition may be inherited, probably due to the inheritance of a weak navicular bone, a too small foot, and/or upright pasterns.

A horse suffering from navicular disease will often point the affected forefoot while at rest. When in motion, the horse will attempt to land on the toe to reduce pain, and the anterior phase of the horse's stride will be shortened, causing a shuffling gait. The use of hoof testers will reveal pain over the middle third of the frog, and the foot will become contracted in advanced cases. Radiographs must always be taken to establish positive diagnosis of navicular disease.

Treatment: Corticosteroid injections into the navicular bursa will provide temporary relief from inflammation and pain, but are not used for long-term treatment. Corrective shoeing, designed to protect the frog from pressure and to aid breakover, will often help relieve the pain of navicular disease by reducing shock. In addition, silicone, or another cushioning substance, should be used between a pad and the sole of the foot to reduce shock by about 20%. The hoof should be put in proper angulation, and the hoof walls allowed to expand. If this conservative therapy is unsuccessful in returning the horse to usefulness, the veterinarian may perform a bilateral posterior digital neurectomy. In this operation, the pain of navicular disease is relieved by severing part of the foot's nerve supply. This surgery will not be successful if the deep flexor tendon has already adhered to the navicular bone, or if coffin joint arthritis is present.

FRACTURE OF THE THIRD PHALANX

A fracture of the third phalanx is usually more prevalent in the forefeet than in the hindfeet. The horse will hold the affected foot off the ground, and use of the hoof testers will reveal uniform pain over the sole of the foot. A third phalanx fracture can also interfere with the action of the flexor and extensor tendons, thereby affecting gait. Increased digital pulse, local heat, and sensitivity to pressure are signs of a fractured third phalanx, but radiographs are used to provide definitive diagnosis. However, the fracture will often not show radiographically until 24 hours have elapsed.

The horse's foot must be immobilized with a corrective shoe and/or plaster cast to permit healing of the fracture. Immobilization for three to six months will prevent expansion of the quarters and thus keep the phalanx from moving. The horse should be rested from exercise for a total period of six to twelve months. If the fracture was caused by a penetrating object, the wound must of course be treated.

A fractured third phalanx does not always heal completely, especially if the fracture line is through the center of the bone. Chronic lameness may result in this situation, and the veterinarian may perform a volar digital neurectomy.

FRACTURE OF THE EXTENSOR PROCESS OF THE THIRD PHALANX

Fractures of the extensor process of the third phalanx are usually seen in a forefoot and are sometimes accompanied by pyramidal disease. Fractures can be caused by excessive pressure on the common digital extensor tendon. The horse will not always react to the use of a hoof tester, but will often react sensitively to pressure over the coronary band. Eventually, the hoof may become V-shaped. Diagnosis of this condition is based on radiographs which show the fracture.

Treatment: Bone fragments must be surgically removed before the fractured extensor process of the third phalanx will heal. After the operation, the horse's foot and leg are placed in a cast for approximately seven days, after which time the repaired area is bandaged for support for about one month. The animal should then be rested for a period of several months.

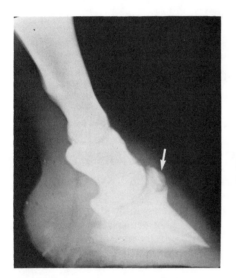

Fig. 6-17 Fracture of the extensor process of the third phalanx.

PEDAL OSTEITIS

Pedal osteitis is the demineralization and/or periosteal proliferation of the third phalanx that occurs as a result of a chronic inflammatory condition of the foot. The inflammation that causes pedal osteitis may result from chronic sole bruising (concussion from work on hard surfaces), from corns, laminitis (particularly road founder), or puncture wounds. Pedal osteitis may also be caused by infection or by poor nutrition. This condition usually affects the horse's forefeet and causes the horse to show pain at the bottom of the foot when examined with hoof testers. Radiographs of the area will reveal demineralization, particularly near the tip of the third phalanx.

Treatment: If pedal osteitis is precipitated by an injury, the initial therapy should be the treatment of wounds incurred during the injury. Corrective shoeing is usually a part of the treatment, and leather or rubber pads with silicone or a hoof cushion between the pad and the sole of the hoof will reduce concussion. Phenylbutazone is often given to control pain; however, the horse will require a period of rest in order to recover completely. If lameness persists, the veterinarian may perform a posterior digital neurectomy.

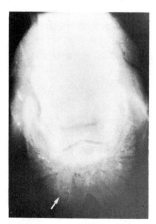
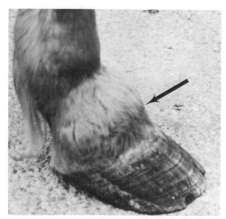

Fig. 6-18   Pedal osteitis.   Fig. 6-19   Pyramidal disease [buttress foot].

PYRAMIDAL DISEASE (BUTTRESS FOOT)

New bone growth on the extensor process of the third phalanx is a type of low ringbone known as pyramidal disease. The cause of this condition is thought to be related to excessive strain on the long digital extensor tendon, causing, in turn, either a fracture or periostitis of the third phalanx. The tendon may tear its attachment on the pyramidal process of the third phalanx, which contributes to the inflammation that causes new bone growth.

A horse with pyramidal disease will usually point the affected foot, walk on the heel, and have a shortened anterior phase of stride. Local heat, pain, and swelling will be apparent at the most forward aspect of the coronary band, and the hair at this area will often stand upright. The foot will eventually contract, and coffin joint arthritis may develop. Radiographs are used to diagnose the periosteal bone growth of low ringbone.

Treatment: Firing and blistering were used as treatment for pyramidal disease in the past, but are no longer considered to be of any real value. In the early stages of buttress foot, corticosteroid injections into the area and immobilization with a cast may prove to be of some benefit, and corrective shoeing to limit the motion of the coffin joint can also be attempted. The veterinarian can perform an anterior digital neurectomy, although there is an accompanying risk of sloughing of the hoof wall. Basically, there is no successful treatment for pyramidal disease.

EQUINE SARCOID

Equine sarcoid is a recurring granulation tissue that usually affects the lower part of the leg. Sarcoid can be a cause of lameness if it occurs as a complication of a wound, or if it is large enough to mechanically affect the stride. Although a sarcoid may appear without a precipitating traumatic incident, it is usually the result of improper wound care and excessive mobility of a healing injury. A virus is believed to be involved in the etiology (causative factors) of this condition.

Treatment: Equine sarcoids can be surgically removed, but they often regrow to an even larger extent. In surgical removal, the sarcoid is excised below skin level and the area pressure bandaged afterwards. The area around the sarcoid should be kept clean, and all hair surrounding the lesion shaved every ten to fourteen days. A corticosteroid-antibiotic ointment should be applied under the pressure bandaging at two to three day intervals. Regrowth will probably occur if pressure bandaging is not carefully maintained until the lesion heals. Fluorouracil, an antimetabolite, is also used topically for about a month to prevent the recurrence of sarcoids.

Cryosurgery is usually quite effective in preventing the regrowth of granulation tissue after its surgical excision. Radiation therapy is also employed in the treatment of this lesion. The administration of a killed virus vaccine prepared from the lesions of a horse with sarcoid may prove helpful in suppressing growth of sarcoids. In addition, the veterinarian may perform skin grafting to cover the area after surgical removal of the granulation tissues.

Pastern

CONTRACTED FLEXOR TENDONS

The flexor tendons of the legs may contract due to injury, nutritional causes, or congenital defects. A nutritional imbalance may cause a young horse (frequently an obese yearling) to develop contracted tendons. Contracted flexor tendons are often associated with epiphysitis in these yearlings. One other cause of contracted flexor tendons is severe pain in one or more joints. In an effort to immobilize the affected joint or joints and alleviate pain, the muscles will contract the tendons. (Congenitally contracted flexor tendons are discussed in "Foal Diseases and Disorders.")

Treatment: In some cases, the initial stages of contracted flexor tendons affecting a young horse may be treated by changing the diet (to correct any nutritional imbalances). Corrective trimming, in which the heel is lowered, and the removal of grain from the diet are often sufficient treatment when the condition is diagnosed early. If the condition is advanced, the veterinarian may decide to perform a desmotomy or tenotomy on the affected tendons (refer to "Surgical Correction of Contracted Tendons").

A horse incurring this condition as a result of a joint injury obviously needs the joint attended to before the tendons can return to normal. Any joint injury should receive immediate veterinary attention.

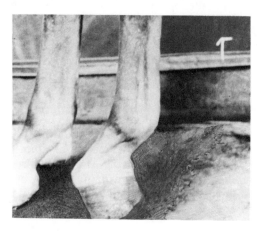

Fig. 6-20 Contracted flexor tendons.

RINGBONE

New bone growth appearing on the surfaces of the first, second, or third phalanges represents a periostitis called ringbone. Ringbone is the result of a traumatic disturbance to the periosteum (the outer fibrous covering of bone) which causes periostitis and new bone growth (exostosis). It may eventually develop into an osteoarthritis or ankylosis of the pastern or coffin joint (refer to "Arthritis"). Poor conformation, e.g., upright pasterns, increases concussion to the foot and predisposes a horse to ringbone. A base-narrow horse will usually have lateral ringbone, while a base-wide horse more often suffers from medial ringbone. It is possible for a wire cut to disturb the periosteum enough to cause ringbone. In some cases, the twisting of an ankle or a severe strain may disrupt the joint capsule and result in ringbone.

Ringbone usually affects the front feet, causing heat and swelling over the area. Radiographs of a horse suspected of having ringbone may show the new bone growth.

The various types of ringbone can be classified as follows:

High: Affects the distal end of the first phalanx and/or the proximal end of the second phalanx.

Low: Affects the distal end of the second phalanx and/or the proximal end of the third phalanx.

Articular (true ringbone): Affects the joint surfaces at the pastern and/or coffin joint.

Periarticular (false ringbone): Does not involve any joint surfaces.

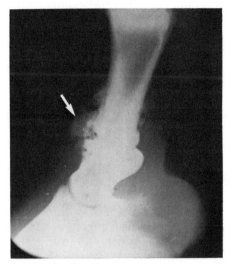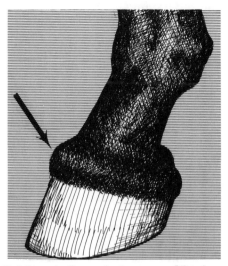

Fig. 6-21 Ringbone is caused by a traumatic injury to the periosteum, resulting in new bone growth.

Treatment: If ringbone is detected in its early stages before excessive exostosis has occurred, a corticosteroid injected into the affected area in conjunction with immobilization of the joint in a cast for at least a month may be adequate treatment. The horse should then be rested for at least four months.

Therapeutic firing and the application of counterirritants will not aid articular ringbone but may be of some use in treating periarticular ringbone. Ankylosing of the pastern or proximal interphalangeal joints can be hastened by surgery, followed by two months' immobilization in a cast.

Periarticular ringbone may respond to the systemic administration of an anti-inflammatory drug such as phenylbutazone, accompanied by a local corticosteroid injection, application of a poultice, and confinement for three to four weeks. Radiation therapy and removal of the new bone growth are two other treatments sometimes successful in arresting periarticular ringbone.

When the coffin joint is affected, ankylosing of the joint is difficult to achieve and the veterinarian may decide to perform a neurectomy. This surgery, however, can cause stumbling and loss of the hoof wall. Actually, no completely satisfactory treatment for articular ringbone exists.

RACHITIC RINGBONE

Rachitic ringbone is a fibrous tissue enlargement of the pastern area that may occur in young horses between six and twelve months of age. In contrast to true ringbone, bone or joint changes are not characteristic of rachitic ringbone. However, the affected horse will be lame and show joint soreness. Rachitic ringbone is caused by a mineral (calcium, phosphorus) and/or vitamin (A, D, and C) deficiency and may involve one or more feet.

Treatment: The horse's diet should be analyzed and the mineral/vitamin deficiency corrected. If this is accomplished soon after the signs appear, the horse should recover from rachitic ringbone in four to six weeks.

Fetlock

WINDPUFFS

Windpuffs, also known as windgalls, are usually a response to trauma and occur when a joint capsule, tendon sheath, or bursa becomes distended with excessive synovial fluid. They can also be caused by hard work or by a nutritional deficiency. Windpuffs do not usually cause lameness unless accompanied by arthritis. Although a windpuff may harden due to fibrosis, there will be no heat or pain at the site of the lesion, and severe heat, pain, and inflammation associated with joint swellings indicate serious joint damage rather than windpuffs.

Treatment: There may be no real need for treating windpuffs, because they do not cause lameness, and the accompanying swelling usually subsides when the horse is rested. Nevertheless, the veterinarian may administer a corticosteroid intrasynovially or drain the joint capsule and apply an elastic support bandage as part of the treatment. Moreover, a young horse with windpuffs may need to have his diet changed or adjusted. If lameness appears as the result of windpuffs, the horse should be rested and treated for arthritis.

OSSELETS

An osselet is defined as traumatic arthritis of the fetlock joint. This problem can be secondary to concussion and, possibly, to upright pasterns. Initially, serous arthritis of the fetlock develops and causes a thickened joint capsule. Stress may then result in an inflammation of the periosteum and ulceration of the joint cartilage. Osselets usually affect the forelimbs and appear in young horses. In the early stages of serous arthritis, the condition is known as "green osselets."

The horse may point the affected foot, and, if both front feet have osselets, the gait will be short and choppy. Heat, swelling, and tenderness will be apparent over the fetlock joint, and the joint capsule may eventually calcify. Radiographs may reveal new bone growth.

Treatment: The primary and most essential therapy for a horse with osselets is rest. Green osselets can usually be treated with ice packs or cold water to reduce the acute inflammation. The veterinarian may inject a corticosteroid into the joint capsule to reduce inflammation and restrict new bone growth. After this therapy, the horse should be bandaged with support bandages for two weeks and rested for at least two months.

Firing may be beneficial in the treatment of chronic osselets if corticosteroids have not been used. After firing, the horse will require a rest of six months. Horses with osselets that respond to corticosteroid therapy are often placed into training too quickly because they appear to be normal, and a recurrence of the disease usually results.

Radiation therapy can also be employed in the treatment of osselets, but it should not be used in conjunction with corticosteroids or firing.

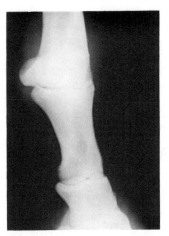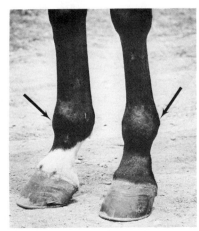

Fig. 6-22 Green osselets are characterized by a thickened joint capsule; note the swelling over the fetlock joint.

SESAMOIDITIS

Sesamoiditis is an inflammation of the proximal sesamoid bones. Inflammation and decreased blood supply cause demineralization of the sesamoids, and in advanced cases, areas of calcification appear in the suspensory ligament and the distal sesamoid ligament. Sesamoiditis is caused by strain to the fetlock joint which results in injury to the attachment of the suspensory ligament to the sesamoid bones. A long, sloping pastern predisposes a horse to this condition because such conformation increases stress on the collateral and suspensory ligaments.

The fetlock joint will be swollen and painful, and the horse will not use the fetlock normally. In chronic sesamoiditis, periostitis and osteitis develop, and new bone growth appears on the sesamoids.

Treatment: Treatment for acute sesamoiditis involves reducing inflammation. This can be aided through the alternating use of hot and cold packs, local corticosteroid injections, and systemic phenylbutazone injections. The horse's leg should be immobilized for two to three weeks in a cast or in heavy support bandages. Corrective shoeing to raise the heel and lower the toe is also employed. The horse will require nine to twelve months rest to recover and prevent a sesamoid fracture.

Volar neurectomy, blistering, and therapeutic cautery have all been used in the treatment of chronic sesamoiditis with little success. Radiation therapy may possibly be of some benefit. Unfortunately, a horse afflicted with sesamoiditis very rarely recovers sufficiently to return to full work.

SUSPENSORY LIGAMENT SPRAIN

Injury to the suspensory ligament causes swelling and pain in the fetlock area. The affected horse will hold the fetlock joint forward with the knee bent and the heel resting lightly on the ground. Frequently, the flexor tendons are injured along with the suspensory ligament. Periostitis and sesamoiditis are two complications of this type of strain. In chronic cases, new bone growth and fibrosis occur.

Treatment: Immobilization of the suspensory ligament in a cast for two to four weeks, in conjunction with daily injections of phenylbutazone for ten days is often used in treating an acute sprain. After the cast is removed, the horse will require elastic support bandages for at least a month and six to twelve months of rest. Anti-inflammatory poultices are often helpful.

Firing and blistering are not very effective in treating a chronic suspensory ligament sprain. However, radiation therapy is sometimes partially successful. The horse may perhaps be returned to work after a year's rest, but should be exercised in elastic support bandages.

The veterinarian may perform a tendon-splitting operation in which he partially severs the suspensory ligament along its length to increase the area's blood supply. After this surgery, the horse will require five to nine months' recuperation time.

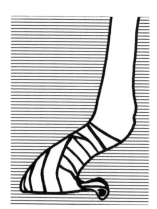

Fig. 6-23 A trailer shoe for a foal with weak flexor tendons can be made from a door hinge.

WEAK FLEXOR TENDONS IN THE FOAL

Occasionally a foal is born with weak flexor tendons. Although this condition is seen more commonly in the hind feet, all four feet can be affected. The flexor tendon weakness results in the foal "rocking back" on his fetlocks until they actually touch the ground (and bear the body weight) and the toe becomes elevated. This is sometimes accompanied by poor conformation such as sickle hocks.

Treatment: Although the tendons may strengthen without treatment, the veterinarian will usually bandage trailers on the foal's feet to provide posterior support. A large door hinge is often used for this purpose because it can be applied to simulate a raised heel. Bandaging will protect the fetlock from abrasion. Treatment usually causes marked improvement of this condition within one week, if damage to the fetlock has not occurred.

TRAUMATIC DIVISION OF THE DIGITAL FLEXOR TENDONS

Trauma resulting from kicking a sharp object or from overreaching can cause division (severing) of the digital flexor tendons. The injury usually occurs between either the carpus or tarsus and the fetlock. If only the superficial digital flexor tendon is severed, the fetlock will drop but will not touch the ground. If both the superficial and deep tendons are cut, the toe will be lifted off the ground and the fetlock will drop when weight is applied to the injured limb. Infection of the tendon sheath is a complication that may cause pronounced swelling and discharge. Obviously, traumatic division of the digital flexor tendon causes severe lameness, which worsens if the suspensory ligament and superficial and deep flexor tendons are cut.

Treatment: If both flexor tendons and the suspensory ligament are cut, the condition is virtually untreatable and euthanasia is normally recommended. When only the superficial flexor tendon is involved, the veterinarian may inject a corticosteroid and antibiotics into the tendon sheath. A cast designed to keep the fetlock flexed is then applied for a period of six weeks.

If both flexor tendons are divided, the veterinarian may attempt surgical correction by suturing the tendon ends together. When surgery is performed, the affected leg is later placed in a cast and the opposite leg bandaged for support to keep it from breaking down.

After the cast is removed, the leg is bandaged and shod with a fetlock-supporting shoe for three to six months (refer to "Corrective Shoeing and Trimming").

TRAUMATIC DIVISION OF THE DIGITAL EXTENSOR TENDONS

Traumatic division of the digital extensor tendons below the hock or between the fetlock and the carpus is primarily caused by wire lacerations. The lateral digital extensor tendon, the common digital extensor tendon, and the long digital extensor tendon are the three structures involved. The horse will be unable to extend the toe and, if forced to walk, the toe will catch the horse's weight causing flexion of the fetlock to the extent that its anterior surface will be forced to the ground ("knuckling over"). In spite of this, the horse will be able to bear weight on the limb if the foot is placed in proper position on the ground. The severity of the injury actually depends on how many of the extensor tendons have been severed.

Treatment: The wound should be cleansed and treated like any other open wound. The tendon sheath can occasionally be sutured, but often it must heal by granulation. The horse should be given antibiotics locally and parenterally to fight infection. The affected leg should be kept in a cast or at least heavily bandaged for four to six weeks, after which time the horse should be shod with a corrective shoe. An appropriate shoe should have an extended toe and metal bar and be bandaged to the foot to keep the toe in extension. Traumatic division of the digital extensor tendons requires approximately four months to heal.

CONSTRICTION OF THE ANNULAR LIGAMENT

The posterior aspect of the superficial flexor tendon is encased in the annular ligament. When trauma, infection, or other injury occurs in this region, fibrous tissue may form and constrict the annular ligament around adjacent tendons. Pressure necrosis of the suspensory ligament and lameness will result if the constriction is severe enough to impede proper sliding of the tendons. Trauma in the palmar or plantar areas, such as from a low bowed tendon, a wire cut, or a puncture wound, can result in constriction of the annular ligament.

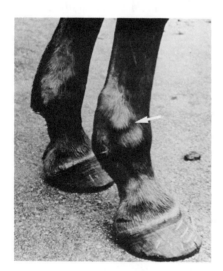

Fig. 6-24 Constricted annular ligament; note the "notch."

After this occurs, adhesions form between the superficial flexor tendon and the annular ligament, and the tendon sheaths of the superficial and deep flexor tendons become distended proximal to the annular ligament.

The superficial flexor tendon will appear thickened and a "notch" will be noticeable at the proximal part of the annular ligament. Exercise will increase the degree of lameness exhibited because it stimulates the circulation and increases the swelling.

Treatment: Surgical resection of the annular ligament and tendon sheath of the superficial flexor tendon is the treatment for a constricted annular ligament. Both structures are cut because of the adhesions that will have developed. After surgery, the horse's leg should be wrapped with elastic support bandages. This treatment is usually successful.

Cannon

BUCKED SHINS (METACARPAL PERIOSTITIS)

Young racehorses often develop bucked shins soon after beginning training. Excessive concussion at this time may cause the periosteum over the metacarpal bones to tear away from the bone, forming a space that becomes filled with blood (a hematoma). Bucked shins can also result from a multitude of microfractures occurring on the metacarpus. The lameness will increase with exercise, and the horse will move with a short, choppy stride. If only one leg is affected, the horse will rest that limb; if both forelegs are bucked, the horse will shift its weight from one side to the other. A warm, painful swelling will be noticeable over the front of the cannon bone. A fracture may occur if the horse is not allowed proper rest after incurring this condition.

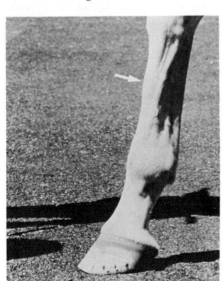

Fig. 6-25 Bucked shins; note the swelling over the front of the cannon bone.

Treatment: The application of cold packs for the first day or two will help reduce inflammation, but rest is also a necessary part of treatment for metacarpal periostitis. Sodium oleate injections into the affected area is currently considered a treatment of choice, and may reduce the convalescent period. Alternatively, the veterinarian may inject a corticosteroid subcutaneously over the area and wrap the leg. After this therapy, the horse will probably require at least a month of rest before being returned to training, even though he may appear sound, since the leg may not be fully healed and stress could result in a fracture.

If a fracture has developed, immobilization with heavy support bandages and a minimum of forty-five days rest is necessary. Counterirritants, firing, and radiation therapy are probably not very effective in treating fractures.

SPLINTS

Periostitis and new bone growth resulting from irritation to the interosseous ligament produces the condition known as splints. Splints on the front legs are most often medial, while splints on the rear legs are usually lateral. High splints (those near the carpal joint) may cause permanent lameness, while other splints usually just constitute a blemish.

Splint formation is the result of trauma to the leg. The trauma is usually from interference or a direct blow, and most often occurs during running or jumping. Consequently, splints are frequently seen on the legs of young horses in heavy training. Vitamin/mineral deficiencies or imbalances (especially in vitamins A and D, or in calcium and phosphorus) as well as poor conformation, such as bench knees, may predispose an animal to this condition.

Heat, pain, and swelling will be noticeable between the second and third, or third and fourth metacarpal bones. If the new bone growth interferes with the action of the suspensory ligament, the horse may become chronically lame. Bone changes may be definitively revealed by radiographs.

Treatment: Conservative treatment of splints consists of a month's rest and the application of hot and cold packs to reduce the acute inflammation that is usually the cause of the lameness. Occasionally, more radical treatments, such as firing and blistering have been tried. Firing, however, only decreases the amount of soft tissue swelling and does not actually reduce the amount of new bone growth. Corticosteroid injections may be of use when administered in conjunction with the application of pressure bandaging. Such injections, when accompanied with a minimum of 30 days of rest, often prevent new bone growth.

A splint can be surgically removed if it is interfering with the suspensory ligament or if it is considered a blemish.

Prevention: If the splint was caused by interference, the horse should receive corrective shoeing to prevent a recurrence. If the splint was believed to be nutritionally caused, the horse's diet should be examined for vitamin/mineral deficiencies or imbalances. Less rigorous training of young horses probably helps to prevent many splint problems.

SPLINT BONE FRACTURES

Splint bone fractures produce signs very similar to those observed in cases of simple "splints," and are usually caused by interference. However, a fracture of the second or fourth metacarpal bone causes a more diffuse swelling than that seen with a splint, and the signs will resemble those seen with desmitis interosseous. The affected area will be hot and painful to the touch, and the horse will show a greater degree of lameness at the trot. Radiographs are necessary to distinguish a splint bone fracture from a simple splint.

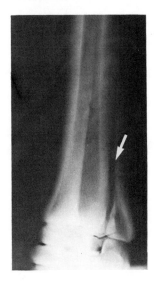

Fig. 6-26   Fractured splint bone.

Treatment: A fractured splint that occurs in the upper third of the bone can be allowed to heal by resting the horse for four to six months. However, splint fractures of the lower third of the bone, or a fracture that does not heal, is treated by surgical removal of the affected bone. When this therapy is used, the horse's leg should be pressure bandaged for a couple of weeks; the horse can usually be exercised within one month.

Although the veterinarian can administer a corticosteroid to reduce the inflammation, this treatment does not heal the fracture and may worsen the periostitis. Injections of sodium oleate have been used locally to stimulate fibrous and fibrocartilaginous tissue to promote faster recovery; the true benefit of this drug, however, remains unverified.

BOWED TENDON (TENDOSYNOVITIS)

Injury to the deep flexor and/or superficial flexor tendons can result in a condition known as bowed tendon. Tendosynovitis, as bowed tendon is also called, usually affects the foreleg, and may be precipitated by the following:

1. long, weak pasterns
2. improper shoeing (shoes that are too long)
3. work on slippery surfaces
4. excessively tight fitting running bandages or boots
5. obesity

In bowed tendon, hemorrhage and inflammation cause swelling and development of adhesions between tendons and between the tendons and tendon sheath. Some tendon fibers tear and the tendon can actually increase in length. The torn fibers may cause necrosis, and fibrous scar tissue eventually forms.

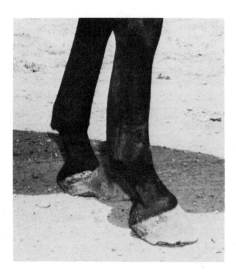

Fig. 6-27   Bowed tendon.

A horse suffering from a bowed tendon will exhibit diffuse swelling over the tendon area and hold the foot with the heel elevated. Heat and pain will also be noticeable over the injured area. Chronic bowed tendon is characterized by a firm, prominent swelling.

There are three classifications of bowed tendons, depending upon location;

High: occurs just below the carpus
Middle: occurs in the middle third of the tendon
Low: occurs in the lower third of the tendon

Treatment: To reduce the acute inflammation and to help stop accompanying hemorrhage, the horse's leg should be treated with cold packs as soon as possible after the injury occurs. An emergency treatment for a bowed tendon involves the immediate cessation of activity and the bandaging of the affected leg with a flexible temporary cast bandage. For best results, this treatment should immediately follow the injury. The veterinarian may administer a corticosteroid parenterally and apply a cast, which remains on the horse for two weeks. Depending upon the amount of improvement shown after the cast is removed, the veterinarian will either apply another cast or a heavy support bandage for one month. Ideally, the horse will need to be rested for a year to recover, and usually does not return to its previous level of athletic ability.

Firing, blistering, and the local injection of counterirritants are not very effective in the treatment of a chronic bowed tendon. The veterinarian may choose to longitudinally incise the affected tendon to increase blood supply to the injured area and accelerate the healing process. After tendon-splitting surgery, the horse will require six to nine months rest.

The horse can also be shod with a raised heel to provide support to the injured tendon. When the animal has recovered enough for mild exercise, swimming will provide good exercise without straining the tendon.

STOCKING UP

Edema and attendant swelling may develop in horses' legs, especially the hind limbs, usually as a result of lack of exercise. Other causes of stocking up include excessive amounts of protein or energy in the diet, diseases such as viral arteritis, and heavy parasitism. Stocking up most often occurs in horses that are normally accustomed to exercise and are subsequently stalled or trailered for an extended period of time.

Normally, when the horse has an opportunity to move about, the spongy material of the frog assists circulation of blood and lymph from the feet back to the heart. When the horse stands idle, however, venous congestion may occur in the lower limbs. An affected animal will appear normal except for a swelling of the lower limbs, which will pit when depressed with the fingers (pitting edema). In rare cases, if the condition is left untreated, the skin may crack and ooze serum.

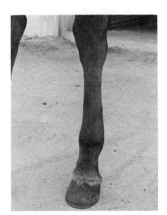

Fig. 6-28 A mild case of stocking up.

Treatment: Preventative care, in the form of regular exercise, proper diet, and a good deworming program (to prevent parasite-caused anemia) are the best solutions for stocking up. As a further preventative measure, support bandages may be indicated when hauling a horse long distances, or if a horse must be stalled without sufficient exercise.

Simple cases of stocking up will usually disappear quickly when the horse is exercised. Since stocking up is a sign of an underlying problem, veterinary assistance should always be sought in persistent cases. The veterinarian may administer a diuretic, such as furosemide, to give temporary relief prior to a definite diagnosis. The diet should be checked for excessive amounts of energy or protein, and a fecal or urine analysis may be done if parasite or kidney disorders are suspected.

Knee

EPIPHYSITIS

Epiphysitis, or "big knee," is an inflammation of the epiphysis resulting from trauma to the epiphyseal plate. The front legs in horses from one to two years of age are most commonly affected. In addition, young racehorses that begin training before their knees have properly "closed" often develop this condition.

Signs include an enlargement over the carpus, occasionally a hot and painful epiphysis, and a slight lameness. The horse with epiphysitis is frequently overweight, and has base-narrow, toe-in conformation. Nutritional imbalances are another cause of epiphysitis, particularly in heavily fed young horses. Radiographs will reveal that the epiphysis in affected horses is wavy, uneven, and open.

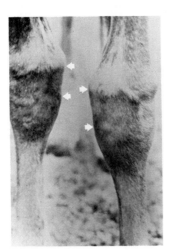

Fig. 6-29   Epiphysitis or "big knee."

Epiphyseal closure of the carpus (knee) may be described as Type A, Type B, or Type C as defined in the following manner:

Type A: Knee completely closed, mature; horse may be trained and raced.

Type B: Knee in the process of closing, slightly open; horse may be lightly trained.

Type C: Knee is open, immature; horse should not be trained.

Some veterinarians and trainers use this classification to help predict the ideal time to begin race training in young horses. It may be that radiographs of the hock region would be more significant in trotters, and fetlock radiographs more significant in horses that run on the flat. Fetlock radiographs can be taken at a younger age (7 to 12 months), while carpal radiographs are taken at an older age (18 to 24 months).

Treatment: If a nutritional disturbance is the cause of epiphysitis, the horse's ration must be corrected. When the horse is simply too heavy for its legs, the diet should be reduced.

Rest is mandatory for young racehorses with epiphysitis. A cessation of training will allow the epiphysis time to close as bone development is completed.

A horse with epiphysitis due to base-narrow, toe-in conformation will recover as the epiphyseal plate closes. However, this type of conformation predisposes the horse to other types of lameness.

RUPTURED EXTENSOR CARPI RADIALIS

Trauma that overflexes the forelimb may result in a ruptured extensor carpi radialis tendon. The muscular portion of the extensor carpi radialis will atrophy, and the veterinarian will be able to palpate the ruptured tendon ends. A horse suffering from this condition will flex the carpus excessively when in motion.

Treatment: If the rupture is discovered soon after its occurrence, surgical repair may be possible. After the tendon ends have been sutured together, it will be necessary to keep the horse in a cast for about six weeks. An older injury may require the surgical substitution of the extensor carpi obliquus tendon for the extensor carpi radialis.

HYGROMA OF THE CARPUS

Hygroma of the carpus is an acquired bursitis over the anterior surface of the carpal joint. Trauma caused by rising from, and lying down on a hard surface, or from striking the knee against a wall while pawing, is the usual cause of carpal hygroma. A similar swelling can result from a synovial hernia of one of the carpal joint capsules.

Treatment: An acute hygroma of the carpus can be treated with three to five corticosteroid injections at weekly intervals. To encourage the formation of adhesions between the skin and underlying tissues, a pressure bandage or spider web bandage should be applied for at least a week. The

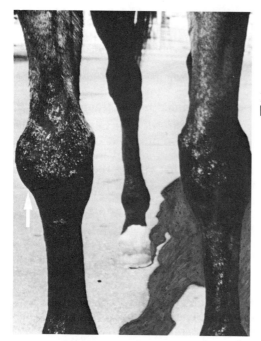

Fig. 6-30 Hygroma of the carpus [capped knee].

a.   **b.**

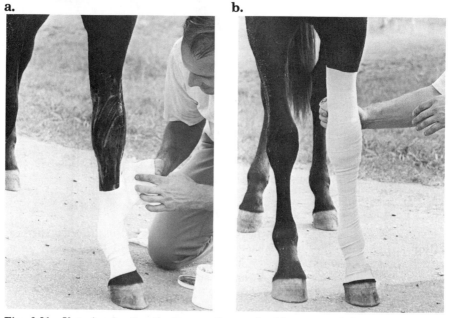

Fig. 6-31 Veterinarian treating a recently acquired hygroma of the carpus. a. Applying a topical medication, then covering the injury with a light layer of padding. b. Applying adhesive elastic wrap as a pressure bandage.

veterinarian may open the hygroma to drain it and may recommend daily swabbing of the hygroma with iodine to facilitate drainage.

A chronic, thickened hygroma of the carpus may be surgically removed. After the operation, the carpus should be pressure bandaged for thirty days and the horse confined to a stall.

CARPITIS (POPPED KNEES)

Carpitis is an inflammation of the carpus, often involving the associated joint capsule, ligaments and bones. Acute carpitis is a serous arthritis resulting from trauma. Bad conformation (calf knees, etc.), poor condition, and excessive work all contribute to the development of carpitis. If not treated, serous arthritis will gradually worsen into osteoarthritis and new bone growth will appear. A horse with carpitis will hold the knee slightly flexed, and the distended joint capsule will cause a noticeable swelling.

Treatment: Acute carpitis may be treated through a series of corticosteroid injections into the joint, pressure bandaging for a couple of weeks, and rest for at least four months. Insufficient rest will frequently cause a carpal fracture.

Although blistering is ineffective in treating carpitis, other forms of counterirritation, such as therapeutic cautery and radiation therapy, are sometimes successful. For example, the horse may be fired after the acute inflammation disappears, as long as the new bone growth does not infringe on the articular surfaces. After firing, a leg paint should be applied for three weeks, and the horse rested for six months.

Bone growth on the articular surfaces can be surgically removed if it is not too extensive. Afterwards, the leg is put into a cast for about a week following surgery, and a pressure bandage is applied for a month. The horse should be confined for four to six weeks and rested for six months.

Forearm

STRAIN OF THE SUPERIOR CARPAL CHECK LIGAMENT

The superior carpal check ligament can be strained by overflexion of the carpus. This may happen when the leg is suddenly extended (straightened) from a flexed position as the horse moves or lunges forward, usually while pulling a heavy load. In acute cases, the carpal sheath will be distended, while in chronic cases, periostitis may be evident.

Treatment: Inflammation of acute strain of the superior carpal check ligament can be treated with corticosteroid injections into the carpal sheath. Afterwards, the horse should be bandaged with support bandages for two or three weeks and confined to a stall for a month. The horse should not be exercised for at least three months.

RADIAL NERVE PARALYSIS

The radial nerve may be inactivated by trauma from a kick or fall. Further, lying on the side for a long time often results in a temporary radial nerve paralysis due to a decreased blood supply. The muscles affected by paralysis of this nerve include the extensors of the elbow, carpus, and foot, as well as the lateral flexor of the carpus.

The horse will be unable to carry the affected leg forward and straighten it enough to accept weight. When the fetlock and pastern are flexed, the horse's elbow will be in a dropped position. The animal will drag the leg and will be unable to lift the foot over obstacles. Eventually, the paralyzed muscles will atrophy. Due to the relaxed state of the muscles, the affected limb will look longer than normal. The horse may suffer further injury because of the inability to use the leg properly.

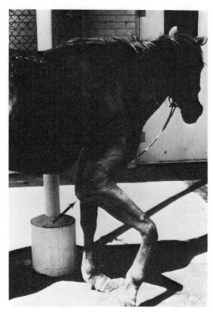

Fig. 6-32   This horse has radial nerve paralysis; note the dropped elbow.

Treatment: The horse should be kept stalled to prevent any other injury from occurring as a result of the paralysis. The veterinarian may choose to apply a lightweight cast to keep the horse's tendons from contracting (refer to "Contracted Tendons"). The cast will also help protect the skin covering the pastern from being worn away as the horse drags his leg. Massage of the affected muscles may aid recovery of the radial nerve.

When the radial nerve is paralyzed because of a fractured humerus, surgical correction will probably be necessary. The veterinarian will free adhesions and remove any bone chips and scar tissue interfering with the nerve. The horse may require as long as six months to recover after surgery. In many cases, radial nerve paralysis is not treatable, and euthanasia becomes the only humane solution.

Elbow

CAPPED ELBOW

Olecranon bursitis, also known as capped elbow or shoe boil, is caused by trauma at the point of the elbow. The trauma may result from the horse continuously lying down with the forelegs folded under the body and the heel pressed against the elbow, from a very high action gait that causes the heel to strike the elbow, or from the horse hitting himself while fighting flies. A soft, flabby swelling will be noticeable over the point of the elbow.

a.

b.

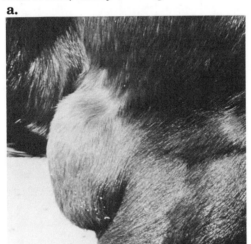 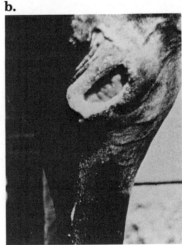

Fig. 6-33 Capped elbow. a. Trauma causes bursitis. b. The opened bursa.

Treatment: The cause should first be determined and corrected. Horses shod with elevated or weighted shoes, or with the heels left too long are often predisposed to this condition. The contents of the bursa can be aspirated by the veterinarian and a corticosteroid injected into the area two or three times a week. In some cases, a single injection of corticosteroid is all that is necessary if the cause is removed.

If the bursa becomes fibrous, surgery may be necessary to completely remove it. After the operation, the horse should be kept cross-tied for ten days to prevent him from lying down and irritating the elbow. To further protect the elbow, an elbow boot or "donut" can be used. A "donut" is a padded roll strapped below the fetlock, which protects the elbow by limiting flexion, and thereby decreases the chance of the horse hitting his elbow with his heel.

Shoulder

SWEENY

Atrophy of the supraspinatus and infraspinatus muscles of the shoulder is called sweeny. A blow to the shoulder from a kick or collision, or a stretching of the nerve due to a sudden, backward movement of the forelimb can cause paralysis of the suprascapular nerve and result in sweeny. The muscles on either side of the scapular spine will waste away, causing the shoulder joint to appear more prominent. When the horse takes a step forward with the affected limb, the shoulder may snap outward as weight is placed on the leg.

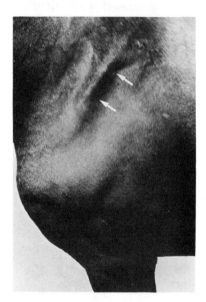

Fig. 6-34 Sweeny; arrows indicate areas of muscle atrophy.

Treatment: Cold compresses and phenylbutazone during the first 24 hours after the injury may help, but there is no proven treatment for a nerve injury. Hot packs, ultrasound therapy, etc., all increase the blood circulation to the shoulder area, but do not aid regeneration of the suprascapular nerve. Likewise, blistering and firing are ineffective in treating this condition.

A corticosteroid, such as triamcinolone acetonide, methylprednisolone acetate, or flumethasone injected directly into the shoulder joint may cause noticeable improvement after the muscle atrophy of sweeny becomes apparent. Acceptable results have been obtained in a group of horses injected two weeks to two months after the initial injury.

Counterirritants are sometimes injected into the shoulder area to stimulate fibrous tissue formation that will improve the shoulder's appearance. This treatment, however, is strictly cosmetic. The horse may recover from a temporary paralysis within a month or two, though observation for six months is necessary to determine whether the suprascapular nerve paralysis is permanent.

Hock

CAPPED HOCK

Bursitis over the point of the tuber calcis is known as capped hock. This condition can be caused by the trauma of getting up and down on hard surfaces or hitting the hock against a wall or fence. An acquired bursa develops in this condition, as it does in capped elbow.

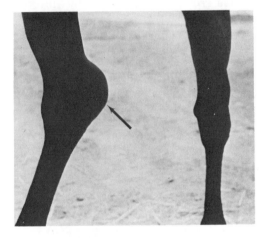

Fig. 6-35   Capped hock.

Treatment: The veterinarian may aspirate the contents of the bursa and inject a corticosteroid into the bursa and surrounding area. A pressure bandage will then be necessary. If injury to the point of the hock is consistently repeated, fibrous tissue will develop into a permanent blemish. Unfortunately, the surgery required to remove this tissue is often disfiguring. After the operation, the horse must be kept in cross-ties to restrict movement, and the hock should be pressure bandaged for ten days to two weeks.

STRINGHALT

Stringhalt is the involuntary overflexion of one or both hocks. Usually, this condition is most pronounced after resting, or when the horse is turned in tight circles. Articular lesions of the hock or stifle, muscle lesions, and nerve lesions are all suspected causes of stringhalt.

Treatment: Surgical correction for stringhalt consists of tenotomy of the lateral digital extensor tendons. (Refer to "Lateral Digital Extensor Tenotomy" under "Surgical Procedures.")

CURB

Curb is an enlargement of the posterior aspect of the fibular tarsal bone, caused by an inflamed and thickened plantar ligament. Horses with poor conformation, for example, sickle or cow hocks, are predisposed to curb because of increased stress on the plantar ligament, but violent exertion that causes extreme hock extension, or trauma from kicking walls may cause curb in horses with good conformation.

A horse suffering from curb will hold the heel of the affected leg up when at rest. The horse's lameness will increase with exercise, and heat and swelling will be noticeable at the hock. When caused by trauma, curb can precipitate periostitis and new bone growth. A chronic curb will often result in a permanent blemish.

Treatment: The veterinarian may inject a corticosteroid subcutaneously into the affected area to reduce the swelling of an acute curb. Rest, anti-inflammatory medications, and cold or ice packs are all part of treatment. Firing and blistering are of doubtful effectiveness in the treatment of curb. These treatments definitely should not be attempted in a case of chronic curb until at least ten days after the termination of the acute inflammation.

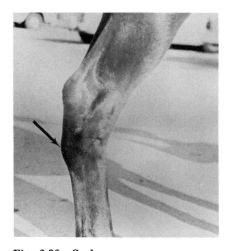

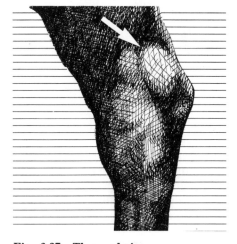

Fig. 6-36 Curb.   **Fig. 6-37 Thoroughpin.**

THOROUGHPIN

Thoroughpin is a tendosynovitis of the deep digital flexor tarsal sheath which occurs at approximately the level of the point of the hock. Since it is usually caused by trauma, thoroughpin is most often found on only one leg. Although a horse with this condition usually goes sound after one or two days of lameness, adhesions between the deep digital flexor tendon and the tarsal sheath occasionally cause an irritation that leads to continued swelling.

Treatment: In a serious case of thoroughpin, the veterinarian can drain the thoroughpin, inject a corticosteroid, and apply a pressure bandage; this treatment may be repeated if necessary. Continuous injections of corticosteroids, however, can degenerate the tendon. Blistering and therapeutic cautery are not satisfactory treatments for thoroughpin.

LUXATED SUPERFICIAL DIGITAL FLEXOR TENDON

When one or both of the attachments holding the superficial digital flexor tendon to the tuber calcis ruptures, the tendon slips out of place, either medially or laterally, and tears due to abnormal force or strain at the point of the hock. There will be some swelling evident at the hock, and the tendon may be seen slipping with each stride the horse takes.

Treatment: Occasionally, the superficial digital flexor tendon will become established in the new, displaced condition, causing the horse to go sound. Otherwise, the veterinarian may surgically replace the tendon and suture the support attachments to the tendon. A bone pin will be inserted to keep the tendon from slipping. After the surgery, a cast will be required for four to six weeks. Counterirritants, applied internally or externally, are not successful in treating a luxated superficial digital flexor tendon.

OCCULT (BLIND) SPAVIN

Occult spavin is characterized by the same signs of lameness as bone spavin, but does not exhibit palpable or radiographical changes (hence the term "occult"). It is sometimes associated with excess fluid in the stifle joint or with a thickened stifle joint capsule. Trauma can cause intra-articular lesions in the form of ulcerated articular cartilages in the hock joint. The animal's unwillingness to completely flex the hock will lower the arc of the foot and cause a shortened stride. The horse's hips will move in a rolling or hitching motion, and the toe on the affected side will wear due to contact with the ground. The horse will also usually respond to the spavin test (refer to "Leg and Foot Examination").

Treatment: Temporary treatment for occult spavin consists of intra-muscular or intravenous corticosteroid injections, or intravenous injections of an anti-inflammatory drug such as phenylbutazone. Blistering, firing, and cunean tenotomy are all useless in dealing with blind spavin.

If the hock is definitely the cause of lameness (instead of the stifle joint), the veterinarian may perform surgical arthrodesis to fuse the distal intertarsal and tarsometatarsal joints to relieve the pain.

BOG SPAVIN

Bog spavin is a distention of the tibiotarsal joint capsule of the hock, and a cause of swelling on the anteromedial aspect of the hock joint. Occasionally, smaller swellings appear on either side of the posterior surface of the hock at the junction of the tibial and fibular tarsal bones. Bog spavin does not usually cause lameness unless it is accompanied by a chip fracture or osteochondritis dissecans (degeneration of the cartilage).

Poor conformation can cause bog spavin, and a horse that is too straight in the hock joint will often develop this condition. In addition, quick stops and turns may lead to this condition in a horse with satisfactory conformation. A vitamin/mineral deficiency or imbalance of calcium, phosphorus, vitamin A, or vitamin D, can result in bog spavin, showing up particularly in horses six months to two years of age.

Treatment: If bog spavin is nutritional in origin, the horse's diet may be corrected by the addition of a vitamin/mineral supplement (refer to the text FEEDING TO WIN). The horse should also be dewormed (refer to "Control of Internal Parasites"). After treatment, bog spavin should disappear within four to six weeks.

If the bog spavin was caused by trauma, the veterinarian will drain the joint capsule and inject a corticosteroid. This therapy may be repeated two or three times at weekly intervals, but should be done only if radiography has revealed no bone changes. The corticosteroid will reduce the synovial lining inflammation and decrease the amount of excess synovial fluid produced. After the injection, an elastic pressure bandage should be applied to the hock area. The horse should receive three weeks of rest after the lameness has gone.

Chronic bog spavin does not usually respond to blistering, firing, or the injection of counterirritants. In fact, the injection of an irritant substance may lead to infectious arthritis (refer to "Arthritis"). None of these treatments should be used in conjunction with corticosteroid therapy. The veterinarian may perform a synovectomy to inactivate the synovial lining of the joint capsule.

Frequent massage, repeated several times daily for prolonged periods of time, may help reduce the swelling.

BONE SPAVIN

Bone spavin is an osteoarthritis that develops into ankylosing arthritis. It affects the medial aspect of the proximal end of the third metatarsal bone, as well as the medial aspects of the third and central tarsal bones. The joints which fuse together are the distal intertarsal and the tarsometatarsal joints.

Poor conformation, in the form of sickle and/or cow hocks, predisposes a horse to bone spavin because it increases stress on the medial aspect of the hock. In addition, a horse with narrow hocks is also likely to develop spavin. Therefore, a tendency to have bone spavin is inheritable. The trauma of quick stopping on hard surfaces can cause bone spavin in a normal horse, as can a mineral imbalance or deficiency.

A horse with bone spavin will "hike" the hip of the affected leg up, in order to lift the foot while flexing the hock as little as possible. The lowered foot arc causes a shortened stride, and the horse will tend to drag the foot, landing on the toe. This causes the characteristic short-toed, high-heeled foot.

The horse will place more weight on the outside of the hoof, and in mild cases lameness will disappear after the horse begins exercise. The spavin test will be positive for bone spavin (refer to "Leg and Foot Examination"), and radiographs will reveal bone changes in the hock joint.

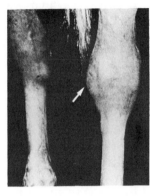

Fig. 6-38   Bone spavin of the hock on the right.

Bursitis of the cunean tendon may cause the same signs of lameness as bone spavin. The veterinarian can inject the bursa of the cunean tendon with a local anesthetic to determine how much of the lameness is due to bursitis. If this injection causes the lameness to disappear, a cunean tenectomy is indicated.

Treatment: Various procedures have been tried in the treatment of bone spavin, but have been successful only about 50% of the time. These treatments include firing over the distal tarsal bones, neurectomy, and blistering (which is useless). Corrective shoeing for bone spavin consists of raising the heels and rolling the toe to encourage breakover at the medial aspect of the horse's toe.

If the lameness is really due to bursitis of the cunean tendon, the veterinarian can perform a cunean tenectomy. This procedure is described in detail under "Surgical Procedures."

The best treatment for bone spavin is either surgically-induced or naturally-occurring arthrodesis (fusion) of the affected hock joint. The veterinarian can destroy the articular cartilage to hasten fusion of the joint. After surgery, the horse must be kept bandaged for two weeks, stalled for four weeks, and thereafter exercised to encourage ankylosis. Usually, the joint fuses completely within five months, although some horses require up to a year for joint ankylosis.

Alternatively, the horse can be continuously worked while receiving pain-relieving medication until the affected hock joint fuses itself. This process can take up to one year.

RUPTURED PERONEUS TERTIUS MUSCLE

Overextension of the hock can rupture the peroneus tertius muscle, thus enabling the stifle to flex without the hock flexing at the same time. This condition can be caused by a horse struggling to free a trapped hind leg, by a fast start from a stationary position, or by a wire cut on the anterior surface of the tibia. The horse will be hesitant to move the hind leg forward when the foot is off the ground. However, when the foot is on the ground, the leg will be able to bear weight and the horse will exhibit little pain. There will be a dimpling of the Achilles tendon, and it will be possible for the hock to be extended independently of the stifle.

Treatment: The only treatment for a ruptured peroneus tertius muscle is confinement for four to six weeks. This should be followed by very limited work over the next few months. Although most of these ruptures heal satisfactorily, overexercising the horse too soon will interfere with a complete recovery.

RUPTURED ACHILLES TENDON

The Achilles tendon may rupture when subjected to excessive stress, for example when a quick stop is made or the hock is overextended. When this occurs, the horse's hock drops and the angle of the joint increases. If both Achilles tendons are torn, the horse will adopt a squatting position. Unless the tendon is completely ruptured, the horse will be able to advance the affected leg and place weight on it.

Treatment: There is no satisfactory treatment for a ruptured Achilles tendon because the muscle ends are not in contact. In addition, a hematoma often fills in the area between the tendon ends, subsequently causing them to calcify and destroy muscle function. The rupture may heal, however, if the horse can be kept for six to twelve weeks in a sling to ease tension of the tendon, with the leg extended and immobilized in a splint or cast. Unfortunately, however, a horse will rarely tolerate a sling. In addition, the horse will require constant supervision while in the sling.

Stifle

GONITIS

Gonitis is a general term used to indicate stifle joint inflammation. Gonitis is most often attributed to chondromalacia (softening) of the

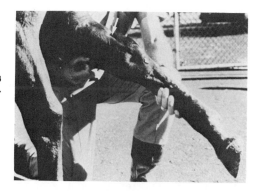

Fig. 6-39 If the peroneus tertius is ruptured, the stifle can flex independently of the hock.

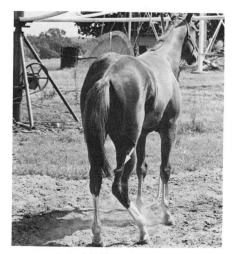

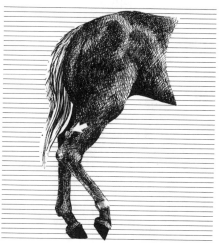

Fig. 6-40 Partial rupture of the Achilles tendon causes a dropped hock.

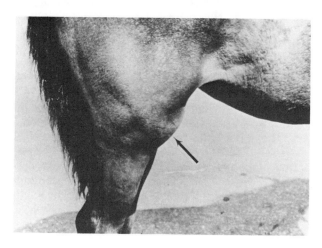

Fig. 6-41 Gonitis.

patella, but can also be caused by the following:

1. partial or complete upward fixation of the patella
2. damage to the medial collateral femorotibial or anterior cruciate ligaments
3. damage to the medial meniscus
4. osteochondritis dissecans (degeneration of the cartilage)

Trauma is usually the precipitating factor in the development of gonitis. To accurately identify the underlying condition, radiographs are necessary. Regardless of the cause of gonitis, there will be distension and thickening of the stifle joint capsule between the middle and lateral, and between the middle and medial patellar ligaments. The anterior phase of the horse's stride will be shortened because of pain associated with forward hindleg motion. To keep the foot off the ground, the horse will flex the stifle continuously or at least hold the foot in a raised heel, fetlock forward position. If one of the ligaments has been ruptured, crepitation will be evident.

Injury to one of the ligaments mentioned above will result in complete incapacitation and osteoarthritis (refer to "Arthritis"). Damage to the medial meniscus will cause constant joint effusion and chronic lameness, while chondromalacia of the patella will result in degeneration of the patellar articular cartilage due to inflammatory disease and/or upward fixation of the patella.

Treatment: There is no effective treatment for rupture of the medial collateral femorotibial or anterior cruciate ligaments, or for injury to the medial meniscus. Likewise, the prognosis for gonitis caused by osteoarthritis is poor. If the condition results from a damaged joint capsule or a slightly injured ligament, the horse may recover if kept stalled for a minimum of one month and confined to a small enclosure for a minimum of two months.

In treatment, the veterinarian may inject a corticosteroid into the joint, but only if the gonitis is definitely not due to suppurative arthritis, as corticosteroids are contraindicated in the presence of infection. Gonitis resulting from suppurative (infectious) arthritis can be treated by intra-articular and parenteral antibiotic injections (refer to "Arthritis").

UPWARD FIXATION OF THE PATELLA

Upward fixation of the patella occurs when the horse's patella catches in the medial condyle of the femur and locks the hind leg in extension. If the catching is only momentary, the horse will appear to have a "hitching" gait.

Poor hind limb conformation involving long, straight legs can predispose a horse to this condition. Other causes include trauma to the extended hind leg and excessive strenuous exercise for an improperly conditioned horse. Ligaments often stretch after the patella has locked, thereby increasing the chance of fixation recurring.

Treatment: When upward fixation of the patella first occurs, the horse is given a sedative and a sideline perhaps used to pull the leg forward and snap the patella back into position. Instead of employing a sideline, the horse may be startled into a sudden, backward movement which will sometimes replace the patella. Firing or blistering the stifle area will not cure this condition; its only effect is to limit extension of the limb by causing pain.

If the horse "hitches" without the patella actually locking, an injection of a strong counterirritant into the origin and insertion of the patellar ligament will sometimes tighten the patella, although this procedure must often be repeated. When upward fixation is present in a young horse, especially in one with poorly developed musculature, the veterinarian may decide to delay treatment until the horse is two years old in the hope that the condition will be outgrown. However, if the patella actually locks the leg in extension, the horse should be treated immediately, regardless of age.

The surgical correction for upward fixation of the patella is a medial patellar desmotomy. This operation is discussed in detail under "Surgical Procedures."

Hip Joint

COXITIS

Coxitis is an inflammation of the hip joint (coxofemoral joint) perhaps resulting from a slip, fall, or an infection. When resting, the injured horse will hold the affected foot in an advanced position with the weight off of it. The gluteal muscles will atrophy with disuse. When in motion, the horse will carry the foot forward and away from the body, often with the toe turned out, causing a gaited movement resembling a dog trot. If the horse is made to turn toward the affected side, the affected leg will give way. The veterinarian may draw some joint fluid for examination and use radiographs to reveal coxitis.

Treatment: The only treatment for coxitis is rest, accompanied by corticosteroid injections in the hip joint. Liniments and other external medications are of little benefit because they do not penetrate deep muscle masses.

DISLOCATION OF THE HIP JOINT

Trauma may cause dislocation of the hip joint to occur when a tired horse catches a foot and tries to free it or when a horse struggles against a sideline. As a result, the femur will move upward and forward, shortening the leg and causing the horse to limit the anterior phase of his stride. There will be swelling and crepitation of the hip joint and the toe and stifle will be turned out while the hock is turned in.

Treatment: Although a horse will not recover to complete working soundness after suffering a dislocated hip, the animal can often be salvaged for breeding purposes. Surgery is necessary to replace the head of the femur, which must remain in place for a period of three months for the muscles to strengthen enough to hold it. The veterinarian may surgically insert a pin to help keep the hip in position.

THROMBOSIS OF THE POSTERIOR AORTA OR ILIAC ARTERIES

The migration of **Strongylus vulgaris** larvae through arterial walls can cause thrombosis of the posterior aorta or iliac arteries. The resulting thrombi interfere with blood flow to the hind limbs, causing lameness. The lameness may disappear with rest, but reappear when the horse is exercised. Sometimes a horse with a small thrombus may be able to exercise strenuously before the onset of lameness, although the signs usually begin soon after the start of work.

Because of the relationship of exercise to the onset of lameness, thrombosis of the posterior aorta or the iliac arteries is sometimes mistaken for azoturia (refer to "Azoturia" under "Myositis"). The horse will sweat heavily and show pain and anxiety. The affected limb will feel cool and have a weaker pulse than the normal leg. If both legs have thrombi, the horse may be unable to support his hindquarters. Furthermore, this condition causes the veins on the affected leg to appear collapsed as compared to those of a normal limb, and the affected leg will not perspire.

Treatment: The veterinarian can sometimes diagnose thrombosis of the posterior aorta or iliac arteries on the basis of rectal palpation. There is no treatment for this condition; however, some horses eventually improve on their own. If the horse's condition worsens, euthanasia is considered the only humane alternative.

FEMORAL NERVE PARALYSIS (CRURAL PARALYSIS)

Paralysis of the femoral nerve affects the quadriceps femoris muscles. Azoturia can cause paralysis of this nerve by affecting the surrounding muscles, while trauma from kicking or overstretching the leg can also result in femoral nerve paralysis.

The affected horse will be unable to bear weight on the limb and will have difficulty in advancing the leg. All joints of the affected limb will be flexed, and the quadriceps femoris muscles will atrophy.

Treatment: Stall rest and massage may be of some benefit in the treatment of femoral nerve paralysis. If the horse begins to show signs of recovery, exercise will discourage muscle atrophy. The nerve will require at least one month to recover.

PELVIC FRACTURE

The pelvis can fracture through the shaft of the ilium, the tuber coxae, the symphysis pubis, or the obturator foramen. Trauma incurred from a horse falling on his side or from fighting a sideline can cause a fractured pelvis.

If the tuber coxae is broken, the hip will appear "knocked down" or flattened, and the skin may be broken by the protruding bone. A fractured shaft of the ilium will cause severe lameness and the horse will not place his foot on the ground. The affected limb will appear shortened, and the horse will exhibit obvious pain. Fracture of the symphysis pubis or the obturator foramen results in a limited anterior stride and halting gait. The veterinarian will diagnose a fractured pelvis on the basis of a rectal examination (refer to "Rectal Palpation"), and by the presence of crepitation and/or a large hematoma. It is possible for an iliac artery to be severed when the pelvis fractures. In this case, the horse will soon die from internal hemorrhage.

Treatment: Depending upon the severity of the case, the veterinarian may elect to surgically remove some of the bone fragments. Otherwise, the horse should be closely confined for a minimum of three months, with the first six to eight weeks spent in a sling (if possible). A fractured pelvis may require up to one year to heal. Consequently, in some cases, euthanasia is the most reasonable alternative.

Back

SACROILIAC JOINT SUBLUXATION (HUNTER'S BUMPS)

Dislocation of the articulation between the vertebral column and the pelvis is most commonly seen in horses used for hunting and jumping. It occurs when the tuber sacrale is pushed upward and forward because of torn ligament attachments, creating the "hunter's bump." At first, the horse will show pain and be reluctant to use the leg. The horse will have a shortened stride and may refuse to jump. The pain eventually decreases, but movement remains partially limited.

Treatment: Sacroiliac joint subluxation can best be treated by complete rest for several weeks. In chronic cases, the veterinarian may inject an irritant and the ventral sacroiliac ligament. This causes the formation of scar tissue, which will help immobilize the joint and facilitate healing. The horse should be gradually returned to exercise.

OVERRIDING DORSAL SPINOUS PROCESSES

Substantial back pain may be caused by overriding of the tips of the dorsal spinous processes. The veterinarian will check for this condition by noting any asymmetry of the pelvis, muscle atrophy of the hindquarters and back, or curvature of the spine. In addition, the veterinarian will note whether the horse flexes its back when the midline is pinched, as a failure to react may indicate the presence of bone lesions. The spaces between the tips of the dorsal spinous processes will be easily palpable in a normal horse, but not in an affected horse. The veterinarian may also inject a local anesthetic into these interspinous spaces and observe the horse's action after exercise to see if the pain has been lessened.

Treatment: To relieve the pain of overriding dorsal spinous processes, the veterinarian can surgically remove a short piece of each of the alternate spines. The horse can be walked within three to four days following this procedure, and gradually be returned to full work. ♞

7

DIGESTIVE SYSTEM

Colic

Abdominal pain in the equine is generally referred to as colic. Colic is a true medical emergency and requires immediate veterinary attention. This condition may result from a variety of primary and secondary causes, many of which are included in the following:

1. parasitism, especially large strongyles (perhaps 80-85% of all colics)
2. nutritional factors such as feed high in fiber or poor in quality; sudden changes in feed; and feed too high in energy
3. improper chewing, caused by poor teeth or mouth injuries
4. systemic disease, accompanied by fever and decreased feed and water consumption
5. circulatory disturbances such as embolism, infarction, and toxemia
6. digestive system infection, resulting in excessive gas production
7. neuromuscular disturbances
8. volvulus or torsion (twisting of the intestine)
9. lipomas (fatty tumors)
10. gastric dilatation caused by grain overload toxicity or bots

The pain of colic is caused either by obstruction of the ingesta, resulting in increased gas production that stretches the intestines, or by hyperactive peristalsis, i.e., spasms in the alimentary canal. (For information on colic in foals, refer to "Colic in Newborn Foals" under "Foal Diseases and Disorders.")

OBSTRUCTION

Obstruction may be caused by the collection of ingesta in the intestines at locations where the intestines turn or decrease in size, or it may be attributed to one of the following occurrences:

1. volvulus or torsion
2. hernia
3. reduced blood supply to the intestine
4. paralysis of the intestine
5. lipomas
6. intussusception (telescoping of the intestine)

The majority of these conditions can be relieved only through early surgical intervention. However, the prognosis in these cases is often poor.

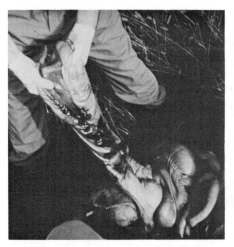 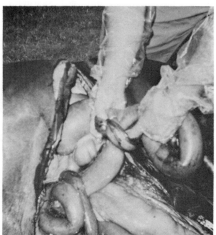

Fig. 7-1 Photograph of twisted intestines. Notice the knotting of the segment.

Fig. 7-2 After the twist is straightened out, the dark areas show the portions that have died from the pressure and lack of blood.

HYPERIRRITABILITY

Spasmodic colic is caused by increased peristalsis (intestinal contractions), and may be the result of an irritation affecting the mucosal surface, the neuromuscular junctions in the intestinal wall, or the central nervous system.

SIGNS OF COLIC

There are several characteristic signs that may be used in identifying suspected colic; these include:

1. lack of appetite
2. unusual attitudes or behavior
   a. biting at flanks
   b. kicking at the stomach
   c. lying down
   d. rolling
   e. restlessness
   f. anxious expression
   g. pawing
3. elevated skin temperature
4. sweating
5. increased and/or thready (weak, uneven) pulse

6. abnormal mucosa color
7. abnormal borborygmi (gut sounds)
8. abnormal feces or lack of feces
9. rising hematocrit (packed cell volume)

The expression of these signs varies with the individual horse and the particular kind of colic involved. However, the veterinarian should be contacted when a case of colic is suspected, as it is impossible to differentiate between mild and serious cases when they first appear. In particular, obstructive colic must be surgically corrected as soon as possible to give the horse its best chance of recovery.

DIAGNOSIS

Auscultating the gut sounds is a valuable tool in diagnosing colic. Increased gut sounds usually indicate spasmodic colic, while decreased or absent gut sounds may indicate obstructive colic (refer to "Auscultation"). The horse's response to pain-relieving medications is a means of evaluating the type of colic present. Simple, spasmodic colics respond well to pain-killing drugs. The veterinarian may also diagnose colic on the basis of rectal palpation, since a lack of feces indicates an acute obstructive colic.

Another procedure that will help indicate the type of colic and the advisability of surgery is paracentesis (puncturing the abdominal cavity with a sterile needle). In obstructive colic, volvulus or torsion will cause the white blood cells and bacteria present in the abdominal fluid to increase in number, and will cause the color of the abdominal fluid to darken (this will be revealed by paracentesis). Fecal material found in the fluid indicates that the intestines have already ruptured, in which case euthanasia is recommended (refer to "Abdominal Paracentesis").

TREATMENT

Suspected cases of colic require veterinary diagnosis and/or treatment. In each case, the horse should be kept calm and relaxed until the veterinarian arrives. A horse that will stand or lie quietly should be allowed to rest. If the animal begins to roll, it should be coaxed to its feet and walked, preferably over a soft, grassy area, to reduce the chances of injury or twisting of the gut. Obstructive colic, which causes severe, unremitting pain, may cause the horse to become extremely violent, in which case the animal's handler should be careful to keep safely out of the way.

Phenylbutazone and pentazocine (Talwin) are often administered by the veterinarian to relieve the pain of colic. The administration of sedatives by the horseman, however, is not suggested since, if the horse goes into shock, such medication will only cause further depression. Dipyrone (Novin), an analgesic anti-inflammatory drug, is also commonly used. The administration of pain relievers and muscle relaxants should be left to the veterinarian. In nearly all cases, mineral oil will be administered through a stomach tube.

In addition, to facilitate elimination, the veterinarian may administer a fecal softener such as dioctyl sodium sulfosuccinate. After this treatment, it is often recommended that the horse be walked until he begins to properly eliminate feces. The hematocrit may be monitored during treatment, as a rise in hematocrit indicates the need for intravenous fluid therapy. The veterinarian may administer as much as 20 liters in an hour. The horse should be carefully watched for at least 24 hours after the signs of colic are relieved, because the condition may recur. The grain ration should be reduced considerably at the next feeding, and bran may be added as a laxative. The horse's feed should then be gradually increased over a period of several days until the normal amount is reached.

SURGICAL INTERVENTION

Depending upon the cause of the obstruction, the veterinarian may be able to massage the obstruction rectally and unblock the intestine. When necessary, the veterinarian will open the abdominal cavity and locate the obstruction. Again depending on the cause, the veterinarian will attempt correction of the obstruction by reducing a hernia, removing an involved piece of intestine, correcting an intussusception, etc. Intestinal anastomosis, the removal of a devitalized section of the intestine, followed by the surgical apposition of the healthy ends, is discussed fully elsewhere in the book. Prompt surgery can possibly save horses afflicted with obstructive colic, depending on how soon the condition is diagnosed and the surgery performed.

PREVENTION

Like many other equine ailments, colic is more easily prevented than treated. A good deworming program is especially essential in controlling the large strongyle populations responsible for verminous colic. It is also important, however, because the larvae of **Strongylus vulgaris** damage the intestinal blood supply, thus causing a predisposition to colic in horses that are stressed.

Horses that colic frequently due to high numbers of migrating larvae of **Strongylus vulgaris** may be helped by one or two tubings with a larvicidal dose of an anthelmintic such as thiabendazole. If two larvicidal doses are given, they are administered two to thirty days apart.

Below is presented a list of preventive measures which, if adhered to, should be beneficial in lessening the occurrence of colic.

1. Follow a regular deworming program.
2. Arrange for regular dental care.
3. Feed on a precise schedule.
4. Feed small amounts three times daily, rather than larger amounts less frequently.
5. Changes in feed rations should be made gradually, over a period of 3 to 4 days.

6. Always feed high-quality rations.

7. Feed the horse hay before grain.

8. Always provide a constant supply of clean, fresh water.

9. During exercise, allow the horse frequent access to water.

10. After exercise, give a hot horse only small amounts of water while cooling out before allowing him free access to water.

11. Have available ample quantities of quality hay, salt, and minerals.

Diarrhea

Diarrhea is a sign of a disease, not a disease itself. It may be caused by infection, overeating, stress, poisoning, etc. The following discussion contains comments on some of the most common causes of diarrhea and their treatment.

PROTOZOAL DIARRHEA

This type of diarrhea is caused by stress that allows the rapid multiplication of **Trichomonas.** It can be peracute, acute, or chronic.

Peracute: This variety causes the horse to have soft feces that resemble cow manure. The affected horse may recover spontaneously within a month.

Acute: With this diarrheal form, the horse has a severe, watery, greenish diarrhea. At first, there are no gut sounds, but a splashing noise eventually becomes audible. The horse with acute diarrhea usually becomes listless and depressed and loses his appetite. Fever will be in the range of 103° to 108°F, and death can occur within 24 hours.

Chronic: This condition causes emaciation and dehydration, even though the horse's appetite may actually increase. Laminitis is a possible development.

Treatment: Acute and chronic protozoal diarrhea should be treated soon after the signs are discovered. Therapy involves the administration of a trichomonacide and fluids and electrolytes. The veterinarian may try to re-establish the normal intestinal flora (bacteria) by giving the horse a mixture of feces from a healthy horse and water via a stomach tube.

SALMONELLOSIS

Salmonellosis is an infectious disease that can cause diarrhea, endotoxemia, septicemia, internal abscesses, abortion, and death. This condition is stress-related and may be precipitated by surgery, deworming, or bad weather. The horse's age, level of nutrition, and parasite load are all factors that affect the development of salmonellosis.

Acute: Acute salmonellosis lasts from 12 to 48 hours and is characterized by depression, anorexia, and a slight temperature. The diarrhea is profuse and watery, perhaps containing blood and shreds of mucosa. The horse will have an elevated pulse (80 to 100 beats/minute) and bluish-colored membranes (refer to "Vital Functions"). A horse suffering from acute salmonellosis may become dehydrated, and may even go into shock.

Chronic: Chronic salmonellosis appears during times of stress. The horse, however, can become a chronic carrier of the disease.

Treatment: A bacterial culture and sensitivity test should be run immediately when salmonellosis is suspected. Treatment of salmonellosis should be begun soon after the signs of the disease appear. The veterinarian will administer oral and parenteral antibiotics, oral and intravenous fluids and electrolytes, and intestinal astringents. Corticosteroids and antihistamines are given for shock. The veterinarian may also decide on fluid therapy for the horse.

COLITIS-X

The suspected cause of Colitis-X is stress, since it commonly precedes the disease's appearance by one or two weeks. Typical stress situations include racing, shipping, affliction with respiratory disease, surgery, deworming, and hot weather. Signs of Colitis-X appear suddenly, and the course of the disease is short. The associated diarrhea is non-bloody and is accompanied by:

1. severe depression
2. weakness
3. dehydration
4. weak, rapid pulse
5. dyspnea (difficulty in breathing)
6. shock
7. bluish-purple mucosa color
8. normal or subnormal temperature

Colitis-X is an extremely serious condition and many affected horses die within 48 hours.

Treatment: The veterinarian will test the horse for dehydration and electrolyte levels, then rapidly administer fluids, electrolytes, corticosteroids, antibiotics, and intestinal astringents.

DIARRHEA ASSOCIATED WITH HEAVY METAL POISONING

The ingestion of certain metals can cause diarrhea and other complications. (For detailed information on poisoning, refer to "Toxic Substances.")

Arsenic Poisoning: Arsenic poisoning may result from ingestion of and/or contamination from dips, sprays, weed killers, paint, or medications containing arsenic. The poisoned horse will have a profuse, bloody diarrhea containing small pieces of intestinal mucosa. Other signs of arsenic poisoning include colic, dehydration, shock, increased pulse, muscle tremors, and dyspnea.

Treatment: Arsenic poisoning must be treated as soon as it is suspected. Unfortunately, once the signs of poisoning appear, there is no successful treatment. Therapy involves the administration of an oily laxative and sulphur (to tie up the arsenic). The horse will require supportive care for recovery (refer to "Basic Care of a Sick Horse").

Lead Poisoning: Lead can be accidentally ingested by the horse through old paint, car batteries, and lead shot. Boiled linseed oil also contains lead, and is meant only for use in paints; it is quite toxic and should never be fed to a horse as a substitute for raw linseed oil. A horse suffering from lead poisoning may be emaciated and develop colic, paralysis, or anemia. He may also become a "roarer."

Treatment: The veterinarian can give the horse several substances that will precipitate the lead and make it unabsorbable. These substances are chelating agents that preferentially bond the metal in a non-ionized soluble substance that is readily excreted in the urine. The drug commonly preferred is calcium-EDTA. In addition, the veterinarian will treat whatever signs have developed, such as colic or anemia.

Mercury Poisoning: Mercury is found in treated seed grain, blistering agents, and antiseptics. A horse poisoned by mercury will suddenly develop diarrhea, depression, and colic.

Treatment: Eggs, milk, and serum can be administered to the horse to tie up the mercury. In addition, the veterinarian will give fluids to protect the horse's kidneys from damage (refer to "Fluid and Electrolyte Therapy").

DIETARY ENTERITIS

Dietary enteritis is a type of digestive upset and is usually caused by either excessive intake of grain, by ingestion of poor quality or spoiled feed, or by coprophagy. The ingestion of too much grain is a serious problem in the equine, and may result in abnormal mucosa color, loose feces containing undigested grain, and even severe colic and laminitis. When the consumption of moldy feed is the suspected cause of enteritis, the horse may develop diarrhea, excessive gas, and may show a loss of appetite. In a severe case of dietary enteritis, central nervous system damage and even death may result.

Treatment: The veterinarian will give the horse mineral oil, antibiotics, antihistamines, fluids, and vitamins.

MYCOTIC (FUNGAL) AND BACTERIAL DIARRHEA

An overdose of oral antibiotics can destroy normal intestinal microorganisms and may allow other microorganisms, such as **Aspergillus**, to rapidly increase. When a horse develops this type of mycotic or bacterial diarrhea, he will usually have a normal temperature and be alert.

Treatment: The veterinarian may give the horse a fluid, made from a healthy horse's feces combined with water, through a stomach tube to restore the normal intestinal flora.

CROUPOUS ENTERITIS

This noninfectious diarrhea is the result of retention of oxalic acid in the horse's blood and may be caused by feeds high in oxalates, such as beet tops. The diarrhea associated with croupous enteritis is watery and often contains bloody streaks. The horse will initially appear restless, but will eventually become depressed. The temperature remains normal. The veterinarian can palpate the thickened intestinal wall resulting from this condition during a rectal examination.

Treatment: Mineral oil and antibiotics, intestinal protectants and astringents are given to a horse suffering from croupous enteritis. The horse should recover within a week to ten days.

OTHER CAUSES OF DIARRHEA

Diarrhea can also be caused by such conditions as infestation with internal parasites, poor teeth, and organophosphate poisoning. If the cause is gastric ulcers, abdominal pain will be one of the prominent signs of illness. In each case, the underlying cause of the disease must be treated (refer to "Control of Internal Parasites," "Dentistry," and "Toxic Substances").

Emaciation

Common causes of emaciation (muscle wasting and weight-loss) are bad teeth, parasites, enteritis, and starvation. These conditions cause emaciation by decreasing the horse's ability to properly digest feed, by hindering the absorption of nutrients, or by interfering with the amount of food the horse can metabolize through direct restriction of feed intake.

STARVATION

Each horse varies in his nutrient requirements according to several factors, among which are:

age	season of the year
sex	pregnancy
work load	lactation
temperament	

Starvation is often caused by an overcrowded pasture situation and by ignorance on the part of the horse's caretaker. For instance, non-aggressive horses may starve if not fed on an individual basis. Parasitism, poor teeth, and disease are often associated with malnutrition.

As lack of feed depletes a horse's glycogen stores, he begins to burn up fat and muscle, gradually weakens, and develops a long, dull haircoat and potbelly. Specific signs of deficiencies may appear (refer to "Vitamins and Minerals"), and infertility in the mare or stallion may develop. Eventually, the animal may go down and die of circulatory failure. (For information detailing feeding of a horse, refer to the text FEEDING TO WIN.)

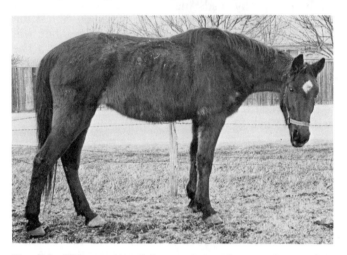

Fig. 7-3 This emaciated horse shows the muscle wasting that is characteristic of this condition.

Treatment: The horse's diet must obviously be increased and improved, but care should be taken to avoid digestive upset and laminitis. To build up an emaciated horse, a high-quality hay should be supplied at all times, and the horse should be gradually introduced to a high-quality grain ration. Since weight gain is desired, the grain should be gradually increased, and the final ration should be greater in amount, and higher in energy content than the maintenance ration.

BAD TEETH

Sharp teeth, root abscesses, and decayed teeth can all cause improper chewing, a process that results in the substantial spilling and wasting of feed. Moreover, improperly chewed grain has not had its hull cracked and so cannot be properly digested. The teeth should be checked when an excessive amount of whole grain is passed in the feces, since this is one of the first signs of dental problems.

Treatment: If the teeth have sharp edges, hooks or points, or if the horse has wave or shear mouth, the veterinarian will file off the offending tooth projections. Broken and infected teeth will have to be extracted (refer to "Floating the Teeth" and "Dentistry").

PARASITISM

Heavy parasitism is a very common cause of emaciation in horses because of the continual reinfestation of the horse that occurs in a normal stable environment. Parasites cause emaciation by interfering with the animal's ability to digest and absorb nutrients.

Treatment: A good deworming program is absolutely necessary for all horses, and is more economical than attempting to feed a parasitized horse enough to keep him in good condition. (Refer to "Control of Internal Parasites" for recommendations on deworming schedules and anthelmintics.)

CHRONIC DISEASE

Heaves, equine infectious anemia, and other chronic diseases may cause emaciation in the horse. For the horse to reverse its emaciated condition, the disease must be diagnosed and treated by the veterinarian.

NEOPLASIA

A neoplasm (cancer) is another cause of emaciation. An abnormal mass may be detected in the abdominal or pelvic cavity by the veterinarian during a rectal examination, indicating the presence of a neoplasm.

Surgical excision of this growth may be possible, or the veterinarian may rely on radiation therapy.

Salivation

Excessive salivation can be a sign of choke, fractured jaw, or several other disorders. The cause of salivation may be as obvious as a foreign object lodged in the mouth, or as obscure as organophosphate poisoning.

CHOKE

Choke occurs when an object lodges in the horse's esophagus. Unlubricated boluses, clumps of dry feed, and pieces of wood or wire are some of the more commonly swallowed objects. Small ponies are especially prone to choke on large boluses. Greedy eaters that bolt their feed are very susceptible to choke, as are older horses with poor teeth. It is sometimes helpful to place several large, smooth stones in the feed bin of a greedy eater. Eating around the stones will slow the animal's rate of feed consumption.

The horse that is affected will swallow repeatedly in an attempt to move the obstruction down the esophagus. Other signs include an anxious expression and walking around in circles. As the condition progresses, saliva and food will come out through the horse's nostrils. If the condition remains for 18 to 36 hours, the horse will become depressed and the tissue around the obstruction will swell. Pressure necrosis may begin to destroy the esophageal wall.

Treatment: Choke caused by grain packed in the esophagus may be corrected spontaneously when saliva is produced and the obstruction softens. The horse should be cross-tied at this time to prevent it from eating or drinking, and if the animal does not recover within a couple of hours, the veterinarian should be contacted. If necessary, the horse may be given a drug to increase salivation. The veterinarian may also administer a drug, such as xylazine, which acts as a tranquilizer and muscle relaxant to reduce esophageal spasms without lowering blood pressure. If the condition persists, a stomach tube can be passed to try and move the mass towards the stomach, or water may be injected down the tube to try and flush the grain away. When choke has continued for more than 24 hours, the horse will require fluids and electrolytes intravenously.

The veterinarian may choose to place the horse under general anesthesia and insert an endotracheal tube before the stomach tube is passed. This method ensures that fluid and grain do not accidentally pass down the trachea and reduces the risk of foreign body pneumonia. Flushing the esophagus with plain water will generally relieve choke in the anesthetized horse.

When the obstruction is lodged near the top of the esophagus, the veterinarian may be able to break up the mass with a surgical instrument.

Because of the risk of scar and stricture formation, which can predispose the horse to future choke, surgical intervention is considered only as a last resort. Similar scar formation may occur in cases of choke that are not resolved for two or three days. This is due to scar formation that occurs when the severely damaged mucosal wall heals. The horse should be given antibiotics during recovery from choke.

FOREIGN BODY IN THE MOUTH

The presence of a foreign body lodged in the mouth may cause salivation by irritating the mucosal lining of the mouth. Cockleburs and awns (plant barbs) from weedy hay are commonly caught in the mouth, but larger objects such as sticks and splinters are also sometimes found. The affected horse will probably be reluctant to eat.

Treatment: The foreign body must, of course, be removed, after which the wound can be flushed with saline solution. Until the wound heals, it should be frequently checked to ascertain that feed is not lodging in the horse's mouth at the wound site.

FRACTURED JAW

The jaw, or mandible, may be fractured by a fall or kick, or by tooth repulsion (refer to "Dentistry"). A fairly common cause of fractured jaws is the horse catching its lower jaw on an object such as a stall latch. When the horse pulls back to free itself, the jaw breaks (usually through the interdental space). Another possible cause of jaw fracture is misuse of a bit.

Signs of a fractured jaw include salivation, swelling, and malocclusion of the incisor teeth. A fractured jaw causes the horse to be reluctant to open its mouth and may cause paralysis of the tongue.

Treatment: Several methods of treatment exist. The veterinarian may wire the teeth or bone fragments together or apply intramedullary nails, screws, or pins to hold the jaw in place. The latter method may damage the tooth buds of a young horse that does not yet have a full mouth.

The veterinarian will remove any bone sequestra (bone fragments minus their blood supply) present. If the fracture is severe, the horse may be fed through an indwelling stomach tube for a week or two. Otherwise, a soft diet can be fed for several weeks.

The horse will require supportive antibiotic therapy during recovery, and the horse's teeth will require frequent checking for signs of uneven wear.

ORGANOPHOSPHATE POISONING

Excess salivation is one of the signs of organic phosphate toxicity. Refer to "Toxic Substances" for more information.

8

RESPIRATORY SYSTEM

Cough

Since a cough is only a sign of an underlying problem, no medication should be administered before the primary cause is identified. A cough often results from an allergy, or from a viral or bacterial respiratory infection. In addition, a cough is often caused by dusty living quarters or feed, and can even result from the migration of internal parasites. Various preparations are available to suppress cough itself, and should only be used in conjunction with the primary treatment. These preparations contain antitussives, expectorants, and antihistamines.

Equine Influenza

Equine influenza is an acute, highly contagious inflammation of the upper respiratory tract caused by the influenza virus A/equi 1 or A/equi 2. This disease is characterized by a dry cough lasting up to three weeks, a moderate to high fever (102-106°F; 39-41°C) for one to four days, and a serous nasal discharge for five to ten days. An affected horse will be depressed, have difficulty breathing, and exhibit muscular weakness and soreness.

In very old and very young horses, influenza may eventually involve the heart. As with any disease, equine influenza increases a horse's susceptibility to other infections, and complications such as a secondary bacterial infection or pneumonia will inhibit recovery.

Equine influenza spreads rapidly among susceptible horses. The disease occurs frequently in young horses after they have been moved to new surroundings and are exposed to a different group of horses.

Treatment: Equine influenza may be prevented by the administration of influenza vaccines. Horses are less susceptible to the disease when they are healthy, well-fed, and protected from chills in draft-free stalls.

A horse with influenza should be kept isolated and provided with individual feed and water buckets. To reduce irritating dust, hay and grain should be slightly dampened before they are fed. The animal should also be kept warm (with blankets if necessary) in a ventilated, dry stall. A minimum of ten days' rest after all signs of disease are gone is essential for a complete recovery.

If a horse with peracute equine influenza has great difficulty breathing, the veterinarian may administer oxygen therapy. In addition, a secondary bacterial infection will require antibiotic therapy. Corticosteroids are administered when shock is eminent, and the horse should receive a balanced electrolyte solution.

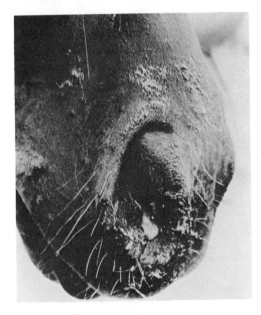

Fig. 8-1 A nasal discharge is a sign of many respiratory ailments, such as influenza or rhinopneumonitis.

Rhinopneumonitis

Rhinopneumonitis is a viral infection that affects mainly young horses (after weaning) and pregnant mares. Occurring most often in late fall and early winter, rhinopneumonitis is not considered exceedingly dangerous in weanlings, though there may be a high incidence of abortions in affected mares. The disease is characterized by fever (102-105°F), nasal discharge, cough, swelling of the eyelids, inflammation of upper respiratory passages, and lack of appetite (all of which will increase in severity after exercise). Like many other respiratory conditions, rhinopneumonitis is easily transmitted from the infected animal to other animals by direct exposure, inhalation of discharges, and ingestion of contaminated materials.

Treatment: When the veterinarian has diagnosed rhinopneumonitis, he may suggest antibacterial treatment to prevent secondary infection and prescribe a period of rest. In the likelihood of an outbreak, the veterinarian may vaccinate all horses which are likely to be affected and quarantine any new horses for a two-week period.

Viral Arteritis

This infectious disease occurs at infrequent intervals and is usually not fatal. However, the disease may still be serious, even if not fatal, since it leads to a partial degeneration of arterial walls (especially small arteries), possibly followed by blood clotting and hemorrhaging. Pregnant mares that are affected usually have a high incidence of abortions. In the case of an outbreak, the veterinarian may vaccinate any exposed horses to prevent the spread of viral arteritis.

Viral arteritis is spread by direct contact with an infected animal, by inhalation of droplets in the air, and by ingestion of contaminated materials and feed. The signs of this disease are common to respiratory diseases and include high fever (102-106°F), nasal discharge, swelling of the limbs and eyelids, excessive lacrimation, coughing, loss of appetite, and stiffness in the horse's gaits. A laboratory examination may be required for complete and correct diagnosis.

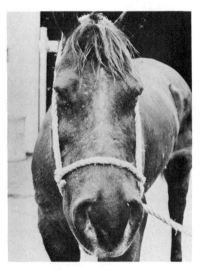

Fig. 8-2 Swelling of the eyelids and head is a typical sign of viral arteritis [swelling of the legs also occurs].

Treatment: Treatment of viral arteritis consists of the administration of antibiotics to prevent secondary bacterial infections, and adequate rest. The affected horse should be housed in warm, draft-free stabling, and rested for several weeks after the signs of the disease have subsided.

Strangles

Strangles is a contagious disease affecting mainly young horses. It is caused by the **Streptococcus equi** or **Streptococcus zooepidemicus** bacteria and is easily transmitted from one horse to another through nasal discharges. However, it may also be indirectly contracted from contaminated feed, pasture, water troughs, etc. The characteristic signs of strangles include the following:

1. swelling of lymph glands in the head and neck
2. a high fever (103-106°F)
3. a thick mucus nasal discharge of yellowish pus
4. stiff extension of the neck
5. hesitancy to eat or drink (due to difficulty in swallowing)
6. a painful, moist cough

Treatment: Immediate treatment of strangles begins with isolating the infected animal(s) and includes antibiotic therapy with penicillin and streptomycin or sulfa drugs to prevent systemic complications.

The abscesses of the lymph nodes associated with strangles are generally not opened surgically, but may instead be encouraged to break and drain with applications of warm compresses. Also, since drainage of the abscesses prompts disappearance of clinical signs, any treatment to prevent their draining may not be recommended.

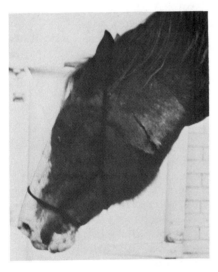

Fig. 8-3 In this case of strangles, the veterinarian surgically incised and drained the submandibular lymph nodes.

There is a strangles vaccine available for disease prevention which can be given to horses on premises where the disease is a problem. Sick, recovered, or exposed horses should not be vaccinated, as an attack of strangles usually produces permanent immunity.

Pneumonia

Pneumonia is an inflammation of the lungs that usually occurs as a secondary complication to a debilitating disease. It often results from the mismanagement of a sick animal. Young horses tend to suffer from acute pneumonia, while older animals usually have chronic pneumonia. Systemic disease, parasitism, malnutrition, and exhaustion are all predisposing factors. A mild, viral, upper respiratory infection may result in pneumonia because of secondary bacterial infection.

Aspiration pneumonia can result from the presence of a foreign body in the lungs. Causes of this type of pneumonia include accidental passage of a stomach tube into the trachea, inhalation of particles of food, and smoke inhalation.

Signs of pneumonia include an elevated temperature (104-106°F), difficulty in breathing, nasal discharge, depression, and cough. The veterinarian will auscultate the lungs to determine the degree of congestion and the stage of pneumonia present. Percussion of a horse with pneumonia will reveal a dull sound. Radiographs will show lung lesions in some bacterial and fungal pneumonias.

Treatment: Good nursing care is of paramount importance in the proper treatment of pneumonia, and the horse should be kept in a warm, dry, well-ventilated stall. The veterinarian may perform tracheal aspiration in order to conduct antibiotic sensitivity tests. Antibiotic therapy should be continued for at least one week after the horse appears normal.

The veterinarian may administer an enzyme solution intra-tracheally to aid the horse in expelling exudates. The use of inhalation therapy or nebulization (misting) will allow the horse to breathe antibiotic and antibacterial agents in droplet form. A horse with pneumonia will require complete rest for two to three weeks in order to fully recover from the disease.

Pharyngitis

Pharyngitis, or inflammation of the pharynx, is a common upper respiratory problem in horses. Pharyngitis often causes abnormal respiration sounds, chronic coughing, and epistaxis, though at times the only disease sign is the horse's inability to perform. Pharyngitis is usually secondary to viral or bacterial infection, and in many cases these infections involve the guttural pouch. A laryngoscopic examination may be used to reveal the thickened and roughened walls of the pharynx.

Possible causes of pharyngitis include viruses, bacteria, stress, changes in airflow patterns, and air pollution, but the exact cause of this condition remains unknown. Because of the high incidence of pharyngitis, some authorities believe that there may be genetic or nutritional causes involved.

Treatment: A variety of treatments have been used with varying degrees of success in the therapy of pharyngitis. Either electrical or chemical cautery is sometimes used to remove any polyps that occur. This procedure increases airflow but does nothing to remedy the disease's cause.

Antibiotic infusions of the guttural pouches have also been employed in treatment. Afterwards, the horse will have a profuse nasal discharge for

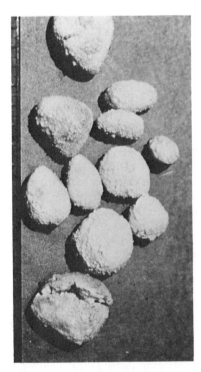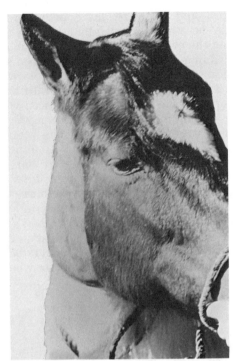

Fig. 8-4 Pus, from a guttural pouch infection resulting in pharyngitis, could harden into masses. These masses were removed from the guttural pouch of the horse shown.

one to two weeks and must be rested (refer to "Draining the Guttural Pouches"). Bacterins made from bacteria and viruses found in the horse's throat may be beneficial.

There is no one specific remedy for pharyngitis, and the attending veterinarian will use treatments that in his experience and estimation may offer relief.

Heaves

This condition may be hereditary or it may be caused by an allergic reaction (such as to mold or dust), by over-exercise without sufficient warm-up, by smog, or perhaps even by psychological problems. Treatment for heaves is designed to relieve the primary signs rather than cure the disease, though therapy conducted soon after the horse develops heaves may alleviate or arrest the condition itself.

Since mold and dust may be causative factors, the horse should not be fed hay. Instead, a complete pelleted ration using beet pulp as the roughage may be fed. If the feces become soft, the beet pulp should be stopped and a low-roughage pellet provided for the horse. The horse should be watched carefully when on pasture, as some lush fields can worsen the condition. If the animal cannot be kept in pasture, he should be stabled in a stall with either damp wood shavings or rubber mats.

Because heaves may have a psychological basis, the affected horse should be treated gently. Many animals with heaves appear nervous and display the signs of this condition when faced with an unusual circumstance (e.g., when moved into strange surroundings).

Treatment: Corticosteroids are often administered in acute cases of heaves and an expectorant, such as an organic iodide, given to relieve signs of bronchitis. A severely affected horse may also require antibacterial injections since infection can contribute to the seriousness of the disease. Heaves caused by allergic reactions sometimes respond to bronchial dilators, but these cannot be administered for long periods of time.

The best prognosis is achieved when good management is provided. The horse should be removed from dusty surroundings, fed a pelleted ration, and worked less. Exercise should be discontinued when the horse experiences difficulty in breathing or when there is coughing.

Epistaxis (Nosebleed)

Epistaxis most commonly occurs in racehorses, either during or after exercise. The bleeding may originate from the horse's lungs or nasal passages. Bleeding from one nostril usually indicates it is nasal in origin, while bilateral epistaxis implies that it originates in the lungs. The precise cause of epistaxis is not known, but may be associated with a rise in blood pressure and increased air flow during exertion which can rupture the fragile capillaries in the nostrils, turbinates and/or lungs. Other potential causes of epistaxis include trauma from stomach tubing or facial bone injury, pneumonia, blood platelet defects, and equine infectious anemia.

The veterinarian can use an endoscope to examine the nasal passages to discover the origin of bleeding. He may insert a needle into the trachea to discover if the blood is coming from a pulmonary hemorrhage; if so, a bloody froth will appear through the needle.

Treatment: Immediate treatment of epistaxis involves packing the nasal passage with a tampon or cotton, but only one nostril should be packed at a time. The veterinarian may flush the horse's nasal passage with an aqueous epinephrine solution. The animal should receive only limited exercise while recovering, as stress could cause a recurrence of bleeding.

Vitamin K and vitamin C are both used in the treatment of epistaxis; vitamin K because it improves blood-clotting ability, and vitamin C because it facilitates wound healing. If a varicose vein in the nasal passage is believed to be the cause of bleeding, the veterinarian can cauterize it.

Furosemide (Lasix) is the diuretic drug most commonly used in treating epistaxis. It is believed to work, at least in part, by lowering the horse's systemic blood pressure and, perhaps, by decreasing blood pressure within the lungs (refer to "Drugs and Related Topics"). ♞

9

CENTRAL NERVOUS SYSTEM

Some of the diseases which disturb the central nervous system of the equine manifest similar irregularities in body functions and behavior. Abnormalities such as muscle spasms, tremors, convulsions, wandering, and head pressing indicate an interruption in the normal function of the central nervous system. The diseases that commonly display these signs are encephalomyelitis, rabies, tetanus, and the wobbler syndrome. (Refer to "Wobbler Syndrome" under "Lameness.") Toxic substances may also cause central nervous system problems. (Refer to "Toxic Substances" under "Drugs and Related Topics.")

Encephalomyelitis

Encephalomyelitis is a viral disease which is transmitted by insect vectors. Insects such as mosquitoes and biting flies become carriers by feeding on an infected host (usually birds or rodents). The infected insect carries the virus in the salivary glands and, after an incubation period, may infect a horse on which it feeds. Because of the method of transmission, encephalomyelitis is more prevalent in the summer when the number of biting insects is greatest.

The three major types of encephalomyelitis that affect equines are: Eastern equine encephalomyelitis (EEE), Western equine encephalomyelitis (WEE), and Venezuelan equine encephalomyelitis (VEE). Of the three types, EEE is the most serious in horses, having a 90% mortality rate, in comparison to the 50% mortality rate of WEE.

All three types of equine encephalomyelitis have similar signs. Usually, the affected horse will exhibit some of the following characteristics:

1. elevated temperature
2. depression
3. blindness
4. muscle tremors
5. paralysis
6. excessive periods of sleep
7. incoordination
8. drooped lips
9. inability to swallow

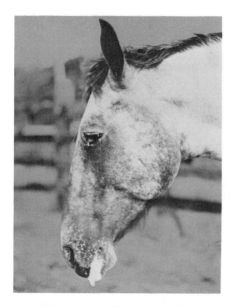

Fig. 9-1 This horse with VEE shows the foaming at the mouth that may result from the horse's inability to swallow.

Encephalomyelitis may additionally cause the horse to exhibit extremely unusual behavior, such as wandering around aimlessly, walking into walls, and attempting to climb trees.

A mild case of encephalomyelitis may run its course in one or two weeks, but acute encephalomyelitis usually results in death within two or three days. The horse will generally have a better chance of recovering if it remains standing. If the animal goes down within the first 48 hours, or remains recumbent for more than 24 hours, the prognosis is poor. Unfortunately, even if the horse survives, in some cases the central nervous system damage is permanent. These horses become "dummies" and are no longer useful as performance animals.

Treatment: There is no specific treatment for encephalomyelitis, besides seeing that the horse gets good nursing care. The veterinarian may administer diuretics and anti-inflammatory drugs, but he will basically provide supportive therapy. The affected horse should be protected from insects and confined to reduce the danger of an accidental, self-induced injury. A sling may be used to keep the horse standing, and an ice pack applied to the horse's head may help relieve pressure and disorientation.

Rabies

Rabies is an extremely virulent disease which results in death. Horses and all other mammals are susceptible to the virus, but domestic dogs and wild animals, such as skunks, bats, foxes, and squirrels, are the major carriers. Since there is such a variety of carriers, and because human immunization procedures are extremely complex and painful, this disease is also a public health hazard.

Although the bite wound, which is the origin of the horse's infection, may show an inflammatory reaction, the signs of the disease may not appear for some time. The incubation period for rabies in horses is anywhere from three weeks to three months, depending upon the location of the bite and the amount of saliva deposited.

The affected animal has great difficulty in swallowing food or water. Extreme caution should be exercised in handling any horse suspected of being exposed to rabies, since a horse that has contracted the disease will characteristically become hyperexcitable, and exhibit aggressive behavior. The horse may bite itself at the wound site, and salivate excessively. Other signs include an increased respiration and pulse rate, muscle spasms, and tremors. Eventually, the animal will experience convulsions and paralysis in the hindlegs. Once the horse becomes recumbent, death follows within a few hours.

Although horses are not routinely immunized against this disease, rabies can be prevented by vaccination, and it may be wise to vaccinate horses in areas where the disease is prevalent (refer to "A Good Vaccination Program").

Treatment: Strict quarantine of suspected cases is strongly recommended since there is no treatment for rabies other than euthanasia. The veterinarian will notify state health authorities, and brain and serum samples will be required to positively identify the disease.

Tetanus

Tetanus, also known as lockjaw, is a disease caused by a neurotoxin produced in the body by **Clostridium tetani** bacteria. This bacterium is a normal inhabitant in the intestinal tract of the horse, as well as in soil. It is anaerobic in nature, meaning that it cannot multiply in the presence of oxygen, and is produced only under anaerobic conditions. The anaerobic environment of some wounds, particularly puncture wounds, provides ideal conditions for the growth of the bacteria.

Since even a minute lesion may be an entry site of **Clostridium tetani** bacteria, a horse should be maintained on a tetanus toxoid immunization program. If an unprotected horse is wounded or subjected to surgery, tetanus antitoxin should be administered prophylactically to provide a few weeks of defense against the bacteria. Provided the horse is on a good tetanus immunization program, only a tetanus toxoid booster will be needed to ensure a high level of immunity.

Tetanus can develop anywhere from a few days to several weeks after an injury has occurred. When infection with the bacteria becomes established, the toxin travels by way of nerve trunks to the central nervous system. The affected horse will be reluctant to move, and when forced to do so, will move stiffly, flexing the joints as little as possible. The tail will be raised, and the head and neck will be held in an extended position. The nictitating membrane, or third eyelid, will protrude and partially cover the horse's eye, which is especially noticeable when the head is elevated. Difficulty in swallowing and breathing are usually evident, and any external stimuli will cause muscular spasms and convulsions. The horse may fall and be unable to rise without beginning another series of muscle convulsions. The heat output by the muscle spasms causes the animal to sweat excessively, although his temperature will usually remain normal until just before death.

Death occurs either from exhaustion, or from respiratory failure when the diaphragm becomes paralyzed. The mortality rate of tetanus is extremely high (approximately 80%), however, animals that recover do not show any signs of permanent damage in the tissues and organs.

Treatment: Veterinary treatment is directed mainly at reducing the muscular spasms and supplying the horse with nutrients. The veterinarian will administer CNS depressants (e.g., tranquilizers, sedatives and general anesthetic solutions), muscle relaxants, massive doses of tetanus antitoxin (sometimes administered intrathecally), and massive doses of antibiotics (e.g., penicillin-streptomycin). Although the antitoxin is ineffective in neutralizing the neurotoxin already attacking the nervous system, it will negate the new toxin being produced by the bacteria.

A horse with tetanus should be kept in a well-bedded, cool, dark stall, away from external stimuli. Feed and water buckets should be elevated to a comfortable height, as the horse will not be able to eat from the floor. The horse should not be given hay or any other feedstuff that may be difficult to swallow. If necessary, nutrients, including water, glucose, and a gruel of soaked pellets, can be given through a stomach tube after the horse has been sedated. In the event dehydration occurs, a saline solution and lactated Ringer's solution can be given intravenously.

Several weeks may be required for treatment of tetanus, and even after the animal has seemingly recovered, care must be taken not to unnecessarily excite the horse and produce a relapse. Besides regular immunization, preventive measures for tetanus should include checking the horse for wounds that could be the entry site of tetanus bacteria, and the cleaning and treating of these wounds.

Euthanasia is, of course, the only alternative for those horses that do not respond to therapy. This perhaps emphasizes that the best treatment for tetanus, and for many other conditions, is prevention through immunization. It is unfortunate that horses are ever lost to this highly fatal disease, since the tetanus toxoid is one of the most effective biologicals that has ever been produced. ◄

10

SKIN CONDITIONS

Skin functions as a protective barrier against external elements, and also acts as a sensory organ and as a regulator of the body's metabolism. Thus, proper skin care is an important element in equine husbandry. Some of the numerous skin diseases that affect horses will be discussed in the following pages. While the majority of the the skin conditions mentioned are commonly seen, a few are rarely encountered in the United States.

Dermatomycosis

The dermatomycotic skin diseases are caused by fungal infections of the horny layer of the skin. These conditions, which include ringworm, sometimes called girth itch, are superficial, contagious diseases. Young animals seem to be more susceptible to dermatomycosis. Fungal infections can be spread by direct contact with an infected horse, or by the use of common grooming tools. An object, such as a brush or a piece of tack, that is able to spread an infection is known as a fomite.

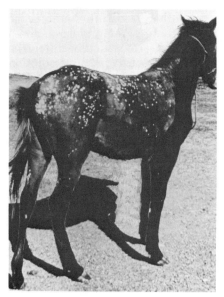

Fig. 10-1 Hair depigmentation is a complication of a generalized fungal condition.

The fungal species involved in dermatomycosis are classified as either ectothrix (meaning that the fungus grows outside the hair shaft) or endothrix (meaning that the fungus grows inside the hair shaft), depending upon the exact fungus involved.

Signs of dermatomycosis include focal lesions, scaling and crusting of the skin, loss of hair (alopecia), and itching (pruritis). A veterinarian is usually able to diagnose this condition by the clinical appearance, but may decide to perform a fungal culture for positive identification of the fungus involved.

FUNGAL CULTURE

The veterinarian will collect scales and hair by scraping the skin. Ideally, the lesions are first gently washed with a nonantiseptic soap, rinsed thoroughly, and dried. The scales and hair, which contain the fungus, are then placed onto a culture medium for growth and subsequent identification.

RINGWORM

Ringworm (**Microsporum trichophyton**) is probably the most commonly seen of the skin conditions caused by fungal infections. It affects both the hair and skin, and can be transmitted either directly by contact between animals, or indirectly by contact with contaminated tack, blankets, etc. Ringworm is most prevalent in saddle and girth areas, where contact with contaminated tack is most likely to occur.

Ringworm is characterized by the following signs:
1. intense itching
2. small, rounded lesions which spread in circular patterns
3. inflammation of the skin accompanied by breaking or shedding of the hair in affected areas.

Dirty, overcrowded stable areas, particularly if warm and damp, are a predisposing condition for ringworm, as are dietary deficiencies. Young, thin-skinned horses are especially susceptible to this skin condition.

Treatment: Dermatomycotic skin diseases such as ringworm will often spontaneously regress, particularly if the horse receives good nutrition and plenty of sunlight. Captan, a herbicide available in garden shops, may be used to treat generalized cases. A solution of one ounce (two tablespoons) of 50% captan to one gallon of water can be sponged over the horse's entire body daily or every other day. A 7% solution of iodine can be used, instead of the herbicide, directly on the lesions every other day. For best results from both these treatments, the crusts should be removed by gentle washing with mild soap before the captan or iodine is applied.

Occasionally, the veterinarian will recommend bathing the horse with a "tamed" iodine-based shampoo. If systemic therapy is considered necessary, the veterinarian may prescribe the oral administration of griseofulvin (Fulvicin). This fungistatic agent is believed to concentrate in the skin to a level that will prevent the further growth of the fungus.

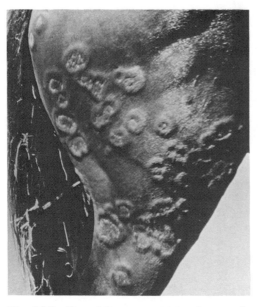

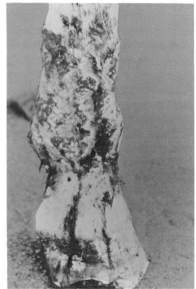

Fig. 10-2 Fungal hypersensitivity has resulted in this severe reaction to a fungal infection [ringworm].

Fig. 10-3 Phycomycosis [Gulf Coast fungus] is a severe fungal infection.

PHYCOMYCOSIS

Phycomycosis ("Gulf Coast fungus") is a localized, systemic fungal infection. It is caused by either **Hyphomyces destruens** or **Entomophthora coronata**. It most commonly affects the legs, especially at the site of an injury, but may be found on the neck, lips, nostrils, or abdomen as well. The lesions caused by phycomycosis are characterized by hard, yellow-grey "leeches" of necrotic matter embedded in exuberant granulation tissue. This disease causes a severe itching that often causes the horse to bite at the lesions. Phycomycosis may eventually infect the tendon sheaths and cause lameness. The veterinarian may perform a biopsy to diagnose this condition. (Refer to "Biopsy" under "Special Techniques.")

Treatment: Early, radical surgical excision is the treatment of choice for phycomycosis. Unfortunately, the disease often recurs. To prevent recurrence, the veterinarian may prescribe the application of DMSO and amphotericin B topically for thirty days after surgery. Another possible treatment is the intravenous administration of trypan blue and red solution or amphotericin B. Neck cradles, cross-ties, and other restraining devices may be required to prevent the horse from chewing and mutilating the affected area.

SPOROTRICHOSIS

Sporotrichosis is a chronic, sporadic fungal infection of the skin and subcutaneous tissues. It is caused by a saprophytic fungus (one that grows on dead or decaying tissue), **Sporotrichum schenckii**. This fungus is usually introduced through a wound caused by a thorny plant. Characteristics of sporotrichosis include subcutaneous hard nodules located along the lymphatics on the medial surfaces of the horse's limbs, particularly the thigh, upper forearm, and chest regions. These nodules eventually ulcerate, producing purulent material (pus) and the animal often loses weight and condition when afflicted with this disease.

Treatment: The veterinarian may treat sporotrichosis with the intravenous administration of sodium or potassium iodides (this treatment may cause abortion), or by the oral administration of an organic iodide. Iodine may be used locally on the ruptured nodules. Griseofulvin may be given orally until all signs of this disease have disappeared.

Bacterial Skin Diseases

Bacteria cause several skin diseases in the horse, one of which, dermatophilosis, is often confused with dermatomycosis.

DERMATOPHILOSIS

This disease, also known as streptothricosis or "rain scald," is a skin condition that is spread mechanically by biting and non-biting flies. Dermatophilosis, caused by **Dermatophilus congolensis**, may be either acute or chronic, and is seen most often in the fall and winter, during extended periods of rainy weather. Prolonged wetting appears to be a predisposing factor in this condition.

The lesions of streptothricosis are usually found on the horse's back, and consist of thick crusts that can be palpated underneath the horse's coat. The skin under the crusts is pink and moist. There may be a lot of skin flaking in the saddle area, which is the site of most chronic infections. The veterinarian will be able to differentiate between dermatophilosis and dermatomycosis by examining one of the crusts microscopically.

Treatment: Streptothricosis often regresses spontaneously with the arrival of dry weather. Protection from rain and vigorous grooming to remove the crusts will hasten the horse's recovery. Antifungal preparations are ineffective in the treatment of streptothricosis, since this is a bacterial, not a fungal, disease. An antibiotic ointment may be applied after removal of the crusts. The systemic administration of antibiotics may hasten recovery.

ULCERATIVE LYMPHANGITIS

Ulcerative lymphangitis is a slightly contagious skin condition characterized by inflammation and swelling of the lymphatics of the lower legs (usually the hind legs). Abscesses which form along the lymphatics may drain pus or lymph, and the horse may subsequently become lame. Culture and sensitivity tests usually reveal the presence of Streptococcus, Staphylococcus, or Corynebacterium bacteria.

Treatment: Since unsanitary stabling conditions contribute to the spread of ulcerative lymphangitis, sanitary measures and clean stabling are important considerations in managing and preventing this disease. For specific treatment, the veterinarian will clip and clean the infected area, then wrap the limb with an antiseptic-treated leg wrap. Antibacterial agents, such as sulfa drugs, may be beneficial, and hot water soaks may be used, if necessary to relieve the swelling. Hydrotherapy and mild exercise may also be helpful in reducing the swelling that accompanies ulcerative lymphangitis.

FISTULOUS WITHERS AND POLL EVIL

Fistulous withers and poll evil are inflammatory disorders of the bursae located at the withers (supraspinous bursa) and the poll (supra-atlantal bursa). Initially, a swelling (possibly attributed to trauma) may be seen in one or both of these areas. Later, a fistula, or draining tract, develops between the infected bursa and a "weeping" lesion on the skin. The veterinarian will diagnose fistulous withers or poll evil by examination and by performing a culture test of the bursal fluid. If infection of the bones is suspected, radiographs may be taken.

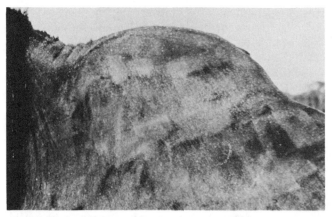

Fig. 10-4 Fistulous withers is an inflammation of the supraspinous bursa.

The two organisms most often cultured in cases of this disease are **Brucella abortus** and **Actinomyces bovis**. Due to the fact that these organisms may cause serious disease in man and cattle, great care is necessary when performing diagnostic procedures and when treating this condition. In all suspected cases of fistulous withers or poll evil, a bacterial culture should be made to identify the causative organism. In a small percentage of cases, fistulous withers or poll evil will be caused by trauma, without any bacterial infection.

The treatment for fistulous withers and poll evil will depend on the size of the lesion, any bony changes present, the causative agent, and the duration of the disease. Treatment for an acute case involves the application of ice packs and anti-inflammatory agents for several days. After this period, heat and counterirritants may be used. The veterinarian may choose to surgically remove the affected bursa and then treat the condition as an open wound. In less severe cases, the veterinarian may administer strain-19 vaccine (a live bacterial vaccine) as part of treatment. This vaccine is given in three doses, at two week intervals.

If the bursa has already ruptured, it should be cleaned with antiseptics, after which the horse may be given antibiotics and oral sodium iodide. In severe cases, where the bones are involved, the veterinarian may have to surgically remove the affected spinous processes. The horse will usually have to be kept isolated during treatment, which may be for six months or more.

Parasitic Skin Conditions

Parasitic skin conditions are caused by a wide range of factors, from mange mites to black fly bites. Insect related skin problems may be serious in the spring and summer months, because of the increased insect population, and regress or disappear during the fall and winter seasons.

HABRONEMIASIS (SUMMER SORES)

Habronemiasis is a skin condition caused by the infestation of Habronema larvae in wounds, moist areas around the eyes, and the sheath. These larvae are deposited in these areas by house and stable flies (**Musca domestica** and **Stomoxys calcitrans**). Habronemiasis is characterized by the accumulation of pus in the lesions, which granulate slowly and then suddenly enlarge with proud flesh. The affected tissue will be reddish-brown in color, protruding, and hemorrhagic (bleeding). There will be a greasy, coagulated exudate over the areas, and the horse will suffer from an intense itching.

The sores may be irregular or circular in shape, and small, calcified areas may develop in the lesions. When habronemiasis affects the eye area, conjunctivitis is a frequent complication, and can cause a swelling of the eyelids and impaired vision. This granular conjunctivitis particularly affects the third eyelid and medial canthus.

The lesions may apparently heal with the onset of cold weather, only to reappear when the temperature reaches 70°F or higher. The larvae are passed in the feces of the horse, then ingested by fly maggots. After the fly matures and eventually lights on a horse, the larvae are transmitted to the horse. The veterinarian will diagnose this condition by the characteristic appearance of the summer sores and occasionally, by a biopsy of affected tissue.

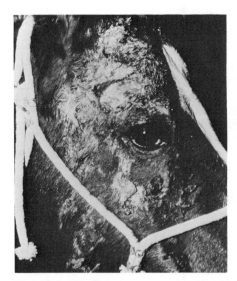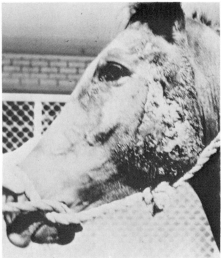

Fig. 10-5   These lesions are caused by Habronema larvae which are deposited by infected flies in skin wounds and moist places such as the eyes.

Treatment: Organophosphates, either orally or intravenously, are administered to kill the larvae. Trichlorfon is administered either intravenously or topically in a paste with DMSO and an antibacterial agent. Some veterinarians will inject an organophosphate directly into the lesion. Cryosurgery, however, is currently the preferred treatment for habronemiasis.

The proud flesh resulting from habronemiasis is controlled through surgical excision, pressure bandaging, and the use of corticosteroids. Bandaging the treated areas will shorten the required healing time and

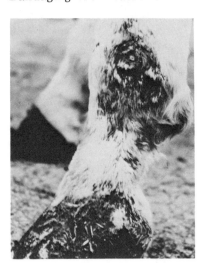

Fig. 10-6   The presence of Habronema larvae can cause the development of "summer sores."

prevent reinfestation. Fly control is extremely important in the prevention of reinfestation. Roll on insecticide and repellents may be used conveniently around the eye area, pastes on the sheath, and sprays and wipes for more general coverage.

ONCHOCERCAL FILARIASIS

Onchocercal filariasis is the infestation of the horse with a nematode, **Onchocerca cervicalis**. Infected sandflies carry the microfilaria and infect the horse when they bite. The presence of these nematodes causes a recurrent, seasonal disease characterized by intense itching, scaling, and hair loss. Onchocercal filariasis occurs mainly on the horse's face, neck, shoulders, and ventral midline. It usually affects horses over four years of age. This is because no signs are seen until the microfilaria begin to die, and since they have a life span of one to three years, affected horses are usually over four before signs of the disease appear.

Periodic ophthalmia may be caused by the presence of onchocerca in the eyes. Another result of this condition is depigmentation (vitiligo) of the skin.

Treatment: Treatment is directed at killing the microfilaria only, since there is no safe method of removing the adult nematodes. Since the adults may live as long as fifteen years, treating this condition is a continuing process. The oral administration of diethylcarbamazine (Caricide) at 3 gm/day for three weeks will kill the larvae. The horse will require a corticosteroid during the first five days of this treatment, due to skin reactions to the dying larvae.

a.

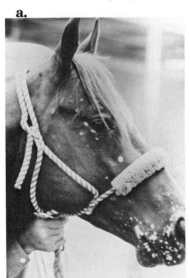

b.

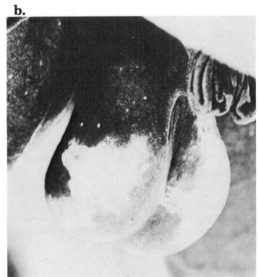

Fig. 10-7   Depigmentation may result from Onchocerca larvae infestation.   a. face b. scrotal region.

VENTRAL MIDLINE DERMATITIS

Ventral midline dermatitis is a skin disease believed to be the result of horn fly bites on the horse's abdomen. It is most commonly seen in horses over four years of age and is characterized by lesions along the abdomen and thorax. The skin will be thickened and scaling, the horse will lose hair in the affected area, and the lesions will ulcerate and develop crusts. Severe itching is another typical sign of ventral midline dermatitis.

Treatment: Treatment for ventral midline dermatitis consists of, first, removing the crusts by cleansing with a mild soap and water. Then an antibiotic/corticosteroid ointment is applied to the lesions twice a day for several days, until healing is completed. A fly repellent should be used frequently around the area, both during healing and afterwards, to prevent a recurrence of this condition.

SCREWWORMS

The screwworm (**Cochliomyia hominivorax**) is the larval stage of a parasitic fly that infests open wounds. Screwworms are occasionally found infesting wounds and/or unclean sheath areas in horses. Attacks by these parasites, which feed on living tissue, cause bleeding and produce a characteristic offensive odor.

Treatment: The following drugs and insecticides are used in the control and treatment of screwworm infestations:

Coumaphos
Ronnel
EQ335
Lindane
Smear 62 (benzene/diphenylamine)

If left untreated, screwworm lesions may be severe enough to seriously disfigure or kill the horse within just a few weeks.

SIMULIIDAE

This insect related skin condition is caused by the bite of the black fly (an insect also known as the buffalo gnat). The bites cause hyperemic (blood congested), hemorrhagic (bleeding) swellings. The afflicted horse will scratch and rub the swellings until there is a loss of skin at the affected areas. The black fly also produces a toxin that is injected into the horse at the time of the bite. This toxin can cause cardio-respiratory problems due to its ability to increase capillary permeability. The increased capillary permeability causes a loss of fluid from the circulatory system into the tissue spaces and body cavities.

A horse attacked by large numbers of black flies will become listless and depressed. The horse will have difficulty in moving, and may lay down. In severe cases, other signs include increased respiration, elevated temperature, groaning, and heart palpitation. Pregnant mares may abort after receiving numerous black fly bites. In extreme cases, the affected horse will die within several hours.

Treatment: In areas near swiftly running water, where there are large numbers of black flies, horses should be protected from the insects by frequent applications (two or three times daily) of insecticide/repellents. Since **Simuliidae** are day biters, horses can be stabled during the day as an added measure of protection.

AURAL PLAQUES

Aural plaques are commonly found on the inner surfaces of a horse's ears. The lesions are grey or white plaques that may initially resemble dandruff and eventually appear wart-like. This condition is not a fungus, and is thought to be caused by the bite of black flies. Aural plaques are usually seen in horses over one year old, and they appear to cause a horse little, if any, discomfort. When the crust of the plaque is removed, pink skin is visible underneath. These lesions will persist indefinitely.

Treatment: There is no specific treatment for aural plaques. They do not respond to the application of antifungal preparations, antibiotics, corticosteroids, etc.

WARBLES

Warbles, which is infestation by the **Hypoderma** species of fly, often occurs in the area of the withers, and is characterized by swelling underneath the skin. This condition is caused by the burrowing of the warble ("cattle grub"), and is most often found in horses kept with cattle. Usually, the affected horse will have only one or two lesions.

Hypoderma bovis and **Hypoderma lineatum** most often affect young horses, and animals in poor condition. During the spring, the larvae reach the back area and may make a breathing hole in the horse's skin. Due to the fact that the horse is not the natural host for warbles, most of the larvae fail to develop normally and do not complete a life cycle.

Treatment: The larva usually must be removed for the swelling to subside, so the veterinarian will often surgically open the breathing hole and carefully extract the grub. If the larva dies while still beneath the skin, severe infection and inflammation may result.

Once the larva has been removed, the horse should recover quickly. In areas of the country with a high degree of warble infestation, the veterinarian may recommend that the horse receive treatment with an organophosphate after fly season.

MANGE

Mange is a parasitic skin infection induced by mites. In the horse, three types of mange are most frequently seen; sarcoptic, psoroptic, and chorioptic. Sarcoptic mange, the most common type, is characterized by the formation of small, hairless patches and dry scabs. The intense itching that occurs with this condition may cause the horse to rub against objects, which results in a thick, wrinkled skin.

Psoroptic mange is very contagious and easily transmitted, especially in warm weather. Horses with thick haircoats are most susceptible to this type. Scabs found on horses with psoroptic mange are more moist than the ones associated with sarcoptic mange.

Chorioptic mange usually affects the fetlocks and lower legs, particularly of the hind legs, and breeds with long hair in the fetlock area are most susceptible to infection with this type. The itching caused by mites living on the skin surfaces may cause the afflicted animal to stomp its feet and bite at the affected areas.

Treatment: Good nutrition and proper hygiene are important considerations in the treatment and prevention of mange. When infections do occur, lindane is often used in dips or sprays. To be most effective, the treatment should be used on all affected horses at the same time.

Allergic Skin Conditions

Allergic skin conditions are caused by the horse's allergic reaction to a substance such as a plant, fly bite, etc. Treatment always involves removal of the offending agent, if possible, or protecting the horse from insects.

ALLERGIC DERMATITIS

This is a chronic, seasonal disease that is due to the horse's allergic reaction to the bite of the sandfly, **Culicoides** species. Also known as "Queensland itch," allergic dermatitis causes a severe itching that results

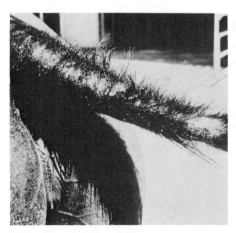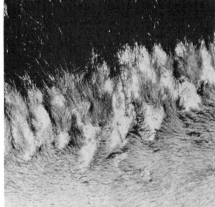

Fig. 10-8 An allergic reaction to the bite of the sandfly [Culicoides species] causes severe itching which may result in a "rattail" appearance[left]. The horse will also rub the mane area [right].

in the horse trying to constantly scratch affected areas. Eventually, hair loss and a thickened "elephant hide" develops.

The veterinarian may use hair and skin scrapings to diagnose allergic dermatitis.

Treatment: Treatment for this skin condition involves the administration of antihistamines to reduce the allergic reaction to the bites. Corticosteroids will reduce the severe itching.

If the horse has developed a secondary bacterial infection due to trauma caused by rubbing the affected areas, the veterinarian may apply an antibacterial ointment. Treatment with diethylcarbamazine may possibly reduce the horse's allergic response. A horse with a demonstrated allergy to the bite of sandflies must be protected from these insects through the use of insect repellents and protective stabling.

URTICARIA

Urticaria (hives) is an acute allergic skin reaction to an ingested or inhaled food or drug. It may result from insect bites, antibiotics, hormones, etc., and is due to increased capillary permeability. Urticaria has a rapid onset, sometimes accompanied by a slight fever, and is characterized by multiple round, flat-topped wheals. Severe attacks may result in a coalescing of a number of hives, and the horse may experience intense itching.

This skin condition may last for a few hours or for several days, and is more common in thin-skinned horses.

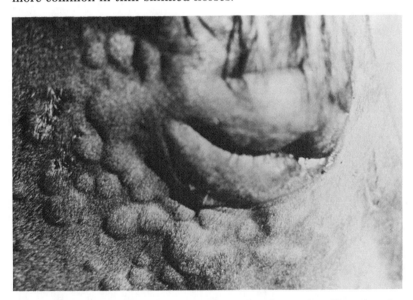

Fig. 10-9 Urticaria [hives] result from an allergic reaction. Note that the eyelids are swollen shut.

Treatment: Urticaria will usually spontaneously regress after the cause of allergy is removed. The veterinarian may administer corticosteroids and antihistamines to alleviate the horse's allergy signs. In cases of chronic urticaria, where the cause of the reaction is unknown, a complete examination and case history will be necessary.

PHOTOSENSITIZATION

Photosensitization is caused by hypersensitivity to the sun. This hypersensitivity results from photodynamic substances that are deposited in non-pigmented areas of the skin and activated by the sun's ultraviolet rays. Therefore, this condition only affects the white-skinned areas of the horse. Signs of photosensitization include the following:

1. a marked line between pigmented and non-pigmented areas
2. the appearance of small, firm nodules
3. a distinct odor
4. dried, cracked skin that may slough

PRIMARY

In primary photosensitization, the phototoxic agent is absorbed into the circulatory system from the digestive tract after the horse has ingested a photodynamic agent. Plants that contain photodynamic agents include red and white clover, alfalfa, and buckwheat. (These plants contain these agents only when fresh, not when dried into hay.) In addition, certain drugs, such as phenothiazine, are photodynamic.

HEPATOGENOUS PHOTOSENSITIZATION

Hepatogenous photosensitization is the result of a liver malfunction and may be congenital. In this form of the disease, the photodynamic agent naturally contained in bile reaches the circulatory system when the bile duct becomes blocked.

Treatment: The affected horse should be removed and/or protected from sunlight. A darkened stall, combined with a change of diet (to eliminate the plant source of the photodynamic agent), may be sufficient therapy.

Steroid lotions applied to the lesions may be beneficial. In addition, the veterinarian may recommend the application of a sunscreen product, such as 0.5% potassium permangenate, to help screen out the sun's ultraviolet rays.

In cases of hepatogenous photosensitization, the veterinarian may prescribe laxatives and change the horse's diet.

CONTACT DERMATITIS

Contact dermatitis is caused by the horse's dermal reaction to an irritating substance that comes in direct contact with the horse's skin. There are two types of contact dermatitis, of which the more common is primary contact dermatitis. This condition usually occurs as a result of continued irritation from either body excretions or wound secretions. However, it may also be caused by accidental contact with acids or irritating drugs, such as blistering agents and counterirritants.

Allergic contact dermatitis, which is generally a less severe condition, is caused by contact with certain irritating plants, insect repellents, bedding, soap, etc.

Signs of contact dermatitis occur on the head, legs, lower body areas and, in cases of allergic dermatitis, on areas that are touched by tack. Signs of this skin condition include itching, redness, vesiculation (the formation of blisters), and crusting. These characteristics are almost always more severe with the primary type of contact dermatitis than with the allergic type.

Treatment: The affected areas should be gently cleansed with a mild skin cleanser (such as pHisoHex: Winthrop), and a gentle astringent applied. A protective ointment may be used to guard the areas from further contact with irritants, while a cream or bath oil (such as Alpha Keri: Westwood) can be applied to soothe the skin and relieve itching. Of course, the use of an irritating chemical (i.e., blistering agents, counterirritants) should be discontinued if it is the cause of the dermatitis.

DIETARY ECZEMA

Dietary eczema is a skin condition in which moist patches may appear on the skin, accompanied by skin sloughing and hair loss. The horse may also "stock up." Horses fed high-concentrate rations containing high levels of protein may develop this condition, particularly if the horse is thin-skinned.

Treatment: Since dietary eczema is diet related, the horse's ration must be adjusted to eliminate the cause of this condition. Variations of well-balanced rations can be tried until a suitable diet is found.

The affected areas should be clipped, then cleansed with a medicated shampoo. The veterinarian may also administer corticosteroids and antihistamines to reduce the allergic signs.

Viral Skin Conditions

The most frequently encountered viral skin condition in horses is cutaneous papillomatosis, commonly known as warts.

WARTS

Warts are epidermal growths that may be either congenital or acquired in origin. They are caused by a virus, and are most often found on the lips, abdomen, and inner ear surfaces. Warts are benign growths. They are much more common in young horses about 9 to 15 months of age.

Treatment: Warts often spontaneously regress, and are not usually removed unless they interfere with eating or secondary changes occur. If removal is desired, the veterinarian may surgically excise the warts, use caustic chemicals, apply thermal cautery, or use cryosurgery. An autogenous vaccine sometimes effective against warts can be administered. This vaccine is given in two doses at two week intervals; the warts should begin regressing within three to five weeks. Daily applications of an oil, such as castor oil, may help soften the warts and speed their disappearance.

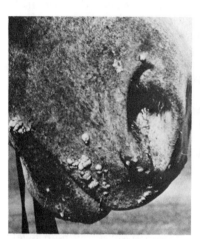 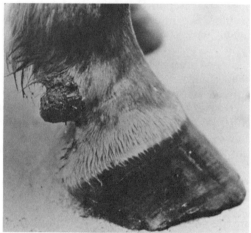

Fig. 10-10 Warts, caused by a virus, may regress spontaneously.

Fig. 10-11 Equine sarcoids, which are viral in origin, frequently recur after surgical removal.

EQUINE SARCOID

A sarcoid is a benign fibroblastic tumor, usually occurring on the horse's head, legs, shoulders, and ventral midline. Sarcoids are verrucous (wart-like) and fibroblastic (proud flesh-like) and are thought to be caused by a virus. Their occurrence is usually associated with a previous injury.

The veterinarian will perform a biopsy to diagnose a sarcoid, examining both normal and abnormal tissues for comparison.

Treatment: Sarcoids can be surgically removed, but frequently recur. The application of a topical antimetabolite, fluorouracil, may help prevent recurrence, but also delays healing of the lesion. This substance must be applied for 30 to 90 days, until the lesion has healed completely. Without this treatment, sarcoids recur about 50% of the time.

Some veterinarians use electrocautery to remove the sarcoid, and post-surgery radiation is sometimes employed to reduce the chances of regrowth. An irritant cathartic, podophyllum, can be applied to the lesion daily (after surgery) to prevent recurrence. This irritant will cause cellulitis in normal skin; however, when used for this purpose, it causes the formation of a black scab which eventually drops off, leaving the lesion healed.

The preferred treatment for a sarcoid is removal by cryosurgery. This treatment most successfully prevents recurrence of the lesion (refer to "Cryosurgery"). Recently, a vaccine has shown preliminary promise in preventing the recurrence of sarcoids.

Cutaneous Neoplasms

The following skin conditions are all tumors; some are benign, while others are malignant and therefore more serious in nature.

MELANOMAS

Melanomas are dark brown or black tumors that may be either hard or soft in texture, and single or multiple in number. They are usually about 1 to 2 cm in size, and are located in the anal, tail, throat, and eyelid areas. Melanomas are most frequently found in grey horses, and in horses over six years of age (80% of grey horses over 15 years old will develop melanomas). These tumors tend to grow slowly for years, then metastasize (spread) quickly and begin to show malignant characteristics.

Treatment: Due to the fact that melanomas tend to be malignant and metastasize, the prognosis for this condition is poor. However, if the tumor has not yet begun to spread, the veterinarian may attempt to surgically remove it. Unfortunately, recurrence is frequent.

FIBROMAS

Fibromas are benign, connective tissue tumors. They vary from hard to soft, and are usually located just beneath the skin's surface. Rubbing from halters, saddles, and harnesses frequently causes fibromas to occur at pressure points.

Treatment: Because fibromas are benign, no treatment is necessary for medical reasons. However, if desired for cosmetic reasons, the veterinarian may surgically remove the fibroma.

KELOIDS

Keloids are a variation of a hard fibroma. They are benign tumors that often develop from scar tissue, particularly on the lower leg; however, they may grow from normal-appearing tissue. A keloid has a raised, smooth surface.

Treatment: Keloids may be removed surgically. Like sarcoids, they tend to recur, so chemical therapy (as described under "Sarcoids") is necessary after surgery to help prevent regrowth.

SQUAMOUS CELL CARCINOMA

Squamous cell carcinomas are highly malignant cancers that appear around body openings and on non-pigmented skin. These neoplasms bleed easily, and occur most often on the breeds of horses with lightly pigmented skin.

Treatment: Squamous cell carcinomas must be removed, due to their highly malignant nature. This can be accomplished through radical surgery, radiation therapy, or cryosurgery. As with sarcoids, cryosurgery is the most successful method of treatment. There is less chance of a squamous cell carcinoma recurring after removal by cryosurgery than with other treatments. Occasionally, a vaccine is used in the therapy of a squamous cell carcinoma.

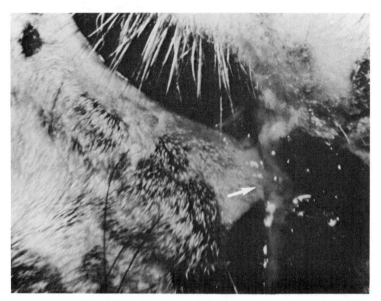

Fig. 10-12 Squamous cell carcinoma at the inner corner of the eye.

Other Skin Conditions

Under this heading are found some common skin conditions that do not easily fit under any of the more specific headings.

SEBORRHIC DERMATITIS

Seborrhea is a skin condition that results in scaling of the skin covering the neck and mane. As this condition worsens, the skin will become oily and may have a rancid odor. Later, the skin will be thick and crusted.

Seborrhea is believed to be due to either an overproduction of sebum (an oily substance secreted by the skin), or to abnormal keratinization (skin production). It is usually secondary to another dermatitis.

Treatment: Since seborrhea is frequently secondary in nature, the original skin condition must be treated first to effect a cure. The horse will require good, general nursing care, particularly since this is a condition which requires treatment over an extended period of time.

The crusts resulting from seborrhea should be removed, and the horse bathed frequently with a medicated shampoo containing one or more of the following medications:

sulfur
hexachlorophene
coal tar
selenium sulfide
salicylic acid

The shampoo should remain on the affected skin for ten to fifteen minutes before rinsing for maximum benefit.

After bathing, wet dressings should be applied to the exudating areas, and a mild antibiotic ointment may be applied to the skin between shampooings. Liberal applications of a cream or lotion (such as Alpha Keri), covered with plastic wrap, may be effective in treating large areas. The medications and bathings may have to be continued for several weeks or even months.

GREASE HEEL

Grease heel is a relatively uncommon dermatitis that is also known as scratches, mud fever, and cracked heels. Grease heel is a form of eczema and may be related to seborrhea. This skin condition is characterized by scratch-like lesions that appear at the heel and pastern area (usually of the hind legs). These lesions ooze serum and eventually become crusty. Granulation tissue may develop in the affected areas, and swelling and lameness may appear in severe cases of grease heel.

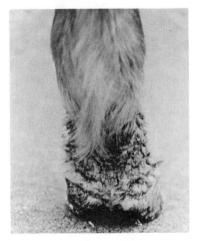

Fig. 10-13 Grease heel, also known as "scratches."

Wet surroundings and unsanitary conditions are believed to predispose a horse to grease heel, particularly if the horse has long, feathering hair in the pastern area. Cuts on the legs are also primary sites of grease heel infection. Dirt particles may cause an irritation that develops a secondary bacterial infection, resulting in grease heel.

Treatment: Treatment for grease heel involves thoroughly cleansing the affected areas, clipping the long hair, and applying a topical antibacterial ointment. Heat packs may be used to relieve swelling, or the veterinarian may administer an anti-inflammatory drug until the swelling goes down.

After application of the ointment, the area is bandaged. This treatment is repeated about every other day until the lesions have completely healed.

ANHIDROSIS

Anhidrosis is the partial or total loss of the ability to sweat. The cause of this condition, which results in the coat becoming very dry, is unknown. Anhidrosis affects horses that have been moved from a temperate area to a hot, humid climate. Initially, the horse will sweat excessively after exercise; eventually, the horse progressively loses the ability to sweat, until only a small area under the mane is still able to perspire.

Anhidrotic horses compensate for the lack of sweating by increased urination to remove surplus body fluids, and by increased respiration. If such a horse is exercised, it may run a fever of 105-108°F, and collapse in respiratory and cardiac failure.

Treatment: An acute case of anhidrosis is treated by replacing lost fluids with physiological saline solution to replenish lost electrolytes. Wetting the coat with water, and blowing fans on the horse, to help him cool off, may also be beneficial (refer to "Hyperthermia" under "Shock").

A horse with anhidrosis will recover upon return to a more temperate climate. The addition of salt to the horse's diet will hasten the animal's recovery.

VITILIGO

Vitiligo is the skin condition characterized by the loss of pigmentation. This lack of the pigment melanin may be due to heredity or, at least in part, to nervous conditions. It may also be caused by onchocercal filariasis. Vitiligo is not associated with any injury or swelling of the skin.

Treatment: A horse with vitiligo must be protected from the sunlight due to its lack of protecting pigmentation. There is no treatment for vitiligo that will restore the lost melanin.

11

EYE CONDITIONS

When a horse suffers an eye injury or develops an eye disease, a complete ophthalmic examination, conducted by a veterinarian, is often necessary to determine the extent of the injury and the subsequent vision impairment (refer to "Eye Examination"). The horseman should contact his veterinarian when any of the following indications of eye injury or disease appear:

1. excessive tearing
2. keeping the eyelids closed
3. pus accumulations around the eyelids
4. whitish color or opacity in the eye
5. tumors near the eye
6. dull or cloudy appearance of the eye
7. protrusion of the nictitating membrane

Eye injuries and disorders should be diagnosed and treated by the veterinarian, or under the direct supervision of the veterinarian.

Blepharospasm, epiphora, photophobia, and protrusion of the nictitating membrane are signs of eye disease that are not specific to any one condition. Each of these should be treated by first diagnosing the specific cause of the problem.

Blepharospasm

Blepharospasm is contraction of the orbicularis oculi muscle, causing the eyelids to be tightly closed. This condition is secondary to another ailment, such as an irritation of the eyelids, conjunctiva, or orbit. Regardless of its nature, the underlying cause must be treated and cured in order to correct blepharospasm.

If the precipitating cause is a minor one, the blepharospasm may be relieved by the topical application of a local anesthetic. This therapy cannot be continued for an extended period of time, however, because a topical anesthetic may cause changes in the cornea or cause drug hypersensitivity. In addition, there is an increased chance that the horse will injure the cornea if it is desensitized. When the cause of blepharospasm requires a lengthy healing period, the veterinarian may block the auriculo-palpebral nerve to reduce the pain.

Epiphora

Epiphora is excessive tearing. In the horse, tears should drain down through the nasolacrimal duct, and not out onto the face. Therefore, the presence of tearing indicates a condition such as blockage of the nasolacrimal duct or the presence of a foreign body in the eye (refer to "Obstruction of the Nasolacrimal Duct").

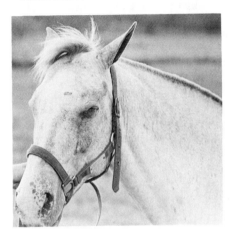

Fig. 11-1   A horse suffering from photophobia will exhibit blepharospasm.

Photophobia

Photophobia (fear of light) is the inability to tolerate light; a horse with photophobia will usually keep the eyes tightly closed in an attempt to avoid light. This condition may be a sign of any one of several different eye ailments and possibly, of systemic disease as well (i.e., many horses with systemic ailments cannot tolerate strong light).

A horse with photophobia should be kept in a darkened stall. The veterinarian will attempt to locate the condition's cause and treat that problem.

Protrusion of the Nictitating Membrane

Protrusion of the nictitating membrane (third eyelid) may be caused by one of the following conditions:

1. severe pain associated with eye disease
2. the presence of a foreign body in the eye

3. a neoplasm affecting the third eyelid

4. tetanus

5. dehydration

The underlying cause of a protruding nictitating membrane must be diagnosed and treated for this condition to be corrected.

The underside of the nictitating membrane should be checked for the presence of a foreign body. A minor injury of this nature can be treated, by the veterinarian, by the removal of the object and the application of a topical antibiotic ophthalmic ointment.

Neoplasms (tumors) affecting the nictitating membrane may be treated by the complete surgical removal of the third eyelid or by cryosurgery. In addition, the veterinarian may prescribe radiation therapy as postsurgical treatment for this condition.

If the underlying cause of the protruding membrane is dehydration, the veterinarian will administer fluids and electrolytes, and of course, the disease responsible for the dehydration must also be treated. If tetanus is the suspected cause of this condition, the veterinarian should be contacted immediately.

Eye Conditions
Caused by Trauma

The following eye conditions are the result of trauma to the eye, such as that resulting from a direct blow or the presence of a foreign object in the eye.

CORNEAL ULCERATIONS

Corneal ulcerations can be detected with the use of fluorescein dye strips; when one of these is applied to the eye, any ulcerated area will be temporarily dyed green.

Treatment: The veterinarian may block the auriculo-palpebral nerve to relieve the blepharospasm which may accompany a corneal ulceration. Most of these injuries respond to the application of an antibiotic ophthalmic ointment and a cycloplegic drug (one which paralyzes the ciliary muscles, allowing the eye to dilate), such as atropine. This treatment should be repeated three or four times daily until healing is completed.

Minor corneal ulcerations often heal within 36 hours, but deeper damage may require ten days to two weeks for proper healing. If an ulcer is slow to heal, the veterinarian may cauterize it with iodine, then protect it by suturing the eyelids together (refer to "Tarsorrhaphy"). When this procedure is used, the horse's eye must be medicated through a subpalpebral medication system (refer to "Subpalpebral Medication System"). Alternatively, the veterinarian may bandage the eye with a stockinette placed over the head.

In the final stages of healing, a corticosteroid may be cautiously used, by the veterinarian, to help reduce scarring of the cornea. Corticosteroids are not used topically to treat ulcerated areas of the cornea during the acute stages, since these drugs can complicate the healing process and cause loss of vision. Loss of sight can also occur when medication prescribed for one specific condition is administered indiscriminately to other horses with eye problems.

If the corneal ulceration does not respond to treatment, the veterinarian may find it necessary to remove the eye, a procedure known as enucleation.

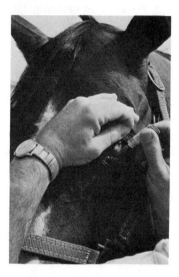

Fig. 11-2 Veterinarian applying an ophthalmic ointment to the eye.

CORNEAL LACERATIONS

Corneal lacerations tend to be more serious injuries than are corneal ulcerations. The cornea may be either lacerated partially, or completely punctured. A superficial laceration is similar to a corneal ulcer. With deeper lacerations, the aqueous humor may escape through the tear and globe may collapse; part of the iris may protrude through the tear in the cornea and vision will be lost.

Treatment: The veterinarian will first cleanse the laceration with physiological saline solution, then either replace any exposed piece of iris back into the globe, or surgically remove it. The veterinarian then flushes the anterior chamber of the eye with antibiotics and epinephrine. If the laceration is less than 72 hours old, the veterinarian may be able to suture it.

Mydriatic drugs are administered to keep the pupil dilated, and a topical antibiotic ophthalmic ointment is applied several times daily for two or three weeks. The veterinarian may also administer antibiotics and corticosteroids systemically.

HEMORRHAGE INTO THE ANTERIOR CHAMBER

Hemorrhage into the anterior chamber of the eye may result from a blow to the eye, and is a condition known as hyphema. Signs of hyphema include corneal edema, blepharospasm, and photophobia.

Treatment: The veterinarian will administer mydriatic drugs to dilate the pupil and thus prevent synechia (adhesions between the iris and the cornea or lens). The hemorrhaging blood must first clot, then the clot retract and finally be absorbed, before this type of injury will be completely healed, a process which requires 4 to 6 weeks. The veterinarian will also prescribe corticosteroids, both topically and systemically, to help prevent the formation of fibrin and facilitate the removal of red blood cells from the aqueous.

LUXATION OF THE LENS

Luxation (dislocation) of the lens is sometimes caused by trauma, although it may also result from old age, recurrent uveitis, or a congenital defect. Glaucoma often develops in a horse that has a luxated or subluxated (partially dislocated) lens, because the displacement of the lens may cause a rapid increase in the intraocular pressure.

Treatment: The veterinarian may be able to surgically remove the luxated lens, thus preventing a recurrence of glaucoma and perhaps salvaging some of the horse's vision. However, the prognosis for a luxated lens is poor.

Eye Conditions Affecting the Eyelids

The following conditions, entropion and ectropion, affect the eyelids of the horse. These may be either congenital, or due to an injury or irritation.

ENTROPION

Entropion is the inversion of the eyelid and lashes and usually involves the lower eyelid. This condition may be congenital, or the result of blepharospasm caused by an irritation, such as from conjunctivitis, A horse with entropion will often blink frequently. Epiphora and discharges from the eye are two other signs of this condition.

Treatment: The horse's eye should first be checked for the presence of a foreign body that could be irritating the eye and causing this condition. If the condition is congenital, it may sometimes be corrected by the veterinarian simply turning the foal's eyelid into its proper position. If this is unsuccessful, the veterinarian may surgically remove an elliptical piece of skin from under the involved eyelid, then suture the wound together. In approximately two months, it should be possible to determine if the operation has been successful.

ECTROPION

Ectropion is the eversion (outward rolling) of the lower eyelid, which exposes the conjunctiva and results in chronic conjunctivitis. This condition may be congenital; it can be caused by an injury to the eyelid (one in which scar tissue everts the eyelid); or it can result from paralysis of the facial nerve. Epiphora and keratitis (inflammation of the cornea) are two complications often seen with ectropion.

Treatment: Ectropion caused by paralysis of the facial nerve may correct itself spontaneously within four to six weeks. If the condition does not spontaneously improve, or if it is congenital or the result of scar tissue, the veterinarian can remove the extra slack in the lower lid by surgically excising a triangular piece of the lid and suturing the remaining skin together.

Congenital Eye Defects

The most severe congenital eye defects are anophthalmus (absence of an eye) and microphthalmus (presence of an abnormally small eye). Both of these conditions may be inherited and there is no treatment available. Coloboma is a congenital structural defect of the iris, in which the iris contains holes, or the pupil is of an abnormal size or shape. Detachment of the retina is another congenital condition. This is a severe defect of the fundus that is usually present at birth, although it may also result from inflammation or infection. The most common congenital eye defect, however, is opacity of the lens (cataracts). Cataracts appearing between birth and one year of age are considered to be congenital. They are sometimes associated with lesions in the retina, which may not be visible due to the opacity of the lens.

With the exception of cataracts, there is no practical treatment for any of these congenital defects. (The treatment for cataracts is covered later in this chapter under that heading.)

OBSTRUCTION OF THE NASOLACRIMAL DUCT

Young foals are sometimes born without a distal (lower) opening to the nasolacrimal duct, a congenital defect known as atresia of the nasolacrimal duct. Blockage of the nasolacrimal duct, which may occur in a horse of any age, may be due to obstruction by a foreign body or conjunctivitis. Signs for these two conditions are similar, and include epiphora and conjunctivitis; in foals with atresia, these signs appear within two to six weeks after birth.

Treatment: Blockage of the nasolacrimal duct due to foreign debris is corrected by backflushing the duct (refer to "Irrigation of the Nasolacrimal Duct"), while atresia may be surgically corrected by opening a distal outlet (refer to "Correction of Nasolacrimal Duct Atresia").

General Eye Conditions

The following eye conditions may be due to more than one cause, so treatment varies with the veterinarian's diagnosis of the underlying condition.

DETACHED CORPORA NIGRA

The corpora nigra is the eye structure that reduces the amount of light that enters the horse's eye. If part of the corpora nigra becomes detached, it may interfere with the horse's vision.

Treatment: If there is only a slight detachment, no treatment is necessary. In more severe cases, the veterinarian may surgically remove the tissue.

CONJUNCTIVITIS

Conjunctivitis, which is an inflammation of the conjunctiva, is one of the most commonly occurring eye conditions. Depending upon the underlying cause, conjunctivitis may be either acute, chronic, primary, or secondary, and it may be accompanied by a serous, mucous, or purulent (pus-containing) discharge.

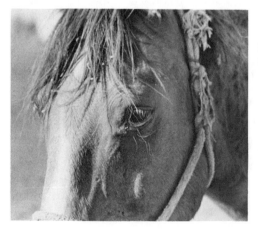

Fig. 11-3 Conjunctivitis with epiphora [tearing].

Acute conjunctivitis may result from the presence of a foreign body or from obstruction of the nasolacrimal duct. This type of conjunctivitis is sometimes accompanied by a mucopurulent discharge.

Primary conjunctivitis may be due either to bacterial infection or infestation with the nematode **Thelazia californiensis**. There is usually epiphora and erosion (ulceration) of the eyelids. Systemic disease may cause the appearance of chronic secondary conjunctivitis.

Granular conjunctivitis may result from Habronema larvae deposited in the eyes by flies. This conjunctivitis most often affects the nictitating membrane. Larvae migrating partially down the nasolacrimal duct, and then eroding through the duct to the skin, may cause a circular skin lesion seen over the area of the nasolacrimal duct.

Treatment: Acute conjunctivitis can be treated with applications of a topical antibiotic ophthalmic ointment and a corticosteroid, three or four times daily over a period of seven to ten days. Chronic conjunctivitis will require a longer period of treatment, from four to six weeks. This extended period of treatment requires the use of a subpalpebral system of medication.

Primary conjunctivitis resulting from an infection is treated by applications of a topical antibiotic. If due to infestation of **Thelazia californiensis**, the veterinarian will anesthetize the eye with a local anesthetic and remove the nematodes with forceps. The veterinarian may also apply an organophosphate insecticide to facilitate removal of the nematodes.

Granular conjunctivitis from Habronema larvae is treated by surgical or cryosurgical removal of the lesions involving the medial canthus and nictitating membrane, or by systemic administration of organophosphates.

RECURRENT UVEITIS (MOON BLINDNESS)

Recurrent uveitis, also known as periodic ophthalmia or "moon blindness," is one of the most common inflammatory conditions affecting the eye. One or both eyes may be involved, and signs include epiphora, photophobia, clouding of the cornea, and pus accumulation. The iris may appear dull or grey, and the pupil may be abnormally small. A horse with recurrent uveitis may also show blepharospasm.

A veterinarian can diagnose this condition by administering an intravenous injection of fluorescein dye. The dye will appear as a green color in the eyes of an affected horse. The exact cause of recurrent uveitis is unknown, but leptospirosis, onchocerciasis, **Toxoplasma gondii** infections, and a riboflavin deficiency are all suspected causes. Uveitis refers to the inflammation of the uvea (vascular structures of the eye, including the iris, ciliary body, and choroid), while recurrent refers to the continual recurrence of attacks. Each attack permanently impairs the horse's vision until the horse eventually becomes blind from a complication such as degeneration or opacities of the vitreous, detachment of the retina, cataracts, posterior synechia, or glaucoma.

Treatment: Treatment of recurrent uveitis is symptomatic. The veterinarian will administer cycloplegic drugs, such as atropine, to alleviate the pain and help prevent synechia by dilating the pupil. If the horse is feverish, the veterinarian will also give systemic antibiotics. Corticosteroids may help prevent future attacks, when given topically, systemically, and subconjunctivally, but they should not be used if any corneal ulcerations are present.

If onchocerciasis is believed to be the cause of the condition, the veterinarian may prescribe diethylcarbamazine to kill the microfilaria. This drug is given orally, in the feed, for three weeks. Since diethylcarbamazine does not kill the adult parasites, this treatment must be repeated at intervals.

The affected horse should be kept in a darkened stall while suffering an attack of recurrent uveitis. Hot compresses may be applied locally to the eye to help relieve the pain of an attack.

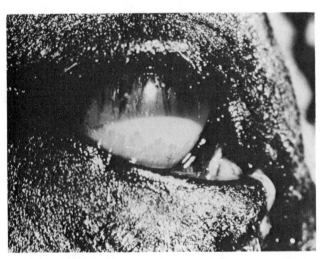

Fig. 11-4   Recurrent uveitis with hypopyon [purulent material in the anterior chamber of the eye].

GLAUCOMA

Glaucoma is an increase in the intraocular pressure. It may be a congenital condition, or occur as the result of trauma such as luxation of the lens. Glaucoma is often accompanied by corneal edema and mild blepharospasm.

Treatment: Treatment for glaucoma consists of the administration of long-acting miotics (drugs which constrict the pupil). If the cause of the glaucoma is a luxated lens, the veterinarian may surgically remove the affected lens.

CATARACTS

Cataracts are opacities of the lens, and may be either congenital, primary, or secondary. Primary cataracts develop independently of any other disease process and may be due to trauma, while secondary cataracts are associated with recurrent uveitis or systemic disease.

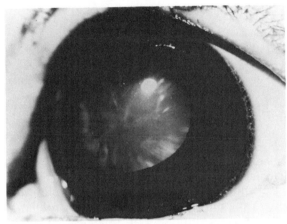

Fig. 11-5 Cataract, showing the cloudiness characteristic of this condition.

Treatment: Cataracts caused by trauma can be treated with corticosteroids and mydriatics, or removed by the veterinarian, if necessary. After surgery for cataracts, the horse will require subpalpebral medication to reduce post-surgery inflammation.

In young foals, congenital cataracts may be aspirated (surgically removed by suction), a treatment with a reported 60 to 80% success rate.

NEOPLASMS

Neoplasms may develop on the eyelids and nictitating membranes. Sarcoids most often affect young horses, while malignant melanomas are common in grey horses. Older light-skinned horses with little pigment around the eyes are especially susceptible to squamous cell carcinomas (refer to "Skin Conditions").

Treatment: The veterinarian will remove the neoplasm, using surgery, radiation therapy, or cryosurgery. Radiation therapy can be used successfully to treat squamous cell carcinomas, but is relatively ineffective in the treatment of sarcoids. Both sarcoids and squamous cell carcinomas tend to recur after surgical removal, and squamous cell carcinomas and malignant melanomas both metastasize (spread throughout the body) in the latter stages of development.

Cryosurgery is the preferred method of removing neoplasms, as there is a greatly decreased chance that the lesion will recur when this treatment has been used. Regardless of the method employed to remove the growth, the veterinarian will attempt to preserve the horse's vision and eyelids.

12

LIVER AND KIDNEY CONDITIONS

Liver

Hepatitis (inflammation of the liver) is generally secondary to septicemia, viremia and toxemia. Cirrhosis of the liver, known as chronic interstitial hepatitis, may also occur in horses. Hepatitis occurs in association with diseases such as equine infectious anemia, viral arteritis, azoturia, streptococcal infections, and leptospiral and clostridial infections. It may also be the result of chemical intoxications such as lead, copper, arsenic, nitrates, phosphorus, and carbon tetrachloride. In addition, hepatitis may occur following grazing on certain plants such as Crotalaria, Senecio, alsike clover, locoweeds, and lupines. In the case of plant poisonings, the pyrrolizidine alkaloids (which are of plant origin) are usually responsible for changes in the liver.

Hepatitis may be suspected upon seeing jaundice (yellowing of the mucous membranes or white skin areas), associated with a loss of condition or coordination, and an inability to work.

Treatment: Treatment for hepatitis consists of diagnosing and alleviating the cause. The veterinarian will administer dextrose, DL-methionine, B complex vitamins, and corticosteroids.

SERUM HEPATITIS

Serum hepatitis is an acute toxic inflammation of the liver, characterized by loss of appetite, intense icterus (jaundice), and central nervous system disturbances. It is an uncommon disease, probably viral, which occurs following the use of biological products derived from serum, when horses carrying hepatitis have been used in the serum production. Examples of such products are:

1. tetanus antitoxin
2. pregnant mare serum
3. antivenom
4. equine encephalitis antiserum
5. normal horse serum
6. blood transfusion

The disease may occur 40 to 70 or more days after injection. Because of this long latent period (time between exposure and onset of the signs of disease), it may be difficult to relate the cause to the disease unless good records have been maintained.

Acute liver damage occurs as the result of serum hepatitis. The disease is highly fatal, with death occurring in 80% of the cases, usually within 12-48 hours of the appearance of disease signs. The horse that survives will recover by the fourth day.

Treatment: Treatment for serum hepatitis consists of administering mineral oil and neomycin to empty the intestinal tract, which prevents endotoxemia. Vitamin B complex, glucose (for its liver-sparing effect), and systemic antibiotics (for control of secondary infection), are also used. Water intake is maintained with intravenous fluids and electrolytes are given if dehydration is apparent. Active cases should be isolated because of the danger of insect transmission.

Serum hepatitis may be prevented by avoiding serum products whenever possible. For example, a tetanus toxoid booster program, with pregnant mares given a toxoid booster 1 month prior to foaling, is far superior to relying on tetanus antitoxin in a hit or miss fashion as injuries occur.

Kidney

Due to today's improved diagnostic techniques, kidney disease in the horse is now found to be more prevalent than once believed.

Nephritis (inflammation of the kidney) is caused by toxic irritant substances classified as endotoxins (produced within the body) or exotoxins (produced outside the body). Endotoxins include toxins from bacterial and viral infections, as well as from metabolic disorders.

Exotoxins include chemical toxins and plant toxins. Some chemical toxins are copper, lead, mercury, arsenic, carbon tetrachloride, tetrachlorethylene, chlorinated hydrocarbon insecticides, phenol and phenothiazine derivatives, and sulfonamides. Sulfonamides should always be used under supervision because they are contraindicated in an animal with kidney problems or inadequate water intake.

Kidney problems are commonly associated with founder and azoturia. Kidney problems may be suspected with chronic weight loss, discoloration of the urine, excessive water drinking, frequent urination, or no urine output. Soreness over the loin is generally a sign of myositis and should not be confused with the signs of kidney disease.

A veterinarian is required for the diagnosis and treatment of kidney disease. The veterinarian will perform a physical exam and urine clearance tests to identify the area of the kidney involved and determine a prognosis. With proper treatment, the kidney can regenerate if the damage is not too severe. ♞

13

TRAUMA

The most common traumatic injuries encountered in horses are cuts and lacerations of soft tissues and fractures of bones. These particular conditions are covered elsewhere in this book. In the present section, three conditions associated with trauma are discussed:

1. hematomas
2. cellulitis
3. burns (including frostbite)

Hematomas

A hematoma is formed by the collection of escaped blood from a ruptured blood vessel. Although hematomas can occur in any damaged tissue, subcutaneous hematomas (located just below the skin) are the most commonly encountered kind in horses. Common causes include a kick from another horse, or collision with a stationary object.

Treatment: Swelling associated with hematomas is usually soft at first, and can be treated with twice daily applications of ice packs. The ice is applied for periods of fifteen minutes at a time, and this treatment may be continued for several days. The veterinarian may decide that a particular hematoma should be allowed to heal naturally, although a lump of fibrous tissue may remain beneath the skin. Alternatively, he may surgically incise the hematoma, ligate (tie off) the ruptured blood vessel, and remove the **accumulated fibrin clot.**

Surgical correction is usually not attempted until the hematoma is at least one week old. Active bleeding can continue during this time, and additional hemorrhage may result if the hematoma is lanced too soon after formation. Also, there is a considerable risk of infection after the hematoma has been opened, since the collected blood makes an ideal medium for proliferation of infectious organisms.

The veterinarian will incise the hematoma along its lowest edge, allow the more fluid contents to drain by gravity, and remove the blood clot along with any fibrous tissue lining the hematoma cavity. He may place a Penrose drain in the cavity and suture the uppermost part of the incision. The bottom suture holds the drain in place where it exits from the cavity, and a small portion of the drain is allowed to protrude from the wound.

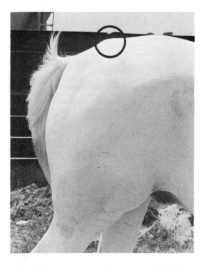

Fig. 13-1 Hematoma.

Antibiotics, such as penicillin and streptomycin, are normally administered for a five to seven day period, after which the sutures and drain tube are removed.

As an alternative treatment, the veterinarian may choose to pack the cavity with gauze soaked in iodine to destroy the fibrous lining; the pack may be removed after two days. Nitrofurazone solution, or hydrogen peroxide, may be used in daily flushings, and the horse can be given antibiotics to help prevent infection. After surgery, spraying the area with warm water or applying a moist heat pack will aid in reducing the stretched skin. The horse should receive mild exercise daily to facilitate draining of the hematoma.

Other locations where hematomas can occur include the subdural space of the spinal cord and brain. Hematomas can develop in this region from an injury, such as a severe blow to the head and neck. Treatment is supportive, and includes administration of antibiotics in conjunction with anti-inflammatory agents, such as phenylbutazone or corticosteroids. Fluids containing diurectics such as mannitol, are given to relieve edema in the brain. Even with treatment, prognosis for this condition is often grave.

Hematomas involving the uterus and vagina may occur at parturition. Given time, these usually regress spontaneously. The veterinarian usually discovers this condition through rectal palpation or vaginal speculum examination. He may recommend that there be a short delay before the mare is rebred.

Cellulitis

Cellulitis is a serious condition resulting from a virulent infection which spreads from a wound to the surrounding subcutaneous connective tissue and tissue spaces. It is characterized by hot, painful swelling accompanied by fever, depression, and loss of appetite. In addition, the bacteria will produce gas which is trapped under the skin. Cellulitis may develop into toxemia or septicemia. Small, infected puncture wounds are often the source of cellulitis.

Treatment: Cellulitis requires prompt veterinary attention. Massive doses of parenterally administered, broad-spectrum antibiotics will be required to combat the infection. The veterinarian may incise any dependent (one which is hanging down), inflamed part to encourage drainage. Cold water hydrotherapy and supportive therapy may also be recommended.

Burns

Burns may be caused by friction, heat, cold (frostbite), chemicals, and electric shock.

Note: When giving emergency care to burns of any type, remember that, after cleansing, the burn should not be treated with substances such as bacon grease, flour. alcohol, iodine, or baking soda.

Dressings that will stick to the wound are also unsuitable, since they will cause additional tissue damage when they are removed.

ROPE BURNS

The most commonly occurring burns are frictional burns caused by rope abrasions. These friction burns are often located near the pastern or fetlock where hobbles and rope restraints are commonly placed. Such

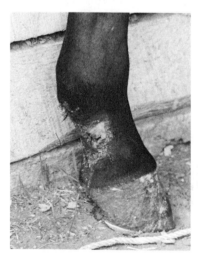

Fig. 13-2   The most common type of burn caused by friction is a rope burn.

wounds should first be washed with water and covered with a nitrofura-zone ointment. The injury is then covered with a non-stick gauze pad and bandaged with a pressure bandage to prevent swelling. When the bandage is changed, it should be carefully removed to avoid pulling dried exudate from the wound and causing further tissue damage.

SMALL BURNED AREAS

When burns occur over less than 10% of the horse's body, the charred debris can be removed from the burned area with a gauze pad soaked in a pint of sterile water to which a tablespoon of salt has been added. Mild soap and water may also be used for this purpose. Treatment of the burn involves cleansing the injury and applying an antibiotic ointment on a non-stick pad before bandaging. An emergency dressing of gauze soaked in warm tea can be applied to the burn before bandaging if no antibiotic ointment is available. When the dressing is in place, the area should be bandaged and the bandage changed every other day.

Systemic antibiotic therapy is necessary for several days. Special regulation of the horse's diet is not required in cases of very small burns.

LARGE BURNED AREAS

Major surface burns extending over 10% of the body area are the most serious type of burns because they involve the loss of large amounts of fluids and often lead to shock and infection. Because of this, and because treatment for very large burns may be extremely difficult, it is often recommended that a horse with burns over 50% of its body be euthanized.

When major burns occur, or when infection or shock develops from minor burns, veterinary assistance should be obtained immediately, and emergency treatment should be directed towards keeping the horse warm and encouraging it to drink water.

The following saline solution may be used to cleanse the burned areas:

1 teaspoon table salt
½ teaspoon baking soda
1 quart of sterile water

The burned horse should receive fluid therapy equal to 10% of its body weight the first day of treatment and 5% the second day. Antibiotics are needed to prevent and control infection.

Since a horse with severe burns has a greatly increased metabolism, special attention must be given to providing a high-quality diet in frequent feedings. Wasting away, dehydration, and severe systemic infection due to extensive damage to the protective skin barrier are serious complications in burn victims.

PREVENTION OF FLUID LOSS

An immediate consideration with severe burns is protection of the skin from further fluid loss. This can be accomplished either by covering the entire burned area with a large, dampened bandage (a sheet may be used), or by applying a hydrophilic (water-absorbing) antibiotic ointment and covering the burn with a thick layer of absorbent material (such as a combine dressing) under a gauze bandage. This bandage should be left in place for seven to ten days, during which time the horse must be prevented from biting or chewing the area.

Another method of treatment for a large burned region involves blowing a stream of warm air over the burned area until it forms a crust. This procedure usually requires one or two days and the crust lasts about two weeks.

Another possible treatment (by the veterinarian) consists of the application of a mixture of salicylic acid, tannic acid, and alcohol to seal the skin. However, this solution is very drying, and if the skin becomes excessively dry, lanolin and cod liver oil should be applied to the dry areas. The veterinarian may prescribe astringent packs as treatment for granulating areas that may appear on the burned region. These packs should be applied for 20 minutes twice daily for three days. Since this procedure may also dry the skin, mineral oil can be used as a skin softener, if necessary, and the astringent packs applied only every other day.

CHEMICAL BURNS

Chemical burns usually result from contact with substances such as phenols (creosote), alkaline compounds (quicklime), or acids. Burns of this nature must first be neutralized before other therapy can begin. The following list contains some common chemicals that produce burns and their neutralizing agents.

Chemical	Neutralizing Agent
alkaline	acetic acid (half and half mixture of vinegar and water)
phenol	alcohol
acid	sodium bicarbonate (1 tsp. baking soda per pint of warm water)
unidentified chemical burns	saturated (highly concentrated) solution of sodium bicarbonate or sodium thiosulfate

If the horse has come in contact with one of these chemicals, apply the corresponding neutralizing agent immediately. After neutralization, the injury can be cleansed with mild soap and water, washed with an isotonic saline solution (1 tsp. salt to 1 pint of warm water), and treated with a wet pack soaked in saline solution or sodium thiosulfate solution.

FROSTBITE

Frostbite is a burn caused by excessive cold, and is most frequently found in young, sick, or injured horses living in climates with very cold winters. Horses that are ill and lying on wet ground are particularly susceptible. The area most often affected is the ears, but the tail and feet can become frostbitten as well.

To help prevent frostbite, the horse's legs should not be washed any more than necessary during the winter months. When they are washed, they should be dried immediately. Of course, young, sick, or injured horses should not be left outside in severe weather to lie on wet ground. Horses that are pastured outside during the winter should be well fed and healthy and should not be pastured on water-logged ground.

In treating frostbite, the affected area should not be rubbed with snow or massaged, as either action will only increase the extent of the damage. Instead, the affected area should be soaked in warm (110-115°F) water for 15 to 20 minutes and/or covered with blankets for warmth.

ELECTRICAL BURNS

Burns caused by electrical shock occur as the result of horses being struck by lightning or when horses come in contact with electrical wiring. Electrical shocks that occur in the stable and barn areas are usually caused by faulty wiring or wiring that is too easily accessible to the horse.

In burns caused by electrical shock, treatment for shock may be the most immediate concern, and the veterinarian should be contacted immediately. After the horse has been treated for shock, the veterinarian will treat the burned areas as described above. ♞

14

SHOCK

Failure of the circulatory system, commonly known as shock, can be caused by severe loss of blood, severe trauma, or other serious conditions. In shock, the blood flow through the capillaries of vital organs is inadequate and the arterioles are constricted. The following conditions are major causes of shock:

1. loss of blood
2. infection (septicemia)
3. pain
4. allergy
5. thermal and chemical burns
6. colic or excessive diarrhea
7. surgery
8. hyperthermia
9. injection reaction

Regardless of the initiating cause, once shock begins, circulatory inadequacy is the inevitable result. Because of circulatory deficiency, irreversible shock leads to cellular death in the vital organs due to tissue hypoxia (lack of oxygen). The treatment of shock or impending shock requires immediate veterinary supervision.

Mechanism of Shock

A slightly decreased blood volume (mild hypovolemia) results in an increase in both cardiac output and respiratory rate. (Cardiac output is the amount of blood pumped by the heart per minute, i.e., the product of stroke volume times heart rate.) The heart is stimulated and many small blood vessels are constricted. This action reduces blood flow to less vital tissues such as muscles and skin in an attempt to maintain near-normal blood flow to the most vital tissues, especially the heart and brain. If circulatory compensation is effective, hemodynamics (circulatory control) will quickly return to normal. However, if the compensating action is ineffective, constriction of the arterioles will be increased in an attempt to maintain pressure in the arterial system. The muscles, kidneys, skin, intestines and other large organs will receive decreased amounts of blood.

Then, because the insufficient blood level will have deprived these areas of oxygen, the cellular metabolism will change from aerobic (oxygenated) to anaerobic (unoxygenated) metabolism. In turn, anaerobic metabolism will result in the accumulation of lactic and pyruvic acids in the tissues, which causes intracellular acidosis and kills the tissue cells. Metabolic products are released into the blood and cause coagulation. The amount of blood returning to the heart is decreased, causing increased difficulty in maintaining cardiac output (since the stroke volume is decreased).

Acidosis will depress the body's natural infection barriers, allowing for subsequent development of toxemia and septicemia. Depression of the brain and heart occurs and death may eventually result.

Detecting Shock

Abnormalities in normal vital functions may be indicative signs of impending shock. For example, lengthened capillary refill time may indicate an inadequate cardiac output. The mucous membranes will be cool and pale and the tongue may appear dry and shriveled. A "shocky" horse will have a low pulse pressure and, usually, a lowered body temperature. In response to acidosis and anoxia, respiratory and heart rates increase in an attempt to compensate for the increased acid production and oxygen deficiency. The arterial pulse will be weak, "thready," or nonpalpable. Urine output will be lowered due to decreased blood supply to the kidneys. In addition, the mental depression of shock may be followed by rapid collapse and loss of consciousness.

Treatment: The horse suffering from shock requires administration by the veterinarian of a large volume of fluids, up to 40-60 liters total, with 12-15 liters administered immediately (within the first hour) and rapidly. These fluids are administered intravenously under pressure to raise the central venous pressure toward normal. Large amounts of corticosteroids, given intravenously, are sometimes helpful in the treatment of shock.

Shock caused by extensive blood loss can be treated by replacement of the animal's lost blood with an equal volume of donor blood. If a large volume of blood is not available, one-third of the blood loss can be replaced by transfusion of donor blood, supplemented by enough fluids to restore the volume loss. Hypotension (low blood pressure) not caused by an actual blood loss may respond to treatment with large quantities of fluid such as lactated Ringer's solution given intravenously. Sodium bicarbonate is often added to the fluid solution to aid in correcting the acid-base imbalance (i.e., acidosis), that accompanies shock.

Because natural barriers to infection may be depressed or destroyed, broad-spectrum antibiotics are often given. The horse should be kept warm (not hot) with blankets, coolers, leg bandages, etc. In addition, any electrolyte solution given should first be warmed to the horse's body temperature.

The horse should neither be sedated nor fed orally while in shock. The effective treatment of a horse in shock necessitates the continuous evaluation and monitoring of the horse's condition by the attending veterinarian.

Anaphylactic Shock

Anaphylactic shock is an acute systemic allergic reaction that occurs when a substance called an antigen (foreign protein) is administered to an animal that has been previously exposed to the antigen and acquired a sensitivity to that antigen. Such a reaction occurs rapidly and may be seen following a drug injection, vaccination, insect sting, or following ingestion of certain plants. It is actually a violent exaggerated response of the immune system and produces severe allergy-related signs such as vascular collapse, urticaria, and bronchiospasm. A veterinarian should be contacted immediately if anaphylactic shock is suspected. If left untreated, anaphylactic shock can terminate in death in a matter of minutes.

Treatment: Early treatment consists of prompt administration of epinephrine (adrenalin), which may be repeated at 15 to 20 minute intervals. Antihistamines are also given intravenously whenever the reaction is severe or not satisfactorily responsive to epinephrine. Later treatment includes fluids for vascular volume expansion, corticosteroids in large doses, and vasoactive and inotropic agents (i.e., those that increase the contractility of the heart).

Hyperthermia

Hyperthermia is a state of abnormally high body temperature. High environmental temperature and/or overexertion can cause hyperthermia, which results in exhaustion. If severe, heat exhaustion becomes heatstroke. Hyperthermia is considered under shock because it will result in shock if left untreated. Signs of hyperthermia include the following:

1. weakness
2. rapid breathing
3. heavy sweating
4. elevated temperature (105-108°F)
5. collapse

Treatment: The most important therapy for heatstroke or heat exhaustion is rapid cooling of the horse's body. This should be done immediately while waiting for the veterinarian's arrival. The animal should be placed in the shade or under an improvised shelter and sprayed with lukewarm or cool water. Once the horse's temperature has decreased to 104°F, spraying should be stopped to avoid occurrence of shock.

Immersion in cold water, in a pond or stream, is not suggested, as drowning can occur due to the animal's weak and debilitated condition.

Ice packs applied to the head will help the horse recover his sense of orientation, and ice applied to the feet will aid in preventing laminitis, a possible sequela to hyperthermia. The horse can also be treated with a cold water enema. If possible, the animal should stand where there is a breeze, or electric fans can be used in a stall.

Most horses will become very thirsty and will attempt to drink a large amount of water within 15 minutes of the beginning of treatment. Water should be available but intake should be controlled in order to prevent laminitis. The veterinarian may administer fluids intravenously to replenish the horse's body fluids.

The grain rations of horses with hyperthermia should be reduced to help prevent laminitis, but all affected animals should be allowed plenty of water, salt, and hay. Heatstroke or heat exhaustion requires a seven to ten day recovery period, during which the horse should be gradually reconditioned. After an attack, a horse will often be unable to perform strenuous exercise while the weather remains hot. ◆

15

ANEMIA

Anemia is an abnormal condition of blood, characterized by a deficiency of hemoglobin and/or erythrocytes (red blood cells). Important causes of anemia include loss of blood (hemorrhage), breakdown of red blood cells (hemolysis), and the decreased production of red blood cells (decreased erythropoiesis). Poor nutrition, parasitism, and blood diseases may contribute to the development of anemia. Medical management of anemia is complicated by, first, the need to differentiate the type of anemia present and, second, by the need to monitor the hematologic response of the equine patient to therapy. Although diagnosis and treatment should be left to the veterinarian, the horseman may be involved in treatment procedures. In addition, he should be well aware of the following:

1. the signs of anemia
2. the signs of regression of the anemic state
3. how to prevent anemia

Inadequate amounts of blood, hemoglobin, or red blood cells results in poor transport of oxygen from the lungs to the body tissues. The lack of oxygen (hypoxia) leads to tissue degeneration, a rapid irregular pulse, weakness, and shortness of breath. Other signs of acute anemia include staggering, apathy, lowered surface temperature, pallor of mucous membranes, and finally, collapse or debilitation. Signs of chronic anemia include: loss of appetite, depression, some amount of weakness, decreased physical performance, pale mucous membranes, and general malaise.

Clinically, the severity of anemia may be determined by comparing the following measurements to normal values:

1. hemoglobin concentration
2. packed cell volume
3. total red blood cell count

These measurements are covered in "Hematology."

Hemorrhagic Anemia

This fairly common type of anemia is caused by an actual decrease in blood volume, either due to acute blood loss from trauma, or due to chronic blood loss, as from parasites. Blood loss can also occur through internal hemorrhage caused by an ulcer, neoplasm, abscess, etc. The signs of hemorrhage include the following:

1. pale mucous membranes
2. rapid pulse
3. evidence of bleeding
4. cold limbs
5. weakness
6. depression

Hemolytic Anemia

Destruction of an excessive number of erythrocytes circulating in the bloodstream causes hemolytic anemia. The red blood cells may be destroyed by a poison (e.g., lead or a phenothiazine overdose), by a blood parasite (e.g., babesiasis), by a viral infection (e.g., equine infectious anemia), or by an antigen-antibody reaction (e.g., neonatal isoerythrolysis). The signs of hemolytic anemia include the following:

1. pale mucous membranes
2. icterus (jaundice)
3. lowered packed cell volume and hemoglobin levels
4. hemoglobinuria (hemoglobin in the urine)
5. hemoglobinemia (excessive hemoglobin in the blood plasma)
6. elevated temperature

Nutritional Anemia

A wide variety of factors can influence red blood cell production, such as minerals, vitamins, and protein. Minerals involved in hematopoiesis include iron (primary importance), copper, cobalt, and perhaps selenium. Important hematopoietic vitamins include B_{12} (cyanocobalamin, primary importance), folic acid (pteroylglutamic acid, primary importance), niacin (nicotinic acid), riboflavin, B_6 (pyridoxine), C (ascorbic acid), and perhaps E. Protein deficiency can also result in inadequate hematopoiesis and, thus, nutritional anemia. Diagnosis involves complicated laboratory procedures.

Treatment

Treatment for hemorrhagic anemia is directed towards arresting hemorrhage and restoring blood volume in acute cases. Therapy includes blood transfusions (in foals, after cross-matching of blood types) and fluid and electrolyte therapy (in foals and adult horses). Antibiotics, hematinics (agents containing iron, copper, cobalt, vitamins C and E, and the B complex vitamins), and corticosteroids may also be administered. Follow-up treatment may involve a high-protein diet for several weeks. Blood loss from chronic causes requires specific therapy. For example, it would be of little value to treat a heavily parasitized horse with a hematinic, if the worm burden was not first reduced. After deworming, however, a vitamin/mineral supplemented high-quality ration would be quite beneficial.

The primary cause of hemolytic anemia must be identified for proper treatment to begin. Once the cause has been determined, the veterinarian can start therapy. For instance, in cases of hemolytic anemia caused by neonatal isoerythrolysis, blood transfusions from a suitable donor may be required.

Treatment of nutritional anemia is directed at replacing the deficient nutrient and correcting future feed rations.

HEMATINIC DRUGS

Hematinic drugs are exceptionally useful when the exact cause of the anemia is known. Treatment should be based on a clear understanding of the indications and limitations of each agent and, as mentioned, should be considered a veterinary procedure only. Some commercial over-the-counter (nonprescription) products contain excessive amounts of cobalt, copper, B complex vitamins, and even some "tonic" agents, whose actual benefits are not known. The usefulness of such remedies has not been determined.

A more rational approach is the proper balancing of feed rations, supplementation (when needed) with appropriate amounts of vitamins and minerals, rigid parasite control measures, and use of specific hematinic agents as prescribed by the veterinarian.

Equine Infectious Anemia

Equine infectious anemia (EIA) is an infectious viral disease characterized by a hemolytic anemia, depression, intermittent fever, and edema. It may be spread by biting insects or by careless, unsterile injection technique. Horses under stress are particularly susceptible to EIA. This disease has an incubation period of two to four weeks, and can be either acute, subacute, or chronic in form.

ACUTE

The acute form of equine infectious anemia causes a sudden rise in temperature (to 105-108°F), depression, weakness, and a rapid pulse. Other signs include discharges from the nose and eyes, heavy perspiration, and colic. The horse will either recover or die, usually within a five or six day period. Pregnant mares affected with acute EIA abort.

SUBACUTE OR CHRONIC

A horse with subacute or chronic equine infectious anemia will exhibit much milder signs of the disease than a horse with an acute case. Often the only indications of the disease will be poor condition and weight loss. The horse with a subclinical case of EIA may suddenly run a fever of about 105°F, then apparently recover, but will become chronically affected. The horse may be clinically normal for an undetermined period of time until another attack, which is frequently precipitated by stress. Laboratory testing will reveal a lowered packed cell volume (PCV), hemoglobin concentration (Hb), and red blood cell count (RBC). (Refer to "Hematology.") A horse with chronic EIA may live for several years.

INAPPARENT CARRIERS

An inapparent carrier of equine infectious anemia will show a positive result on the agar-gel immunodiffusion test (commonly known as the AGID or Coggin's test). These horses do not show any signs of the disease, nor do they seem to be infective to other horses in the same pasture. At present, it is not known if an inapparent carrier could infect other horses with EIA; it is also not known under what conditions such a horse could become infective. Controversy over this point exists at the present time because many authorities claim that the enforcement of current laws enacted to eradicate the disease are more costly than the final loss due to EIA fatalities. There is a great need for research that will enable the infective carriers to be distinguished from the noninfective, inapparent carriers.

COGGIN'S TEST (AGID)

The Coggin's test (agar-gel immunodiffusion test) is widely used to identify carriers of equine infectious anemia. It works by detecting the presence of antibodies against the disease. A horse recently exposed to EIA may test negative due to the insufficient time to produce antibodies, and a seriously ill animal about to die may test negative due to a depletion of antibodies. (Refer to "Coggin's Test" under "Special Techniques.")

TREATMENT

There is, at present, no treatment for equine infectious anemia. Under the current laws (which vary from state to state), positive carrier horses are often branded, quarantined, or euthanatized. ▰

III.SPECIAL TREATMENTS & PROCEDURES

16

SPECIAL TREATMENTS

The Stomach Tube

The use of a stomach tube provides a thorough, safe way for the veterinarian to administer liquid medicines. **Because the stomach tube is introduced through a nostril, the technique requires a veterinarian's skill and a complete and thorough understanding of the anatomy and function of the upper respiratory and digestive tracts. Improper technique could damage the nasal turbinates and cause bleeding through the nose or allow foreign material into the lungs.**

The stomach tube should be constructed of fairly stiff plastic or rubber so that it will not fold back on itself, and should have a smooth, beveled end to allow for easier passing. A three-quarter inch tube is suitable for adult horses, whereas a three-eighths inch diameter tube is best for ponies or foals. A urinary stallion catheter makes a good stomach tube for newborn foals.

Procedure: Passing the stomach tube is considered a "veterinary only" procedure. The following description is offered for educational purposes only.

The end of the tube should be lubricated with water, mineral oil, or preferably, surgical lubricant to make passage smoother and less irritating. The horse may also be fed a handful of grain, before the stomach tube is passed, to produce saliva and lubricate the pharynx and esophagus.

The horse will probably need to be restrained with a twitch while the stomach tube is passed. After initial insertion of the tube, the head should be held in a partially flexed position to encourage the horse to swallow when the tube touches the pharynx. The tube should be held against the bottom surface of the nasal cavity as it is passed; it should not be forced, for too much pressure can cause it to bend backward. As the tube is introduced into the esophagus, it should encounter a slight resistance; consequently, if no resistance is felt, the tube has probably been passed into the trachea. When this occurs, the horse will usually cough and show some signs of discomfort from the tube's misplacement.

The veterinarian may check the position of the tube by visualizing it as it passes through the esophagus in the jugular furrow (the esophagus is usually visible on the left side of the neck). A slight bulge should be observable in this furrow as the rounded tip of the tube is advanced down the esophagus into the stomach. When the tube is correctly positioned, a bubbling noise should be audible from the stomach when air is blown into the tube.

Administration of Medicine: Medicine can be poured through a funnel into the tube using gravity flow, introduced with a dose syringe, or, in the case of large quantities, pumped with a stomach pump. Before removal, the tube should be rinsed through with water and allowed to completely drain. This precaution will prevent irritating substances or water from accidentally seeping into the laryngeal area as the tube is removed.

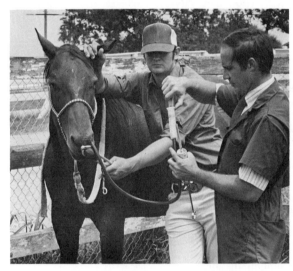

Fig. 16-1 The veterinarian is administering an anthelmintic through a stomach tube. Note that the horse is adequately restrained for this procedure.

Force is not desirable when removing the tube; instead, it should be held against the floor of the nasal cavity and slowly withdrawn. During this procedure, the thumb should be held over the end of the tube to prevent any residual medicine or water from leaking out.

Floating the Teeth

Floating (filing) the horse's teeth is a necessary part of proper dental care. Horses' teeth grow continuously and often wear unevenly. This often results in the development of sharp edges which may lacerate the cheeks and tongue. Signs that a horse's teeth require floating include quidding (rolling feed into balls and dropping them from the mouth), tilted head position, thin condition, and unchewed grains of feed in the feces. (For specific information on the correct procedure of floating the teeth, refer to "Dentistry.")

Flushing (Irrigation) of the Nasolacrimal Duct

Irrigation of the nasolacrimal duct becomes necessary when the canal is obstructed with mucus, dust, or some other substance. Two similar procedures are used to accomplish this: nasolacrimal and lacrimonasal irrigation. The simpler of these methods is nasolacrimal irrigation, which can generally be conducted with the horse restrained by a twitch.

Nasolacrimal Procedure: The lacrimal canal opens on the border of the upper and lower eyelids at the inner corner of the eye, where its opening slits are very narrow (about 2 mm in length). At its other end, the canal terminates at openings in the nasal cavity, close to the juncture of the skin and mucous membrane; the nasolacrimal duct is irrigated through these openings.

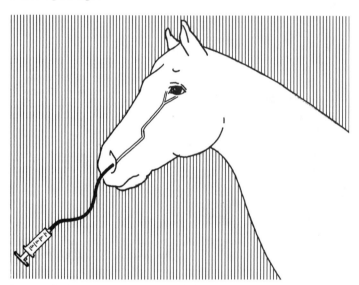

Fig. 16-2 Flushing the nasolacrimal duct. The tubing has been inserted into the lower opening of the duct.

Irrigation requires a #8 rubber catheter (or polyethylene tubing) for dislodging the obstruction, and a 10 cc syringe for injecting saline solution. For treatment to be most effective, the horse's head should be positioned in good light and held so that the nasolacrimal duct is clearly in view. The veterinarian will then gently insert the tubing into the opening and inject saline solution through it to dislodge any obstruction present. This procedure can be repeated if necessary. After the obstruction is removed, the injected solution will escape through the canal's opposite opening in the upper and lower eyelids, pour over the edge of the lower lid, and run down the horse's face.

Lacrimonasal Procedure: If an obstruction is not successfully removed by the nasolacrimal method, the lacrimonasal technique can be tried. The veterinarian will use a local anesthetic and the horse should be adequately restrained during this procedure. Occasionally, a general anesthetic or a tranquilzer is required before the procedure can be implemented.

After properly anesthetizing the area, the veterinarian will insert the tubing into the duct at either of the lacrimal openings near the inner corners of the eyelids (usually on the lower eyelid). The tube is usually inserted to the point of the obstruction before the saline solution or mineral oil is injected through it. Sometimes irrigation of the duct is most successful when used in conjunction with a probing motion.

Horses kept in dusty surroundings are especially prone to tear duct blockage and may require irrigation more often. Irrigation will also improve the animal's appearance by enabling tears to follow their normal path through the nasolacrimal canal. Otherwise, the tears flow over the lower lid and down the face where they collect dust, debris, and cause irritation.

Suturing

Suturing is the process of joining the apposing edges of a wound together to promote healing. In wound treatment, suturing is often desired because it promotes first intention healing, allows for minimal scarring, and decreases the injury's healing time. Most incisions and some lacerations can be sutured provided certain measures are taken to minimize infection, remove dead tissue present, and satisfactorily immobilize, protect, and support the injury.

CRITERIA FOR SUTURING

An injury suitable for suturing by the veterinarian should:

1. be less than 10 hours old
2. be clean
3. be located in an area of little movement
4. not be extensive in size
5. be free of dead or dying tissue
6. have a good blood supply
7. have a minimum amount of bruising
8. have few bacteria present

Suturing of an injury that is more than 10 hours old may not be desired because of the increased risk of infection. This much elapsed time between the wound's occurrence and suturing would allow for a rapid bacterial growth, which would only be sealed inside the wound by suturing. Large injuries should not be sutured because of the extent of damaged tissue and diameter of the wound. The sutures in this type of wound would be under severe tension with the wound edges in apposition, and could cut through the skin and cause sloughing due to pressure necrosis and restricted blood supply.

TYPES AND PATTERNS OF SUTURES

The suture pattern employed depends on the wound and its location. Some commonly used sutures include the following:

1. Continuous suture: a series of uninterrupted stitches knotted at each end of the suture line; used in areas not requiring a great deal of strength.
2. Simple interrupted suture: separate stitches tied individually for greater strength; if one suture fails, the entire suture line will not fail.
3. Mattress suture: either horizontal or vertical
4. Inverting suture: used in gastrointestinal and uterine surgery; patterns include Lambert, Connell, and Cushing
5. Subcuticular suture: used to prevent skin scarring
6. Purse-string suture: used to prevent the recurrence of a prolapse or to close a small puncture site.
7. Retention suture: applied at a distance from a wound sutured closed under excess tension to transfer strain from traumatized tissue to healthy tissue; includes button and quill sutures.

The selection and use of the suturing material depends on the wound, its location, and of course on the type of suture to be used. Some materials used are non-absorbable, meaning that they must be removed after the wound has sufficiently healed; examples of these materials are silk, polyamide non-absorbable synthetic polyfilament (Vetafil: S. Jackson, Inc.), linen, nylon, and stainless steel. Braided silk, linen, and nylon are used only in noncontaminated wounds because they are capable of carrying infections into the body, which could produce a chronic discharge from the wound. There are also absorbable suturing materials, such as cutgut and polyglycolic acid suture (Dexon), which are dissolved by the body's tissue fluids during healing.

Procedure: Suturing is normally conducted after the horse has been chemically restrained and the injured region anesthetized. The veterinarian can give the horse a tranquilizer (such as Acepromazine) and inject a long-acting local anesthetic into a cleansed site near the wound edges before proceeding with the preliminaries of inspecting and cleansing the wound.

Initially, the veterinarian will examine the injury to remove foreign matter and determine whether a joint cavity has been penetrated. He will remove dead or contaminated tissue and debris and undermine (tunnel

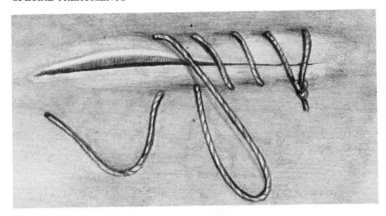

Fig. 16-3   Types of sutures.   a. Continuous suture.

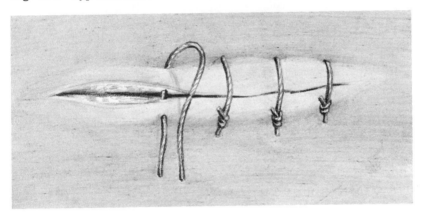

b. Interrupted suture.

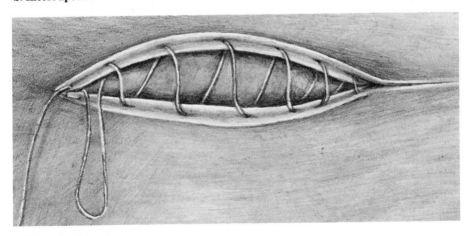

c. Subcuticular suture.

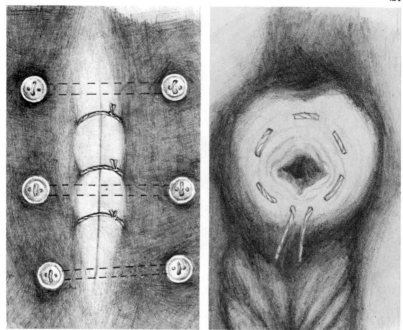

Fig. 16-4 **a. Button suture; the buttons relieve some of the tension on the suture line.**
b. Purse-string suture; this is most often used around the anus to prevent the recurrence of a prolapsed rectum.

under) the skin at the wound edges to make it moveable over the subcutaneous tissue. It is usually necessary, also, to trim the wound edges or scrape them with a scalpel to freshen them and make them bleed. This extensive preparation is necessary to prevent infection, decrease tension on wound edges and sutures, and ensure a good blood supply to healthy tissue to promote first intention healing.

Before suturing is performed, the wound is normally packed for protection with suitable medication and gauze sponges. The surrounding area is clipped, shaved, and rinsed with an iodine solution or similar antiseptic. The veterinarian will then remove the packing, scrub the surrounding skin with surgical soap, and rinse the wound with physiological saline solution. An antiseptic is also painted on the skin encompassing the wound area and the injury sometimes is dusted with nitrofurazone powder.

The veterinarian may delay suturing when the wound is more than a few hours old, when there is swelling, or if he suspects that contamination is present. In such cases, the horse may be given systemic antibiotics and anti-inflammatory agents, and a nitrofurazone ointment may be applied topically. The wound can then be covered with plastic, wrapped with a support bandage, and left for two or three days, after which time suturing can be attempted with reasonable hope of success.

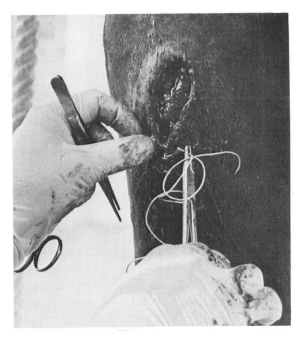

Fig. 16-5 Wound suturing procedures.

a. Suturing the wound.

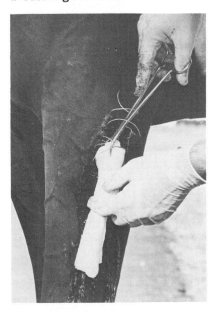

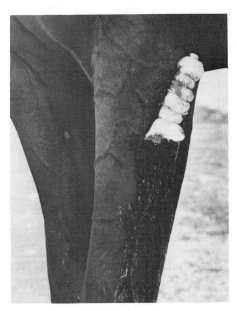

b. Applying a gauze roll to provide pressure support to the suture line.

c. Finished suture.

PROTECTION OF SUTURED AREAS

The suture line will require adequate protection and support to prevent excessive movement and subsequent reinjury, inhibit infection and edema, and control seepage of serum. To help accomplish this, the veterinarian can stitch a roll of gauze against the suture line to support it and to prevent a serum pocket from forming under the skin. If not provided with protection and support, the wound may split open (dehisce).

The horse should be given a tetanus antitoxin or toxoid injection (according to his vaccination program) and some systemic antibiotics to prevent and control infection. It is extremely important to confine the horse and limit movement. In addition, neck cradles, sidesticks, and bibs are often used to restrain the horse from chewing on the sutured area.

Plastic Surgery

Techniques such as Z-plasty and W-plasty are used to minimize or reduce scarring, as well as to cosmetically repair old scars. These techniques work by freeing skin so it can be stretched across underlying tissue, thereby covering the defect without placing undue tension on suture lines.

Additionally, skin grafts donated from other areas of the body (autogenous grafts), may be used to encourage skin growth across large beds of granulation tissue. Pinch grafts consist of small circular plugs of skin that are taken from another area on the horse's body with a biopsy punch and transferred to the wound area. A mesh graft is a technique in which a pattern is cut into the skin that allows it to expand horizontally to cover an increased area.

Corrective Shoeing and Trimming

The purpose of corrective shoeing and trimming is to preserve or return the hoof to its natural form. Corrective shoeing deals both with congenital and acquired defects affecting the horse's movement, and is used to correct faulty gaits and their harmful effects. For corrective shoeing to be successful, each horse must be considered individually, since two horses with the same fault may require totally different corrective measures.

Usually, the least severe corrective measure that will suffice is best. For this reason, sometimes corrective trimming alone will be adequate to treat a young horse. However, as a horse matures, the faulty gait becomes permanent to the extent that corrective shoeing and trimming will usually only modify, not correct, the defect.

TYPES OF CORRECTIVE SHOES

The types of corrective shoes discussed below have certain common characteristics, and are used for one of the following purposes:

1. to ensure proper breakover at the toe
2. to provide better traction
3. to provide support
4. to offer pressure
5. to provide protection to the hoof

The horse should be "gaited" (led through the various gaits) to see how the foot lands, where the weight is placed, and where the toe breaks over. This will enable the veterinarian and farrier to determine the defect in gait and decide on a suitable corrective shoe. The shoe should be applied only after the hoof has been leveled by trimming.

Roller Toe Shoe: This shoe allows the horse's hoof to break over at the center of the toe more easily. It can be made by filing off the bottom edge of a shoe at the point where it aligns with the horse's toe.

Full Roller Shoe: This shoe permits the hoof to break over more easily in any direction. It can be made by filing off the outside branch of the shoe all the way around.

Bar Shoe: A full-bar shoe has a bar from heel to heel which can apply or decrease pressure on the frog. A half-bar shoe has a half bar from the heel or branch which increases frog pressure. The bar of either shoe should press in about one-quarter inch on the frog to increase pressure.

Rocker Toe Shoe: This shoe causes easier breakover at the toe. The horse's hoof must be trimmed back at the toe to fit the shoe.

Rim Shoe: This shoe has a wedge-shaped rim around the bottom outside of the web. This type is used to provide extra traction and to correct conformational defects such as base-narrow, toe-out.

Heel Calks: These are projections on the heel of the shoe that provide extra traction. They are also known as jar calks, block heels, and heel stickers, depending upon their shape.

Toe Grab: This is a wedge-shaped bar on the ground surface of the toe of a shoe. It increases traction and is used on some racing shoes.

Trailer Shoe: This shoe has extensions on either one or both heels. These extensions, which are one-half inch long or less, extend outward and backward. A trailer shoe may be used to correct a conformational defect, such as base-narrow, toe-in (pigeon-toed).

Extension Shoe: This shoe has a metal projection from the toe which facilitates breakover at the center of the toe. This shoe can be made by welding a piece of metal to a regular shoe.

Toe and Quarter Clips: These are metal projections on the outside, hoof-bearing surface of a shoe. These clips are applied to shoes worn by horses with cracked hoofs, since they help prevent the crack from enlarging and also reinforce the hoof wall.

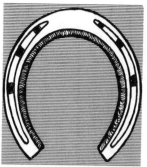

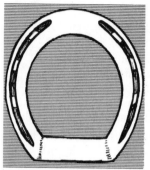

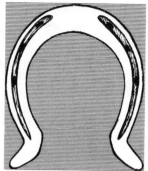

Fig. 16-6 a. Full rollermotion shoe.

b. Full-bar shoe.

c. Plate shoe with trailers on both heels.

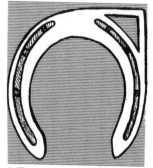

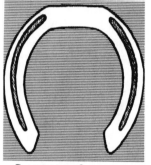

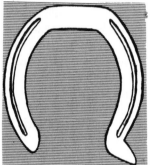

d. Toe-extension shoe.

e. Square-toe shoe.

f.   Square-toe shoe with trailer.

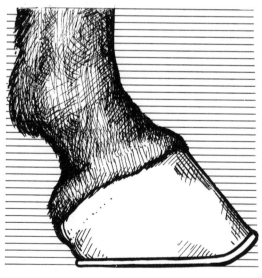

g. Rocker-toe shoe.

CONDITIONS REQUIRING CORRECTIVE SHOEING

The following conditions often require corrective shoeing and trimming. These defects may be treated by a variety of corrective shoes, most of which work by causing breakover at the center of the toe and/or by supporting and raising a portion of the hoof wall. In some cases, hoof pads will be used to cushion the sole and protect the foot. These pads may be made of leather, rubber, or plastic. A full pad covers the entire sole, while a rim pad is only as wide as the horse's shoe.

Base-wide, toe-out (splay-footed): The horse wears off the inside wall of the hoof, from heel to toe, causing the foot to be unlevel. The outside wall should be trimmed to level the foot, regardless of whether the horse is to be shod. A leather rim may be used with the shoe if the hoof is especially uneven.

Half-rim Shoe: This shoe has a one-quarter inch rim (or welded rod) on the outside edge of the inside branch. It causes breakover at the center of the toe while raising the inside of the foot.

Square-toe Shoe: This shoe has a square toe that is fitted flush with the toe of the hoof. The shoe's square edges will force breakover at the center of the toe.

Toe-extension Shoe: The extension is applied to the inside of the toe to cause breakover at the center.

Base-narrow, toe-out: The foot breaks over the outside of the toe, causing the outside hoof wall to be lower. The hoof must be leveled before the shoe is applied. The same types of shoes used for **base-wide, toe-out** are used for this condition, with their corrections reversed.

Half-rim Shoe: The rim should be on the outside edge of the outside branch, where it will cause breakover at the center of the toe while raising the outside of the foot.

Square-toe Shoe: The square toe forces center breakover.

Toe-extension Shoe: The extension is applied to the outside of the toe to help force center breakover.

Short Outside Trailer Shoe: This is a square-toe shoe with a trailer extension turned out at a 30° to 40° angle. The trailer strikes the ground first and turns the foot in.

Base-narrow, toe-in (pigeon-toed): The feet are usually off-level, and the outside toe and wall are worn down. The same shoeing used for **base-narrow, toe-out** is applied.

Base-wide, toe-in: The inside toe and wall are worn down, so the foot should first be leveled.

Half-rim Shoe: As described for **base-wide, toe-out.**

Contracted Heels: Frog pressure should be increased. If the horse does not require shoeing, frequent proper trimming may be enough to increase frog pressure and aid foot expansion. Rasping or grooving the hoof can also help foot expansion. Vertical grooves (parallel with the foot axis) can be made at the quarter, or the quarter area may be rasped (thinly at the bottom, weight-bearing surface and a bit deeper at the coronary band) with a farrier's file.

Half-bar Shoe, Full-bar Shoe, T-bar Shoe: These shoes all work by putting increased pressure on the frog.

Slipper Shoe: This kind of shoe has tapered walls which tend to expand the foot when weight is placed on it.

Chadwick Spring: A Chadwick spring puts constant outward pressure on the heels to aid in expansion. This device should be used with a full leather pad.

Sidebones: This condition requires a corrective shoe that is rolled on the affected side. A suitable shoe can be made by grinding off the outside edge of the ground surface of a regular shoe.

Ringbone: A full roller motion shoe is applied after the toe is shortened.

Navicular Disease: The quarters and heel can be filed to help expand the hoof. It may be helpful to use silicone rubber or retread rubber cut to shape and covered with a pad to cushion the horse's foot. A shoe with slippered heels can be applied to aid foot expansion.

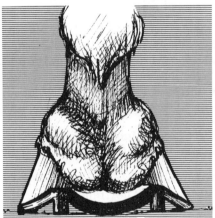

Fig. 16-7   Slipper shoe.

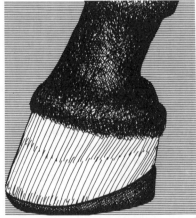

Fig. 16-8   Corrective shoeing may be used for navicular disease with a rolled toe and raised heel.

Interfering: If interference is difficult to detect, chalk can be put on the hoof and shoe to pinpoint where the interference is occurring.

Square-toe Shoe: This shoe if used for horses that strike the inside area of the fetlock on the forelegs.

Extension Shoe: An inside extension of the toe is used for horses with **base-wide, toe-out** conformation that interfere.

Half-rim Shoe: A shoe with a half-rim on the outside branch is applied if the horse has **base-narrow, toe-out** conformation.

Trailer Shoe: A shoe with a trailer extension on the inside of the shoe may be used on a horse with **base-narrow, toe-out** conformation that interferes.

Square-toe Trailer Shoe: An extra-light square-toe shoe with an outside trailer can be used on a horse which strikes the inside of the fetlock on the hind legs.

Flat Feet: Any trimming should be limited to the sole and wall. Pads may be necessary. The corrective shoe should cover the entire wall and white line, and be full length.

Forging: Since forging occurs when a hind foot strikes the bottom of a front foot, the breakover of the back feet must be slowed, or the breakover of the front feet quickened.

Rocker-toe Shoe: This shoe will speed breakover of the front feet.

Square-toe Shoe: This shoe will slow breakover of the hind feet.

Laminitis: The foot should be trimmed to as near normal a shape as possible (trimming will be necessary more often than for a normal horse). Leather or rubber pads can be used to protect the sole, and shoes with wide webs may also be helpful. The hoof wall can be rasped or grooved (as described under "Navicular Disease") to aid expansion of the quarters. Acrylics may be used to reshape the hoof (refer to "Acrylic Hoof Repair").

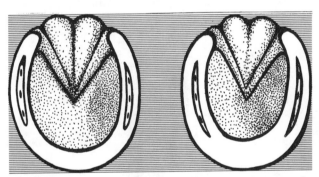

Fig. 16-9   Wide-webbed shoe [left]; compare it to the normal web shoe [right].

Toe and Quarter Cracks: The area of hoof wall on both sides of the crack should be cut away to protect it from bearing weight. An inverted triangular pattern, or a groove perpendicular to the crack, can be rasped into the hoof wall to help stop the progress of the crack up the wall.

Half-bar Shoe: This shoe can be used to put pressure on the frog. It should be adjusted so that the bar is pressing in one-quarter inch on the frog.

Toe and Quarter Clips: For toe cracks, the shoe should have toe clips on both sides of the crack to help support the hoof wall. In cases of quarter cracks, quarter clips will immobilize the crack and help keep the shoe in place if part of the hoof wall has been cut away.

Nerve Blocks

Nerve blocks are used both as diagnostic aids during examination and as anesthetics during surgical procedures. The following are the most frequently conducted nerve blocks:

AREA OF THE BODY	NERVE BLOCKED
leg and foot (lameness exam)	posterior digital nerve sesamoid block palmar or volar nerve ring block
teeth (tooth repulsion)	infraorbital nerve
eye (surgery)	auriculopalpebral nerve
hindquarters and tail (surgery)	epidural block

For more information about each nerve block, refer to the procedure in which the block is performed; for example, nerve blocks of the leg and foot are discussed under the heading "Leg and Foot Examination."

a.   **b.**

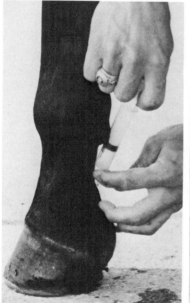 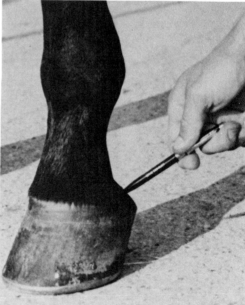

Fig. 16-10   Posterior digital nerve block.   a. Local anesthetic is injected into the nerve.   b. The area is tested to determine the block's effect.

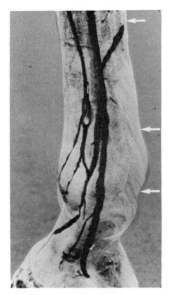
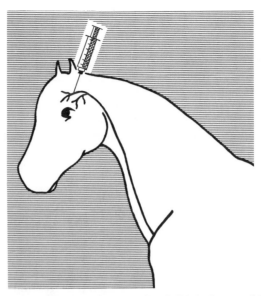

Fig. 16-11   The nerves supplying the foot have been outlined. Digital nerve blocks
are usually performed in sequence from the lower to the upper position [left].
Fig. 16-12   The auriculopalpebral nerve is blocked to desensitize the eye [right].

Casts

Immobilization of injured limbs is an important method of therapy used
in the treatment of wounds, strains, sprains, and fractures. A cast can often
accelerate the healing process and reduce aftercare by limiting movement
of the injury. Casting is exclusively a veterinary procedure, and serious and
even fatal injury can result from improper cast application.

WOUNDS

Restricting movement is beneficial for inflammatory conditions because
it helps prevent or reduce swelling and decreases scar tissue formation.
Wounds below the carpal (knee) and tarsal (hock) areas are sometimes
covered by casts because injuries in these regions are slow-healing and
often form proud flesh if the wound is not properly immobilized.

Procedure: Before a cast is applied, the wound is thoroughly cleansed
to aid in avoiding infection. An ointment, such as nitrofurazone or
chlorhexidine, is applied to the cast padding. Cast padding is placed on the
injury in such a way that uneven pressure on the limbs is prevented, and it
is held in place by conforming gauze bandaging. It should extend
approximately three inches above and below the cast. Two layers of cotton
are next wrapped over the cast padding and held with more gauze, after

which plaster of paris bandages are placed over the cast padding. If the veterinarian considers extra support necessary, metal braces may be applied to the cast and additional plaster bandages layered over them. When a neglected wound requires casting, a compression bandage and Stockinette (under the cast) is indicated.

The horse should be closely watched for 24 hours following application to detect any swelling below or within the cast. A foul odor emanating from the cast and the horse's chewing on the cast are both indications that veterinary help should be immediately acquired and the cast removed. Otherwise, the cast is normally removed after several weeks. After removal, the wound can be treated with nitrofurazone or other appropriate wound dressings.

SUPPORT OF TENDONS AND LIGAMENTS

A cast can also be used for support of a tendon or ligament, to help prevent contraction or stress. For this purpose, the casting method will be different from that used for wound protection.

Procedure: The limb is first covered with orthopedic stockinette, then wrapped with quick-setting plaster of paris bandages to cover inclusively the area from the sole to above the injury. Orthopedic felt is then used in rings around the leg at the top and bottom of the cast to prevent chafing, and plaster splints are placed on the front and back surfaces of the leg for additional support. Additional plaster bandages are rolled around the limb, and the cast is rubbed thoroughly to encourage adhesion of all layers.

FRACTURES

Thorough immobilization for a fracture is necessary; however, some slight weight on the fractured ends may encourage proper callus formation.

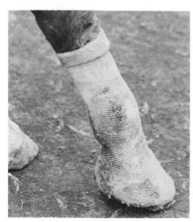

Fig. 16-13 Completed cast.

The cast must extend over at least one joint on either side of the break, and preferably over the entire limb. Such a cast should reduce pain caused by muscle spasm, stimulate healing, prevent movement of bone fragments, and encourage quicker restoration of the damaged leg. A walking cast is suitable for fractures below the knee or hock and allows the horse to bear some weight on the leg during convalescence.

TYPES OF CASTING MATERIALS

Materials suitable for use on a fractured limb include plaster of paris, plaster/resin, and fiberglass. Different plaster of paris bandages have different "setting up" or hardening times. Moreover, the hardening times of these bandages are affected by water temperature (warm water decreases the time), the amount of minerals contained in the water (hard water decreases the time), and by the quantity of water used (less water decreases the time). The advantages of plaster of paris are that it is inexpensive, easily applied, and unlikely to cause allergic reactions. The disadvantages of this material are that it requires a lengthy "setting up" period, crumbles when exposed to water, and makes a very heavy cast.

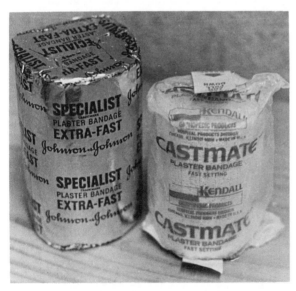

Fig. 16-14 Commercially available plaster bandages for casting.

The second type of cast, made from plaster/resin, is, like the plaster of paris cast, inexpensive, but is also much lighter and more water-resistant. The resin compound, however, is corrosive and must not be allowed to contact the horse's skin during application. This cast is applied by first making a light plaster cast from two plaster bandages rolled over a layer of cotton and orthopedic felt. Four inch rolls of fiberglass, that have been dipped in a polyester-resin-catalyst mixture, are then added over the plaster cast until three to five layers have been built up. Instead of dipping the fiberglass bandages in the mixture, the plaster cast can first be painted with the compound, and then the fiberglass bandages added onto the plaster cast until the necessary thickness is attained. With either of the above methods, another fiberglass bandage is wrapped tightly over the entire cast to compact the layers. This type of cast requires about 30 minutes to dry, but the process can be hastened by using a heat lamp or by increasing the amount of catalyst used in the mixture.

The third kind of cast for fracture immobilization is the pure fiberglass cast. This cast is stronger than a plaster cast; in fact, it can withstand 125-150 pounds pressure per square inch compared to only 50-60 pounds per square inch for plaster. Furthermore, it is much lighter and more water-resistant. The greatest disadvantage is the high cost of the cast material and the ultraviolet light required for construction. Also, some horses may develop an allergic reaction to the resin that is used in its construction.

The fiberglass cast is applied in much the same way as are the other types. A stockinette is rolled over the horse's leg before orthopedic felt is wrapped on, and sponge rubber or a similar material is used to pad any bony prominences. Three to five layers of cast material are then applied to encase the leg from the hoof to the top of the limb. The cast is cured layer-by-layer under an ultraviolet light.

a.

b.

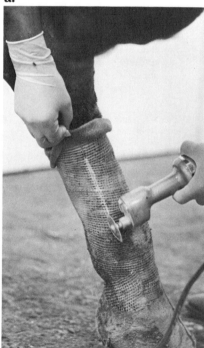 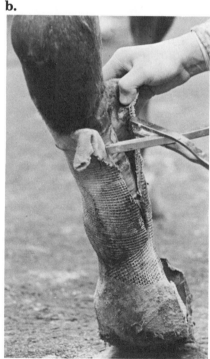

Fig. 16-15 Removing a cast. a. A Stryker saw is used to cut the cast. b.The cast is then pried off.

EMERGENCY IMMOBILIZATION

Quick-setting, temporary casting materials and plaster-impregnated bandages are available and can be kept on hand for use in emergency situations. They are used to provide temporary support to an injured limb until adequate veterinary care can be secured. For example, a bowed tendon acquired on a trail ride might respond more favorably to treatment if the leg received immediate support. Such a temporary cast, however, should be checked and replaced as soon as possible by a veterinarian. Otherwise, pressure necrosis or swelling could occur from improper application.

When a horse has a suspected broken leg and no veterinary help is immediately available, a temporary support should be devised for the limb. This may be successfully done by first applying a bandage to any open wound to keep contamination to a minimum, and then wrapping several pillows around the leg, secured by very tight elastic bandages. A splint made from 1 inch by 4 inch boards or from broomsticks can then be placed on the medial and lateral surfaces of the leg and wrapped within the bandage (refer to "Bandaging").

Laboratory Techniques

HEMATOLOGY

Blood serves as a transport medium within the body of horses and other animals, and has the following functions:

1. carries digested nutrients from the alimentary canal to body tissues
2. transports oxygen (O_2) from the lungs to tissues, and carbon dioxide (CO_2) from tissues to the lungs
3. removes other metabolic waste products from tissues to excretory organs
4. translocates hormones and related substances to target organs and tissues
5. regulates the body's acid-base balance and temperature
6. maintains a constant state of hydration of body tissues
7. defends the body against invading microorganisms

These functions are mediated by both the cellular and liquid components of the blood, resulting in a favorable "micro-environment" within the horse's tissues. This uniform environment within body tissues is referred to as homeostasis; homeostatic conditions are essential to the proper functioning of all body organs. Maintenance of homeostasis in individual tissues is essential for optimum physical performance of the animal as a whole. Hematologic (blood) characteristics are of considerable importance in general equine husbandry, as well as in specialized areas of physical performance of horses, since certain hematologic characteristics have been associated with superior athletic performance of horses. In addition, the blood is an excellent indicator of an animal's state of health. Signs of illness can sometimes be detected earlier by hematologic changes than by changes in the physical appearance of the animal.

The present section considers some of these aspects and reviews basic equine hematology in relation to good health and disease. Due to the introduction of numerous technical terms, the following list of definitions is provided.

DEFINITIONS

Hematology: the scientific study of blood and blood-forming tissues.
Corpuscles: formed elements of blood; the blood cells.
  a. Erythrocytes: red blood cells, RBCs; they contain hemoglobin and transport oxygen from the lungs to tissues, and carbon dioxide from tissues to the lungs.
  b. Leukocytes: white blood cells, WBCs; they participate in infection control and allergic reactions; different types of WBCs are lymphocytes, neutrophils, monocytes, eosinophils, and basophils.
  c. Thrombocytes: platelets; they participate in blood clot formation.
-cytosis: suffix used to describe an increased number of blood cells, e.g., leuko**cytosis**, erythro**cytosis**.
-penia: suffix used to describe a decreased number of blood cells, e.g., leukocyto**penia**, erythrocyto**penia.**
Hemoglobin: Hb, the iron-containing pigment of RBCs that normally complexes with oxygen and carbon dioxide, and abnormally with carbon monoxide (CO); indicates the oxygen-carrying capacity of the blood.
  a. Oxyhemoglobin: the specific form of Hb when combined with oxygen.
  b. Carbaminohemoglobin: combination of Hb and carbon dioxide.
  c. Carbonmonoxyhemoglobin: combination of Hb and carbon monoxide.
  d. Methemoglobin: oxidized form of Hb; it cannot transport oxygen; is produced by certain toxins.
  e. Myoglobin: a form of Hb, but localized in muscles.
Packed Cell Volume: PCV. "Hematocrit" indicates the percent volume of packed red blood cells in whole blood after centrifugation, and is a good indicator of the hematologic status of the horse; used as an indicator of physical conditioning.
Hematopoiesis: production of new blood cells, e.g., erythropoiesis.
Erythrocyte Sedimentation Rate: ESR; rate at which RBCs sediment out of blood.
Blood Plasma: the fluid portion of blood in which the cells are suspended; it contains fibrinogen.
Blood Serum: the liquid which separates from the blood after clotting; plasma minus cells and clotting factors.
Fibrinogen: a soluble protein in blood plasma; the precursor of fibrin.
Fibrin: an insoluble protein in blood that forms the essential matrix of a blood clot.

Thrombin: an enzyme present in shed (but not in circulating) blood that converts fibrinogen to fibrin for clot formation; (thromboplastin is the precursor of thrombin).

Plasma Proteins: soluble proteins identified as albumin, globulin fractions and fibrinogen.

Gamma Globulins: contain most of the sites of plasma antibody activity.

Coagulation: clot formation; a process whereby blood components undergo characteristic changes into a gelatinous mass or clot.

Hemoconcentration: an increase in the relative amount of blood cells and/or a decrease in the fluid component of blood; can result in an artificially high PCV.

Bilirubin: breakdown product of Hb; formed in the liver and gives plasma its yellow color.

Icterus Index: a measure of the yellow color of blood plasma; reflects liver function.

Anemia: a reduction in circulating red blood cells, hemoglobin, or both; different types depending on cause (etiology).

Polycythemia: physiologic opposite of anemia, or increase in the number of blood cells.

Hematinics: drugs used to stimulate production of red blood cells.

GENERAL ASPECTS

When the hematologic status of an individual horse is evaluated, the veterinarian will consider the fact that blood values are subject to very rapid changes. These variations can be within "normal limits" for the equine species and represent physiologic responses, or they can be abnormal due to pathologic conditions. For example, a considerable percentage of the total red blood cells (RBCs) within a horse's body are not circulating in the bloodstream, but are stored in the spleen. If the horse is excited, epinephrine (adrenalin) released from the adrenal gland can constrict the spleen, causing the release of RBCs into the circulation, thereby increasing the RBC count, hemoglobin concentration, and packed cell volume (PCV). Thus, the physical and emotional state of the horse must be considered when blood samples are collected for hematologic evaluation, and attempts should be made to provide uniform and familiar environmental conditions when the blood is withdrawn.

In addition to environmental influences, differences among breeds are also responsible for a large proportion of the variation of normal hemograms (blood pictures) in horses. The light breeds (hot-blooded horses), particularly the Thoroughbred, tend to have higher RBC counts, PCV, and hemoglobin than do the heavy breeds (cold-blooded horses). Age and sex differences have also been identified. Stallions, in general, have higher RBC values than do mares or geldings. There usually are little differences between 3 year olds and older horses, but 2 year olds, especially 2 year old geldings, seem to have lower values than do older or younger horses.

The high and low extremes of the range of hematologic values in horses are primarily useful for diagnosis of disease conditions such as anemia. However, the extremes are so wide that considerable variation can occur within these limits and still be designated as "normal." This does not necessarily mean that such changes are inconsequential, however, because they may have influence on physical performance capabilities, as will be discussed subsequently. The horseman should be well aware of those varied factors that can influence hematologic values.

BLOOD VOLUME

The total blood volume status of a horse is important for the proper interpretation of other hematologic factors, such as PCV, hemoglobin concentration (Hb), and RBC count. Since these values can be affected by changes in blood volume, they may be misleading if blood volume is abnormal. For example, if the fluid portion of the blood volume has been abnormally reduced (e.g., by abdominal edema or severe dehydration) without a corresponding change in the number of blood cells, then hemoconcentration will yield an artificially high PCV. Hemoconcentration is unlikely to occur in horses except in cases of severe illness; nevertheless, the preceding example illustrates the danger of overemphasizing one hematologic parameter to the exclusion of others. Due to the complexity of determining blood volume, this procedure is usually confined to research or complicated diagnostic tests. Unless severe dehydration signs are apparent, it is usually assumed that blood volume is normal when routine blood values are determined.

The average blood volume in horses varies from 60 to 70 ml of blood per kg (2.2 lb) of body weight in draft horses and ponies; from 60 to 80 ml per kg in saddle horses; and from 100 to 110 ml per kg in the hot-blooded (Arabian descended) equine breeds.

ERYTHROCYTES

Red blood cells in the normal adult horse are produced in the marrow of long bones and flat bones, especially the ribs. Erythropoiesis (RBC production) is a continual process and counterbalances the physiologic breakdown of "worn out" RBCs after their tenure (about 140 days) in the blood. Erythropoiesis can be accelerated by certain conditions, such as anemia and hypoxia. The red blood cells are specialized structures that transport oxygen from the lungs to all body tissues. Importantly, the process of oxygen transport supplies the muscles with the oxygen needed for energy utilization to meet the horse's requirements during athletic competition. The critical importance of red blood cells to equine management is therefore obvious.

The number of erythrocytes (as well as other cell types) in blood is measured microscopically, by counting the number of cells in a certain area of a blood smear, and expressing the volume-corrected value as the number of cells (in millions) per cubic mm (ul) of blood. The RBC count gives an indication only of the number of red blood cells and not the size of the cells. New automated counting devices have replaced individual counting in many laboratories. The red blood cell count remains fairly constant in an individual horse maintained under unchanging environmental conditions. However, the count can rapidly change as the horse's physical or emotional state changes. For example, a horse may have a RBC count of 8 million per cubic mm at rest, but this value could increase to 10 or 11 million per cubic mm during physical exertion. This example serves to further validate the need for standardizing blood collecting procedures when serial blood samples are evaluated.

The RBC count in horses can vary from 5 to 10 million in draft horses and ponies, and from 7 to 14 million in the light breeds.

HEMOGLOBIN

Hemoglobin is the iron-containing pigment present in RBCs that is responsible for the red color of blood. Hemoglobin is directly responsible for transporting oxygen to muscles and all other tissues. As with the RBC count and PCV, hemoglobin is a direct indicator of the hematologic status of an animal, and a low hemoglobin value indicates anemia.

Oxygen consumption by the horse's body increases with work. The increased release of RBCs into the circulation and the activated cardiovascular system are methods used by the body to increase oxygen availability. As RBCs pass through the pulmonary (lung) circulation, oxygen of inhaled air combines with the hemoglobin of the red blood cells. Oxygen is then released as the RBCs pass through small blood vessels of the tissues. Each gram of hemoglobin can carry only a certain amount of oxygen (1.36 ml). Thus, the amount of hemoglobin present in the blood is a direct determinant of the oxygen-carrying capacity of the blood, and has been used as an index of physical conditioning status. For these reasons, hemoglobin analysis is considered an important hematologic procedure.

Hemoglobin concentration is measured in grams per 100 ml of blood. Most horses have normal hemoglobin concentrations between 13 and 15 grams per 100 ml. The value of cold-blooded horses is somewhat lower, from 12 to 13 grams, whereas the hot-blooded breeds have higher values, from 13 to 19 grams. Since hemoglobin is contained in RBCs, the wide range in normal concentrations is due to the same factors affecting RBC counts and PCV.

PACKED CELL VOLUME

PCV is the percent volume of packed red blood cells in whole blood after centrifugation. This value is obtained by centrifuging blood (with an anticoagulant) in a small calibrated centrifuge tube called a hematocrit.

After centrifugation, the red blood cells precipitate to the bottom of the tube, and the height of the red cell column is read from the calibrations on the tube. A thin layer of leukocytes (white blood cells), the buffy coat, is present on top of the packed red blood cells. (The hematocrit tube has now been largely replaced by a "microhematocrit," which is a small capillary tube.)

Since the PCV is a direct reflection of the amount of RBCs in the blood, it is comparable to the RBC count and hemoglobin concentration in relation to hematologic status. In fact, the PCV gives an indication of both the number and size of the red cells, while the RBC count only indicates the number of cells.

The average PCV for most horses is about 35%; however, it may be as high as 45 to 50% in conditioned Thoroughbreds. The pronounced variation of PCV among "normal" horses is related to the same previously discussed factors that affect RBC counts and hemoglobin, i.e., sex, age, state of physical and emotional activity, breed, physical conditioning status, etc. Even small changes in physical activity can be reflected in the PCV. In one study, a 4% increase was observed in a horse when the blood sample was collected by a veterinarian rather than by the usual groom. Another study found that exercise, pain, fever, and excitement can result in a 30% or larger increase in PCV.

HEMATOLOGIC RESPONSES TO TRAINING

The hematologic status of horses has been found to reflect changes in physical activity, especially changes associated with prolonged intervals of intense athletic training. Importantly, differences among horses in their hematologic response seem to have some relation to their ability to perform in a superior manner. That is, it has been suggested that blood values can be used as an index to differentiate "winners" from "nonwinners," in that winning animals usually exhibit higher than average RBC, PCV, and hemoglobin values. This is not an absolute law, however, and much research needs to be done in relation to hematologic effects of physical training. Nevertheless, the potential importance of such a relationship bears discussion.

In horses placed in training after returning from pasture rest, the greatest increase in blood values was seen in those animals that started the training period with PCV less than 40%. These horses had average increases of 2.4 million RBC per cubic mm, 2.8 gm hemoglobin per 100 ml, and 7.3% PCV after 10 to 12 weeks of training. This increase in blood values during training was later confirmed in another study of Thoroughbreds in Australia. When 50 metropolitan race winners were checked, 41 (82%) had hemoglobin concentrations greater than the breed average. Of the 9 horses below the average, five were two year olds, an age group recognized as normally having lower blood values than other ages.

While attempting to establish the range for normal blood values in Thoroughbreds in Australia, researchers concluded that optimal and suboptimal levels within the normal range could be indicative of racing performance capabilities. For example, a study of Thoroughbred winners during three racing seasons confirmed that they have higher blood levels than horses in the general population. Higher values were also obtained in winners on metropolitan tracks than in winners on country tracks where the standard of racing is lower. Further, these researchers also concluded that the need for high blood values (RBC and hemoglobin) increased as the distance of the race increased because of higher demands on the body.

Several precautions should be considered when blood values are determined in performance horses. Due to the "normal" variability of blood parameters, results from one blood sample should be interpreted cautiously.

For example, suppose the blood pictures of two horses, after twelve weeks of training are as follows:

	RBC	Hemoglobin	PCV
Horse A	11.8	18.4	47
Horse B	11.4	17.9	45

Since horse A has a higher RBC, hemoglobin value and, importantly, PCV than horse B, an initial conclusion might be that horse A is further along in training than horse B and is more likely to be a winner. However, values from both horses are higher than the breed average, and it would be rather tenuous to select horse A based on this one hematologic evaluation. This example can be extended by assuming that another blood test was also made twelve weeks earlier at the beginning of training. At that time, values were as follows:

	RBC	Hemoglobin	PCV
Horse A	11.0	17.9	45
Horse B	10.2	16.0	39

Thus, during the twelve week training period, values increased as follows:

	RBC	Hemoglobin	PCV
Horse A	+0.8	+0.5	+2
Horse B	+1.2	+1.9	+6

In relation to increases in blood values during training, horse B actually showed a much greater increase than horse A. Thus, horse B seems to be demonstrating a more pronounced hematologic response to training than does horse A, and could be closer to his peak performance capabilities. In any case, such examples clearly indicate the need for carefully controlled evaluations of blood pictures in equine athletes.

Finally, one important aspect that should not be overlooked when blood values/physical performance relationships are evaluated is the fact that, although studies have shown that race horse winners usually have higher blood values than the breed average, this does not mean that all horses having high values will be winners!

ERYTHROCYTE SEDIMENTATION RATE (ESR)

The ESR is the rate at which RBCs fall in their own plasma under standard laboratory conditions. The ESR is quite rapid in horses, when compared to other species, and quite variable. RBCs of horses, for example, fall from 2 to 12 mm in 10 minutes and from 15 to 40 mm in 20 minutes. This rate is generally increased in anemia and decreased in polycythemia; however, the significance of such changes are not known. At this time, it is doubtful that ESR has any diagnostic value in predicting performance capabilities.

LEUKOCYTES

The white blood cells (WBC), unlike the RBCs, do not permanently reside within the bloodstream, but travel into body tissues to perform their functions. There they fight infections and are involved in immunologic responses.

The WBC count is expressed as the number of cells per cubic mm of blood. The average normal value in hot-blooded breeds is about 9,000 cells per cubic mm, with a range of 5,000 to 14,000. In cold-blooded horses, the average is about 8,500 and the range is 6,000 to 12,000.

Changes in WBC counts are used to diagnose bacterial and viral infections. During the first day of a bacterial infection, a transient leukopenia (decreased number of cells) may be detected, since circulating WBCs leave the blood to attack the bacterial invaders at the infection site. The WBC count quickly increases, however, as WBC production accelerates later in the infection process. A moderately severe bacterial infection may cause an increase in the WBC count to 15,000 to 17,000 cells per cubic mm of blood. A leukocyte count of 35,000 or more may accompany a severe bacterial infection. An increased WBC is commonly referred to as leukocytosis. Viral infections are usually accompanied by leukopenia.

BLOOD UREA NITROGEN TEST (BUN)

The BUN test measures the amount of urea nitrogen present in the horse's blood. In a normal horse, the amount will be about 10 to 20 mg urea nitrogen per 100 ml of blood, or 10 to 20 mg%.

A low blood urea nitrogen level can be a sign of liver damage. The BUN level can increase in cases of severe diarrhea, dehydration, and shock, due to hemoconcentration. When the kidneys are incapable of excreting urea, or when the blood flow through the kidneys is decreased, the blood urea nitrogen level will become elevated.

THE COGGIN'S TEST (AGID TEST)

The agar-gel immunodiffusion (AGID) test, the official test for equine infectious anemia (EIA) throughout the United States, is commonly called the Coggin's test after its inventor.

The Coggin's test detects the presence of antibodies against equine infectious anemia, not the actual presence of EIA virus itself. Therefore, it can accurately identify a positive horse only after the animal has developed antibodies against the disease, or, after a required time period of approximately two to six weeks following infection (the incubation period). In addition, the test does not differentiate between active antibodies developed as a result of infection and passive antibodies acquired by a nursing foal from the colostrum of its infected dam. The Coggin's test is also incapable of distinguishing between infective carriers and noninfective, inapparent carriers. Controversy over the use of this test exists at the present time because many authorities claim that enforcement of current laws aimed at eradicating EIA is far more costly than the actual loss due to EIA fatalities.

Procedure: Only authorized laboratories are allowed to perform the AGID test, and these institutions use a standard antigen and antiserum for testing. Basically, the Coggin's test checks for the presence of antibodies through an antigen-antibody reaction. A small, shallow dish, known as a "petri dish," is filled with agar, a nutritive medium, and seven "wells" are cut into the agar. Standard antigen is placed into the center well, and standard antiserum is put into alternate surrounding wells. The remaining wells are then filled with the sample serum from the horse to be tested. The dish is incubated for two to three days and then read by a skilled technician. If there is any question concerning the test's negative or positive results, the sample is sent to the National Animal Disease Center.

Because of the known positive antiserum used in alternate wells, there will be definite precipitin lines at those points. If there are also definite lines at the other wells, the horse is considered to have tested positive for EIA. The absence of a line indicates the horse does not have any antibodies at the time of the test, and is therefore considered negative. A weak precipitin line could be caused by developing antibodies, or it could be a result of seepage from the adjacent wells. In this case, another test should be conducted in two weeks. Other lines crossing the agar that do not cross the control precipitin lines or that do not join it smoothly are caused by antigen-antibody reactions different from EIA.

Usually, if the horse tests positive for the presence of EIA antibodies, he may be retested soon afterwards as a double-check. If this test is also positive, current state regulations must be observed.

A high percentage of foals from mares infected with the EIA virus will not be infected. However, it should be realized that colostral antibody acquired from the mare may mask the true status of the foal until approximately 6 months of age.

CROSSMATCHING BLOOD TYPES

Blood transfusions are sometimes given to horses that have a decreased blood supply, whether due to hemorrhage, shock, burns, infectious disease, or isoerythrolysis. Like humans, horses have different blood types that involve a variety of factors, making certain types of blood incompatible. When two blood types are incompatible, the donor blood contains antigens that are not naturally present in the recipient's blood. The recipient develops antibodies that attack these foreign antigens, resulting in hemolysis (destruction of red blood cells). Fortunately, naturally occurring antibodies against blood antigens are rare, and a first transfusion is usually safe even if the blood is not crossmatched. However, if a horse requires more than one transfusion, has had a transfusion in the past, has produced an icteric (jaundiced) foal, or is suffering from isoerythrolysis, it should not receive a transfusion without crossmatching.

In an emergency situation in which crossmatching cannot be done, the chances of incompatibility can be reduced by not using any of the following types of horses as donors:

1. horses that have received non-crossmatched blood transfusions in the past
2. mares that have had foals with isoerythrolysis
3. horses that have been vaccinated with vaccines prepared from equine tissue, such as tetanus antitoxin

The donor animal should also be healthy and possess a normal hematocrit (packed cell volume) and hemoglobin level.

Procedure: Crossmatching involves mixing the recipient's red blood cells with the donor's serum (major test), and the donor's red blood cells with the recipient's serum (minor test). Any agglutination, or clumping, that results is a sign of incompatibility and indicates that the transfusion should not be made. Both major and minor tests should be negative (i.e., without clumping) before a transfusion is given. However, if another donor is not available, blood that gives a positive minor test can be used.

A more accurate test, called the Coombs' test, may be necessary in diagnosing neonatal isoerythrolysis in foals. Some of the foal's cells are washed with saline solution to remove plasma and placed in rabbit anti-horse globulin, procured from a rabbit that has been sensitized to horse globulin. In this test, agglutination, or clumping of the cells, means that the foal's red blood cells are coated with horse globulin and the foal has the disease. Using the mare's serum in place of the foal's red blood cells, this test can be employed before parturition to predict whether the foal will be born with neonatal isoerythrolysis.

Blood Transfusion

Blood is collected from a donor horse, mixed with an anti-coagulant and administered intravenously to the recipient horse. The blood can be withdrawn from the donor at a rapid rate (perhaps one gallon within ten minutes) if necessary, and then slowly given to the recipient horse. During administration, the blood is strained through a filter integral to the infusion apparatus.

A foal with isoerythrolysis is usually given blood at the same time that some of its own blood is removed in order to quickly rid the foal's body of antibodies causing the condition. Horses usually are not given more than twenty percent of their blood volume in a transfusion. Because of the volume of blood required, transfusion is often impractical except in the case of foals.

MARE IMMUNOLOGICAL PREGNANCY (MIP) TEST

The MIP test diagnoses pregnancy in mares by detecting the presence of pregnant mare's serum gonadotropin (PMSG). This test is about 97% effective from 40 days to 100 days of pregnancy. The ability of the MIP test to determine the presence of the gonadotropin is due to hemagglutination inhibition. Red blood cells coated with gonadotropin will agglutinate in the presence of antibody to that hormone. The gonadotropin in the pregnant mare serum inhibits the agglutination process, resulting in a positive test identical to a control test run without antibodies.

Procedure: Serum from the mare to be tested is placed into two test tubes, one for a control and the other for a sample. Several reagents are added to the test tubes, then the two tests are allowed to sit for two hours. If a doughnut-shaped ring (identical to the one in the control tube) is present in the sample tube, the test is positive for pregnancy. Any clumping or matting of cells, however, indicates a negative result.

URINALYSIS

When making a urinalysis, the veterinarian will determine the volume, specific gravity, color, odor, and sediment of the urine for indications of the state of health of the horse's urinary system.

VOLUME

A horse should excrete between 3000 to 9000 ml of urine in a 24 hour period. An abnormally high volume can be an indication of the following diseases: diabetes, pyometra, renal disease, salty diet, or chronic nephritis. An abnormally low urine volume may indicate one of the following: dehydration, fever, diarrhea, decreased water intake, poisoning, cardiac decompensation, glomerular nephritis, bladder atony or rupture, or urethral spasm.

SPECIFIC GRAVITY

The specific gravity usually varies with the volume of urine, and a normal range would be 1.025 to 1.050. Specific gravity may increase in cases of dehydration, fever, severe hemorrhage, or acute nephritis. It may decrease if the horse is suffering from pyometra, chronic nephritis, polydipsia, or polyuria. In addition, some drugs have an effect on the specific gravity of urine.

COLOR

The urine of a horse varies in color from yellow to brown. The color may be altered by the presence of hemoglobin, red blood cells, bile pigments, and some drugs. If blood is present when the horse first begins urinating, the veterinarian will suspect it is of urethral origin, while blood appearing at the end of urination is probably the result of cystitis (inflammation of the bladder). Renal bleeding causes a smoky, bloody urine, and liver disease causes a dark brown urine. A port-wine color may be due to hemolytic jaundice or a protozoal disease. Obstructive jaundice will cause a yellowish-green urine.

ODOR

Any abnormal odor will be noted by the veterinarian. An unusual odor may be the result of ketone bodies, drugs, bacteria, or pus in the urine.

SEDIMENT

The veterinarian will examine the urine sediment microscopically to identify debris such as parasite eggs, epithelial cells, bacteria, etc.

CULTURING THE URINE

If an infection is suspected, the horse's urine can be cultured to detect the presence of infectious microorganisms. A sensitivity test will also be performed to help determine suitable antibiotic therapy.

HAIR ANALYSIS

Analysis of a horse's hair can aid in the assessment of the overall mineral balances within the body. Hair analysis is considered more accurate than blood or urine analysis because the hair is more stable than either blood or urine, and does not change in mineral content as quickly or as often (it is possible for the horse to have a 10 to 15% deficiency in total body content of a certain mineral and still have a normal blood level).

The analysis will reveal regional differences in mineral content of the soil and water which are reflected in the hair. Minerals that can be detected through hair analysis include the following:

calcium	iron
sodium	copper
zinc	manganese
potassium	phosphorus
magnesium	

Procedure: A hair sample is clipped from the underside of the mane. The sample is washed, dried, and dissolved, then analyzed with an atomic spectrophotometer to determine the mineral content.

URINALYSIS REPORT

Owner _____

Address _____

No. _____ Species _____ Age _____ Sex _____

Object _____ Date _____

	NORMAL HORSE	SAMPLE
Amount in 24 hours	3000 to 4000 ml	
Specific gravity	1.025 to 1.050	
Reaction	alkaline	
Color	yellowish brown	
Translucency	turbid	
Consistency	viscid	
Total solids parts per 1000:	50-120	
Chlorides	8-14	
Sulphates	2-3	
Phosphates	.05-.2	
Urea	20-40	
Uric acid	trace	
Hippuric acid	4-8	
Indican	.1-.2	

ABNORMAL CONSTITUENTS
Albumin _____
Sugar _____
Bile _____
Hemoglobin _____

CRYSTALLINE CONTENT
Calcium carbonate _____
Calcium oxalate _____
Triple Phosphates _____

MICROSCOPIC EXAMINATION
Epithelial cells _____
Leukocytes _____
Blood _____
Casts _____
Spermatozoa _____
Bacteria _____

Fig. 16-16   A urinalysis report form.

BIOPSY

A biopsy is the removal and microscopic examination of body tissue. This technique is used by veterinarians as an aid in the diagnosis of some illnesses, and can be performed in a variety of ways, depending upon the location of the organ to be biopsied. Some of the most often performed types of biopsies are discussed below. Regardless of the specific purpose of the biopsy, the horse should be given either tetanus antitoxin or tetanus toxoid after the procedure, and should be watched for one or two days for signs of excessive bleeding.

UTERINE

This type of biopsy is often performed on infertile mares as a routine diagnostic procedure.

The veterinarian will insert the biopsy forceps into the vagina, then through the cervix into the uterus. The forceps are used to remove a piece of endometrium tissue.

a.   **b.**

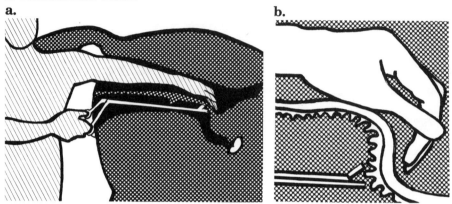

Fig. 16-17   Uterine biopsy. a. Position of the veterinarian's arm in the rectum, directing the biopsy forceps towards the uterine wall. b. Closeup showing the uterine wall being pressed into the open biopsy instrument.

SKIN

A skin biopsy is performed to diagnose skin diseases, to determine optimal therapy, and to indicate prognosis. A veterinarian may do a skin biopsy if any of the following conditions are present:

papules	neoplasms
nodules	unusual skin lesions
persistent ulcerations	unresponding skin diseases

The veterinarian may completely remove the suspected lesion (total excision), or just take a sample of all areas of the lesion.

The area involved is prepared as for surgery and a local anesthetic is administered. A biopsy punch or scalpel blade is used to remove a small piece of affected skin. The veterinarian will then suture the wound.

LIVER

An aspiration biopsy is the type often performed on the liver. An area on the horse's right flank is clipped, shaved, and prepared as for surgery. The veterinarian will administer a local anesthetic, then make a small incision at approximately the fifteenth rib. The trocar and cannula are then inserted into the incision, through the pleura and diaphragm. The trocar is removed (leaving the cannula in place) and a syringe is attached to the cannula. The cannula is then pushed deeper, into the liver, then rotated while the syringe is withdrawn. This procedure removes a core of liver tissue by suction. The veterinarian will suture the skin incision after removal of the cannula.

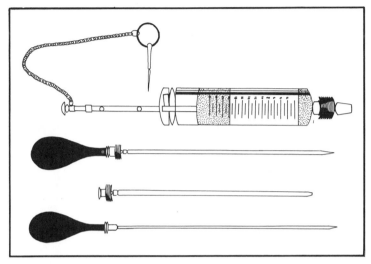

Fig. 16-18 Liver biopsy instruments. From top to bottom: syringe, trocar with cannula inserted, trocar and cannula separated.

CULTURE AND SENSITIVITY TESTING

In order to administer the most effective antibiotic for a specific infectious disease, the veterinarian will culture the infectious organism to discern what antibiotics are useful in treatment. Basically, sensitivity testing involves inoculating a growth medium with the bacterial culture taken from the infected horse, adding an antibiotic to the medium (in the form of discs containing an antibiotic, for instance), and incubating the culture. After a period of time, the results are observed and interpreted by the veterinarian.

The absence of bacterial growth around a disc of low antibiotic concentration indicates a bacterium sensitive to that antibiotic. A zone of no bacterial growth around a higher concentration disc is a sign of a moderately sensitive microorganism, while the presence of bacterial growth indicates a resistant organism.

There are other types of sensitivity tests as well. For example, there is a test based on the ability of bacteria to reduce the hemoglobin in red blood cells, thus changing the color of a blood solution from bright red to dark red. Bacteria inhibited by an antibiotic to which they are susceptible will not be able to reduce the hemoglobin in this test. The veterinarian will inoculate several tubes of the blood solution with the bacterial culture and add antibiotic discs to all but the control sample. Within one hour, the results of this test should be obvious, since the tube of blood solution containing an antibiotic effective against the bacteria involved will remain a bright red.

ABDOMINAL PARACENTESIS

Abdominal paracentesis, the perforation of the abdominal wall to collect samples of peritoneal fluid, may be used by the veterinarian as a diagnostic aid in various conditions. For example, it may be indicated in one or more of the following:

1. acute and chronic cases of colic
2. traumatic injury to the abdomen
3. possible inflammatory and noninflammatory conditions involving the peritoneal cavity
4. complicated births
5. rupture of the urinary bladder in foals
6. peritonitis

The fluid samples taken may be especially valuable in diagnosis of colic, because discoloration of abdominal fluid occurs early in the course of the disease. If serosanguineous (both fluid and blood) fluid is recovered, surgical intervention may be necessary.

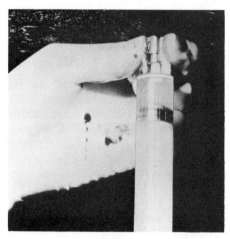

Fig. 16-19   Performing abdominal paracentesis.

Procedure: Abdominal paracentesis is performed with a small trocar after the site on the abdominal midline has been aseptically prepared. This area is locally anesthetized, and the horse restrained by application of a twitch and by an assistant holding up the foreleg on the side away from the operator. If necessary, the animal may have to be tranquilized. At the site of the operation, the abdominal wall is 2 cm to 6 cm thick. When collected, normal fluid is transparent and amber in color. Abnormal fluid color, however, will vary according to the horse's condition; a dark brown sample, for instance, is associated with a ruptured stomach, and a sample the color of blood usually means internal bleeding. Normal peritoneal fluid also contains numerous white blood cells but not many red blood cells. When acute or chronic inflammation is present in the abdominal cavity, the normal cellular contents will change in ratio to each other.

TRACHEAL ASPIRATION

Aspiration of the trachea is employed in the diagnosis of pneumonia and emphysema. The tracheal washing collected in this manner can be inspected for the presence of bacteria or viruses. Culture tests can then be done to identify the type of bacteria present, and sensitivity tests can be performed to help the veterinarian choose the proper antibiotic for treatment. Transtracheal aspiration is especially helpful in initial cases of herd pneumonia. This technique allows samples to be obtained as close as possible to the lung, thus eliminating contamination.

Procedure: After preparing the surgical site, the veterinarian will incise the sternocephalicus muscles of the neck over the midline, halfway down the neck. Of course, the area has already been injected with a local anesthetic before the incision is made. A large diameter needle is passed into the trachea between two of the tracheal rings, then a piece of flexible polyethylene tubing is passed through the needle into the lumen of the trachea. This tube is directed down the trachea to the point at which the bronchi divide (the horse will probably cough at this time), and a volume of sterile physiological saline solution is injected into the tube. This solution is then aspirated immediately as the polyethylene tubing is removed slowly. The material collected is used to inoculate culture media, usually a tube of nutrient broth and a blood agar plate.

Enemas

An enema is the injection of a liquid into the rectum. In the horse, enemas are used most often in the treatment of

1. flatulent colic
2. spasmodic colic
3. impaction colic in the adult
4. meconium retention in the foal

Additionally, cold water enemas are sometimes employed in treatment of hyperthermia, to help lower body temperature.

FLATULENT AND SPASMODIC COLIC

If the horse has flatulent or spasmodic colic, the veterinarian may give an enema of up to two gallons of warm, soapy water or dioctyl sodium sulfosuccinate (DSS), a stool softener, through a funnel and hose inserted about two feet into the rectum. The solution is given slowly, using only the force of gravity to move the liquid into the rectum; after this, the horse is walked until he defecates.

IMPACTION COLIC

In the case of an impaction, the veterinarian will usually first attempt to locate and massage the impaction to break it up via rectal palpation before the cold water enema is given. A cold water enema of up to two gallons of liquid is required in this treatment, though mineral oil and other medications may also be administered first by stomach tube.

MECONIUM RETENTION

Several substances, including soap, glycerine, and mineral oil, are used in enemas given to relieve meconium retention in foals. All enemas administered to foals suffering from meconium retention should be given with a soft rubber hose that is inserted a maximum of two inches into the rectum. A special guard, constructed to prevent the hose from going too far into the rectum, may be used. Caution should be observed when administering an enema to a young foal to avoid injury.

One type of enema frequently given to foals consists of two ounces of glycerine administered with a dose syringe. Another useful type consists of two pints of warm water with either soap or three ounces of dioctyl calcium sulfosuccinate (Surfak: Hoechst-Roussel) dissolved in water. Other enemas used with foals include a solution of four ounces of mineral oil (liquid paraffin) given every three or four hours until the meconium is passed. The commercial enemas are very useful to have on hand. A commercially available four ounce phosphate enema with prelubricated applicator tip (such as one made by Fleet) can be given soon after the foal is standing and has nursed.

Procedure: To administer an enema to a foal, the following procedures should be performed.

1. Hold the foal upright, but do not insert any fingers into the rectum to remove the meconium; they can cause serious damage.
2. Do not force the tube.
3. Hold the funnel, and attached end of the rubber tube, up to allow the liquid to flow into the rectum by gravity. No other force should be used.
4. Administer the enema slowly; rapid administration of the solution could cause serious injury or death.

Rectal Palpation

Rectal palpation is often used to detect estrus, pregnancy, or suspected pathology of the abdominal cavity (such as an impaction). It should be done only by a veterinarian or other experienced person, as improper palpation technique frequently results in rectal wall perforation, peritonitis, or fetal damage. In addition, palpation is quite useless if done by someone who lacks detailed knowledge of the anatomy being examined. For instance, a person inexperienced in palpation could easily mistake a fecal ball for an ovary, or the bladder for a developing pregnancy.

Procedure: The horse's tail should be wrapped and tied out of the way (refer to "Bandaging"), and the animal restrained if necessary (refer to "Restraints"). A twitch is usually sufficient restraint for a horse, although breeding hobbles or a bale of hay (placed behind the hind legs) may be required. The palpator should be wearing a clean obstetrical sleeve, preferably of rubber, which is less irritating to the mucosal lining of the anus than is plastic. First, the horse's hindquarters and anus are washed with a mild soap and water, then both the rectal area and the glove are lubricated. Mineral oil, a sterile lubricant (KY Jelly: Johnson & Johnson), or a nondetergent soap can be used for this purpose. Before inserting the gloved hand, the operator should form a wedge with his fingers; this wedge is then slowly introduced into the anus. In a case of impaction, the mass should be carefully dislodged and removed by hand, a procedure that can take up to 30 minutes. Sometimes, with an extremely hard, impacted fecal ball, the rectum should be flushed with an enema before palpation.

When palpating a mare to detect estrus, the same washing and entering procedure is employed. The palpator can either gently remove the feces from the rectum, or "submarine" his hand carefully underneath them, along the floor of the rectum. The arm will have to be inserted up to the shoulder, and the hand moved slowly in a "paddling" motion. Using this

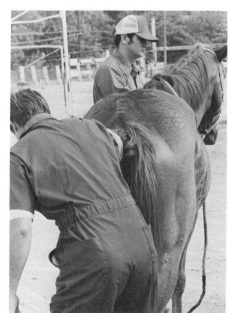

Fig. 16-20 Veterinarian performing rectal palpation.

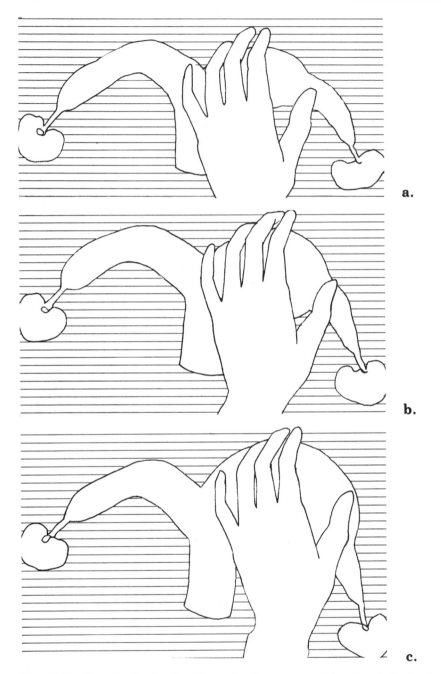

Fig. 16-21   Rectal palpation for diagnosis of pregnancy. The size of the fetal sac is shown in relation to the hand.   a. 33 days.   b. 42 days.   c. 60 days.

paddling movement, the operator should locate the pelvic brim, then reach over it to feel the uterus. The uterus can then be palpated along each horn to an ovary which will be approximately the size of a walnut. There will be an indentation on one side of the ovary, known as the ovulation fossa. During estrus, a follicle, usually at least 1 cm in diameter, is present at one end of the ovary. Towards ovulation, the follicle enlarges until it reaches a size somewhere between 1.5 and 7 cm, moves towards the fossa, and becomes soft.

Locating a follicle, and following it through development and maturation, will help determine the mare's state of estrus. Of course, there is a wide variation between mares.

Examining The Mare

VAGINAL SPECULUM EXAMINATION

A mare can be examined with a vaginal speculum to aid in the diagnosis of estrus or pregnancy. There are two main types of speculums, the Caslick speculum, which is stainless steel, and the plastic fiber speculum. These instruments are about eighteen inches long and one and one-half inches in diameter. When used to inspect different mares, the speculum is sterilized between uses in an autoclave. Incorrect procedure and unsanitary technique are important causes of infection.

Procedure: In preparing for a speculum examination, the mare is restrained in the same way as for rectal palpation, and the external genitalia are washed with water and an antiseptic lubricant and protectant (such as Viscogen: Haver-Lockhart). Cotton should be used for this cleansing procedure and thrown out after use, instead of a reusable sponge which could spread infection. A clean, lubricated speculum is then inserted into the vagina, and changes in the cervix noted. The use of a flashlight enables the veterinarian to perform a better inspection.

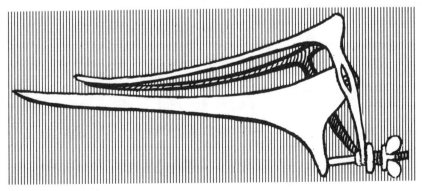

Fig. 16-22 Vaginal speculum.

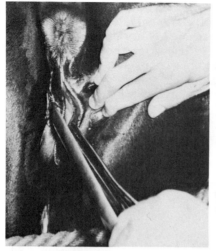

a.

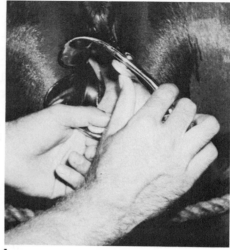

b.

Fig. 16-23 Speculum examination a. Inserting the speculum. b. Opening the speculum. c. Shining a light into the vagina to facilitate the examination.

c.

If the mare is not in heat, the cervix will be small and white, protruding into the vagina, with thick secretions. When the mare is in estrus, the cervix will be darker in color, with striations ranging from pale pink to red. The cervical folds and secretions will also be thinner. Immediately prior to ovulation, the cervix will be three to four times its size when not in heat. The cervix will be relaxed and lying on the bottom of the vagina, with a red color and viscous fluid secretions. During pregnancy, the cervix, now tight and pale in color, will be completely sealed by thickened secretions.

CERVICAL AND UTERINE PROCEDURES

Bacterial infection of the reproductive tract is a common cause of physical infertility in the mare. It can even be present in maiden mares, and usually prevents the mare from conceiving. A mare infertile due to infection must be placed on a program of treatment as soon as possible, since chronic, well-established infections respond very slowly to medication.

CERVICAL AND UTERINE CULTURES

Since an infected mare may not have a vaginal discharge or an irregular estrus cycle, a cervical or uterine culture is necessary to diagnose the infection. For the best results, the culture should be done when the mare is in full heat, because the cervix will be dilated at this time, allowing the collection of a good sample.

The sample of cervical secretions for the bacteriological culture is collected by the veterinarian or technician with a sterile cotton swab placed through a sterile speculum. This swab is next streaked on bacterial growth medium in sterile test tubes, which are then incubated.

A uterine secretions sample is taken at the same time as the cervical culture, with special sheathed swabs. The swab is inserted into the cervix as far as possible, and rubbed over the uterine mucosa.

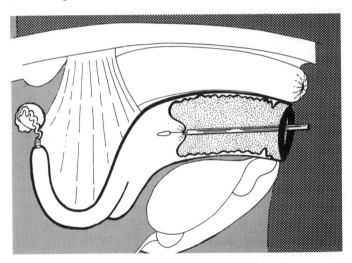

Fig. 16-24 Cervical culture. The swab is inserted through a sterile casing placed in the cervical opening.

Although a positive culture indicates that the mare is infected, a negative culture does not necessarily mean that she is not. To avoid having false negatives, the cultures should be taken at ovulation and one or two days afterwards.

If the mare is infected, treatment consists of a Caslick operation (if pneumovagina is the cause of the infection), sexual rest, and antibiotic therapy during estrus. The medication is usually given both topically and parenterally, and sometimes enzymes are added to the antibiotics.

CURETTAGE

Curettage, the scraping of the uterine mucosa, is another method of therapy that may be successful, particularly with chronically infected mares. First, any feces are removed from the rectum, and the vulva and surrounding area are cleansed. The veterinarian will introduce one hand into the rectum to guide the other hand, holding the curette, into the uterus. The curette is used to scrape each section of the uterus body and horns 10 to 15 times. Curettage should increase the mare's hormonal activity, and will not usually damage the uterus.

After treatment, cultures should be continued at each estrus until negative results are obtained twice in a row. At this time, an attempt at breeding the mare can be reinstituted.

UTERINE INFUSION

A uterine infusion is frequently employed as a treatment for physiological causes of infertility in the mare. It works by increasing the hormonal activity in cases of irregular heat cycles or ovulation, incomplete opening of the cervix, chronic abortion, and false pregnancy.

In this procedure, the veterinarian administers 500 cc of antibiotic-treated physiological saline solution into the uterus through a pipette, by the force of gravity. The vulva should first be washed with soap and water before the lubricated, gloved hand of the veterinarian is inserted into the vagina. The cervix is then dilated gradually by the index finger, and the plastic pipette (one of the type used for artificial insemination), attached to the bottle of saline solution, is slid along the finger. The infusion is instilled, and the mare will probably come into estrus within three to four days. If necessary, the veterinarian may repeat the saline infusion. For

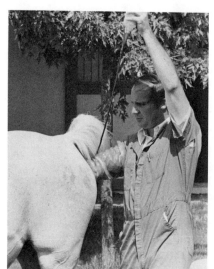

Fig. 16-25   Veterinarian performing a uterine infusion.

instance, the mare may receive three infusions, at two day intervals. The number of infusions required varies with the individual animal.

Endoscopy

The veterinary use of an endoscope is invaluable in the diagnosis of upper respiratory diseases, intestinal disorders, and certain neoplastic lesions. There are two types of endoscopes available; the rigid tube, and the flexible fiberoptic type. The first type is portable, but it is more difficult to pass (it may cause nosebleed), while the latter kind is better tolerated by the horse, is more easily passed, and yields a larger field of vision.

Endoscopy of the pharynx can reveal signs of pharyngitis, scar tissue and polyps, in addition to other disorders that may block the upper airway. Air movement and swallowing can also be studied with the endoscope. The flexible type of endoscope may be used to evaluate the condition of the glottis and soft palate. The horse should be tranquilized and restrained with a twitch (refer to "Restraints") before the endoscope is passed.

Laryngeal hemiplegia (roaring) can be detected by observation of the arytenoid cartilages, since an impairment of their retraction suggests paralysis of the laryngeal nerves. Arytenoid cartilage cysts, vocal cord polyps, and epiglottis entrapment are some of the other conditions that can be diagnosed with the fiberoptic endoscope.

The endoscope can be utilized in the examination of the trachea. Tracheoscopy can detect tumors, exudate from the lungs, and stenosis, a collapse or scarred narrowing of the windpipe.

The rigid endoscope is used to view the interior of the guttural pouches, since it is difficult to insert the flexible fiberoptic endoscope into the Eustachian tubes, although the long slit-like openings into the pharynx may be easily viewed. A diagnosis of exudate, inflammation, hemorrhage, and lesions from diphtheria can be made.

Procedure: An endoscope may be put through a trocar that has been inserted into the abdominal cavity. Once the peritoneal cavity has been inflated with oxygen, the abdominal viscera (organs) can be examined, thus aiding the diagnosis of ovarian disease and other ailments. In such a situation, the endoscope can be used to collect a biopsy sample, withdraw fluid, or inject medication. Cystitis or the formation of urinary calculi may be discovered through an endoscope passed into the bladder through the urethra (a rigid tube endoscope is used for mares, and a flexible fiberoptic one for stallions and geldings).

A flexible endoscope can be placed through the cervix to allow the veterinarian to examine the uterus. The endometrium will be visible only if the uterus is insufflated with air. The endoscope may be used to facilitate a uterine biopsy and to aid in finding the exact cause of reproductive failure in problem mares.

Radiography

Diagnosis and prognosis of possibly injured areas are greatly aided by radiographs. They can differentiate between bony and fibrous swellings, as well as determine the nearness of a bone growth (such as a splint) to a joint. Radiographs, also referred to as X-rays, can locate fractures and bone chips, or identify periosteal injury better than other means of diagnosis. They are particularly useful for the discovery of nondisplaced fractures or small fractures at joints. Some veterinarians use radiographs of the epiphysis to estimate the stage of epiphyseal maturity in racehorses. Radiographs of the lungs can be taken to help diagnose respiratory disorders. In addition, a radiograph is a permanent record that can be used later as a reference to a previous injury. A radiological examination is used to confirm a tentative diagnosis resulting from a thorough physical examination. It is intended to augment, not replace, a careful physical examination.

Procedure: Ideally, before taking a radiograph of the foot, the veterinarian will remove the shoes, and pare the sole and frog. The sole, hoof wall, and coronary band are carefully cleaned to remove any dust or radiopaque substance (such as a blister or iodine) that would make confusing shadows on the X-ray. Bandages and leg wraps are also removed.

The hoof may require rasping and/or trimming to ensure an even and uniform shadow. This is particularly important when radiographing quarter cracks and keratoma, especially in horses with elongated hoofs.

In cases of suspected navicular disease, the veterinarian will pack the sole, frog, and bars with a substance (such as lanolin, soap, or clay) that will fill in any air pockets or irregularities in the sole that may cause shadows on the radiograph.

The veterinarian is also able to radiograph draining tracts by first injecting a radiopaque substance, such as iodized oil, into the sinus or fistula. This contrast medium will clearly outline the tract and may reveal the presence of a foreign object that is radiolucent (such as a wood splinter) and does not normally appear on an X-ray. An injection of a radiopaque substance can also be made directly into a joint for arthrography, to enable the veterinarian to X-ray a joint lesion.

Radiation Therapy

The intent of radiation therapy is to destroy malignant cells while affecting normal cells as little as possible. This is possible because neoplastic and inflammatory cells are killed more readily than normal, healthy cells. Radiation therapy causes deep tissue inflammation as it destroys abnormal growths and already inflamed cells. Radiation increases the amount of oxygen available in the cells, thereby also increasing the tissue's susceptibility to the therapy. Tissue that is completely oxygenated is about three times more susceptible to radiation than is unoxygenated tissue.

Besides being used in the treatment of neoplasms such as melanomas and carcinomas, radiation therapy can also be used for acute and chronic inflammations. Radiation reduces swelling, pain, and heat by destroying a large number of leukocytes which are present at the site of inflammation. It is successful in smoothing excess bone growth, but will not cause immediate improvement. If the horse's lameness disappears rapidly, nerve endings in the area have probably been damaged by the radiation. Since radiation acts somewhat like a counterirritant, it can encourage the reabsorption of calcium from bone as it increases circulation and available tissue oxygen.

Other conditions that respond well to radiation therapy are chronic lamenesses, such as those caused by exostosis, chronic traumatic arthritis, osteoarthritis, periosteal new bone growth, and other lesions located around joints. It has been used with varying degrees of success in cases of fibrosis, calcification, bucked shins, ringbone, tendinitis, navicular disease, and tumors.

Procedure: Radiation can be administered in a variety of ways; the main sources are X-rays, beta particles and gamma rays. Radiation penetration is increased as its wavelengths become shortened. A machine with a higher kilovoltage provides shorter wavelengths, resulting in more powerful radiation. X-ray units designed for therapy instead of for diagnosis emit more energetic radiation. These units are usually heavy and are not really portable. Because the X-ray machine is stationary, any movement of the horse will cause a change in radiation intensity; therefore, other methods of radiation may be employed.

Gamma rays, another source of radiation, are photons of electromagnetic energy that penetrate deeper and are more energetic then X-rays. A commonly used source of gamma rays is Cobalt-60, which can be applied directly to the treatment area. The isotopes, in the shape of needles, tubes, or seeds, are placed inside metal containers and taped to the horse. The horse's movements will not have any effect on the intensity of gamma ray radiation applied in this manner.

Still another form of radiation therapy is beta particle treatment. Decay of certain radioactive isotopes results in the release of electrons called beta particles. Typical sources of these electrons are strontium-90 and radon-222, which are usually mounted in silver inside a lead-lined box. Beta particles are typically applied to superficial lesions since 95% of the radiation is absorbed in the top 4 mm of tissue. Examples of conditions that can be successfully treated this way are corneal and mucosal lesions.

The total dosage of radiation given depends on the condition being treated, its size and depth under the skin, the sensitivity of surrounding tissue, and the horse's general condition. Ideally, the irradiated area is little larger than the area requiring treatment.

Administering a full amount of radiation at a single treatment has a more potent effect than does giving one-half the same amount at two treatments. This division into smaller equal amounts (called fractionation) provides the safest method of using radiation, though there is a period of some recovery by cells between treatments. Consequently, malignant tumors are better treated with fewer fractionated doses.

Because radiation does produce deep inflammation and reduces bone density, a horse should be completely rested for 60 to 90 days after treatment of joints, bones, and tendons to produce the most satisfactory results. Additionally, another 60 to 90 days should be allowed before the horse returns to racing condition. Exercise before this time could cause a fracture. When used to treat bone disorders, the results from radiation therapy cannot be properly evaluated for one to six months after treatment.

Radiation therapy should be carefully applied, as severe consequences can result from improper use. Anemia, for instance, should be treated before radiation therapy begins. Tissue necrosis, dermatitis, and hair loss are some of the indications of overdosage. When immature epiphyseal plates are exposed to radiation, it is possible for growth of the horse to be stopped. In addition, a horse with infected skin lesions that are exposed to radiation should receive antibiotics to prevent the spread of bacterial infection which could be encouraged by radiation therapy.

Electrocardiography (ECG)

Electrocardiography is a method of studying the heart through graphic records of the electric current produced by excitation of the heart. These elctrocardiograms can be analyzed and related to racing performance and clinical signs of heart disease. If this information is collected from enough horses, normal patterns can be determined, which would allow the detection of abnormal values which may indicate heart disease. Valvular malfunction, shunts, flow rates, and pressure changes will not be detected by an electrocardiogram.

The major waves of the ECG are P, Q, R, S, and T. The P wave designates the depolarization (excitation) of the heart as it goes from the sinoatrial node through both atria. The time needed for the movement of the excitation process (from the sinoatrial node, through the atrioventricular node, and into the ventricular muscles) is represented by the P-R interval. Depolarization of the ventricular musculature causes QRS, where R is any upward deflection, Q is a downward deflection before R, and S is a downward deflection after R. If there is no upward wave, the segment is simply called QS. The interval between the end of QRS and the beginning of the T wave is labeled S-T. T itself is the point designating the repolarization.

These waves are picked up through leads attached to the horse with electrodes in various positions. If the placement of the electrode is altered, the wave will be recorded differently. Any change in the heart position will also affect the electrocardiogram. In addition, individual animals differ in their ability to conduct the waves. Therefore, in order to have comparable ECGs, the position of the electrodes, limbs, and body must be kept constant, and there should be no excitement causing the horse's heart to beat more than 40 times per minute.

EVALUATION OF THE ECG

When the veterinarian is evaluating an electrocardiogram, he will measure the deflection and duration of the waves, and determine the heart rate. He can also calculate the "heart score," which is the arithmetic mean of all the QRS duration values from each standard limb lead. Some authorities believe that the higher the heart score, the more successful will be the performance of a racehorse. The veterinarian will also note any signs of arrhythmia, displacement, etc., revealed by the ECG. An example of desired values for a successful racehorse would be a slow heart rate (30 to 35 beats per minute), a long P-wave duration (.14 to .16 second), a short P-R interval (less than .40 second), a high heart score (.120 second or more), and a long Q-T interval (.54 to .58 second).

This information can then be used to determine the size of the horse's heart and the normality of its electrical conduction. A larger heart is considered to be directly related to the heart score. Of course, an abnormal electrocardiogram would be a disadvantage for the animal. Besides their use as an evaluation of racehorses, ECGs can also be used for such applications as the determination of altitude effects on horses.

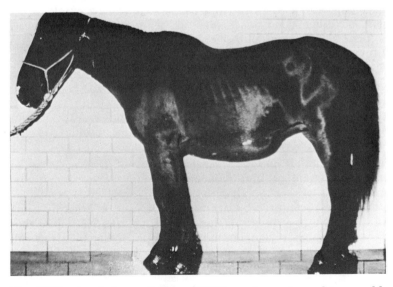

Fig. 16-26   An electrocardiogram [ECG] may be performed to reveal heart disease, as in the case of this horse with congestive heart failure.

Therapeutic Cautery (Firing)

Therapeutic cautery, or firing, is the practice of applying a red-hot iron to a chronic or subacute inflammation to produce hyperemia. It is thought to increase the blood supply and thereby assist healing of the chronic condition through counterirritation. The increased blood circulation is believed to promote healing, while the resulting fibrosis acts as a pressure bandage, applying even pressure to the underlying tissue. Opponents of firing maintain that the period of forced rest needed after this treatment (6 months) is what really causes rehabilitation.

Firing supposedly shortens the recuperation time for an injury, but it also reduces mobility, often reverses mineralization, and may calcify the tissue surrounding a joint. The excessive fibrous scar tissue produced through firing, along with the other side effects, restricts the horse's range of movement, thereby increasing the chances of further trauma.

Before attempting cautery or any other method of therapy, a veterinarian must first consider the duration of the injury, how soon it was diagnosed, conformation of the horse, age, any complicating lamenesses, the type of work to be performed by the horse, comparative performance before and after treatment, and the length of usefulness expected after recovery. Firing has the advantages of being less expensive and easier than other methods of producing counterirritation, such as radiation and ultrasonics.

Firing can be used with the greatest amount of success in treating the following conditions: soft tissue injury around joints, tendons, and ligaments; carpitis; chronic arthritis; and osselets. It can be employed in the treatment of other conditions, such as tendosynovitis, tendinitis, sesamoiditis, bone spavin, and splints, although it is of uncertain value in these conditions. Firing should never be done under the following conditions:

1. near open wounds
2. on the flexor surface of a joint
3. in areas of infection, dermatitis, or acute inflammation
4. if the area has recently been injected with a corticosteroid
5. on young or weak horses

In addition, firing should not be used as a preventative measure to strengthen the joints, tendons, and ligaments of young horses; scar tissue resulting from firing is weaker than healthy tissue.

Although therapeutic cautery appears to be successful in treating some ailments and in hastening recovery, it does have some disadvantages; skin necrosis, tetanus, wound infection, laminitis, arthritis, and synovitis are all possible results of firing. All of these aspects will be considered by the veterinarian and will be discussed with the horseowner before a decision to fire is made.

There are two types of firing; pinfiring (also called point or punch firing) and linefiring (also called feather firing). The latter method is rarely used because it disrupts the skin's blood supply and is not as effective as pinfiring. Linefiring is done with a knife-like blade, one-eighth inch wide, which is used to make lines one-half inch apart. Pinfiring can be done with the use of an ether firing iron, handmade iron, or with an electrical cautery. The electric cautery instrument is the best choice, as it has interchangeable points, and is silent and portable.

Procedure: The horse is fired while standing, and a tranquilizer administered if necessary. First, the area to be fired is clipped, washed, and rinsed with a skin antiseptic. A local anesthetic, such as procaine or lidocaine hydrochloride, is then administered. The firing iron should be red-hot, and is not pressed deeply into the flesh, as this could penetrate bone or a joint capsule. If the iron is allowed to remain in contact with the skin for too long, or if the holes are spaced too close together, severe tissue necrosis will occur.

a.   **b.**

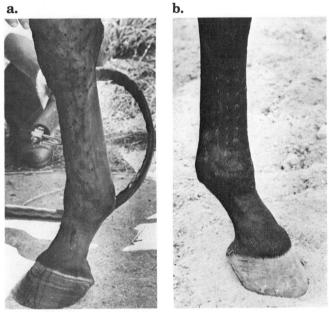

Fig. 16-27 Therapeutic cautery. a. Firing the leg; note the spacing of the fired points. b. Scars remaining after the wounds resulting from firing have healed.

Blisters are often used after firing to encourage inflammation and scurfing of the skin, but this treatment is exceptionally painful. The tissue necrosis caused by blistering requires an extended healing period. Instead of a blister, a soothing leg paint, such as iodine/glycerine/phenol or liquid nitrofurans, can be applied. This paint should be applied daily to the legs for three weeks, during which time it acts as a germicidal agent, as well as increases the irritation. The legs should be kept wrapped with cotton. After firing, the horse should be rested for 6 months.

Another method of firing involves the injection of chemicals into the afflicted area. Injections can be administered by the veterinarian either subcutaneously or supraperiosteally, and the injections should be made about one inch apart. This technique causes less pain and tissue damage, and also works by increasing blood circulation. These injections should be done only after the skin has been prepared as for cautery firing, and the treated area should be bandaged afterwards. The horse will need to be rested for six weeks after this treatment.

Deep Heat Therapy

Deep heat therapy refers to the application of heat so that it penetrates two to five inches below the body surface. This is accomplished by conversive heat, developed in tissues by resistance to high-frequency electrical energy or soundwaves. This treatment is meant to encourage the reabsorption of swelling. The dilation of blood vessels caused by heat increases the metabolism, temperature, and oxygen supply of the area. Heat should not be used in cases of infection, as it causes greater vessel permeability and increased toxin absorption. At least 24 to 48 hours should have elapsed since the time of injury before any traumatized area can be given heat therapy. In any case, because of possible side effects, deep heat therapy should not be used without advice from a veterinarian.

DIATHERMY

Diathermy is the heating of body tissues due to their resistance to the passage of high-frequency electromagnetic radiation through the body. Shortwave diathermy uses a frequency of 10 to 100 million cycles per second and a wavelength of 3 to 30 meters, while ultrashortwave refers to treatment using wavelengths of less than 3 meters. This therapy will penetrate about two inches below the skin, and raise the temperature five or six degrees. The electrical energy passes from one electrode to the other through the horse's tissues, causing a rise in tissue temperature that varies with the impedance of the electricity. Tissues with a high fluid content will heat more, while fatty tissues, bone and tendons will heat less. An important caution to remember is that bone pins or screws may heat up enough to cause bone damage. A major disadvantage of diathermy is the possibility of an electrical short-circuit shocking the horse.

ULTRASONICS

Ultrasonic therapy consists of the production of heat through high-frequency soundwaves (20 to 500 kilocycles) passed through the body. These soundwaves are converted from electricity by a crystal in the ultrasound instrument. This heat is capable of reaching the joint of a bone or limb, and is used in the treatment of arthritis, nervous system lesions, trauma, bursitis, tendon injury, and myositis. Ultrasonic therapy gives a pulsating heat that causes a massage-like effect and relieves pain. It can penetrate three to five inches below the skin surface and raise the tissue temperature five degrees. There is less chance of bone necrosis with ultrasound than with diathermy, but the high temperature may possibly cause some damage.

The area to be treated should be clipped, shaved, and covered with mineral oil. The head of the machine is then applied to the part for five to ten minutes while being constantly moved. This continual movement is necessary to prevent an accumulation of heat under the head of the instrument.

Ultrasonic treatment can spread cancer, so it is not used in such cases. This type of treatment may cause bone demineralization and should not be used for two to three days after a trauma occurs, as it may lead to hematoma or seroma if employed earlier. Since ultrasound produces an inflammation, it should not be applied in conjunction with radiation therapy which also causes a long-lasting inflammation.

Acupuncture

Acupuncture is a "surgical" procedure that consists of the insertion of needles into certain points of the body. It has been used in mainland China for the last 3,000 to 5,000 years as a disease treatment, and for the last 15 years as an experimental method of anesthesia. Acupuncture has been tried as therapy for virtually any condition one wishes to name, such as the following:

1. diarrhea
2. heaves (emphysema)
3. colic
4. laminitis
5. constipation
6. liver dysfunction (hepatitis)
7. navicular disease
8. respiratory and pulmonary diseases
9. torticollis (wryneck)
10. arthritis
11. radial and facial nerve paralysis
12. glaucoma

The actual benefits derived from acupuncture are not discernible at this time. Evaluation of responses to acupuncture in horses has been done on a subjective, rather than objective, basis. Thus, it is usually difficult, if not impossible, to accurately evaluate the true benefits, or even results, of acupuncture studies in horses. Acupuncture is still considered a highly controversial area.

17

SURGICAL PROCEDURES

Management of the Equine Surgery Patient

Before deciding on any surgical procedure, the veterinarian will have considered the horse's history, carefully examined the animal, and run the tests required to correctly diagnose the horse's condition. Elective surgery (surgery that is not necessary to save the animal's life) should only be performed when the horse is in good physical condition. For instance, to avoid excessive stress, a weak, heavily parasitized and anemic colt should not be castrated until it has improved in general health.

The veterinarian must also exercise judgement in deciding precisely when to operate. Although unnecessary surgery should not be attempted, neither should the horse's condition be allowed to deteriorate to the point where it will have a difficult time surviving the stress of surgery. Before commencing actual surgical preparation, the owner and veterinarian will discuss the surgery, its expected outcome, and any risks involved.

Surgery may be done with the horse in a standing position (under local anesthesia and sedation) or recumbent (under general anesthesia), depending upon the procedure and the veterinarian's personal preference. If the horse is under a local anesthetic, care should be taken to ensure that the horse is not forced into an uncomfortable, strained position. This could not only lead to pinched nerves or muscle cramps, but will probably also cause the horse to struggle. In situations where general anesthesia is employed, the horse must be positioned in such a manner that facial or radial nerve paralysis will not result from pressure on the nerves. Ample padding and careful positioning of ropes and halters are required to protect against nerve injury.

When attempting aseptic surgery, the surgeon (and any assistants), his instruments, the horse, and the environment must be clean, and as free from bacteria as possible. Of course, if operating under field conditions, the veterinary surgeon will not be able to maintain the cleanliness possible in a veterinary hospital where he will have control over the environment, but he still observes the basic rules of sterile technique.

SURGICAL PREPARATION

Although it is admittedly impossible to clean skin to the point of sterility, the horse should still be groomed and clipped, as the skin and haircoat are major sources of bacterial contamination. The area immediately surrounding the surgical site is first washed with a surgical soap such as povidone-iodine (Betadine: Purdue Frederick) or pHisoHex, then rinsed and wiped with alcohol (or a similar defatting agent) to remove skin oils and fats. Before shaving around the injury or surgical site, the veterinarian can pack a wound with a sterile gauze pad soaked in physiological saline solution to help keep hair out of the injury during clipping. An antiseptic, such as tincture of zephiran or Betadine solution is then painted or sponged on the area from the proposed line of the incision to the outer edge of the shaved area.

If the surgery must be performed in a place other than a veterinary hospital, such as a pasture or barn, the location should be as free of dust, debris, and insects as possible. A casting pad (which can be made of straw covered with a tarpaulin) should be provided for an operation in which the horse is in a recumbent position. Adequate lighting must be available, and outside disturbances should be eliminated, or at least kept to a minimum.

The veterinarian will prepare himself for the procedure by scrubbing his nails, hands, and arms with surgical soap. The veterinary surgeon will usually wear sterile surgical gloves.

STERILIZATION OF SURGICAL INSTRUMENTS

The surgical instruments, such as scissors and scalpels, must be sterilized, either chemically, with moist heat, or with gas sterilization. Chemical sterilization is accomplished through the use of commercially available disinfectant solutions, and takes from three hours to a full day. Instruments sterilized in this manner must be rinsed before being used in surgery, as some disinfectants irritate body tissues. Chemical disinfection will be unsuccessful if there is any organic matter, such as blood, adhering to the instruments.

An autoclave provides a superior means of sterilization by using moist heat under pressure, and takes far less time (fifteen minutes at 250°F) than chemical methods. Boiling water alone (212°F for thirty minutes) will not kill all spores and bacteria, but its efficiency can be increased by alkalizing the water through the addition of sodium carbonate, which also decreases the time required for sterilization to fifteen minutes.

Gas sterilization, using ethylene oxide gas, takes twelve hours, and the instruments should not be used for at least six hours after sterilization.

ANESTHETIZING THE HORSE

When a horse is to undergo general anesthesia, feed is usually withheld the night before the scheduled operation; however, the horse is usually allowed limited access to water. The surgical site, especially in leg surgery, may be clipped, scrubbed, and wrapped the day before. The horse is given a tranquilizer or another preanesthetic agent while he is still quiet in the stall area. After the preanesthetic agent has had time to take effect, the horse is moved to the surgery area. His mouth is rinsed thoroughly with plain water, using a dose syringe. Next, anesthesia is induced with a short-acting barbiturate, such as thiamylal sodium. Care is taken that the horse is not injured as he goes down.

Then, an endotracheal tube is inserted through the mouth into the trachea, and the animal may be placed on a gas anesthesia machine (those using halothane gas are most common). Variations of the above procedure will, of course, be seen when other anesthetic agents are used.

The ideal place for a horse to recover (wake up) from general anesthesia is on mattress-type padding in a dark, quiet, padded room. The horse may need assistance to steady him when he first regains his footing. Sometimes it is necessary to hold the horse down by sitting on his neck and covering his eye if the animal shows a tendency to thrash about. The horse can be released and helped to his feet when he is a little more awake. When the horse first rises, it may be necessary to have one person take hold of the halter while another person takes hold of the tail until the horse regains stability.

The Head and Neck

DENTISTRY

The horse's teeth are composed of four substances;

1. the soft pulp that fills the inner cavity of the tooth
2. the dentine, a hard yellow-white material that forms the bulk of the tooth
3. the enamel, a very hard blue-white substance which covers the dentine in several layers and makes up the outer "white" portion of the tooth crown
4. the cement, a bone-like substance which cements the root of the tooth into the jawbone

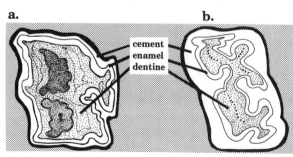

cement
enamel
dentine

Fig. 17-1 Occlusal surfaces of the cheek teeth. a. Maxillary. b. Mandibular.

a.   b.

Horses' teeth are often neglected and do not receive proper dental care. This is unfortunate, for although equines tend to have far less trouble with tooth decay than do people, they do have some dental problems, particularly between the ages of one and one-half to four years of age. It should, therefore, be common practice to have the horse's teeth checked at least annually at vaccination time and to initiate preventive dental care when necessary.

DENTAL PROBLEMS

In the horse, the most frequently encountered conditions include: sharp teeth edges, retention of deciduous teeth (caps), wolf teeth, and dental caries.

Sharp Teeth Edges

Because of the uneven surfaces necessary for grinding roughages, the horse's normal side to side mastication, and the fact that the upper jaw is wider than the lower, the enamel often wears unevenly and causes sharp points on the inside edges of the lower teeth and the outside edges of the upper teeth.

In old horses, arthritis can lead to a condition called "shear mouth" in which the sharp edges become so exaggerated that they can cut the opposing gums. Another result of uneven wear usually found in older horses is "wave mouth," a condition in which the surfaces of the back molars are shaped into wave-like forms. A horse with wave mouth should have dental care at least twice a year.

Irritation of the gums may occur when decay or breakage causes a tooth to wear more quickly than the normal wear rate. Of course, the horse's teeth are continual eruptors and grow throughout the animal's entire life; therefore, when breakage occurs, the opposing tooth must be floated to prevent penetration of the opposite gum and the alveolar periostitis that would result. The tooth opposing an empty socket will also require periodic dentistry to prevent it from growing too long (a condition called step mouth).

At other times, projections on the anterior premolars, called hooks, cut the cheeks and tongue and cause the horse to resist his bit. These projections, too, will have to be floated to prevent abrasions.

Floating the Teeth

Sharp teeth edges, shear mouth, hooked projections, and those conditions caused by irregular wear can be treated through filing the teeth with a dental float. Floating, as this procedure is called, is most successful in removing sharp edges, but may also be useful in correcting other conditions as well.

Floating is best accomplished with the horse effectively restrained. The horse's mouth can be held open either by pulling his tongue to the side between the cheek teeth or by using a speculum. Often, the horse will open his mouth sufficiently when the float is introduced at the interdental space.

To prevent injury to the mucosal surfaces of the cheek, the halter should be held away from the cheek as the teeth are floated. A few strokes with the float are usually sufficient to remove most projections, and those that require extensive floating should be attended to when the horse is anesthetized.

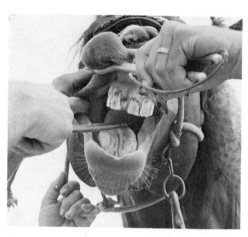

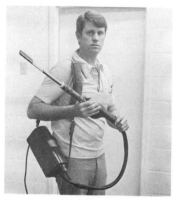

Fig. 17-3 Portable electric tooth float. This float has the advantage of requiring less effort when floating numerous horses' teeth.

Fig. 17-2 Floating the teeth; note that the cheek is held away from the teeth to avoid injury to the mucosa.

The objective of floating, in attempts to correct such conditions as "wave mouth" and "shear mouth," is to file the teeth into as close an approximation of a normal mouth as possible. Because lengthy tooth projections are sometimes encountered, the veterinarian may use compound cutting forceps to remove the long edges before they are filed.

Wolf Teeth

Wolf teeth are the small round teeth that sometimes grow in front of the second upper premolars and cause irritation in the horse's mouth. This may be especially apparent when the bit is first introduced, as correct placement may be impossible. Wolf teeth usually erupt at five to six months of age and are not replaced by permanent teeth.

The veterinarian can remove wolf teeth by giving the horse an infraorbital block and loosening the teeth with a root elevator or specially constructed wolf tooth elevator.

Retained Caps

Retention of deciduous, or temporary, teeth occurs frequently in young horses, particularly in three year olds. There is, in this condition, a recessed gum line and a noticeable line between the deciduous tooth (i.e., the cap, or baby tooth) and the permanent tooth, and if not removed, the cap can cause pain and severe swelling in the sinus area of the upper jaw and bumps along the outer edge of the lower jaw. Moreover, when the deciduous tooth is firmly in place, the permanent tooth may become impacted and grow backwards into the nasal sinus. To prevent this, the cap will have to be removed.

The veterinarian can remove the retained cap by prying the tooth out with a root elevator or twisting it out with a bone cutter or molar extraction forceps. A mouth speculum is required to adequately expose the molars for this procedure, and a 2% procaine solution can be injected locally as an anesthetic if the horse resists having the cap removed.

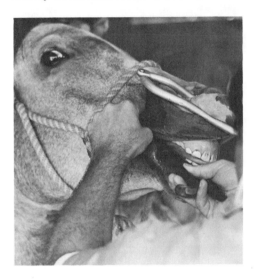

Fig. 17-4 A retained cap can be removed by a veterinarian.

Dental Tartar

Excessive tartar formation is not often a problem, but when it does occur, it should be treated. The veterinarian can do this by cracking off the excess tartar with dental forceps and removing remaining tartar fragments with dental scalers.

EXTRACTION AND REPULSION OF TEETH

Teeth that have fractured, abscessed, or decayed must be removed by the veterinarian. Abscesses often result when food particles wedge between the cap and permanent tooth, causing decay and infection. Infection caused by lodged food particles can also inflame the periosteum lining the alveoli around the fourth, fifth, and sixth cheek teeth and cause a purulent discharge from the nostrils.

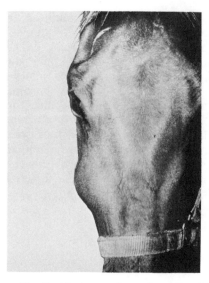

Fig. 17-5   An infected tooth can cause profuse swelling and may necessitate removal by repulsion.

Teeth that are decaying should be removed to prevent infection from spreading to healthy teeth. Unfortunately, unless a decayed tooth has loosened in its socket, it is unlikely that it can be removed by extraction, even with forceps. When a tooth has been extracted, however, the alveolar cavity must always be examined to ensure that all tooth fragments have been removed. The socket should then be rinsed with a mild antiseptic and packed with antiseptic-soaked cotton or gauze. Following this, the horse should be maintained on a diet of soft feed (mashes) for a few days.

Teeth that are not loose enough to be extracted must be repulsed. In this process, the veterinarian opens a hole through the horse's jaw to the tooth (trephining) and uses special instruments to knock the tooth out. Repulsion, of course, is conducted only when the horse is under general anesthesia.

Repulsion requires a great deal of skill, for the trephining site must be carefully chosen to avoid injury to the nasolcarimal duct and lacrimal canal. Furthermore, repulsion very often requires several firm, properly directed blows to force the tooth out, as many teeth removed in this manner have long roots. After the tooth is repulsed, the socket is checked to determine if there are tooth fragments remaining, then packed with cotton or gauze soaked in antiseptic. The veterinarian may prefer to use a plug made of dental wax to prevent food from lodging in the socket until granulation tissue fills the area.

Tooth repulsion is an exacting task because of its inherent risks; these include jawbone damage, injury to the facial nerves and arteries, and, as mentioned previously, damage to the nasolacrimal duct and lacrimal canal. In spite of these risks, however, the horse that has periodontal disease, dental caries, or a fractured tooth should have the offending tooth/teeth removed.

TRACHEOSTOMY

A tracheostomy is a surgical procedure in which an opening is made into the trachea to provide an air passage when, for some reason, the normal airway has been blocked.

EMERGENCY TRACHEOSTOMY

In a serious emergency situation, when a horse is unable to breathe due to a tracheal obstruction, whether caused by a strangles abscess, a snakebite near the nostrils, etc., it might be necessary to perform a tracheostomy before the veterinarian's arrival, in order to save the horse's life. If the horse is having great difficulty in breathing, and the gingiva is bluish in color, it is better to perform a tracheostomy and risk infection than to have the horse suffocate to death within minutes.

Procedure: An assistant should try to hold the horse's head and neck fixed in an extended position during this procedure. A clean, sharp knife is used to make a vertical incision into the trachea, about five inches below the larynx. Two or three of the cartilages should be severed, then the opening is held open by some sort of tube, such as a piece of rubber hose.

An emergency tracheostomy is, of course, only a temporary measure, and the veterinarian should still be contacted immediately.

PERMANENT TRACHEOSTOMY

Sometimes a horse requires the installation of a permanent tracheostomy tube. In this situation, the veterinarian will incise the trachea over the fourth to sixth tracheal rings while the horse is in a standing position with the head and neck extended. An ovoid tube (three-quarter inch to one and one-half inch in diameter and usually made of brass) is positioned through the tracheal incision, and the flange of the tube is sutured to the surrounding skin.

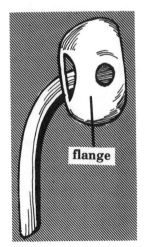

flange

Fig. 17-6 **Temporary tracheostomy tube. The tube is inserted between the two tracheal rings. The flange is held in place with gauze or tape tied around the horse's neck.**

A permanent tube is kept closed with a stopper, except during exercise, to keep out foreign debris. A horse that has had a tracheostomy should be protected from dust, mud, and water, which could get into the lungs through the tracheal opening. If the tissues and cartilage are greatly inflamed, the operation may be repeated at a lower location along the trachea.

ROARING OPERATION

Roaring (laryngeal hemiplegia) is a progressive disease, in which the laryngeal muscles are unable to hold the vocal cords to the side. The only treatment is early surgical correction. The most frequently used operation, a laryngeal ventriculotomy, can be performed with the horse either standing (after having been administered a tranquilizer and a local anesthetic) or under general anesthesia. Allowing the horse to remain standing prevents inhalation of blood, but the tracheal tube used when the horse is under general anesthesia also prevents this from occurring.

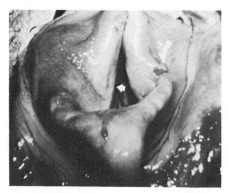 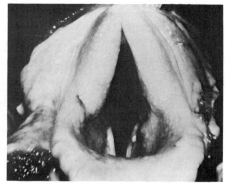

Fig. 17-7 Abnormal larynx of a horse that requires a roaring operation [left]: note the sagging laryngeal fold [arrow]. Compare this larynx to the normal one [right].

Procedure: During this procedure, the veterinarian will strip the mucosal lining from the afflicted laryngeal saccule (usually the left one, although some veterinarians prefer to strip both ventricles). A laryngotomy tube can be sutured in place for the first day following surgery, and bleeding can be minimized by medicated gauze packs. Packing and cleansing of the wound is necessary for three to five weeks, and the horse will require antibiotics for several days after the operation. During the first 36 hours after stripping, edema can be prevented (to an extent) by tying the horse's head high. The wound should be allowed to heal as an open wound, a process that will take three to five weeks, and the horse must be kept stalled for two to two and one-half months, at which time the success of the surgery can be evaluated.

The fibrous tissue formed during healing contracts and pulls the vocal cords to the side of the larynx, thereby correcting the condition. Best results are received from this operation if it is performed soon after the horse is diagnosed as a "roarer," when the chances of recovery are approximately 70%. The longer the horse suffers from laryngeal hemiplegia, the less likely it is that surgical correction will be successful.

A related therapy for roaring is the addition of a laryngeal prosthesis to replace the atrophied laryngeal muscle caused by the damage to the recurrent laryngeal nerve. The elastic prosthesis consists of a braided section of Lycra, which holds the arytenoid cartilage and the vocal cord out of the way of the flow of air. After this treatment, the horse is administered antibiotics for five days and kept stalled for six weeks.

Before the horse undergoes laryngeal ventriculotomy, or if edema develops during that operation, a tracheostomy can be performed to assist breathing (refer to "Tracheostomy").

OPENING THE FACIAL SINUS (TREPHINING)

An infection of the frontal sinus may result from a respiratory disease (such as influenza), parasites, cysts, or tumors. When infection occurs, the affected sinus will appear swollen and have a dull sound upon percussion. The horse will have a nasal discharge from the nostril on the same side as the infected sinus. To treat sinusitis, the veterinarian can open the frontal sinus (trephining) to allow it to drain.

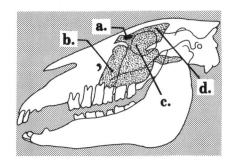

Fig. 17-8 Anatomy of the nasal sinuses. a. Recommended site for trephining frontal sinus. b. Anterior maxillary sinus. c. Medial canthus. d. Frontal sinus.

Procedure: The horse is placed under general anesthesia before the veterinarian makes a circular skin incision over the anterior turbinate portion of the frontal sinus. A trephine is worked through the nasal bone, until the isolated plug of bone comes away in the instrument. This completes the opening into the sinus cavity.

The sinus is irrigated daily with a substance such as hydrogen peroxide, warm saline solution, nitrofurazone solution (Furacin), potassium permanganate solution, iodine, or enzyme solution. To maintain the opening, gauze is either passed entirely through the passage or used to plug the trephined hole. The flushing is continued until the sinusitis clears, and the horse may be exercised after flushing to encourage drainage.

Once the infection has been eliminated, the gauze may be removed and the opening allowed to heal. Within a few months, usually only a small scar will remain.

DRAINING THE GUTTURAL POUCHES

Chronic pharyngitis is often associated with a guttural pouch infection of bacterial or fungal origin. The horse will often exhibit epistaxis and difficulty in swallowing, as well as a cough. In addition, pus draining from the nostrils when the horse lowers its head may originate from the guttural pouch. Although this condition may improve spontaneously, the position of the guttural pouches and the shape of the pharyngeal opening often hinders drainage, and the guttural pouches must be flushed.

Procedure: An endoscope is used to visualize the opening into the guttural pouch, through which the veterinarian passes a plastic catheter. The pouch is then flushed with a disinfectant and/or antibiotic solution (e.g., enzymes, acriflavine, nitrofurazone, or iodine).

Although a single irrigation may suffice, flushing may be repeated as often as necessary. If irrigation is to be continued over a period of several days, an indwelling catheter can be inserted into the guttural pouch. This can either be a regular straight catheter sutured to the horse's nostril or a catheter with a spiral end. The spiral will hold the catheter in place when placed into the pouch. If the horse has a fever, the veterinarian will administer antibiotics.

The nasal discharge may continue for several weeks. If the pus hardens into chondroids, the veterinarian may have to remove them by opening the guttural pouches from the outside.

CORRECTION OF NASOLACRIMAL DUCT ATRESIA

A foal may be born with a congenital defect in which the nasolacrimal duct does not extend completely and open into the nose. In this condition, the foal lacks the lower opening to the duct, which should be located on the nasal cavity floor, where the skin joins the nasal mucosa. Atresia of the nasolacrimal duct is usually suspected when a young foal has persistent epiphora (tearing), and the condition must be surgically corrected.

Procedure: A piece of small-diameter polyethylene tubing is passed into the duct from the upper puncta (opening), and is extended the length of the duct. The veterinarian will palpate the tubing where it stops and make the incision at that point. The mucosa of the duct and that of the nostril are then sutured together, and a piece of polyethylene tubing is left in the duct to hold it open. This catheter should remain for approximately one month; meanwhile, the area is treated with topical application of antibiotics and corticosteroids.

TARSORRHAPHY

Complete tarsorrhaphy (closing of the eyelids) is sometimes temporarily employed in therapy of corneal ulcers and lacerations, as well as after surgery of the cornea or inner eye. When closed, the eyelids give adequate support to the cornea and cause a desirable mydriasis (dilation of the pupil). In addition, tarsorrhaphy combined with subpalpebral (under the eyelids) medication allows the medicine a lengthened period of contact with the eye.

a.   **b.**

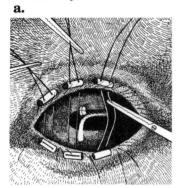 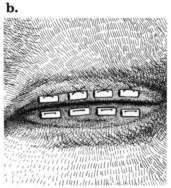

c.

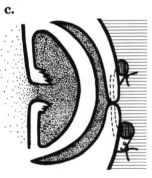

Fig. 17-9 Tarsorrhaphy. a. Suturing the eyelids together. b. Appearance of the eye after surgery. c. Cross section of the eye; note the sutures do not touch the cornea.

Procedure: A tarsorrhaphy can be performed with the horse under general anesthesia or locally anesthetized and tranquilized. The surgery involves using a non-absorbable suturing material to make four to six interrupted mattress sutures in the eyelid, but not through it. If the sutures were to perforate the lid, the cornea could be damaged by abrasion. To reduce tension, rubber tubing or buttons can be used in the suture pattern, thus allowing the sutures to remain in place without excessively cutting into the eyelids if swelling occurs.

After a tarsorrhaphy, eye ointments can be administered through the suture line at the corner of the eye. When medicating the horse, which is done at frequent intervals, approach the horse (whenever possible) from the animal's good side. If it is necessary to approach the horse from his blind side, always announce your arrival.

SUBPALPEBRAL MEDICATION SYSTEM

During recovery from eye surgery, or in the treatment of severe ocular diseases, topical medication must be repeatedly applied to the horse's eye. Since it is often difficult to accomplish this with an excited animal, the veterinarian may install a subpalpebral medication system.

This system is easy to use and ensures that all of the drug reaches the horse's eye. In addition, there is much less chance of the horse resisting treatment, thus the likelihood of injury to the horseman, veterinarian, or horse is reduced.

Procedure: A subpalpebral medication system consists of a piece of plastic tubing surgically implanted through the upper lid of the eye to be treated. It may be positioned with the horse under a general or local anesthetic, and is held in place at the upper lid by a small flange in one end of the tubing. The other end of the tubing is taped to the horse's forehead and extended over the poll to the level of the withers on the opposite side of the body. A syringe is used to inject medication through the tubing.

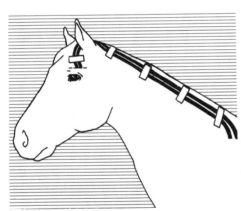

Fig. 17-10 A subpalpebral medication system is used when ophthalmic medications must be administered over an extended period of time.

Some swelling may appear around the tubing at the eyelid, and the tube may cause itching. However, a subpalpebral medication system may be left in place for several weeks, usually with no harm to the horse.

Abdominal Surgery

LAPAROTOMY

A laparotomy is a surgical opening into the abdominal cavity. This approach is used for ovariectomies, Caesarean sections, correction of intestinal torsions or intussusceptions, and various other abdominal procedures. An approach can be made either through the midline of the abdomen, just off the midline but parallel to it (paramedian), or through the flank, depending upon the reason for surgery and the veterinary surgeon's preference.

LATERAL LAPAROTOMY

The flank approach is sometimes chosen because the weight of the viscera (abdominal organs) does not interfere with the surgical wound's healing, as is the case with a midline incision. If the flank approach is used, the operation is usually conducted with the horse in a standing position, after sedation and the administration of a local anesthetic.

Procedure: The area between the last rib and the point of the hip is surgically scrubbed and prepared for surgery. After the incision is made, the muscle fibers can be separated in one of two ways.

The first method, which is less time-consuming, involves making a simple incision through all of the muscle layers, parallel to the one already made through the skin. With the second method, called a "grid" incision, the fibers of each muscle are split along their natural direction. When a "grid" incision is made, a large skin incision is required to allow proper exposure and separation of the underlying muscles. This technique, while slower in execution, has the advantage of making an incision that requires less suturing, as the muscle layers will adhere naturally after the operation. If a single incision was made through all of the muscle layers, each muscle will be individually sutured to avoid the formation of serum pockets or necrotic tissue.

MIDLINE LAPAROTOMY

If an especially large incision is needed (as for a Caesarean section), a midline laparotomy is often performed. In most colic surgeries, a midline laparotomy is the best approach allowing adequate visualization of the intestinal tract. Of course, good surgical exposure is always important, but it is especially required for such tedious procedures as removing an obstruction in the intestine, or removing a dead portion of the intestine and suturing the viable sections of the intestine back together.

Procedure: The horse will be under general anesthesia and in dorsal recumbency for this operation. The incision is made through the skin immediately over the linea alba (the linea alba is a white tendinous band of tissue that connects the abdominal muscles and indicates the anatomic midline of the abdominal wall). The skin incision is continued through the underlying subcutaneous tissue and linea alba; then the peritoneum is carefully incised to avoid accidental damage to the intestines.

After the incision is sutured, the veterinarian will prescribe antibiotics for an extended period of time. Of course, tetanus antitoxin or a toxoid injection will be administered according to the horse's vaccination program. The veterinarian will recommend that the horse's activities be restricted for at least a few weeks. Initially, exercise is generally limited to a period of hand-walking, as prescribed by the veterinarian.

ENTERECTOMY AND INTESTINAL ANASTOMOSIS

Enterectomy is the removal of a devitalized segment of the intestine, and intestinal anastomosis is the resectioning of the healthy portions of the intestine that remain. These procedures become necessary when intussusception, strangulated hernia, torsion, volvulus, or obstruction cause necrosis (death) of a section of the intestine.

Procedure: The veterinary surgeon will first perform a laparotomy to open the abdominal cavity and locate the affected portion of the intestine. After the damaged tissue is isolated, the ingesta is massaged away from the site of resection. The dead tissue is removed, and care is taken to ensure good blood supply to the remaining intestinal ends.

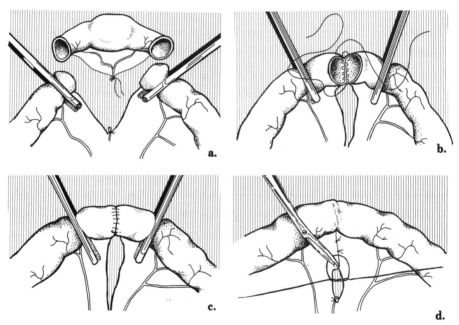

Fig. 17-11 Intestinal anastomosis. a. The devitalized section of intestine is removed. b. and c. The intestinal wall is sutured. d. The mesentery is sutured.

The two healthy portions of the intestine are sutured together, and the defect in the mesentery is repaired. If gas accumulates in the intestine during surgery, the veterinarian may insert a needle into the bloated area to relieve the pressure.

A horse suffering from a condition that requires intestinal anastomosis should receive immediate veterinary attention, for shock and intestinal necrosis can occur within one or two hours. Fluid therapy and prevention and treatment of shock are extremely important because the horse is very susceptible to shock. Peritonitis is also frequently a complicating factor.

Genito-Urinary System

CASTRATION

Most male horses are castrated between the ages of one and two years to prevent the development of secondary sexual characteristics (such as a crested neck), to improve their disposition, and to prevent the propagation of undesirable inheritable traits (such as poor conformation). As with any elective surgery, the horse to be castrated should be in good general health and on a good deworming program. Anemia, malnutrition, infectious disease, parasitism or other similar conditions are reasons for postponing the castration. Any pre-existing scrotal or inguinal hernias should be noted and repaired at the same time.

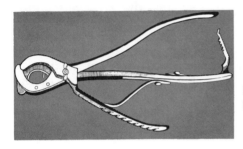

Fig. 17-12 Emasculator used to perform castration.

Procedure: Simple castration can be performed with the horse in either a standing, a lateral recumbent, or a dorsal recumbent position. When in the standing position, the horse is tranquilized or sedated, and a local anesthetic is usually administered by injection directly into the testicles. The horse should also be restrained with a twitch (refer to "Restraint of the Horse"). The scrotum and sheath are cleansed with surgical soap (such as Betadine or pHisoHex) and painted with an antiseptic solution (refer to "Surgical Preparation"). The veterinarian stands at the left flank of the horse, immobilizes the horse's testicles in his left hand and makes two incisions through the scrotum, each five inches long and one-half inch on either side of the medial raphe (midline). The testicles are then freed from surrounding tissue, and an emasculator is applied to the spermatic cord (taking care to avoid the scrotal vein) of one testicle at a time. The veterinarian may choose to make only one incision, removing both testicles through the single opening. Although the standing procedure is the quickest way to castrate a horse, it is also the most dangerous for the veterinarian.

If the horse is restrained in lateral recumbency, a general anesthetic is used, often in conjunction with a muscle relaxant. In the lateral position, the horse is first cast and the upper hind leg is flexed and tied by a sideline (this allows the veterinarian good access to the scrotum). The actual castration is performed in the same manner as with the standing position, with either a "closed" or an "open" technique. With the open method, the tunica vaginalis is incised at the same time as the skin, or in separate incisions, before the testicles are removed. With the closed method, the testicles are removed while still covered by the tunica vaginalis. The closed technique greatly reduces the chance of an intestinal prolapse from occurring in a horse with a tendency to herniate. However, the open technique is favored by some veterinarians since it allows a better view of the testicles and spermatic cord.

When the horse is in dorsal recumbency, under general anesthesia, both hind limbs are tied in a flexed position to give the veterinarian the greatest degree of safety. While this method does permit greater ease in dealing with any complications, it takes the most amount of time and involves a higher level of risk for the horse. The actual castration procedure is carried out as described above unless one or both testicles are undescended. In this case, an incision is made over the external inguinal ring and the retained testicle is retrieved from either the inguinal canal or just inside the abdominal cavity with a pair of long, curved sponge forceps. Alternatively, the veterinarian may make the incision into the abdomen, anterior to the inguinal ring, and retrieve the testicle through this incision, instead of through the inguinal ring. When an incision is made, either over the inguinal ring or anterior to it, the veterinarian will suture the incision after completing the castration.

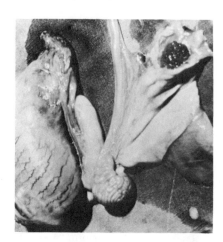

Fig. 17-13 Testicle after its removal. The tail of the epididymis must be completely removed or the horse may still retain some stallion characteristics, a condition known as "proud cut."

To encourage proper drainage of the incised scrotal area, the veterinarian will not suture the scrotal incisions. After castration, the horse should receive tetanus antitoxin or a toxoid injection, and be exercised twice daily for a short period of time. This will encourage proper drainage of the surgical site and keep swelling at a minimum. If the horse is kept on pasture, it should be examined periodically for excessive swelling or bleeding. If excessive hemorrhage occurs, the veterinarian should be contacted.

CASLICK'S OPERATION

A Caslick's operation is the surgical procedure used to correct an enlarged vulval opening of a mare suffering from pneumovagina. Pneumovagina can be caused by faulty conformation, in which the vulva tilts forward causing air to be forced inside (this condition is most often noticed in either lean racehorse mares or in old mares in poor physical shape), by an injury which lengthens the opening, or by the stretching of the tissues that naturally occurs at foaling.

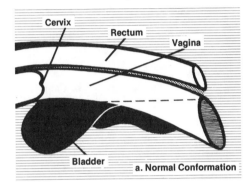

Fig. 17-4 Caslick's operation. a. Normal conformation. b. Abnormal conformation requiring suturing; note that the opening of the vulva is above the level of the pelvic floor [dotted line]. c. A strip of mucosa is removed from the upper opening of the vulva. d. The cut surfaces are then sutured together.

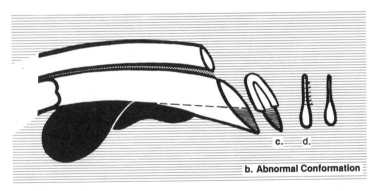

Procedure: A Caslick's operation can be performed on a standing mare, using a local anesthetic. In this procedure, a narrow strip of mucosa is cut away from both lips of the vulva, and the two surfaces are sutured together. The extent of the suturing, and the resultant shortening of the vulval fissure, is individually determined by the conformation of the mare. Ideally, the mare's vulva should be at an angle of 80°, and the opening should begin beneath the pelvic floor. The veterinarian will close the upper commissure to the extent needed to approximate this ideal. After operation, the surgical site should be kept clean, and the stitches removed in about one week. A culture taken a few weeks after suturing should not show any infection.

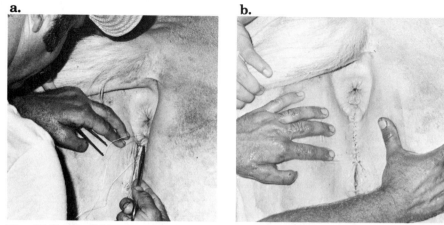

Fig. 17-15 Caslick's operation.   a. Suturing the vulvar lips together.   b. Completed Caslick's operation.

Before breeding the mare, or performing a speculum examination, a breeding stitch or cross-stitch of umbilical tape or doubled 0.6 Vetafil should be taken at the bottom of the closure to ensure that the suture line is not torn. Prior to breeding, all mares should be examined for a Caslick's operation. If the mare is tightly closed, she must be opened to permit live cover. The lips of the vulva can then be closed with wound clips until ovulation occurs, after which time the mare is resutured. About two weeks prior to the mare's calculated foaling date, an episiotomy (re-opening the vulva) is necessary to prevent ripping of the vulva at parturition. Artificial insemination is used rather than live cover in some mares that have undergone a Caslick's operation.

RECONSTRUCTION OF A RECTOVAGINAL FISTULA

During parturition, it is possible for the foal's hoofs to lacerate the rectovaginal wall. Depending upon the severity of the injury, a first, second or third degree perineal laceration may result. First degree refers to abrasions of the vaginal mucosa, second degree to injury to the submucosa of the vagina, and third degree to a rupture of the rectovaginal septum. In some cases of third degree lacerations, the foal is actually delivered through the fistula and anus. Attention during parturition and correction of dystocia (abnormal foaling) can help prevent a rectovaginal fistula.

If the injury is discovered during foaling, it can be repaired immediately. Otherwise, because of edema and bacterial invasion, a waiting period of at least three to four weeks will be required before the veterinarian can surgically reconstruct the area. A convenient arrangement might be to postpone the treatment until the foal has been weaned. Meanwhile, the damaged area should be kept clean and protected from insects. The mare should be immunized against tetanus, and may receive antibiotics as well.

Parasite control and adequate nutrition are also important to keep the mare in good condition for the surgery.

Procedure: The bulk in the mare's diet should be reduced by a gradual change in ration to soften her stools and reduce straining.

The surgery, which may be performed with the mare in a standing or recumbent position, involves reconstruction of the shelf of tissue dividing the rectum and vagina. The veterinarian places the sutures so that they do not protrude through the rectal mucosa, where they would cause irritation and straining, then sutures the perineal area between the anus and vulva.

After surgery, the mare should be maintained on a soft diet for at least two weeks. In six weeks, the veterinarian will perform a speculum examination to check the condition of the mare's reproductive tract. Artificial insemination may be conducted from this time on (providing the examination reveals nothing abnormal), but natural breeding should not be attempted for at least four to six months, depending on the outcome of the procedure.

OVARIECTOMY

Ovariectomy is the surgical removal of an ovary, and is performed either as treatment for an ovarian abnormality, or to cause sterility. A granulosa cell tumor is the most common reason for an ovariectomy. However, this type of surgery may also be indicated in other types of tumors, ovarian hematomas and abscesses, cysts, or in nymphomania. A granulosa cell tumor produces androgen causing infertility, lameness, abnormal muscle development, colic, anestrus, and personality changes. This tumor usually affects a young mare which has never cycled, and is most often discovered through rectal palpation. A granulosa cell tumor is quite large but rarely metastasizes (spreads throughout the body).

Abscesses, hematomas, and cysts may also be revealed by palpation. These abnormalities may vary considerably, depending upon the season, etc. In nymphomania, the ovaries are usually small and firm, and the mare often displays abnormal behavior.

In cases of granulosa cell tumor, if the other ovary is normal, removal of the affected ovary will often cause the mare to begin cycling normally. After surgical correction, the mare is often able to conceive and maintain pregnancy. Occasionally, however, the mare will still remain sterile. Other types of tumors, hematomas, and abscesses require only the removal of the affected ovary. Both ovaries must be removed from a mare with nymphomania (spaying).

Before performing a unilateral ovariectomy, the veterinarian may analyze a blood sample for hormone concentrations, as an aid both in determining whether the mare will return to fertility after surgery and in deciding on a program of hormonal therapy. The veterinarian will decide on the surgical technique to be used after considering the mare's temperament and physical condition, the type of abnormality involved, and the size of the affected ovary.

Procedure: If the mare is debilitated or crippled, the veterinarian may decide on a standing approach so that the animal will not require general anesthesia. When using this approach, the ovary may be removed either through the vaginal wall or through the flank. Only a small ovary may be removed through the vaginal wall (a procedure known as colpotomy) and this technique is contraindicated if cervical, uterine or vaginal infection is present. In this procedure, the veterinarian will make an incision through the vaginal wall, then insert a chain ecraseur. This instrument is looped over the ovary and used to amputate it. When a colpotomy is performed, the mare will require a Caslick's operation after surgery. If the flank approach is used, the veterinarian will make a vertical incision through the skin and underlying muscles, from just in front of the point of the hip down to the fold of the flank. In this procedure, the veterinarian may also use the ecraseur.

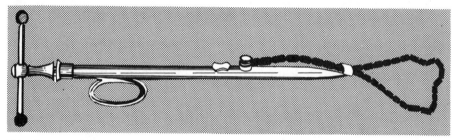

Fig. 17-16   Chain ecraseur used for an ovariectomy.

If the tumor is large, or the mare is temperamental (due to nymphomania), the veterinarian may choose to place the animal under general anesthesia and remove the ovary or ovaries through a midline incision. This method is best for very large granulosa cell tumors, but a dorsally located ovary may be difficult to remove using this approach. In this case, the flank approach may be preferred.

Regardless of the exact procedure used for an ovariectomy, the veterinarian will administer a tetanus toxoid or antitoxin injection and will prescribe antibiotics for several days following surgery. The mare will also require a low-bulk diet to avoid straining, and grain should be added gradually to her ration over a period of several days. Controlled exercise, as recommended by the veterinarian, will help reduce edema.

If the ovary was removed through the vagina, the mare should be restrained in cross-ties for 36 to 48 hours to reduce chances of herniation.

Correction of Hernias

Approximately two to five percent of all young foals develop umbilical or scrotal hernias, which are usually present at birth or appear within a few weeks. Although the tendency to herniate is considered inheritable, improper management practices at parturition can also be responsible. For example, breaking the umbilical cord too close to the body wall can cause an umbilical hernia. Other causes of acquired hernias are poor nutrition, constipation with excessive straining, foal diarrhea with straining, and infection of the umbilical cord.

TYPES OF HERNIAS

The sac of a hernia is composed of an inner layer of peritoneum (lining of abdominal cavity) and an outer layer of skin. The hernial contents may consist of intestines, omentum, or both. There are two major types of hernias; the reducible hernia, in which the contents of the hernial sac can be easily pushed back into the body cavity, and the irreducible type, in which adhesions form between the protruding contents and the sac, preventing the hernia from being pushed back into the abdominal cavity. If not corrected, irreducible hernias can develop into strangulated ones that cause a reduced blood supply to the area, necrosis of part of the intestines, and eventually result in peritonitis and the horse's death. This can also occur with reducible hernias, should a loop of intestine drop through the hernial ring and swell so that the hernia is no longer reducible.

UMBILICAL HERNIAS

Many small, reducible hernias without adhesions will eventually close spontaneously without surgical correction. Therefore, reducible hernias should be checked often for adhesions, and, if none are found, a period of six months to a year should be allowed for spontaneous correction. If the hernial ring is larger than two fingers in diameter, however, or if adhesions have formed or heat has developed in the area, surgery should be performed to correct the hernia.

Several methods of correction exist, including conservative treatments as well as surgery. Belts to encircle the abdomen and application or injection of counterirritants have both been employed (with questionable results) in the past to facilitate closure of small umbilical hernias. Clamps and skewers have also been used when the hernial ring was less than three inches in diameter and the sac contents were considered reducible.

Surgical Reduction

For open reduction of an umbilical hernia, a foal is placed in dorsal recumbency under general anesthesia. After removal of the skin covering the hernial sac, the sac is either inverted into the abdomen by the veterinarian or completely removed, and interrupted overlapping mattress sutures are sewn into the fascia on either side of the sac and pulled tight, causing one edge of the hernial ring to overlap the other. The margin of overlap is sutured down with continuous or simple interrupted sutures to give additional support to the suture line, then the skin edges are apposed (sutured together) using the suture pattern the veterinary surgeon prefers.

If the herniated area is considered to be especially weak, the veterinarian may insert a piece of stainless steel or polyethylene mesh on either the inside or outside of the abdominal cavity. The mesh patch is larger in diameter than the ring and is sutured to the body over the ring before the skin is closed to give additional support to an area where muscles and muscle sheaths are abnormally thin.

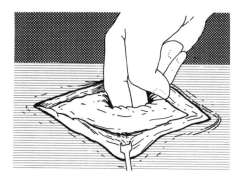

Fig. 17-17   Replacement of umbilical hernia prior to trimming muscle edges and suturing the defect in the abdominal wall.

SCROTAL HERNIAS

Scrotal hernias will not disappear spontaneously and always require open surgical reduction. Since scrotal hernias that are present congenitally or develop soon after birth are believed to be hereditary, colts with this condition are usually castrated at the same time the hernia is reduced.

Surgical Reduction

In this surgery, the horse is placed in a dorsal recumbent position under general anesthesia, and an incision is made through the skin over the superficial inguinal ring through which the testicle and hernial sac are lifted free of the scrotum. The veterinarian will hold the testicle in such a manner as to keep the spermatic cord taut, then twisting it, he will force the contents of the sac back through the hernial ring into the abdominal cavity. The twisted sac is tied with a ligature, then opened and the testicle removed. The external inguinal ring is closed by suturing to give additional support to the body wall. Following surgery, a drain tube is sometimes placed in the scrotum for a few days.

A strangulated scrotal hernia requires an emergency procedure, but is otherwise corrected in much the same way described above, with the exception that reduction will be more difficult. It may be necessary to remove necrotic or dead tissue, and antibiotics as well as drain tubes will be indicated for at least a few days following surgery.

In any routine castration, the veterinarian will check for an undiagnosed scrotal hernia prior to surgery. Otherwise, evisceration could occur following the normal castration technique, and an emergency hernia repair, often requiring resection of the intestines, would be required to save the horse. Vigorous antibiotic treatment to prevent peritonitis would be necessary after surgery.

As with all surgical procedures, the correction of a hernia should be accompanied by administration of tetanus antitoxin or toxoid, depending upon the horse's immunization program.

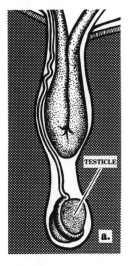

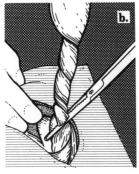

Fig. 17-18 Surgical correction of a scrotal hernia. a. Scrotal hernia. b. The scrotum is twisted, forcing the intestine back up into the abdominal cavity. The testicle is then removed.

Orthopedics

CHIP FRACTURES

All horses, especially those that are raced and heavily trained, are subject to orthopedic (bone) disorders and, particularly, injuries. Certain injuries result in bone fracturing and chipping. Chip fractures of the fetlock, sesamoids, and carpus are usually caused by trauma associated either with excessive strain, with overextension of the limb, or with fatigue. Such conditions are frequently encountered in racing and training, particularly in the young horse.

FETLOCK

Chip fractures of the fetlock usually occur because of trauma as the horse's leg strikes the ground. The condition is directly related to weight-bearing capabilities, stress, force and motion, and indirectly related to overextension of the joint and overall fatigue. The horse with a typical fetlock fracture will be most noticeably lame when put into a trot, and the lameness will become more pronounced with continued exercise. There may be heat over the surface of the joint area, and palpation or flexion of the fetlock will cause pain. Palpation may reveal some crepitation in the joint as well. For a correct diagnosis, the veterinarian will have to radiograph the injured area. Treatment for a chip fracture of the fetlock includes topical applications of a DMSO/corticosteroid mixture, the use of a "sweat," and rest. Since horses with a chip fracture frequently have arthritis or ringbone as well, the chip is not surgically removed unless it is specifically identified as the cause of lameness. Surgical removal of the chip may reduce mobility of the joint.

SESAMOID

Fractures of the sesamoids are most common in racing horses. Though they may be congenital, such fractures are more often the result of stress and fatigue associated with extended running. Fractures of the proximal sesamoids are caused specifically by stress when the foot lands in an unbalanced position. An animal with a sesamoid fracture may be very noticeably lame during the acute stages of the injury. Prevailing signs accompanying the lameness include swelling, heat and pain in the affected area. The lameness may cause the horse to carry his injured leg more rigidly, and he may hesitate to put any weight on the limb. An attending veterinarian will base his diagnosis on present physical signs and on radiographs of the area.

Suggested treatments will depend on the size of the injury, the time lapse between injury and start of treatment, and the owner's intended future use for the animal. If the fracture is not too severe and the horse is not to be raced, the leg may heal if it is placed in a cast. The cast must be worn for three to four months because the area heals slowly. During this period the horse will have to be confined. This lengthy recovery period will allow the fractured bones to reunite and heal properly. Good results can be anticipated if the cast is applied immediately after the injury occurs. An alternative treatment for horses not to be raced is the securing of the fracture with bone screws. For fractures that are greatly displaced or slow to heal, surgical removal of the chips will probably be necessary, but only if the fractured bone constitutes less than one-third of the total bone area.

CARPUS

Like other fractures, carpal injuries are caused by trauma to the area, often as a result of overextension of the leg. The carpal joint, when injured, will swell and there will be local heat, pain (when the joint is flexed), and lameness. Radiographs and careful palpation of the joint are necessary for correct and specific diagnosis. Again, treatment by surgical removal of chips or by use of bone screws is possible, depending on the amount of damage and elapsed time since the injury occurred. After surgery is completed, a support bandage is wrapped around the limb from hoof to forearm. Then, after five to seven days, it is removed. The veterinarian may recommend that the horse's leg be manually flexed and extended as physical therapy. Exercise will be prescribed by the veterinarian.

STAPLING THE EPIPHYSIS

Angular deformities of bones constitute problems in all breeds of horses. Such deformities may be congenital (affecting young foals) or acquired (the result of hard training before the bones have completed development). Deviations in the proper closure (development) of the epiphysis can be corrected either by the application of a cast or by stapling. Generally, casts are useful only on foals less than two months of age. After two months, stapling is more successful and is therefore preferred. Stapling of the fetlock joint must be done before six months of age. In the case of the carpus or tibia, staples must be put in place by fifteen months of age.

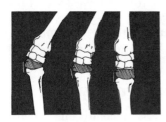

Fig. 17-19   The staple prevents deviation of the convex side of the leg, allowing the concave side to grow and straighten the leg.

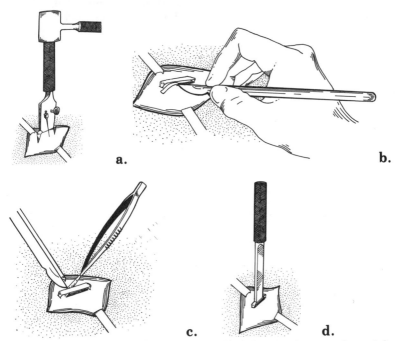

a.

b.

c.

d.

Fig. 17-20   Stapling the epiphysis.   a. Inserting a staple over the epiphyseal line, which is marked by a needle.   b. Cutting the soft tissue under the staple.   c. Removing the soft tissue.   d. Placing the staple in the bone.

Although this procedure may require several months to be effective, variations in time needed for correction depend on the seriousness of the deviation, the number of staples used, and the type of staples inserted. The principle of stapling is that the metal staple will prevent further deviation on the convex side, while the concave side grows continuously and thereby straightens the leg.

Procedure: Before the surgery is performed, radiographs of the area are made and the epiphyseal line is located by probing with a needle. With the horse under general anesthesia, the staples are placed so that they cross the epiphyseal line, uniting the bones. The number and size of staples used depends on the size of the horse. To help prevent strain and lessen the chance of staple movement, a bandage should be applied to the area after surgery. The animal should be confined for four weeks to prevent straining the leg. As soon as the leg is straight, the staples should be removed to avoid the chance of overcorrection. Corrective trimming of the hoof during this recovery time is important, for it will keep the hoof wall straight and hasten the foal's recuperation.

MEDIAL PATELLAR DESMOTOMY

Upward fixation of the patella (knee cap) is a condition, sometimes hereditary, that mainly affects young horses. When the horse's hind leg is extended, the part of the patella between the middle and medial patellar ligaments catches on top of the medial condyle of the femur, locking the leg in extension. Occasionally, the patella will catch only momentarily, particularly when the horse is making a sharp turn towards the affected leg. The "hitching" that results can be mistaken for the jerking gait of stringhalt.

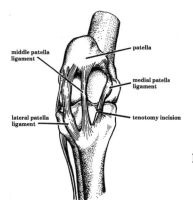

Fig. 17-21   Medial patellar desmotomy.

Procedure: The cutting of the medial patellar ligament, an operation known as a desmotomy, is the treatment of choice for this condition. The surgical site is shaved and scrubbed with an antiseptic and a local anesthetic is injected into the area. Usually, this surgery can be performed with the horse tranquilized and in a standing position. A small incision is made over the middle patellar ligament, through which a knife is placed underneath the medial patellar ligament. The knife blade is turned so that its sharp edge is against the ligament, which is then severed. Since conformation often causes upward fixation of the patella, both legs should probably be operated on at the same time. If necessary, a suture is used to close the small skin incision. The horse should be given tetanus antitoxin or toxoid, and confined for a week to ten days. The horse will require four to six weeks of rest to become accustomed to the loss of the ligament.

LATERAL DIGITAL EXTENSOR TENECTOMY (STRINGHALT CORRECTION)

An involuntary, spasmodic flexion of one or both of the horse's hind legs, particularly at the beginning of exercise after a rest period, is called stringhalt. This disorder may be caused by nerve damage, but the exact cause is unknown. Tenectomy (removing the tendon) of the lateral digital flexor tendon will frequently relieve this condition, at least partially.

Procedure: The horse is often operated on while in a standing position, under local anesthesia, but a fractious animal may have to be put under general anesthesia and placed in a lateral recumbent position. The skin over the surgical site should be aseptically prepared. The tendon is cut in two places; where it joins the long digital extensor tendon, and where it becomes muscle. It is then completely removed, and the two skin incisions are sutured. These sutures should be removed in one week to ten days, and the horse should be exercised during the recovery period (which can be several weeks). If stringhalt recurs after surgery, the veterinarian may remove an additional piece of the lateral digital extensor muscle. Often the surgery will be performed on both hind legs even if only one leg seems to be affected, because generally this condition will eventually affect both legs.

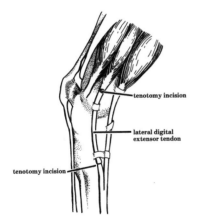

Fig. 17-22 Lateral digital extensor tenectomy.

Another form of treatment, much less commonly used, involves the administration of drugs which decrease skeletal muscle tone. This is supposed to prevent involuntary movement by reducing the number of repetitive nerve impulses that are causing the flexor spasms. However, drug therapy of stringhalt is generally ineffective.

CUNEAN TENECTOMY (CORRECTION OF CUNEAN TENDON BURSITIS)

Bursitis of the cunean tendon produces the same signs of lameness as bone spavin, and the two conditions are frequently confused. In cases where the horse becomes sound after injection of a local anesthetic into the cunean bursa, the true cause of lameness is bursitis. A cunean tenectomy can be performed to remove the section of the cunean tendon that rubs against the spavin area. This surgery may return the horse to soundness.

Procedure: The surgical site is prepared and a local anesthetic is administered. One to one and one-half inches of the cunean tendon is removed, through a skin incision, then the skin is sutured. These sutures can be taken out in ten days to two weeks, and the horse should be rested for two months or more.

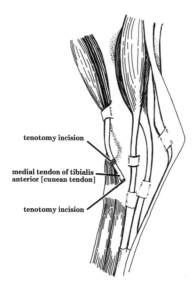

tenotomy incision

medial tendon of tibialis anterior [cunean tendon]

tenotomy incision

Fig. 17-23   Cunean tenectomy.

Another surgical procedure, called the Wamberg operation, is sometimes used to cut the nerves around the area of exostosis (excessive bony growth), thereby reducing pain. A diamond-shaped cut is made around the spavin, through all of the surrounding tissues. The subcutaneous tissues and skin are sutured and the area bandaged. Postoperative exercise will be prescribed by the veterinarian.

SURGICAL CORRECTION OF CONTRACTED TENDONS

Contracted tendons may be either congenital or acquired. When congenital, due to cramping in the uterus, the foal will often spontaneously improve within a few days. Sometimes splints and casts are used in more severe cases. In older foals, this condition may result from oversupplementation, particularly with a high-protein diet. Young horses that have previously been provided with just a maintenance diet and are switched to a highly supplemented, high-protein feeding regime are most susceptible to contracted tendons. Actually, the tendons do not contract; instead, the cannon bone (third metacarpal bone) and/or radius outgrow the flexor tendons. In older horses, contracted tendons may occur as a result of scarring and shortening of a healed cut tendon, or as a result of shortening of tendons due to long-term disuse of an extremely lame leg.

Accelerated growth of the cannon usually occurs at three or four months of age. In this condition, because of the disproportional length of the cannon, the inferior check ligament pulls on the back of the third phalanx, causing the foal to go up on its toes. In two or three weeks, the foal develops a club foot as the toe wears away. Although this condition does affect both fore and hind legs, it will be more noticeable in the front. Eventually, the hoof wall may separate from the sensitive laminae, resulting in a dished foot similar to that seen with laminitis. If the condition continues uncorrected, the foal may suffer degenerative joint disease, due to the abnormal pressures that the short pastern bone transmits to the third phalanx.

Contracted tendons due to extremely rapid growth of the radius usually occur between the ages of 9 and 28 months (16 months is the average). Within three weeks of onset of the condition, the foal will begin "knuckling over." The superior check ligament's attachment to the pastern bones will cause the fetlock joint to snap forward at every stride. As with the condition caused by overgrowth of the cannon bone, accelerated growth of the radius is due to the young horse being fed a very high-quality, highly supplemented diet. Unless the signs of contracted tendons are recognized early and dietary adjustments are made, both forms of contracted tendons may occur in the same horse due to accelerated growth of both the cannon bone and the radius.

Procedure: A change in diet may correct very mild cases of contracted tendons; however, if the foal has developed club feet or is "knuckling over," surgery is necessary. In cases where the foal has arthritis in association with the contracted tendons, it will not return to complete soundness after surgery.

If the contracted tendons are due to the growth of the cannon bone, the veterinarian may perform an inferior check ligament desmotomy, in which the ligament is cut in two. This operation, which is done about halfway down the length of the cannon bone, will result in an immediate correction of the condition. The legs are bandaged for one day following surgery and, of course, the foal receives either a tetanus antitoxin or toxoid injection. Within four to six months, scar tissue will repair the ligament. To prevent a recurrence of this condition, the foal should not be returned to the high-protein diet.

In cases where the radius is the cause of the contracted tendons, a surgical correction known as a superior check ligament desmotomy can be performed, if the condition is severe enough to cause the foal to "knuckle over." The veterinarian will sever the superior check ligament one-third of the way up the radius. This operation will not result in an immediate improvement, because of the other associated tissues which have shortened due to the contracted tendons. A cast is applied following surgery, but it must be removed daily for physical therapy. A corrective shoe with a toe extension can be applied to help stretch the shortened tissues. Within 48 hours, the horse should show noticeable improvement. If the operation does not appear to have corrected the condition within a week, the veterinarian may decide that an inferior check ligament desmotomy is also required.

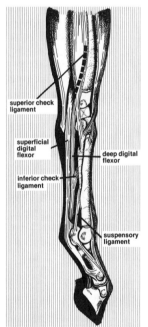

superior check ligament

superficial digital flexor

deep digital flexor

inferior check ligament

suspensory ligament

Fig. 17-24 Contracted tendons due to accelerated growth of the cannon or radius may be surgically corrected by an inferior and/or superior check ligament desmotomy.

The veterinarian may choose, in some cases, to perform a tenotomy to correct this condition, instead of a desmotomy. In this operation, one of the flexor tendons is completely or partially severed through a skin incision. Support bandages or casts are used postoperatively. In addition, procedures exist for tendon lengthening as well as tendon stretching by cutting notches along the length of the tendon.

FLUSHING OF A JOINT (ARTHROCENTESIS)

Successful treatment of an infected joint often requires flushing of the joint (arthrocentesis) to wash away cartilaginous material, fibrin and purulent debris that reduce the lubricating ability of the synovial fluid.

For this procedure, the horse is placed under general anesthesia in lateral recumbency. The skin surface over the joint to be flushed is prepared as for any other major surgical operation. Sterile technique is used throughout the procedure. The drainage needle, equipped with a stopcock, is passed into the lower or outermost part of the joint space, which is then drained of excess fluid. Sterile saline solution (warmed to the horse's body temperature) is introduced into the joint through another needle inserted into the upper or innermost portion of the joint space. The drainage needle is kept closed while the solution is introduced under pressure until the capsule is distended. Then, the stopcock is opened and the joint allowed to drain. This procedure is repeated several times in succession. Before beginning the flush, the veterinarian may aspirate a sample of synovial fluid to submit for laboratory analysis.

The veterinarian may choose to flush the joint with an antibiotic or enzyme solution in addition to the saline solution. If necessary, this procedure can be repeated until the infection appears to be under control. The skin incisions (from the needle insertions) are sutured closed, then the joint is bandaged. The veterinarian may immobilize the horse's limb with a cast and the horse will also be given tetanus antitoxin or a toxoid injection.

Arthrocentesis is particularly effective in horses with joint diseases that are characterized by lameness which regresses with rest and recurs with exercise. This type of condition often requires only one flushing treatment. In cases of infectious (septic) arthritis, flushing of the joint should be followed with heat therapy and exercise, in order to keep the joint mobile. It is important that the infection be controlled before heat treatment is initiated, because heat will increase the horse's circulation and spread infection.

ANKYLOSING A JOINT (ARTHRODESIS)

Surgical ankylosing of a joint, known as arthrodesis, is sometimes necessary in the treatment of bone spavin, ringbone, and other chronic arthritic conditions. In this procedure, the veterinarian uses a drill or bone chisel to surgically remove at least 60% of the articular cartilage of the involved joint(s). This treatment causes the joint's bone surfaces to gradually fuse, relieving the horse of pain, but of course does not return soundness to the animal because the involved joint is no longer functional.

Procedure: The horse is placed under general anesthesia in a lateral recumbent position, and the veterinarian uses a drill to remove the joint surfaces. (For bone spavin, these would be the distal intertarsal and tarsometatarsal joints, while the pastern joint would be treated in a case of ringbone.) The hole is flushed out with sterile saline solution, and may be packed with cancellous bone chips from the tuber coxae to hasten fusion of the joint. The incisions are then sutured, and a bandage (for bone spavin) or cast (for ringbone) applied. The horse should receive tetanus antitoxin or toxoid, and, if necessary, analgesics and antibiotics.

If the ankylosis was performed for treatment of bone spavin, the horse should be kept stalled for one month. After ten days, the sutures are removed, and the bandage is taken off in two weeks. The horse may be exercised after one month to hasten the ankylosis, and by four to twelve months the joints will have completely fused.

If the pastern joint has been ankylosed, a trailer shoe is often applied for the first month following surgery to support the horse's fetlock. For the joint to completely fuse, a cast will be required for a period of two months.

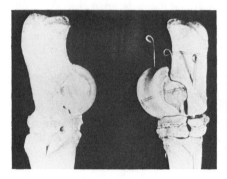

Fig. 17-25 The hock joint of a horse with bone spavin eventually becomes ankylosed, a process that can be hastened by arthrodesis. The fused hock is shown on the left, while a normal hock is on the right.

The Foot

ACRYLIC HOOF REPAIR

Cracks in the hoof wall are classified as heel, toe, or quarter cracks, depending upon location. Conditions that predispose the hoof to cracks include excessive wall growth, improper trimming, thin hoof walls, and exceedingly dry hoofs. Dry hoofs occur when the hoof's natural moisture is drawn out, as happens when a horse continually stands in dry stalls or is out on pasture in drought conditions. Another cause is the practice of rasping or sanding the hoof wall itself to make it smooth or to make it conform to an ill-fitted shoe. This destroys the periople, a structure which helps preserve the hoof's moisture, and causes the hoof to be brittle and to be more likely to crack on concussion.

Hoof cracks should always be treated in order to prevent them from splitting the entire length of the hoof wall and to prevent infection from developing in sensitive inner structures and causing lameness. Acrylic repair of simple cracks is usually successful unless infection is already present or unless the crack is so deep that it penetrates into sensitive inner structures, making acrylic repair hazardous. A deep crack could seriously damage the hoof and require extensive treatment to prevent infection and lameness. In less serious cases, however, an acrylic material can often be used to replace the portion of original hoof wall that has cracked or deteriorated. Repair should only be attempted by a skilled and knowledgeable person.

REPAIRING HOOF CRACKS

A part of the bottom of the hoof wall is usually cut away (as in a toe crack) on both sides of the crack to remove the area's weight-bearing responsibilities and thereby stop further crack expansion. Similarly, a section is drilled or filed from the hoof at the top of the crack to limit its upward expansion. The crack is then stripped out down to the sensitive laminae and enlarged. Small holes are next drilled on both sides of the crack and laced with umbilical tape or stainless steel wire to provide a reinforced base for the application of the acrylic filler and to help prevent further crack expansion. After lacing is complete, the catalyst is applied before the acrylic is applied and allowed to harden. The filler material may then be rasped after it hardens to blend more evenly with the hoof wall.

a.

b.

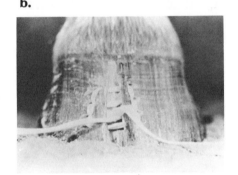

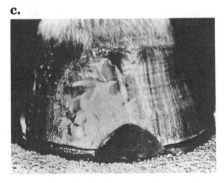

c.

Fig. 17-26 Acrylic hoof repair. a. Holes are drilled on either side of the defect. b. Umbilical tape is laced through the holes. c. An acrylic compound is applied to fill in the defect. In this case, a shoe with a toe clip has been applied to provide more support to the affected area.

If the crack occurs at the heel or quarter area, the bottom section of the hoof wall behind the crack may have to be filed away from the shoe to prevent the cracked area from bearing any weight. When this is necessary, the open area between the hoof wall and shoe must be cleaned daily to prevent accumulations of dirt from exerting pressure on the hoof.

REPLACING THE HOOF WALL

If the bottom of the hoof wall has broken off, leaving a space between the hoof and shoe, acrylic is often used to replace the missing portion of wall. Both soft and hard acrylics are used in this repair; soft acrylic to replace areas of the frog that have worn away, and hard acrylic to patch the hoof wall itself. Hard acrylic sets up in only ten to fifteen minutes and is extremely durable, making it an excellent choice for hoof wall repair.

To patch the wall, the veterinarian will mix the substance and apply it to the damaged hoof a little at a time. He will then patch the acrylic into the area between the shoe and hoof, from outer wall to sole, and sometimes pour warm water over the patch to reduce the setting-up time (heat quickens the process and cold retards it). Afterwards, the acrylic can be rasped to conform with the shape of the hoof. Since the material's final hardness makes later nailing impossible, any nails that are to be driven must be implanted in the patch before the acrylic has completely set up.

CORRECTIVE SHOES FOR REPAIRED HOOFS

Corrective shoes are often used to aid the recovery and reconditioning of the hoof after it has been treated with acrylic materials. For a horse with a toe crack, the corrective shoe should have clips placed on each side of the crack to help hold the patch in place and keep the crack from expanding. If the hoof is cracked at the quarter or heel, a full or half-bar shoe with clips to immobilize the crack can be used (refer to "Corrective Shoeing and Trimming").

NEURECTOMY

Neurectomy is the surgical sectioning of the sensory nerve supplying a certain part of the body (thus removing all sensation from the area). Neurectomy of the posterior digital nerve is most commonly performed on horses with navicular disease, although it is also used in treatment of conditions such as a broken third phalanx. Because this operation leaves the heel area of the hoof numb, the horse feels no pain from the navicular bone and therefore is no longer lame.

Complications can occur following a neurectomy, as neuromas often develop in the ends of cut nerves. In fact, in approximately ten to fifty percent of these cases, the neuromas become exceedingly painful and can cause lameness. There is also a risk of stumbling gaits and hoof sloughing following this procedure; puncture wounds will also be a serious problem since the horse will be unable to detect pain in the foot. Approximately 80 percent of the horses receiving proper postoperative care show improvement from navicular disease lameness after a neurectomy. However, a neurectomy should be chosen only after more conservative treatment (such as corrective shoeing) has been tried.

Procedure: This surgical procedure can be performed while the horse is either standing or in a recumbent position. If standing, the horse is first tranquilized, and a local anesthetic is administered just below the fetlock. After a one and one-half inch long incision is made, approximately one-half inch of the posterior digital nerve is removed. At this time, the veterinarian will also check for alternate accessory nerve pathways. Between fifty and seventy percent of all horses have these extra nerve branches, and if the branches are not also dissected, the horse may remain lame after the operation. The veterinarian will suture the incision and repeat the procedure for the nerve on the opposite side of same foot to complete the operation. The veterinarian may perform epineural capping (a procedure in which the cut nerve endings are covered) to prevent the formation of neuromas.

A pressure bandage, changed on alternate days, is necessary for one week following the neurectomy, and after ten days the sutures can be removed. The horse should then be allowed an additional four to six weeks of rest. After a neurectomy has been performed, the horse should be given tetanus antitoxin or a tetanus toxoid injection, depending on whether or not the animal is on a regular program of immunization.

To help prevent neuroma formation, the horse should not be exercised sooner than six weeks, and the wound should remain bandaged until it has completely healed. Corticosteroids or phenylbutazone injections may prevent further growth of the neuromas.

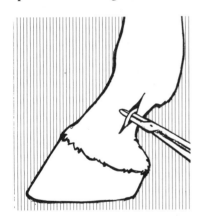

Fig. 17-27 Elevating the digital nerve with forceps prior to performing a posterior digital neurectomy.

Cryosurgery

Cryosurgery is the use of extreme cold to remove sarcoids, squamous cell carcinomas, and other neoplasms. This is accomplished by lowering the cells' temperature to -20°C or less, which kills the more rapidly growing cells (cancer or pigment cells) by forming and dissolving ice inside and outside the cells, and by changing electrolyte concentrations. The cryogen, or freezing substance (in this case, liquid nitrogen), damages the proliferating cells and destroys the venules, capillaries, and arterioles supplying blood to the area. In addition, there is a possibility that cryosurgery causes an immune response (as does vaccination) and stimulates the body's defenses against the tumor by increasing the horse's level of antibodies. Cryosurgery was originally developed from the technique of freeze branding (the use of excessive cold to permanently mark a horse). As in freeze branding, cryosurgery kills pigment-producing cells and leaves a loss of hair or hair color at the surgery site.

Aside from its use in the treatment of sarcoids and squamous cell carcinomas, cryosurgery has been successfully employed in treating cases of melanomas, habronema granulomas, fibrous granulation tissue, and myosarcomas. In therapy for most conditions, cryosurgery causes regression of at least 95% of all treated lesions (as compared to approximately 50% for conventional therapy), and does so without causing hemorrhage, pain, or development of proud flesh. In addition, there is little risk of infection.

A disadvantage of cryosurgery, however, is that, although liquid nitrogen is a readily available and inexpensive cryogen, the cryosurgery unit itself can be expensive and inconvenient for field use. Of course, cryosurgery also tends to be less satisfactory when performed on large, deep tumors, as the thickness of such lesions retards the depth of freezing.

Procedure: Although the procedure for cryosurgery is less painful than other types of surgery (due to the quick withdrawal of heat from the horse's body), the animal is usually tranquilized and a local anesthetic administered. To ensure even contact between the sarcoid and the cryogen, the area to be treated is cleaned and shaved, after which the surrounding skin is protected from the cold with a surgical lubricant or petroleum jelly-covered gauze. Microthermocouple needles (used to measure temperature change) are inserted into the lesion where they will not directly contact the cryogen. The liquid nitrogen is either sprayed onto the tumor with a spray attachment, or a closed-end probe is used to apply the cold. Large sarcoids over 2 cm in diameter are treated with larger spray applicators.

Treatment with the cryogen is continued until the lesion's temperature is reduced to approximately -25°C. The area is allowed to thaw to 0°C at this time, then is refrozen to the -25°C reading again. This "quick-freeze, slow-thaw, quick-freeze" method has been demonstrated to be the most successful technique in cryotherapy, as it causes the greatest amount of cryonecrosis (tissue death due to cold). After cryosurgery, the tumor will usually desiccate and slough within ten days, and the remaining lesion will scab over and heal by second intention (granulation) healing in approximately four to six weeks. Larger lesions, of course, may require a longer period to heal.

If a sarcoid removed by cryosurgery reappears, the veterinarian may repeat the freezing procedure. Sometimes, however, and most frequently in the treatment of large growths, a combination of surgery and cryosurgery may be elected. If so, the lesion is first surgically removed, then its base and surrounding band of tissue are frozen.

Euthanasia

The life of an animal with a curable condition should never be terminated. Unfortunately, the owner of a horse will sometimes be faced with an animal in extreme pain caused by an incurable condition. After veterinary consultation, the decision to euthanatize the horse may be reached.

Procedure: The method most commonly used today for euthanasia in horses is a chemical injection. Chemical injectables have been found to be very reliable in causing death without pain in a very short period of time. Since these chemicals are smooth acting, the horse does not struggle; this minimizes the psychological effects.

Other methods of euthanasia, such as electrocution and shooting, are greatly discouraged except for certain rare, emergency situations. None of the above methods are perfect and all of them can be mishandled. Therefore, these procedures should be conducted only by trained personnel.

Necropsy

A necropsy (i.e., post-mortem examination) of a horse serves to increase knowledge of disease processes, aids in positive diagnosis of otherwise unexplained deaths, and indirectly suggests improvements in management and health care.

Necropsy may reveal the following to the veterinarian:

1. confirm or refute diagnosis of primary disorder
2. cause of death in instances of sudden death
3. unsuspected additional problems in the horse
4. the reason a specific course of treatment failed
5. a malicious act in a case of sudden death
6. the need for immediate treatment of other horses

For example, if the necropsy provides a positive diagnosis of a contagious disease, an effective program of preventive treatment can be introduced to exposed horses. Even aborted fetuses should be necropsied so that the cause of abortion may be learned and future abortions prevented. The result of the necropsy on an aborted fetus may suggest a change in breeding management.

Procedure: The necropsy should be performed as soon as possible after death to avoid confusion of pathological lesions with postmortem changes. The veterinarian usually begins the examination by checking the body for skin lesions and for signs of trauma caused by a struggle. He then examines the body for signs of disease processes, such as congested blood, localized edema, and gaseous odors. Gingiva (gum) color is also noted, for it may help indicate the type of condition that affected the horse (e.g., pale mucous membranes suggest anemia or hemorrhage, while yellowish membranes may indicate icterus).

The veterinarian additionally examines all viscera (internal organs) and, in many cases, the spinal cord and brain. When infectious disease is the suspected cause of death, bacterial or fungal cultures are submitted to a diagnostic laboratory for testing, and a drug sensitivity test is performed. The results of sensitivity tests aid the veterinarian in choosing a course of prophylactic (preventive) treatment for other exposed horses. In some instances, virus isolations may also be attempted.

Tissues that are sent to the diagnostic laboratory for testing purposes may vary depending on necropsy findings, but often include the following:

1. blood and urine samples collected prior to or sometimes after death
2. fecal samples
3. stomach contents
4. tissue samples from various organs, including the liver, lungs, kidney, intestines, heart, and brain

Plants and feedstuffs are also submitted to the laboratory when they are suspected as possible sources of toxicity.

IV. DRUGS
& RELATED TOPICS

18

BASIC CONCEPTS OF
DRUG THERAPY

The proper therapeutic use of drugs in a species such as the horse represents an exceptionally exact and complex science. Thorough basic training is required to understand the fundamental principles of drug therapy, and extensive clinical training and applied experience is needed to effectively implement drug therapy. Most horsemen are well aware of these facts. The summation of drug concepts presented in the subsequent chapters can by no means be substituted for professional training. Instead, this information is offered as a supplemental aid to the overall, proper husbandry of the horse. The horseman will be performing a serious disservice to himself and his horses if the material in the following chapters is used in attempts to avoid care by a veterinarian.

On the other hand, the horseman is routinely confronted with the need to administer drugs in the form of liniments, leg braces, insecticides, deworming preparations, etc., and also various other more complicated medicinals that may be prescribed or dispensed by the veterinarian. Because of the serious and even fatal complications that can be accidentally produced by the administration of even "safe" drugs, the horseman should be aware of the complexities and, particularly, the limitations and precautions of rational drug therapy in the horse.

The present chapter considers some of the basic concepts of drug therapy in horses, and includes various definitions that may prove useful. The indications, limitations and contraindications for individual drugs and groups of drugs are presented in the following chapters. An attempt is not made to consider the hundreds of different drugs that are available. Instead, an attempt is made to present relevant information about selected drugs and representative drug groups that have practical importance to the horse owner, trainer and handler. Included are those drugs and drug preparations that are routinely administered by the horseman in everyday husbandry, training and conditioning situations. In addition, drugs that are restricted by law to be used by or under the supervision of a veterinarian are also included in order to familiarize the horseman with certain drugs and therapeutic procedures that may be administered or prescribed by the veterinarian.

Definitions

Drugs are defined as those chemical substances or mixtures of chemical substances used for the cure or prevention of diseases or signs of diseases. In other words, the term drug is used to designate those chemical substances used to promote or safeguard health. A large portion of the benefits derived from drug therapy can be attributed to the development of the youngest of the medical sciences, Pharmacology, which is defined as "the scientific study of drugs and their actions in living organisms."

One of the most important practical advancements resulting from the emergence of Pharmacology is the dominance of "rational drug therapy" over "empirical drug therapy." Empirical drug therapy is based only on experience and tradition, and its definition can be summarized as follows: "if a drug works (or seems to help), use it." Rational drug therapy, on the other hand, is now the basis for a true clinical science; it is founded on:

1. a thorough understanding of normal bodily functions (physiology)
2. knowledge of disease processes (pathology)
3. knowledge of abnormal bodily functions (pathologic physiology)
4. a comprehension of the actions of drugs in the body (pharmacology)

Due to a lack of complete understanding of many bodily functions and drug actions, some empirical therapies are still useful. However, the practical importance of rational drug therapy to the horseman is the recognition that drugs should never be used indiscriminately, but should be reserved for use in specific diagnosed conditions where there is a rational basis for their use.

General Aspects

The subdisciplines of pharmacology include:

1. the study of the sources of drugs (pharmacognosy)
2. the fate of drugs within the body (pharmacokinetics)
3. the mechanisms whereby drugs affect bodily functions (pharmacodynamics)
4. the use of drugs in the treatment of disease (pharmacotherapeutics)
5. the adverse or poisonous actions of drugs (toxicology)

Although equine pharmacotherapeutics is the primary concern of this section, several basic aspects of pharmacology deserve brief consideration due to their practical importance in the treatment of different conditions of horses.

DRUG SOURCES

A wide variety of therapeutically used drugs are now chemically synthesized in the laboratory (e.g., phenylbutazone, acetylpromazine, chloramphenicol). However, many useful drugs are obtained from animal, plant and mineral sources. Mineral based agents include the various iron preparations used in treating anemic conditions. The solutions of electrolytes (for example, sodium chloride) used in fluid replacement therapy are mineral source drugs as are certain of the astringents (e.g., silver nitrate), disinfectants (e.g., sodium hydroxide), laxatives (e.g., magnesium sulfate) and various other types of medicines. Animal source drugs include hormones (for example, insulin), vitamins (A and D from cod-liver oil) and antisera (tetanus antitoxin). Plant materials have provided medicinally active products since the times of primitive man. Digitalis is an important plant-source drug, as are atropine and opium. Antibiotics are metabolic by-products or microorganisms that have been found to be exceptionally helpful in treating infections of pathogenic (disease producing) bacteria.

DRUG PREPARATIONS

Aqueous solutions consist of a water-soluble drug of mineral, plant or animal origin dissolved in water. "Solutions for injection" are sterilized aqueous solutions. Fixed oils, such as peanut oil, are sometimes used to suspend an insoluble drug for intramuscular injection. Aqueous suspensions are comprised of insoluble drugs that are thoroughly mixed and suspended in water. Emulsions, for example, are aqueous suspensions of insoluble liquids. Usually, an emulsifying agent is added to assist in dispersion and suspension of the insoluble liquid. Mixtures refer to a suspension of an insoluble solid substance in water. Magmas are dense viscous mixtures of a finely ground solid and a liquid, such as milk of magnesia. Extracts are prepared from plant materials by soaking the plant in a solution of liquid until the active ingredient is extracted into the liquid. Tinctures are alcoholic extracts.

Drugs that are insoluble in most solvents often can be administered in solid form. Powders, for example, are finely-ground solids used for topical application and, when packed into hard gelatin capsules, for oral administration. Tablets for oral administration are made by compressing powder into solid objects of either round, discoid or oblong shapes. Pills are similar to tablets but often contain a sticky ingredient for cohesiveness, and are often coated with a thin shell for protection. If the protective shell is resistant to breakdown by the acidity of the stomach contents, the pill is referred to as an enteric-coated pill and it passes into the small intestine before it dissolves. A bolus is simply a large tablet used for oral administration of drugs to large animals, or for use as a suppository. Suppositories are used for conveyance of drugs into body openings such as the rectum and vagina.

Liniments are liquid preparations of active drugs dissolved (in solution) or suspended (as a mixture or emulsion) in water or dilute alcohol. Emulsified oils are often included in liniments intended for external application to the horse's limbs in conjunction with a vigorous massage.

Lotions are mild, usually soothing liquid preparations comprised of an insoluble drug suspended in water. Ointments are viscous, semiliquid preparations used for local application to mucous membranes or skin. Ointments are commonly prepared by incorporation of an active drug into solid fats, petrolatum or paraffin. External dosage forms of medicine are covered in the chapter on "Skin and Mucous Membrane Preparations."

PHARMACOKINETICS

The fate of drugs within the body can be subdivided into:

1. absorption of drugs from administration sites
2. distribution of drugs into bodily tissues
3. breakdown (metabolism) of the drug by body tissues
4. elimination (excretion) of the drug from the body

Drugs are absorbed from administration sites due to their passage through the cells of small blood and lymph vessels. In this manner, drugs enter the bloodstream and are circulated throughout the body. Drugs differ in their ability to be absorbed. For example, neomycin is an antibiotic that is poorly absorbed from the digestive system. Administered orally, neomycin could be helpful in treating bacterial diarrhea of foals but would be virtually useless in treating infections of bodily tissues since it would not be effectively absorbed from the gut. For such reasons, recommendations of drug companies should always be followed when different routes of administration are considered.

After absorption into the blood, drugs can:

1. be distributed evenly throughout the body
2. be concentrated within certain tissues
3. be restricted from entry into certain regions
4. follow a variety of the above three pathways

For example, antibiotics that are chemically similar to streptomycin do not enter the brain due to their inability to penetrate the "blood-brain barrier." Thus, such drugs are of little value in treating infections of the central nervous system. Some drugs (e.g., certain of the barbiturates) are so fat-soluble that they are distributed throughout fatty tissues of the body.

As drugs are circulated through the liver, they can be metabolized (their chemical structure changed by enzymes) into water-soluble metabolites that can be excreted by the kidneys into the urine and, thereby, be eliminated from the body. Some drugs (e.g., kanamycin) do not undergo metabolism within the body but are excreted unchanged in the urine.

DRUG ADMINISTRATION

One of the most common routes of administering a drug is by mouth. The oral route is usually fairly easy and does not require sterile preparations such as are necessary for injection into bodily tissues. However, effects of the drug may not be obtained for an hour or longer after oral administration due to slow absorption from the gastrointestinal tract.

Parenteral refers to routes of administration other than by the gastrointestinal tract. This term is usually reserved to designate the injection of a drug into bodily tissues with use of a needle and syringe. Important parenteral routes in horses include subcutaneous, intramuscular and intravenous, as shown in the accompanying illustration. Importantly, administration routes affect the availability of a drug in the blood and thus, tissue sites. For example, after intravenous injection, the concentration of the drug in the blood reaches a very high level almost immediately, but decreases quickly as the drug is rapidly distributed into other tissues and is subjected to metabolism and excretory pathways. After intramuscular injection, the maximum blood concentrations are obtained more slowly than after intravenous injection; however, blood levels are maintained for a longer interval. Absorption of a drug is even slower after oral or subcutaneous administration, but the drug may be available in the blood for a longer interval than with either intravenous or intramuscular injection. Thus, selection of a particular administration route is dependent in part upon whether a brief and intense (as with intravenous) or a moderate and prolonged (as with intramuscular) duration of action is required.

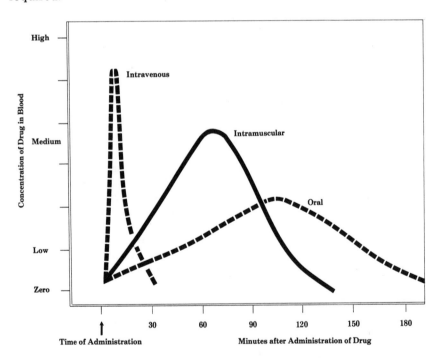

Fig. 18-1 Concentrations of drugs in the blood after different routes of administration.

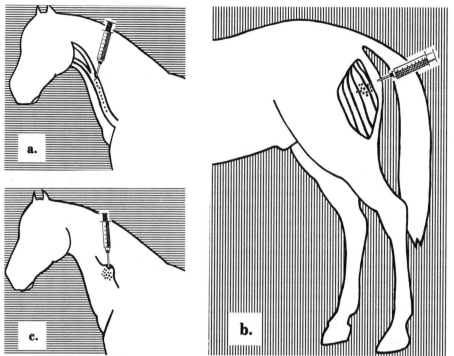

Fig. 18-2 Parenteral routes of administering drugs in horses. a. Intravenous injection; the drug is administered directly into the blood stream. b. Intramuscular
injection; the drug is administered into the muscles, then absorbed into the blood
stream. c. Subcutaneous injection; the drug is administered under the skin, then
absorbed into the blood stream.

FACTORS AFFECTING DRUG RESPONSE

Although responses to drugs can usually be accurately predicted, all
animals do not identically respond to the same drug even when the drug is
administered in the same dosage and by the same route. In other words,
there is biological variation in relation to drug effectiveness. Several factors
have been identified which can directly affect the responsiveness of an
animal to a drug.

For example, the condition of the digestive system can have considerable
impact on the absorption of a drug after oral administration. The rate and
extent of absorption of a drug is usually more pronounced in a fasted
animal, than when administered to the same animal after a meal. Diarrhea
tends to decrease the effectiveness of an orally administered drug due to a
more rapid rate of passage through the digestive tract. However, if the
intestinal lining is severely inflamed and engorged with blood and lymph,
as occurs in enteritis, then drug absorption can be enhanced. Constipation
may cause enhanced absorption of a drug due to delayed movement
through the gut.

As in adult horses, drug dosage in foals is determined primarily by body weight. However, young animals can neither metabolize nor excrete drugs as effectively as can adults. Therefore, dosages are usually decreased in young foals. Doses may also have to be somewhat reduced in old horses due to the slowing down of many bodily functions that occurs in the aged.

Several general precautionary considerations should be remembered when broodmares are treated with drugs. For example, purgatives should not be administered during pregnancy due to the danger of producing abortion or rectal or vaginal prolapse. Diarrhea can be produced in the nursing foal if the dam is administered certain purgative drugs. There are few important sex differences in responses of mares, geldings, and stallions to drugs (except, of course, the sex hormones). However, a tranquilizing agent used in the past caused several instances of permanent relaxation of the penis in stallions.

The temperament of an individual animal can exert considerable influence on drug effectiveness. For example, a "high-strung" horse usually requires a greater dosage of nervous system depressants (such as a tranquilizer or anesthetic agent) than do other, more tractable horses. Conversely, an excitable animal usually responds excessively to a central nervous system stimulant and, in some cases, may become uncontrollable.

The general condition of an animal's health is an important determinant of drug effectiveness. In severely ill and debilitated horses, for example, drug effects may well be accentuated. Dosages should be reduced accordingly and drugs should be administered particularly slowly and carefully in such cases.

Drug interactions can occur when more than one drug is administered simultaneously or, in some cases, within a few days of each other. If two drugs produce opposite effects on the same organ, their interaction is one of antagonism, and they can cancel each other's actions. Conversely, if two drugs produce identical effects, their interaction is called synergism, and a marked potentiation of the actions of both drugs can result. Careful records of drug usage should always be maintained and consulted in order to prevent drug interactions. The veterinarian should always be advised of any drugs, insecticides or environmental chemicals to which the horse has recently been exposed.

PURCHASING AND ADMINISTERING DRUGS

The useful and often life-saving benefits that can be derived from the appropriate use of drugs in modern equine husbandry are, of course, unequivocal. Unfortunately, however, drugs and chemicals are often considered as a panacea (cure-all), especially by inexperienced people, and little attention is directed toward learning the specific indications, limitations and contraindications of a particular drug. Because of such specificities, the use of highly potent drugs in horses should routinely be considered as a veterinary-only or veterinary prescribed and supervised procedure, as continually emphasized and explained throughout this book.

However, a practical exception to this philosophy is the fact that veterinary care is not always immediately available. Furthermore, veterinary care is not always necessary in handling many conditions commonly encountered by the horseman, e.g., certain parasite infestations, superficial abrasions, general health conditioning and various other aspects of proper herd management. Thus, the horseman is often confronted with the need to purchase nonprescription (over-the-counter) drugs, chemicals and supplemental aids. Obviously, the purchase of such preparations should be conducted in a knowledgeable and comprehensive manner, in order to obtain the proper drug in an economical fashion. Once the drug has been purchased, administration by the proper route and dosage remain critically important considerations. Furthermore, those drugs prescribed and dispensed by the veterinarian for administration by the horseman represent an important management responsibility, since correct administration of the prescribed dosage becomes the horseman's responsibility.

For the various reasons outlined above, the following discussion summarizes some of the basic aspects that should be considered when over-the-counter drug preparations are purchased and, importantly, when drugs are administered to horses.

SPECIFIC DRUG THERAPY

When a medication is purchased, the buyer should first clearly understand the specific purpose for which the substance was intended; what the chemical will and will not do. For instance, antibiotics are not effective against viral infections, but, on the other hand, they are often useful in preventing secondary bacterial infection. Also, a vitamin/mineral supplement may be useful in maintaining a good health status in heavily worked animals, but most certainly will be of little, if any, benefit to an emaciated horse suffering from severe internal parasitism if the parasite load itself is not first removed. Thus, the specific indications and limitations of a drug should always be considered when a particular medicinal preparation is purchased. Specific aspects of the use and/or abuse of drugs in horses are discussed in the individual drug chapters of this book.

Only drugs that are specifically recommended for horses should be used. Topical medications, especially dips, must be intended for use on horses, since the emulsifiers and dispersing agents used in the formulation of the product will partially determine which species can be treated with the medication. In addition, whether an injectable is oil or water-based affects the route of administration.

DRUG MANUFACTURERS

The concentrations and formulations of basically similar drug preparations may be somewhat different depending upon the particular manufacturer. A neomycin solution from one drug company, for example, may not be exactly the same as that produced by another pharmaceutical firm. Concentrations of the active ingredients may vary, and completely different vehicles may be used. The product label should be examined to determine the actual ingredients and, importantly, their concentration. In this manner, valid comparisons can be made with other available products before buying.

Concentration particularly varies in such injectables as vitamin B complexes and antibacterial agents. What seems to be a less expensive injectable, on a bottle-to-bottle basis, may contain such a small concentration of the active drug that it is actually more economical to buy a higher priced preparation that contains a more highly concentrated drug.

For example, Product A is a 100 ml vial of a streptomycin preparation that costs $10.00, but it contains only 25 mg of streptomycin per ml of solution (i.e., a total of 2,500 mg). Product B is also a 100 ml vial of streptomycin from another drug company: it costs $20.00 but contains 100 mg of streptomycin per ml (i.e., a total of 10,000 mg). The actual cost of streptomycin in Product A is $1.00 per 250 mg. The actual cost of streptomycin in Product B is $1.00 per 500 mg. Obviously, the more economical preparation is Product B, even though the 100 ml vial of Product B costs more than the 100 ml vial of Product A.

Also, it is entirely possible that a new and less well-known company may offer a comparable product at a more economical price than does a well established drug firm. On the other hand, well established companies may have greater quality control and better reputations for a dependable product than do newly established manufacturers. All of these points should be evaluated by the horseman, particularly when selecting preparations from the highly competitive "over-the-counter" market where scores of liniments, hoof dressings, antiseptics, etc., are highly advertised in attempts to attract the horseman's attention.

CALCULATING DOSAGES

The specific dosage of a particular drug is dependent primarily upon the potency of the drug and, secondarily, upon the biological characteristics of each individual equine patient. For instance, it is unlikely that a 500 pound pony and a 1,000 pound horse would both need the same total quantity of medication for identical ailments. It is more likely that on a per pound of body weight basis, the same "weight of drug per pound of body weight" would apply to both animals. In the majority of commonly used drugs, this indeed has proven to be basically true.

The dose of most drugs, therefore, is usually expressed as a certain number of mg of the drug per pound (or mg per kg, 2.2 lbs) of body weight. For example, the dose of drug A may be 10 mg per lb (or 22 mg per kg) of body weight. Some drugs are expressed as "units" rather than weight, e.g., the dose of vitamin B may be 100 units per lb of body weight.

The above discussion initially may seem at odds with the common (but technically incorrect) practice of expressing "dose" as ml (cc's) of a drug per horse. This practice actually indicates what total volume of a particular drug solution has been calculated to be administered, but does not indicate the actual dose of the active drug ingredient. For example, an individual might state that the dose of tetracycline in a 400 kg (880 lb) horse is "10 cc's." However, tetracycline product A may contain 100 mg of tetracycline per ml of the drug solution; whereas, product B may contain 200 mg of tetracycline per ml of the drug solution. Thus, if a "10 cc dose" (or 10 ml dose) of tetracycline was used, a two-fold error could be made in the administered amount of tetracycline, depending on whether product A or B was used.

Rather, total dosage (and thus, volume of drug solution) is calculated according to the "mg of drug per kg of body weight" basis, as recommended by the drug manufacturer for each individual drug. For example, if the dose of tetracycline is set at 5 mg of tetracycline per kg of body weight (5 mg/kg), the volume of any drug solution to be administered to any horse can be calculated as follows:

EXAMPLE 1:

[a] **Manufacturer's Recommended Dose:** 5mg/kg
  Body Weight of Horse: 400 kg (880 lbs)
  Concentration of Drug in Solution: Product A = 100 mg/ml

[b] **Total mg of Drug per Horse:**
  = dose (in mg/kg) x body weight (in kg) = mg
  = 5mg/kg x 400 kg = **2,000 mg**

[c] **Total Volume of Drug Solution to be Given to the Horse:**
  = total mg ÷ drug concentration (in mg/ml) = ml
  = 2,000 mg ÷ 100 mg/ml = **20 ml**

EXAMPLE 2:

[a] **Manufacturer's Recommended Dose:** 5mg/kg
  Body Weight of Horse: 400 kg (880 lbs)
  Concentration of Drug in Solution: Product B = 200 mg/ml

[b] **Total mg of drug per Horse:**
  = dose (in mg/kg) x body weight (in kg) = mg
  = 5mg/kg x 400 kg = **2,000 mg**

[c] **Total Volume of Drug Solution to be Given to the Horse:**
  = total mg ÷ drug concentration (in mg/ml) = ml
  = 2,000 mg ÷ 200 mg/ml = **10 ml**

From the above examples, it can be seen that "10 cc's" (ml) does, indeed, represent the proper "amount" (not dose) of this drug that should be given to the 400 kg horse, if product B is used. However, if a 10 ml "dose" of product A was used, then only 50% of the correct dosage would be administered to the horse. Obviously, therefore, dosage of a drug in mg/kg remains constant, whereas, the total volume of drug solution to be given to any individual horse depends upon body weight of the horse and the concentration of the drug in any particular drug preparation.

Dosage recommendations for individual horses may vary somewhat depending upon the health status, age, temperament, lean-fat ratio of the body, etc.; however, it should be remembered that, with some exceptions, drug doses are generally expressed as "a weight unit of the drug per weight unit of the horse" (e.g., mg/kg, mg/lb, mg/100 lbs, etc.). Exceptions to this rule include: inhalant anesthetics and gases which are administered as a percentage of inhaled air, and relatively inactive compounds like kaolin-pectin and mineral oil which are commonly given as "ounces or quarts per horse."

DRUG RECORDS

Accurate and adequate records of the administration of any drug should be carefully maintained since this information may be useful in later treatment of the horse (refer to "Importance of Good Health Records"). Drugs should not be mixed without the knowledge and approval of a veterinarian, since some drugs given together act quite differently than when administered separately. A medication should not be used for a purpose different than that for which it was originally intended. An injection of a drug will not automatically cure the horse of an illness, and may even harm the animal, unless that specific drug is required in the treatment of that particular ailment. Therefore, for example, a horse with a nasal discharge may not be benefited by the same antibiotic preparation the veterinarian prescribed for another horse with a respiratory disease.

CARE OF DRUGS

Drugs should be properly maintained in the stable pharmacy since they often lose their effectiveness if not stored according to package directions. It is a waste of time and money to administer a drug if it has not been stored correctly, and an improperly stored drug may actually be harmful to the horse.

Drugs are an invaluable aid in the treatment of many of the ailments affecting horses if properly prescribed and administered. It is the horseman's responsibility to ensure that any drug he gives to his horse is appropriate for the horse's condition, is the correct dosage, and is administered in the proper manner.

19

SKIN AND MUCOUS MEMBRANE PREPARATIONS

Treatment of abnormal skin conditions of horses represents an important therapeutic consideration for at least two major reasons. First, dermal (skin) problems are very common in horses and, second, simple treatable skin problems of horses can easily develop into serious, complicated and sometimes debilitating disorders if not promptly identified and properly treated.

Several kinds of drug preparations are employed for their local action upon the skin and mucous membranes. If such preparations are applied with reasonable care, their medicinal effects are usually relatively simple and localized to the site of application. However, problems can occur. For example, "overdosage" of a moderately irritating drug can occur if the skin is bandaged improperly tight for too long a period. This can cause overintensification of the irritant effect. Necrosis and sloughing of the skin can occur, resulting in an unattractive scar and perhaps in limited movement of the affected part of the limb. Also, local application of a drug in powder form usually has a very limited and superficial site of action. However, the same drug incorporated in a penetrating ointment could have a penetrating action and could even be absorbed into the bloodstream, resulting in systemic toxicity.

Although these examples represent extreme cases, they nevertheless have been encountered. Moreover, they explain why even relatively simple problems such as skin disorders require prompt attention and, in many cases, treatment by a veterinarian.

Specific Preparations

Drugs that are used for their local effect on skin and mucous membranes can be placed into several different catagories depending upon the response of the target tissues to the drugs, as follows:

EMOLLIENTS

These agents are used to soften, soothe, lubricate and protect damaged

444

skin surfaces. Bland ointments serve as protective emollients. However, active drugs can be incorporated into ointments for specific therapeutic purposes. Emollients include natural and synthetic fatty substances, vegetable and hydrocarbon oils and waxes.

Cod-liver oil is a fish oil rich in vitamins A and D that is sometimes used as a base for eye medications and soothing ointments. The vegetable oils include cottonseed oil, corn oil, theobroma (cocoa butter), olive oil and linseed oil. These plant-source oils are used externally as bases for preparing various liniments and ointments and have been used as protective agents for burns. If administered internally, the oils are usually laxative and purgative (for example, castor oil and linseed oil). Natural oils, due to their rancidity problems, are being replaced in modern medicine to a large extent by synthetic agents.

Lard and lanolin are animal-source fats sometimes used as ointment bases and emulsifiers. Lanolin is used more commonly and can absorb over 50% of its weight in water. Although lanolin has the disadvantage of occasionally causing allergic reactions, it does assist in drug penetration to the skin.

The hydrocarbon derivatives are important emollients and the most representative of this class is soft paraffin (white petrolatum, petroleum jelly, Vaseline) and mineral oil (liquid petrolatum). Mineral oil is used as a liniment base and, when administered internally, as a stool softener. Soft paraffin is frequently used on burns and abrasions. Paraffins retard the evaporation of body moisture from skin surfaces, and also prevent air and water from reaching damaged tissues. The ability to retard fluid loss is an important part of burn therapy. (Refer to "Burns" under "Trauma.")

Waxes are used as ointment bases. They can be obtained from natural sources such as beeswax or from synthetic sources such as emulsified wax. Collodions are solutions of nitrated cellulose in a mixture of alcohol and ether. When applied on the skin, the alcohol and ether evaporate, leaving a protective covering similar in appearance to skin. This film is waterproof and can be used to protect small superficial, aseptic (clean) and dry wounds.

Glycerin, also called glycerol, is an oil derivative used on chapped dry areas as a wound dressing and as a base for rectal suppositories. Due to its high osmotic pressure, glycerin produces a localized inflow of tissue water (lymph). Lymph drawn into the wound area assists in cleansing the damaged tissue due both to a simple mechanical flushing action and to the influx of lymph-borne antibodies and those white blood cells that phagocytize (engulf and digest) foreign material.

DEMULCENTS

These compounds are used for softening and protecting raw and abraded surfaces, particularly for relief from inflammation and irritation of the mouth and gums. Acacia (gum arabic) is a dry gummy plant extract that readily dissolves in water to form a thick adhesive liquid (mucilage).

Glycerin can also be classified as a demulcent. Silicone and propylene glycol are synthetic compounds used as demulcents and the latter of the two agents is also used as a vehicle for drugs.

PROTECTIVES AND ADSORBENTS

Certain insoluble and finely ground powders can be applied locally as protective and adsorbent agents. By their simple mechanical action, they prevent friction and adsorb secretions such as sweat. Dusting powders, such as talc (magnesium silicate) and kaolin (aluminum silicate) are used externally in the treatment or prevention of skin abrasions. Kaolin, pectin, and bismuth salts are administered internally to soothe irritated mucosal linings of the digestive tract, thereby aiding in the treatment of diarrhea. Calamine and zinc stearate are referred to as "healing powders" for use on skin abrasions. Preparations of these substances dry the application area and adsorb secretions, thereby providing a favorable environment for body mechanisms to fight infections.

ANTISEBORRHEICS

Selenium sulfide suspension and cadmium preparations are used as shampoos in the treatment of the oily flaky skin condition of seborrheic dermatitis and dandruff.

ASTRINGENTS

These agents are used locally to precipitate and coagulate tissue proteins, thus assisting the healing process. Tannic acid, zinc sulfate, silver nitrate and ferric chloride are typical astringents. When applied to damaged tissue, the astringent coagulates proteins forming a protective scab, underneath which healing can take place. Also, slight and superficial bleeding, of a slow seepage type, can be stopped due to the astringent causing coagulation of blood proteins. This local hemostatic action is commonly referred to as a styptic effect. However, it should be remembered that if the styptic action simply covers up hemorrhage at the surface and bleeding continues underneath the scab, harm rather than good may result due to unnoticed blood clot (hematoma) formation within the tissue.

COUNTERIRRITANTS

These compounds are applied to the skin surface for the purpose of producing an acute localized irritation and inflammatory response over the region of an established long-term inflammation. The reasoning which prompts the intentional production of tissue inflammation is based on the theory that acute irritation of the skin will cause increased blood supply to both the newly inflamed area and also to immediately surrounding tissue. The increased blood supply concentrates white blood cells and antibodies, increases inflow of nutrients and improves removal of tissue wastes. Hopefully, the newly increased vascularity and its attendant effects will assist in curing the primary chronic ailment.

However, the proper use of counterirritation is not always a simple procedure, and considerable controversy exists concerning its actual direct benefits. For example, many knowledgeable people believe that the major benefits from counterirritation are actually due to resting the horse during the convalescent period. This rest period, and not the acute inflammation, is believed to be what actually assists the body in repairing the chronic problem.

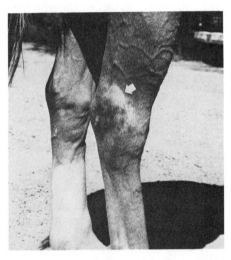

Fig. 19-1 Counterirritants can be used in the treatment of conditions such as thoroughpin [arrow].

In any case, counterirritation procedures and appropriate rest periods have proven helpful for certain conditions, and have been used in the treatment of tendonitis, curb, synovitis, ringbone, bog spavin, side bones, joint inflammation, and others. Some chemical counterirritants commonly used are iodine, ammonia, volatile oils (camphor, mustard, turpentine), cantharides and mercuric iodine.

The two therapeutically useful stages of counterirritation are rubefaction and vesication; the undesirable third stage is pustulation.

RUBEFACTION

A rubefacient action occurs when irritation is mild and only a slight increase in congestion (blood engorgement) occurs. The term itself refers to the characteristic redness of such a congested area. Common rubefacients are weak solution of iodine (2.5% iodine solution in alcohol) and strong solution of ammonia (33.3% solution of ammonia in water). A rubefacient response can be produced by application of one of the above substances in liniment form, accompanied by the friction of a massage. The use of liniments containing an essential (volatile) oil, a rubefacient, or both, should not be used on a working horse since edema and soreness can be associated with the inflammatory response. An antiphlogistic effect refers to a counterirritant effect.

"Tighteners" are rubefacient preparations used to reduce the edema of a tendon sheath or joint capsule. They are applied under cotton bandages and should not sore the skin. An example of this type of preparation could include tincture of belladonna, tannic acid, menthol, camphor and alcohol.

A "sweat" encourages the buildup of moisture on the skin's surface. These products usually contain alcohol and glycerin, and are applied to the horse's legs which are then wrapped with a moisture-proof bandage. Following exercise, a "brace" is often rubbed over the limbs, theoretically to prevent edema of the tendon sheaths and joint capsules. A brace usually contains alcohol as the basic ingredient; other ingredients may include thymol, menthol, ammonia, oil of wintergreen and turpentine. Most likely, the major benefits derived by the horse are due to the massage which it receives during application of the preparation, rather than from direct medicinal effects of preparation ingredients.

VESICATION

Vesication, the second stage of counterirritation, is achieved if the action of a counterirritant is concentrated and prolonged by bandaging the treated area. Vesication is characterized by severe irritation and inflammation, damage to capillaries and by the formation of blisters in superficial layers of the skin (thus, the term "blistering" is often used for this type of therapy). Cantharides and red iodide of mercury are two frequently used vesicants.

Several important conditions constitute contraindications for blistering. Blistering agents should never be used in cases of acute infection, acute inflammation or open wounds. Otherwise, a pronounced worsening of the condition is likely to result. Also, blistering should not be conducted on flexing surfaces of joints, on mucosal linings, in ill debilitated horses, or in horses that have recently been treated with corticosteroids. The area surrounding the surface to be blistered should be protected with an emollient such as Vaseline. The person who applies the blistering compound obviously should not expose his hands to the preparation.

It is quite likely that the beneficial results achieved from blistering occur, at least in part, because of the forced rest period required for the horse while the scurfing and sloughing skin associated with this therapy is allowed to heal. Blistering is a painful process and the horse may have to be tranquilized and restrained to prevent self mutilation of the treated area. The beneficial results and recuperative powers of an adequate rest period should always be considered and tried first, before the complicated and painful procedure of blistering is selected.

PUSTULATION

Pustulation, the third and undesirable stage of counterirritation, is characterized by damage to deep layers of the skin, joint and tendon injury, and permanent scars or blemishes. Pustulation can inadvertently occur if vesication is excessively prolonged, or when too strong a blistering agent is used. It is obvious that counterirritation should never be employed in such a manner that it causes irritation beyond a stage of moderate blistering.

In fact, blistering (and probably even milder forms of counterirritation) should always be administered by or under the supervision of a veterinarian. This is because of the fine line between careful induction of controlled vesication and the disastrous complications of inadvertent pustulation.

CAUSTICS AND ESCHAROTICS

Caustic agents cause destruction of tissues at the application site. If the compound also coagulates cell proteins resulting in formation of a scab that later organizes into a scar, the compound is referred to as an escharotic. Such chemicals are sometimes externally applied to proud flesh in an attempt to remove and prevent regrowth of granulation tissue. Granulation tissue should always be diagnosed and treated by a veterinarian because it is often difficult to distinguish granulation tissue from primary cancers, and granulation tissue can proliferate and spread to adjacent tissue quite rapidly.

Copper sulfate, or bluestone, is one of the most often used caustic chemicals. It is applied to the surface of the granulation tissue which is then bandaged. After the bandages are removed, the outer layers of tissue are sloughed and healing will, hopefully, take place. However, unless this procedure is supervised by a knowledgeable person, granulation can recur to an even greater extent. Silver nitrate and a paste made from sulfur and sulfuric acid are other caustic agents. Extreme care should always be exercised when caustic chemicals are used, since improper use can result in damage to the horse, to the person applying the medication, and even to inanimate objects (leather, plastic, etc.) that may come in contact with the chemical.

The use of caustics in the treatment of granulation tissue is considered in the section on "Cleansing and Treating Wounds."

KERATOLYTIC AGENTS

These compounds are often referred to as "desquamating" agents since they provoke a sloughing of the epidermis (squamous cells) of the skin. Salicylic acid is often used as a keratolytic agent to remove warts, and also to make less superficial layers of the skin more accessible to active medicines (for example, in the treatment of skin fungal infections).

LOCALLY ACTING ENZYMES

Enzymes are substances of biological origin that assist in the breakdown and, in some cases, the liquifaction of tissue proteins. Some locally active enzymes are used to facilitate the spread of an injectable drug. Hyaluronidase, for example, is used principally to increase the diffusion and absorption of injectable fluids and drugs, and also for the breakdown and absorption of blood clots and exudates. Streptokinase and streptodornase are enzymes derived from hemolytic streptococcal bacteria. They are often used together to assist in the breakdown and removal of clotted blood and accumulations of pus. Trypsin and chymotrypsins are proteolytic enzymes extracted from the pancreas of cattle. These preparations are often used alone and in combination for enzymatic debridement (tissue removal) of infected surface areas and open abscesses, and for the purpose of breaking down clotted blood, purulent exudate and necrotic tissue.

Enzymes should not be applied to cancerous areas or used in acute infectious conditions because of the danger of spreading the malignancy or infection.

Other Topical Drugs

A wide variety of drugs are applied to the skin surface for specific medicinal purposes. For example, there are many antibacterial, insecticidal, antifungal, and antihistamine drugs that are incorporated into ointments or other topical preparations for use in treating particular skin conditions. However, to avoid repetition, those drugs will be considered in their respective primary categories. ♞

20

GASTROINTESTINAL DRUGS

Digestive processes in horses can be influenced by many different types of drugs that act through mechanisms ranging from mild stimulation of the appetite to harsh and forceful emptying of the intestines and cecum. Drugs acting on the digestive system (gastrointestinal tract) can be subdivided into the following:

1. digestive aids
2. purgatives and laxatives
3. drugs that directly affect the motility and secretions of the gastrointestinal tract (autonomic drugs)
4. antidiarrhea agents

Digestive Aids

Drugs used for assisting the digestion of feedstuffs have been used for many years. However, their actual benefits are still questionable. For example, "bitters" are a group of bitter tasting drugs (usually of plant origin) that were commonly used in the past as appetite stimulants in both human and veterinary medicine. Their use by physicians is now obsolete, and they are infrequently used in animals. Occasionally, however, drenches and powders containing bitters are employed in attempts to stimulate and improve digestion in convalescent horses. Nux Vomica powder (2-5 grams) and gentian (10-30 grams) have been used as bitters. These types of drugs must be applied orally in powder or liquid form since they are believed to exert their effects by direct contact with the taste buds.

CARMINATIVES

Carminatives are defined as those drugs that, when administered orally, promote the expulsion of fermentative gases from the stomach (eructation) and intestines (flatulence). They have been used to expel gases from the digestive tract in attempts to relieve pain resulting from flatulent colic. In horses, capsicum (red pepper) and powdered root of ginger have been used for carminative effects, as has oil of turpentine (30-60 ml). It should be mentioned though, that a true carminative effect from these or other drugs has never been clearly established.

ANTACIDS

On the other hand, the direct therapeutic benefits of antacids (anti-acids) have been established for a number of years. In humans, antacids are used to neutralize the excess gastric acidity associated with "nervous indigestion" or emotional disturbances. There is little evidence that gastric hyperacidity is a practical problem in horses; however, antacids are sometimes used as protectives to coat the irritated mucous membranes of the stomach and small intestines in animals suffering from gastroenteritis. Calcium carbonate, magnesium oxide, magnesium carbonate and aluminum hydroxide are commonly used antacids.

Purgatives and Laxatives

Purgatives (or cathartics) are defined as those drugs that cause a pronounced intensification of intestinal movements (peristalsis) and, thereby, cause the expulsion of the contents of the intestines. Laxatives produce similar results but their action is milder and less stimulating than that of cathartics. In the past, purgation was a routine supportive treatment for the management of virtually any systemic illness regardless of whether or not the digestive system was involved. Fortunately, this is no longer true and purgatives are now recognized for use only in specific disorders.

In horses, purgatives are used in treating simple impactions of the intestinal tract, nonobstructive constipation and certain types of colic. Laxatives, but not purgatives, are sometimes given to mares to prevent straining during defecation in pregnancy and after surgical repair of rectal or vaginal prolapse. Purgatives should never be used indiscriminately, particularly in severely ill horses, since superpurgation may result, leading to loss of body fluids, dehydration, shock and even death. Purgatives should not be used in pregnant mares because of the danger of producing abortion, and diarrhea may occur in nursing foals if purgatives are used in the dam. Also, and importantly, superpurgation could result in rupture of the intestine if severe impaction or strangulation of the gut exists.

Purgative drugs can be classified into 4 major groups, depending upon their mechanism of action:

1. irritant cathartics
2. intestinal lubricants (also referred to as mechanical stimulants)
3. bulk purgatives
4. drugs that directly activate the smooth muscle of the intestinal walls

Irritant cathartics act by irritating the mucosal lining of the lower intestinal tract and, thereby, cause increased peristaltic movements of the gut wall. Intestinal lubricants coat the mucosal surfaces of the digestive system and ease the passage of ingesta through the tract. Bulk purgatives act by causing an increased influx of bodily fluid into the digestive tract and its contents; the resulting increased fluidity of the ingesta and swelling of the intestines cause increased peristaltic movements and thereby aid the rearward movement of fecal material.

IRRITANT CATHARTICS

These agents include both the mildly irritating vegetable oils (such as olive oil) and the exceptionally active "emodin-type" purgatives. An effective emodin cathartic that has been used in the past, and usually does not produce signs of colic, is cascara sagrada. The usual dosage in mature horses is 10 ml of a 0.2 grams per ml solution, and 6-8 hours is generally required for the effect. Aloe and senna are other types of emodin cathartics; they are now infrequently used in horses due to their tendency to cause signs of colic, superpurgation, enteritis, abortion and, in some cases, kidney damage.

Vegetable oils are the safest of the irritant purgatives. Their laxative action is the result of saponification (soap formation) of the oil within the intestinal lumen. The soap-like substances that result are mildly irritating to the gut lining (as with olive oil) or severely irritating (as with castor and linseed oils). Another product of saponification is glycerin, which coats the feces and promotes defecation by a lubricating effect. Results of administering vegetable oils in horses are usually produced within 12-18 hours. Dosage of castor oil in adult horses is usually from 250-1,000 ml, and 50-100 ml is used in foals.

INTESTINAL LUBRICANTS

These drugs, the mechanical stimulants, are the mildest purgatives and produce only a laxative effect even in large dosages. They are oils and act by softening and lubricating the intestinal contents. Acute and simple constipation, rectal or vaginal prolapse, and colic are indications for the use of lubricants. However, they can delay healing of repaired rectovaginal fistulas and slow absorption of nutrients (carbohydrates, vitamins, fats, and proteins) from the gut. Also, lubricant oils should not be repeatedly used in cases of chronic constipation since the soothing effect of the oil may further decrease intestinal activity.

Mineral oil is the most commonly used intestinal lubricant. It is bland, odorless and indigestible, and is administered by stomach tube in volumes of 250-1,000 ml. Other oils, such as linseed, cottonseed and corn oils can be used; however, they are more expensive than mineral oil and are more irritating. Boiled linseed oil or other industrial preparations of this product should, of course, never be used, due to their poisonous effects.

BULK PURGATIVES

These compounds produce catharsis by increasing the volume of the ingesta resulting in stimulation of peristaltic movements. Such drugs produce their effects either by absorption of water (causing swelling to many times their original size) or by causing an influx of body water into the gut contents through an osmotic effect. Wheat bran mash is an example of a bulk purgative that absorbs water. This laxative is particularly useful in older horses that have a tendency to become constipated, and is also fed to mares in the late stages of pregnancy. Bran also contains a large amount of fiber that acts as needed bulk in the horse's diet.

Magnesium sulfate (also called epsom salts) is an osmotic bulk laxative as are magnesium hydroxide (milk of magnesia), magnesium carbonate and solution of magnesium citrate. The dose of magnesium sulfate is 250-1,000 grams in mature horses and 24-50 grams in foals. Since saline cathartics act by causing the movement of body fluids into the intestinal contents, they should not be used in severely dehydrated horses, as worsening of the animal's condition could result.

Autonomic Drugs

The normal digestive functions of the stomach and intestines are controlled by that part of the body's nervous system called the Autonomic Nervous System. This system is also referred to as the "involuntary nervous system" since it regulates those bodily functions that are not under voluntary control (for example, heart rate, blood pressure, blood flow and, of course, digestion of foodstuffs).

There are two major subdivisions of the autonomic nervous system, the sympathetic and the parasympathetic nervous systems. The stomach, intestines, heart, kidneys and other visceral organs are innervated (that is, they receive nerves) from both the sympathetic and parasympathetic nervous systems. However, each system produces opposite effects on the same organ and, thereby, regulates organ functions in a "push-pull" manner, consistent with body needs at any given moment. Gastrointestinal activity is primarily regulated by parasympathetic nerves.

The parasympathetic nerves regulate the stomach, intestines, and their glands through the release of a chemical from the nerve endings. This chemical is called acetylcholine and, after its release from the nerve endings, it directly stimulates the smooth muscle and secretory glands of the stomach and intestines. The net result is increased peristaltic movements and increased fluidity of the feces. After acetylcholine acts upon its target organs, it is inactivated (metabolized) by those enzymes called the cholinesterase enzymes. These enzymes are important not only because they limit the duration of action of acetylcholine, but also because many drugs (for example, certain cathartics, dewormers and insecticides) inhibit the enzymes and, thereby, prolong and intensify the action of acetylcholine.

Drugs that mimic acetylcholine and act as gastrointestinal stimulants are referred to as "cholinergic" drugs; they are used for their cathartic effects. Conversely, "anticholinergic" drugs block the action of acetylcholine and, thereby, produce an antiperistaltic or "antispasmodic" effect; they are used in the treatment of diarrhea.

STIMULANTS (CHOLINERGIC AGENTS)

Arecoline is a plant source (betel nut) drug that produces a pronounced "cholinergic" effect. That is, it increases peristaltic contractions of the gut, increases gastric and intestinal secretions and, through these effects, produces a pronounced and harsh purgative response. In the past, arecoline has been administered subcutaneously in doses of 40-60 mg to produce a rapid evacuation of the intestinal tract of horses. This nonconservative procedure is now infrequently practiced due to the severity of the reaction and the signs of colic it produces.

Carbachol is a chemically synthesized cholinergic drug used for its purgative effects; it also produces profuse salivation and sweating. In horses, carbachol has been used to treat colic produced by intestinal atony (loss of tone) and simple impaction of the colon and cecum. In these conditions, 1-2 mg doses of carbachol administered subcutaneously every 1-2 hours have been used. However, intestinal lubricants, saline cathartics or other stool softeners should first be administered in order to ease the passage of the fecal material.

Physostigmine is a cholinergic agent used occasionally in horses for its cathartic action. This drug produces its effects by inhibiting the cholinesterase enzymes; that is, physostigmine is a "cholinesterase inhibitor." Therefore, after administration of physostigmine, the acetylcholine released from nerves is not rapidly inactivated (as occurs normally), but actually accumulates in body tissues. The net result is an intensification and prolongation of the action of acetylcholine. Peristaltic movements and intestinal secretions are markedly accentuated; purgation occurs within a relatively short period of time.

Several precautions should always be heeded when physostigmine or any other potent cholinergic-gastrointestinal stimulant is used in horses. First, it should be remembered that acetylcholine (and, therefore, cholinergic drugs) acts upon body organs other than just the digestive system. Therefore, cholinergic drugs used in the treatment of gastrointestinal disorders can cause adverse side effects such as abortion, respiratory distress, bradycardia (slowing of the heart rate), lowered blood pressure, uncontrolled urination, skeletal muscle weakness, and others. Inadvertent overdosage of cholinergic drugs can lead to dysentery, dehydration, prostration and even intestinal rupture and death. In addition, responses to usual dosages of cholinergic drugs can be greatly potentiated if the horse has recently been treated with those dewormers or insecticides that act as cholinesterase inhibitors, such as organophosphates. (Atropine is the primary antidote to cholinergic drugs.) Due to these serious limitations, only use cholinergic drugs under the supervision of a veterinarian.

ANTISPASMODICS (ANTICHOLINERGIC DRUGS)

These drugs block the effects of acetylcholine (and other cholinergic agents) and, thereby, produce relaxation of the smooth muscle of the stomach and intestinal walls and also decrease secretion by gastrointestinal glands. The net effect is a relaxed and quiescent digestive system. Such effects are useful in treating diarrhea, and antispasmodic drugs are routinely used to decrease intestinal spasms occurring from diarrhea and scours. Atropine is a representative antispasmodic; however, intestinal protectants such as kaolin and pectin should also be administered to soothe and coat the intestinal lining. Also, atropine is the primary antidote for cholinergic drug overdosage and poisoning by cholinesterase inhibitors. However, in horses, atropine has on some occasions slowed gastrointestinal activity to such an extent that constipation resulted. Atropine should be used only by the veterinarian.

Antidiarrhea Agents

Diarrhea in horses can sometimes be a relatively simple and temporary problem or, conversely, it can be an extremely serious and even debilitating condition, particularly in young foals. Loose stools are often the result of changes in the diet, and effective treatment includes evaluation of the ration for suspect ingredients such as moldy hay or grain. Horses may develop diarrhea when first placed on a green pasture. This can be prevented by gradually introducing a horse into lush pasture. Foals can scour from drinking too much milk, and milk intake may have to be reduced in addition to treatment with drugs. However, water intake should not be restricted during episodes of diarrhea because water deprivation can worsen the dehydration associated with severe diarrhea.

Severe and complicated diarrhea can be caused by a variety of factors such as bacterial infection of the intestines, insecticide overdosage, internal parasites and ingestion of irritating substances. Therefore, a diagnosis should always be made since diarrhea can recur after supportive therapy is stopped if the primary cause (etiologic agent) of the condition is not corrected with appropriate therapy. In any case, diarrhea should be promptly treated to prevent the development of dehydration and subsequent progression to shock.

Most of the drug products used to treat diarrhea are chemically inert (inactive) and act by coating and protecting the lining of the gut. Kaolin (aluminum silicate) and pectin are such products and when administered together as kaolin-pectin, 2 to 6 ounces 2 to 3 times daily, will usually control simple diarrhea in foals. The carbonate, salicylate and subnitrate salts of bismuth are also used for treating diarrhea, sometimes given in conjunction with small amounts of mineral oil. Adult horses are usually given 15 to 30 grams (one-half to 1 ounce) of bismuth subnitrate; foals are given 2 to 4 grams. Administration is by drench or stomach tube.

Antispasmodics are drugs that prevent excessive peristaltic movements of the intestines; they are frequently used for treating diarrhea and are discussed in the preceeding section.

FIG. 20-1 TABLE 1
DRUGS DIRECTLY AFFECTING THE MOTILITY
OF THE GASTROINTESTINAL TRACT

Drug	Effects	Clinical Use in G-I Problems
Epinephrine(Adrenaline) Norepinephrine (Noradrenaline)	Inhibits Peristalsis	None
Cholinergic Agents Carbachol Pilocarpine Bethanechol	Stimulates Peristalsis	Increase gut motility
Cholinesterase Inhibitors (Cholinergic Effects) Physostigmine Neostigmine	Stimulates Peristalsis	Increase gut motility
Anticholinergic Agents (Antispasmodics) Atropine Scopolamine Propantheline	Inhibits Peristalsis	Decrease gut motility

FIG. 20-2   TABLE 2
TYPES OF CATHARTIC DRUGS

Drug Group	Examples	Site of Action
Irritant	Castor Oil Aloe Cascara Sagrada	Small Intestine Colon Colon
Emollient	Liquid Petrolatum Linseed Oil-Raw	Entire G-I tract
Saline Bulk	Magnesium Sulfate Magnesium Citrate Sodium Sulfate	Small Intestine
Hydrophilic Bulk	Bran Psyllium Methylcellulose	Colon and Small Intestine
Surface Acting Agents	Dioctyl Sodium Sulfosuccinate (DSS)	Colon

21

ANTI-INFECTIOUS
CHEMOTHERAPY

This section pertains to a large number of different types of drugs that are used not to affect normal bodily functions of the horse, but instead, to selectively destroy invading disease-producing organisms such as bacteria and fungi. Therefore, anti-infectious chemotherapy can be defined as the treatment of infectious diseases by the selective use of specific pure chemicals (drugs) that have toxic effects on the infective organism but, hopefully, produce no ill effects in the patient. However, as with all drugs, anti-infectious compounds can produce adverse side effects, especially if they are administered without caution. Nevertheless, these drugs represent some of the most therapeutically useful compounds ever discovered and, in the treatment of many disease conditions, have proven to be truly lifesaving.

This chapter is divided into disinfectants and antiseptics, antibacterial chemotherapy, and antifungal agents. Anthelmintics (dewormers) and insecticides are covered in other chapters (refer to "Control of Internal Parasites" and "Control of External Parasites").

Definitions

Before considering the different drugs, a group of basic definitions is given in order to facilitate discussion of anti-infectious drugs.

Disinfectant: A chemical used to destroy microorganisms present on inanimate objects.

Antiseptic: A chemical applied topically to destroy or prevent growth or reproduction of microorganisms on living tissue.

Sanitization: To effectively reduce the number of microorganisms, especially pathogenic (disease causing) microorganisms.

Sterilization: To completely destroy all microorganisms.

Antimicrobial agent: A drug that destroys or suppresses the growth or reproduction of microbes (microorganisms).

Antibacterial agent: An antimicrobial drug that specifically affects bacteria.

Antibiotic: A substance produced by microorganisms that is toxic to other microorganisms; some antibiotics can now be chemically synthesized.

Bactericidal: Refers to killing of bacteria.

Bacteriostatic: Refers to suppression of the growth or reproduction of bacteria.

Antifungal or Antimycotic agent: An antimicrobial agent that specifically affects fungi.

Antibacterial spectrum: Refers to the "spectrum" or range of different types of bacteria that a drug will destroy. A "narrow spectrum" antibiotic is toxic to only one or a few types of bacteria; whereas, a "broad spectrum" antibiotic is toxic to several or many different bacterial species.

Anthelmintic: A drug used to kill internal parasitic worms or to aid in the removal of such worms (helminths) from the body.

Antiseptics and Disinfectants

These compounds are used most frequently by the horseman to reduce the number of microorganisms, especially pathogenic organisms, in the barn, stall, etc. and, thereby, maintain the horse in a more sanitary environment. The desired goal, of course, is to prevent disease and to decontaminate equipment exposed to diseased horses. Antiseptics are chemicals used topically to destroy or inhibit the reproduction of germs that may have, for example, contaminated a superficial skin abrasion. These agents are also used to sanitize the skin surface prior to surgery of the area. Disinfectants may be chemical or physical in nature, and actually kill the microbes with which they come into contact. Disinfectants as a rule are too toxic to be used on living tissue and are therefore used to kill bacteria on inanimate objects.

Bacteria and other infectious organisms (for example, fungi, worm eggs or worm larvae) can be physically destroyed by direct sunlight, extreme heat, electricity, steam, severe dehydration (desiccation), etc. An autoclave, for example, is used to sterilize surgical instruments by use of steam under high pressure.

The mechanisms whereby disinfectants kill bacteria include oxidation, protein coagulation and inhibition of reproduction. Effective chemical disinfection depends on the following:

1. a thorough cleansing with a good detergent
2. adherence to manufacturer's directions
3. temperature (disinfectants are more effective if applied after heating)
4. thorough application of the disinfectant
5. a lengthy exposure time to the disinfectant product

Heat is a reliable disinfectant, with moist heat more penetrating and, therefore, more effective than dry heat. Ten minutes of boiling in water, preferably repeated 2 or 3 times, will destroy most disease producing germs. Ultraviolet rays of sunlight are also disinfectant.

A usually effective disinfection procedure for a barn or stall includes the following:

1. Thorough sweeping of the inside of the building of all dust and cobwebs.
2. Disposal, such as burning, of all manure and refuse.
3. If the building has a dirt floor, remove top 4 inches of soil, and replace with washed sand or clay and treat with chloride and lime.
4. Remove manure from all barn surfaces.
5. Spray the disinfectant, under pressure, onto all surfaces, especially feed troughs, crevices and gutters; allow adequate exposure time.

Obviously, several precautions must be considered before the preceding procedures are followed. The horses should first be removed prior to spraying the disinfectant. The person spraying the disinfectant should be careful to avoid contamination of his skin, eyes or mouth with the chemical. Importantly, although the disinfectant needs to be in direct contact with feed troughs, buckets, etc. for a lengthy interval, all such feeding and watering utensils should be thoroughly washed before they are used again. Otherwise, trace amounts of the disinfectant could contaminate feed and water, resulting in toxicity to the horse.

A list of some of the most commonly used antiseptics and disinfectants follows.

ANTISEPTICS

Alcohol: Either ethyl or isopropyl alcohol is an antiseptic; methyl alcohol is a poison when ingested and should not be used; alcohol is usually quite effective in a 70% solution. At least 30 minutes exposure time is necessary.

Boric acid: Weak acid and antiseptic that has some anti-bacterial action and is non-irritating to tissues; may be applied to the cornea, on eczema and on moist wounds; use a 2% solution and keep refrigerated.

Coal tar: Antiseptic used in the treatment of skin ailments such as eczema, seborrhea, and ringworm; should be diluted with twenty parts of oil and is too harsh for use on open wounds.

Creosote: A 1.0-1.5% solution is sometimes used topically in minor wound ointments.

Hexachlorophene: Antiseptic with slow antibacterial action that is active against various microorganisms; often used as a surgical scrub on both the operative site and the surgeon's hands.

Hydrogen peroxide: Mildly germicidal antiseptic that mechanically removes purulent and cellular debris from wounds with its effervescent release of oxygen.

Iodoform: Antiseptic and deodorant used in the treatment of seborrhea; mixed with zinc oxide, talc, or kaolin at the rate of 1 part iodoform to 4 or 8 parts inert carrier.

Lugol's iodine: A 5% solution of iodine used in the therapy of skin diseases caused by bacteria, fungi, or parasites; also can be used to prepare the skin before an injection is made; when applied to open wounds may delay healing. Iodine is also frequently used to treat thrush, canker and puncture wounds of the foot.

Pine tar oil: An antiseptic often used in hoof conditioners, it helps prevent hoof wall cracking; it is also used to treat skin diseases and as an insect repellent.

Potassium permanganate: An antiseptic and deodorant; used in a 1:1000 solution to rinse wounds and mouth injuries.

Scarlet red: Antiseptic that stimulates the growth of granulation tissue in open wounds; 4% ointment applied every 48 hours; can cause tissue necrosis and irritation; can augment the growth of proud flesh.

DISINFECTANTS

Carbolic acid: A disinfectant which is the standard of comparison for all others; used as an antiseptic in infected regions in a solution of less than 2%; 5% solution used for disinfection of contaminated buildings; expensive, highly toxic, has a strong odor.

Chlorine: Used as a disinfectant at the rate of 800 parts per million; irritating and promotes excessive granulation tissue if applied to open wounds.

Cresol: A 2% solution in warm water used to disinfect stalls, dirt floors, etc; when saponated (combined with soap) and applied to the horse for five minutes, can help control some skin diseases and lice.

Formalin: A formaldehyde solution used topically on the frog of the foot.

Lye: Also known as soda lye and sodium hydroxide; a disinfectant that can kill viruses and bacteria; use 2% solution made with hot water (1 lb lye to 15.5 gallons), add 2.5 pounds water-slaked lime. Lye is a caustic poison.

Lime: Also known as calcium oxide or quicklime; disinfectant used as a soil sterilant; slaked lime means mixed with water.

Lysol (Lehn and Fink): Commercially available solution of cresol and soap.

Antibacterial Chemotherapy

The use of drugs to treat systemic bacterial infections has been possible only for a relatively short time. Prior to the 1940's, chemicals that were known to kill bacteria were either antiseptics or disinfectants, and they were much too toxic to be administered systemically to man or his animals. Bacterial infections that can now be effectively cured with appropriate antibiotic therapy (pneumonia, for example), quite often terminated in death. The discovery of systemic antibacterial drugs, therefore, represents one of the most important advancements ever made in medical science.

Important advantages of many antibiotic drugs are their selective toxicity for the invading bacterium and their tendency to be relatively nontoxic to the patient. However, the latter advantage is too often taken for granted, resulting in actual "abuse" of antibacterial drugs. Streptomycin, for example, is an antibiotic that is usually safe for the horse when administered in proper dosage and manner. However, if improperly administered in excessive amounts and/or for too long a period, streptomycin can cause several serious and potentially disastrous complications. These include permanent deafness due to damage of the auditory nerve, loss of equilibrium, kidney dysfunction, skeletal muscle and respiratory paralysis, and even depression of the heart. The point is not that streptomycin should not be used; rather, the major practical importance of this example to the horseman is that, although most antibiotics are relatively safe compounds, they can be misused and even produce harm to the horse if not carefully administered.

Many factors have been identified that can contribute and, in fact, are often essential to the successful cure of bacterial infections. These factors can be classified as patient, bacterial and drug factors.

PATIENT FACTORS

An essential aspect of antibacterial chemotherapy that must be remembered is that the use of drugs does not by itself cure the disease. The infection must eventually be overcome by inherent disease defense mechanisms of the horse's body. An antimicrobial agent acts to control the invading organisms, restricts their reproduction and spreading and, thereby, grants assistance and time to the body to dispose of the organisms. If the defense mechanisms of the horse are severely suppressed, the antibiotic will simply delay or temporarily depress the infection. This point is confirmed by the tragic occurrence of "immunoincompetency" that is occasionally seen in children. These infants lack the ability to develop natural immune responses to microbial organisms. Therefore, if they are not maintained in a completely sterile environment, they may eventually succumb and die from germs that may not even be pathogenic in normal children. Antibacterial agents have not been successful in curing these children.

Immunoincompetency occasionally occurs in Arabian foals; however, the practical aspect of immune mechanisms in relation to the present discussion is that any horse may not favorably respond to antibacterial therapy if natural body defenses are depressed. Body defenses include antibodies that inactivate bacteria, and white blood cells that envelope and digest (phagocytize) bacteria. (Antibodies are proteins produced by the body's immune system. Antibiotics are produced by microorganisms). Therefore, when drugs are used to treat infections, care should also be taken to insure that anemia, exhaustion, dehydration or other debilitating changes do not occur and, thereby, inhibit the ability of the body to manufacture and implement its own defense mechanism.

Another important patient factor pertains to the nature of the infectious condition. A large walled-off abscess, for example, is difficult to treat by drugs alone since they poorly penetrate the abscess walls. Thus, the abscess usually has to be surgically incised and drainage established. The presence of a foreign body (splinter, metal filing, etc.) complicates matters since it can act as a reservoir for the organisms where they cannot be reached by effective drug concentrations. Abscesses caused by foreign bodies almost invariably heal over, then drain, and repeat this cycle until the foreign material is surgically removed.

Also, it is often difficult to obtain effective concentrations within the uterus if a drug is administered by parenteral injection. Thus, medicine is sometimes deposited aseptically (in a sterile manner) within the uterine lumen by passage through the vagina and cervix.

MICROBIAL FACTORS

Bacteria can become resistant to a drug. That is, an organism that is initially susceptible to the drug can later develop (through changes in its own metabolic processes) a lack of sensitivity to the drug. Resistance can occur spontaneously but can also be produced. For example, a horse's condition may improve after 2 or 3 days of treatment although a small number of organisms may still exist. If treatment is prematurely stopped, this small colony of germs can reproduce and re-establish the infection. Often, the organisms that survived the initial therapy did so because they were individually more resistant to the drug. Thus, the new and re-established population may be completely resistant.

Resistance can be tested by determining the sensitivity of the bacteria to different antibacterial drugs. After a culture of the organisms is taken from the infection site and grown in a test tube, it can be exposed to various drugs. In this manner, a drug that has been shown in the test tube to be effective against the specific pathogen can be selected for use in the patient. Ideally, whenever possible, isolation, identification and sensitivity testing should be done prior to initiating drug therapy (treatment of the horse with a drug can complicate test tube testing). Depending upon the type and severity of infection, therapy with appropriate drugs can be started by the veterinarian until the results of sensitivity testing are known.

DRUG FACTORS

Depending upon its chemical structure, antibiotics are handled by the body in completely different manners. Tetracycline, for example, is quite effectively absorbed from the gastrointestinal tract, and can be administered orally to treat body infections. Penicillin, on the other hand, is broken down by digestive fluids. Streptomycin, kanamycin and gentamicin are poorly absorbed from the gut. Thus, these compounds are effective in treating systemic infections only when administered parenterally. There-fore, the selection of drugs for clinical use is dependent on a variety of drug factors including the reaction of the drug with blood and tissue fluids and physiologic barriers (blood-brain barrier, placental barrier, intestinal barrier, etc.).

Factors that can influence the storage stability of drugs include moisture, temperature, pH (acidity or alkalinity), oxidizing agents and light. If discoloration of a drug preparation occurs, it should be discarded due to a probable loss of potency (and perhaps development of greater toxicity).

More than one antibiotic (antibiotic combinations) are often given in the belief that if "one is good, two should be twice as good." It is true that in some cases two antibiotics are beneficial. Penicillin and streptomycin, for example, are often effective when given in combination. However, as illogical as it may seem, some antibiotics may actually antagonize one another. Usually, a bactericidal agent can be administered with another bactericidal drug, and two bacteriostatic drugs may be used together. However, if a bacteriostatic and a bactericidal drug are used simultane-ously, the effectiveness of both drugs can be reduced. It is much better to treat infections with a single drug known to be effective rather than to attempt a "shot-gun" approach which can sometimes do more harm than good. Various incompatabilities of several antibacterial drugs are given in an accompanying Table.

INDIVIDUAL DRUGS

Several of the more useful antibiotics and some common applications are summarized below (other useful antibiotics are listed in a Table). Manufacturer's recommendations and instructions from the veterinarian should be closely followed since certain preparations may not be specifically approved for use in horses.

Erythromycin: A stable antibiotic that is readily absorbed into the blood and diffuses well into tissues and fluids; it is used to treat organisms that are resistant to penicillin (mainly staphylococci). Intravenous injections for horses are 4-8 mg/kg of body weight every 12 hours.

Nitrofurazone: A broad-spectrum antibacterial used in treating infections due to Salmonella, and infections from wounds and burns, for which a cream containing 0.2% nitrofurazone concentration can be used.

Neomycin: A medium-spectrum antibiotic used to treat coliform enteritis (oral dose of 4-7.5 grams daily divided into two or four doses), and skin, eye, and ear infections (topical application of 5 mg neomycin sulfate per ml or per gram, in aqueous solution or ointment); too toxic for systemic administration.

Tetracycline: A broad-spectrum drug used to treat various skin and tissue infections (daily intramuscular dose of 2.2-4.4 mg/kg of body weight); 2 grams are often added to 250 cc saline solution for slow intra-venous injection.

Chlortetracycline: A broad-spectrum drug, used in foal septicemia, strangles, transit fever, and various other bacterial infections.

Streptomycin: A narrow-spectrum antibiotic used in treating leptospirosis infections, Corynebacterium equi infections (a cause of pneumonia in foals), and several other bacterial diseases. The usual parenteral dose for horses and foals is 5-10 mg/kg body weight every 3-4 hours; often given in conjunction with penicillin.

Penicillin: A narrow-spectrum antibiotic used to treat strangles (100,000 units penicillin/kg body weight daily for 5 days), joint ill, tetanus, navel ill, and leptospirosis (usually in conjunction with streptomycin).

Ampicillin: A broad-spectrum synthetic penicillin that is active against both gram-positive and gram-negative organisms. This antibiotic has few adverse properties, and is used in the treatment of respiratory, gastrointestinal, and urinary infections. Ampicillin is administered at the rate of 250 mg/100 lbs body weight. Other synthetic penicillins include hetacillin and carbenicillin.

Gentamicin: Related chemically to neomycin and streptomycin, administered intravenously or intramuscularly in the dose of 1-2 mg/kg for treatment of gram-negative bacterial septicemia and urinary infections.

Sulfonamides: Many sulfonamide compounds are available, for example, sulfamethazine, sulfanilamide, sulfaguanidine. They vary from narrow to relatively broad-spectrum depending on the individual compound. Some are absorbed rapidly from the digestive tract, while some are not absorbed from the gut. They are often useful in treating urinary tract infections and, when administered intravenously, in the treatment of strangles.

Kanamycin: An antibiotic chemically related to streptomycin and gentamicin, has been used for purposes similar to gentamicin.

Antifungal Drugs

Fungicides are drugs that destroy parasitic fungi, while fungistatic drugs inhibit the growth and reproduction of fungi. Collectively, these substances are also referred to as antimycotic or antifungal drugs.

There are two major classifications of fungal diseases; superficial infections involving the skin and its structures, and systemic mycosis affecting body organs. Drugs used to treat fungal infections can act either specifically or nonspecifically. Specific antifungal agents include antibiotics such as amphotericin B and griseofulvin. The usual antibiotics used in antibacterial therapy rarely have any antimycotic activity. Specific antifungal drugs can be used to treat both superficial and systemic mycosis. Nonspecific antifungal agents include various antiseptic compounds that are used only for topical application to dermal infections. Benzoic acid, for example, is the primary ingredient of Whitfield's ointment; it is occasionally used topically for ringworm and other dermatomycotic infections. Griseofulvin is administered orally. It is deposited in the new cells of the hair, skin and other dermal structures, thus preventing the fungi from invading the new tissue.

Some of the most commonly employed antimycotic preparations are listed below.

Amphotericin B: (Fungizone: Squibb) This antifungal antibiotic is effective against such conditions as blastomycosis and phycomycosis (Gulf Coast fungus). This drug is highly toxic, and can cause fever, anorexia, hematuria and proteinuria.

Griseofulvin: (Fulvicin, Fulcin: Schering) Used in treating ringworm, dosage 2.5 grams daily, orally, for 2 weeks or 15-20 mg/kg daily for 10-14 days; horses sometimes require treatment for four to six weeks.

Benzoic acid: Used most commonly in the treatment of ringworm; usually in the form of Whitfield's ointment or compound ointment of benzoic acid, containing 6% benzoic acid and 3% of salicylic acid; applied topically.

Copper sulfate: Also known as bluestone; applied topically in an ointment or paste of 5% concentration, or in an aqueous solution of 1-2% applied daily.

Gentian violet: 1% solution in alcohol used for mycotic skin infections; stains the skin.

Iodine: 1-7% tincture employed on ringworm and other fungal infections.

Kopertox (Ayerst): A commercially available preparation of copper napthenate; applied according to label directions in the treatment of ringworm.

Salicylic acid: 10-30% ointments or alcoholic solutions used in the treatment of ringworm; also found in 3% concentration in Whitfield's ointment.

Sulfur: When combined with lime, used as a dip for the control of ringworm and other fungal infections.

Captan: Solution of 1 ounce, 50% captan/1 gallon water; used topically to treat fungal skin infections, such as ringworm. Applied daily or every other day.

Pesticides

Anthelmintics and insecticides may be considered a part of anti-infectious chemotherapy because they are used to destroy invading, disease-producing parasites. Anthelmintics and deworming are covered in depth under "Control of Internal Parasites," while a complete discussion of insecticides and their application is found under "Control of External Parasites."

FIG. 21-1 TABLE 1
INCOMPATIBILITIES OF ANTIBIOTICS

Antibiotic	Incompatibilities
Tetracycline	Calcium salts
Oxytetracycline	Sodium bicarbonate
Chlortetracycline	Sulfonamides Polymyxin B Penicillin G Nitrofurans Erythromycin Chloramphenicol Cephalosporins Carbenicillin
Penicillin G	Tetracyclines Sodium bicarbonate
Lincomycin Kanamycin Gentamicin	Does not mix with other drugs Compatible with some IV solutions
Erythromycin	Carbenicillin Chloramphenicol Tetracyclines Iodides
Cephalothin	Does not mix with other drugs
Carbenicillin	Erythromycin Gentamicin Lincomycin Tetracyclines
Ampicillin	Does not mix with other drugs

22

NERVOUS SYSTEM DRUGS

General Aspects

The nervous system is by far the most highly organized of all the body systems and, in horses and other higher mammals, is estimated to be comprised of more than 10 billion cells. The central nervous system (CNS) is comprised of the brain and spinal cord. The brain, of course, is the site of consciousness and regulates both the voluntary reactions of a horse to its environment and the involuntary functions of its internal organs. The peripheral nervous system consists of motor and sensory nerves located outside of the CNS.

Due to the complexities involved in normal CNS function, it is not surprising that:

1. this system is exceptionally sensitive to the actions of many drugs
2. drugs are used to affect the CNS of horses only under specified circumstances where responses of the patient can be closely monitored by the veterinarian

THERAPEUTIC INDEX

Due to the extreme sensitivity of the CNS to drugs, a small therapeutic index is characteristic of many drugs that are used to affect CNS functions in horses. This means that the therapeutically useful dose often is only slightly smaller than the toxic dose. Compounding this danger is the significant degree of variability of horses to some CNS drugs. A therapeutic dose in one horse may actually represent a toxic dose in another, especially if normal bodily functions are already disrupted by disease.

EXAMPLES OF VARIABILITY

Probably the most well known example of variability of horses to CNS drugs involves the morphine-like narcotics. As their name implies, these drugs produce narcosis (a state of CNS depression resembling sleep) in several mammalian species, including man. In horses, however, narcotics

470

such as morphine can actually produce an apparent and sometimes pronounced state of CNS excitation. This depends on the particular drug, the dosage in which it is administered and the condition of the horse at the time of treatment (refer to "Narcotics").

The "tight-rope walking" that exists between the proper administration of a therapeutically useful CNS drug and the inadvertent production of toxicity with the same drug can further be demonstrated using general anesthetics as examples. Pentobarbital is an injectable anesthetic recommended to be administered intravenously. If pentobarbital is administered orally or subcutaneously to an agitated and excited horse, absorption may be too slow to obtain effective anesthetic-producing concentrations in the blood (and, subsequently, the brain). Instead of obtaining anesthesia or even sedation (as seen in man or the undisturbed horse), a highly excited, struggling and even uncontrollable animal is occasionally seen. This is due, apparently, to the fear and apprehension experienced by the already agitated animal as it senses a loss of voluntary control of its body. This type of reaction is not uncommon and also is often seen in horses as they recover from the effects of barbiturates and certain other anesthetic drugs.

Responses to CNS stimulants are also somewhat difficult to accurately predict and control. For example, a dose of amphetamine that is mildly stimulating to one horse may produce pronounced CNS activation in another. This could result, at best, in a hyperexcited and intractable horse or, at worst, in convulsions, self-inflicted wounds, and death. Although such examples are extreme, they serve to point out the variability in responsiveness of horses to certain CNS drugs.

CAUTIONS REGARDING DRUG USE

For the various critical reasons outlined above, it is emphatically advocated that the horseman not attempt the use of CNS stimulants or depressants unless instructed to do so by, and under the supervision of, a veterinarian. Veterinary CNS drugs are legally sold only to veterinarians, and their use is stringently regulated by federal government agencies. More important in relation to the well-being of the horse is the unequivocal fact that some CNS drugs can quickly kill if they are not administered in a carefully controlled manner. (The probability should also be noted that the use of drugs in attempts to artificially increase levels of performance in horses ultimately results in decreased physical ability.)

Therefore, the present section is particularly not intended to encourage the use of CNS drugs in horses by the horseowner, trainer, or handler. Instead, this section is intended to provide a brief overview of several drugs that may be administered or dispensed by the veterinarian to affect certain nervous system functions in horses.

This section is divided into central nervous system depressants, narcotics, central nervous system stimulants, local anesthetics, and muscle relaxants.

Depressants

The CNS of horses can be depressed to different degrees depending upon the potency of the individual drug and the dosage in which it is administered. Sedatives are those drugs that calm the horse and produce drowsiness by lowering perception and reaction of cerebral brain regions, but which do not necessarily prevent the animal from responding to environmental stimuli. Tranquilizers are drugs that produce a sedative, calming effect by depressing emotional centers of the brain without affecting consciousness. Hypnotics are those drugs that produce a state of CNS depression resembling sleep. Narcotics are usually defined as drugs that can produce a state of CNS depression characterized by deep sleep. However, it should be remembered that in horses, a state of CNS arousal often occurs after administration of narcotics. General anesthetics are drugs that produce a complete loss of consciousness and render the horse insensible to all sensations and pain. Analgesics, drugs that reduce pain, are well known to most people as "pain-killers."

From the preceding definitions, it is obvious that sedation, hypnosis, and anesthesia represent successive and progressively deeper stages of CNS depression. Moderate overdosage of a hypnotic can produce light anesthesia, whereas severe overdosage of an anesthetic (or other CNS depressant) can produce coma and death. All of the anesthetics, sedatives, and hypnotics intensify the effects of each other. Therefore, dosage is reduced if two or more CNS depressants are administered concurrently (e.g., acetylpromazine and a barbiturate).

CNS depressants are used in horses for the following reasons:

1. to produce general anesthesia in support of surgery
2. as a presurgical sedative to reduce stressful reactions to surgical preparation and induction of anesthesia
3. to provide chemical restraint of temperamental and fractious horses during teeth floating, shoeing, transportation, etc.
4. to provide relief from pain
5. to reduce cough
6. to relieve intestinal spasm

Obviously, all CNS depressants are not effective in providing all of these effects. Rather, certain compounds have been found to be useful only in producing certain of these responses in the horse.

GENERAL ANESTHETICS

INHALANT ANESTHETICS

General anesthesia can be produced by intravenous injection or by inhalation of the anesthetic preparation, depending upon the chemical nature of the particular drug. Examples of inhalant anesthetics include chloroform, ether, methoxyflurane, halothane, cyclopropane and nitrous oxide (laughing gas). Nitrous oxide and cyclopropane are gases, whereas the other anesthetics listed above are classified as volatile anesthetics. Volatile anesthetics are in liquid form, but they readily vaporize when bubbled with a gas such as oxygen. The resulting oxygen-anesthetic vapor mixture is inhaled by the animal through a face mask or, more commonly, through a tube placed in the trachea (windpipe). Prior to administration of an inhalant anesthetic, the horse is commonly administered a short-acting intravenous anesthetic in order to allow placement of the endotracheal tube in the windpipe.

INJECTABLE ANESTHETICS

Injectable anesthetics include various barbiturates, chloral hydrate and others. Hundreds of barbiturates have been synthesized; however, only a few have been used to any appreciable extent in equine medicine. The use of barbiturates is somewhat limited in horses due to the hyperexcitability that may be experienced by these animals in the early stages of anesthesia and also as they recover from the effects of barbiturates. In the past, it was even recommended that horses be hobbled before the recovery period to prevent self-injury. However, if the horse is first administered a tranquilizer, a smoother recovery period is usually seen. Barbiturates are now rarely given as the sole anesthetic agent in horses, but are given in conjunction with another general anesthetic, such as halothane.

Phenobarbital and Pentobarbital: Phenobarbital is a long-acting barbiturate used infrequently in horses, but occasionally used in other animal species and humans as a sedative or "sleeping pill." Pentobarbital is an intermediate-acting barbiturate that has been used in small doses for its sedative effects and, in large doses, as a general anesthetic. In horses, pentobarbital is usually administered in conjunction with chloral hydrate or other CNS depressants in order to obtain effective sedation without difficult recovery periods.

Thiopental and Thiamylal: Thiopental (Dipentol: Diamond) and thiamylal sodium (Surital: Parke, Davis) are ultrashort-acting barbiturates. They are used most often by intravenous injection to produce a brief period of anesthesia sufficient to allow passage of an endotracheal tube for administration of an inhalant anesthetic such as halothane. The barbiturates are poor analgesics unless general anesthesia is actually produced. Furthermore, considerable struggling and fighting nearly always occur as the horse recovers from barbiturate anesthesia, as mentioned previously.

Chloral hydrate: Chloral hydrate is one of the original CNS depressants used in equine medicine to produce sedation and relief from pain. It can be administered intravenously in a sterile solution for immediate effect or administered orally which produces CNS depression in 20 to 30 minutes. When a 7% solution is used, intravenous administration can be readily controlled. If some of the solution is accidentally injected outside of the vein, less tissue reaction will occur than if a more concentrated solution is employed. Chloral hydrate is very irritative to tissues, especially in the horse, and sloughing may occur if it is injected outside the vein. The dosage required for acceptable sedation depends on the temperament and physical condition of the horse; however, approximately 300 ml of a 7% chloral hydrate solution for a 1,000 lb horse is usually effective.

Chloral hydrate may cause marked inflammation of the upper alimentary tract (or respiratory tract if accidentally inhaled) if it is administered by drench. Furthermore, if gelatin capsules containing the drug break or dissolve in the pharynx or esophagus, severe pharyngitis and esophagitis may result. The degree of CNS depression occurring after oral administration of chloral hydrate is more variable than after intravenous injection. Another disadvantage of oral administration is that sedation occurs only after 20 or 30 minutes.

Chloral hydrate by itself is not a satisfactory general anesthetic in horses since the dosage required to produce general anesthesia is not too far removed from the lethal dose. In anesthetic doses, this drug severely depresses the respiratory and blood pressure control centers of the brain, and in smaller doses does not have pronounced pain-relieving power. Thus, chloral hydrate is infrequently used as a general anesthetic in horses but is occasionally employed for its hypnotic and sedative action, often as a preanesthetic agent to render the horse less fearful and more cooperative. To obtain such an effect, chloral hydrate has been used in combination with other CNS depressants. For example, chloral hydrate, magnesium sulfate and pentobarbital sodium have been used successfully as an intravenously administered sedative mixture in horses. Chloral hydrate has also been used in attempts to reduce pain resulting from colic.

SIDE EFFECTS

The major side effects of all the general anesthetics are cardiovascular and respiratory depression. If the horse is suffering from respiratory or cardiovascular disease, a usual anesthetic dose of a general anesthetic may further depress the already embarrassed circulatory and respiratory systems. In an attempt to avoid such problems, anesthetics are usually not given by bolus injection of a single precalculated dose. Instead, they are administered in a step-wise fashion, and the responsiveness of the individual horse is continuously monitored until adequate anesthesia is reached.

TRANQUILIZERS

Examples of tranquilizers include meprobamate (Equanil or Miltown), chlordiazepoxide (Librium) and diazepam (Valium). These three drugs are only occasionally used in horses or other animals but are extensively used in human medicine.

In horses, certain drugs that are chemically related to phenothiazine have been found to possess useful tranquilizing properties. Promazine (Sparine) and acetylpromazine (Acepromazine) are such drugs. Promazine and acetylpromazine have been used to provide chemical restraint for minor surgical or diagnostic procedures such as skin suturing, palpation, teeth floating, deworming, etc., especially in nervous, unstable animals. These tranquilizers have also been used to calm fractious horses prior to their transportation and, in some cases, to calm horses suffering from colic pains.

However, in some rare instances horses may experience hyperirritability and respond abnormally to phenothiazine-derivative tranquilizers. Chlorpromazine (Thorazine) in particular seems prone to produce undesirable responses in horses; some animals treated with the drug will fall back on their hocks and then suddenly lunge forward. Promazine is less prone to produce such effects. However, in some cases, horses treated with promazine may respond violently to sudden disturbances such as the rattle of bucket handles.

Acetylpromazine seems less likely to produce adverse reactions than does promazine or chlorpromazine, and acetylpromazine has proven to be an acceptable tranquilizing agent for various purposes in horses. In any case, the use of tranquilizers should be carefully monitored due to the potential for unusual and unexpected responses in the horse. Oral preparations are sometimes dispensed by the veterinarian for the horseman to administer. However, injections of tranquilizers should be done only by or under direction of the veterinarian.

Promazine can be administered intravenously, intramuscularly or orally. The intravenous dose in the horse is from 0.2 to 0.5 mg per lb of body weight; doses higher than the recommended amounts may cause the horse to go down. Accidental injection into the carotid artery (instead of the jugular vein) has been reported to occasionally produce death. The recommended intramuscular dose of promazine in the horse is 0.33 to 0.5 mg per lb. The oral preparation of promazine can be mixed with the feed for administration at the dose level of 0.75 to 1.25 mg per lb of body weight. The best dose should be determined for each horse, starting with the smaller amounts. The tranquilizing effect is usually seen within 3 to 5 minutes after intravenous administration, within 10 to 20 minutes after intramuscular injection and within 45 to 60 minutes after the oral route. The duration of the tranquilizing effect usually lasts for 2 to 4 hours after intramuscular or intravenous injection and up to 6 to 10 hours after oral administration.

The recommended dose of acetylpromazine in the horse is 2.0 to 4.0 mg per 100 lb of body weight, administered either intravenously or intramuscularly. At the present time, an oral preparation of acetylpromazine is not available. Propionylpromazine (Propiopromazine) is a potent phenothiazine derivative tranquilizer that has been withdrawn from the market in the United States because it occasionally produced permanent paralysis of the penis in stallions.

It has been found that phenothiazine derivative tranquilizers may potentiate the toxicity of organophosphate drugs and other cholinesterase inhibitors. Thus, phenothiazine tranquilizers should not be administered to horses recently exposed to such compounds.

Xylazine (Rompun) is an injectable tranquilizer-sedative used in horses to produce sedation and to increase ease of handling prior to minor surgical procedures. It is a rapidly acting, potent drug that can be administered intramuscularly at the dose of 1 mg per lb or intravenously at the dose of 0.5 mg per lb. Recovery of horses from the effects of this drug is usually quiet and smooth.

NARCOTICS

The narcotic drugs include those agents that are chemically and/or pharmacologically similar to opium and morphine. These include opium, morphine, codeine, methadone (Dolophine), heroin and meperidine (Demerol). Narcotics are usually classified as CNS depressants due to their sedative action in man. Nevertheless, they are included as a separate topic for two major reasons that have importance to the horseman. First, horses often respond atypically to narcotics when compared to the responsiveness of man and some other species. Secondly, it is quite likely that certain of these drugs periodically become illegally available for the purpose of "hopping" a horse prior to a physical performance. The horseman should be well aware of the danger to horse and handler involved in such types of drug abuse.

GENERAL ASPECTS

The response to morphine narcotics in several mammalian species is characterized by both an excitatory phase and a depressant phase. The depressant phase is seen in man, and in dogs the depressant phase dominates after a transient excitatory phase. In these species, narcotics produce the classical state of CNS depression resembling sleep (i.e., narcosis), and narcotics have been widely used as exceptionally potent pain-killers and sedatives.

In the horse, however, the excitatory response often dominates and the narcotics can actually produce a net effect of CNS arousal instead of depression. The final response, though, seems to be dependent upon the particular narcotic that is used, the dosage in which it is administered, and the condition of the horse at the time of administration. For example, if the horse is actually injured and suffering from severe pain, narcotics seldom exhibit undesirable excitatory effects. Instead, fairly effective sedation and relief from pain are usually produced. In normal horses, however, morphine drugs may well produce an excitatory response. This response may be minimal in intensity and be characterized by voluntary muscle movements, stamping and neighing. In some cases, however, severe excitation may occur and the horse can become difficult to manage. No doubt, injuries have occurred both to horses and handlers when an uncontrollable, excitatory response to narcotic drugs was encountered instead of an increase in physical performance, as was anticipated.

When narcotics have been used in equine medicine, they have usually been employed in attempts to reduce intense pain associated with fractures, deep lacerations, other serious traumas or severe colic. However, their use in certain types of colic has been questioned since these drugs actually have a spasmolytic (relaxing) effect on the digestive system. Thus, if the horse is suffering from constipation due to impaction, narcotics could worsen the condition by slowing peristaltic movements. On the other hand, abdominal cramping due to enteritis or spasmodic colic is usually relieved by these drugs.

In horses, the narcotics that have received the most use are morphine, meperidine (Demerol), oxymorphone (Numorphan), and dihydromorphinone (Dilaudid).

Morphine: Morphine can usually produce effective sedation and relief from pain if administered in doses less than 200 mg per horse. Dosages greater than 200 mg may well cause the excitatory phase. Most references and textbooks of equine medicine list excitation as an important problem and limiting factor of morphine use in horses. The dose of morphine is usually kept as low as possible in order to avoid the excitatory phase. It has been suggested that doses as low as 60 mg per horse produce good analgesia with a low incidence of CNS arousal. Pretreatment with sedatives seems to reduce the excitatory response to morphine in horses, and chloral hydrate has been suggested for this purpose.

Meperdine: Meperidine (Demerol) is a morphine substitute first synthesized in 1939. This drug has been the most successfully used narcotic in horses, and its effects are basically similar to those of morphine, except that meperidine seems less prone to produce excitatory responses. However, when rapidly injected intravenously, meperidine can cause excitation to occur in horses. The duration of analgesia produced by meperidine is shorter than with morphine, but may last for one-half to two hours. In an experimentally induced form of colic in ponies, the average duration of analgesia produced by meperidine was only 21 minutes.

Meperidine is sometimes used as a preanesthetic sedative in horses scheduled for surgery to correct intestinal conditions causing colic. Meperidine is usually not administered to horses in shock, since this drug produces a fall in blood pressure (hypotension). In combination with acetylpromazine (Acepromazine), meperidine has been reported to produce predictable and safe chemical restraint for minor surgical procedures.

Methadone: Methadone (Dolophine) is not chemically related to morphine but produces some similar pharmacologic effects. Analgesia produced by methadone is equivalent to that associated with morphine, and less sedation is usually seen. The duration of action of methadone is longer than that of morphine or meperidine, and may last for 4 to 6 hours. However, whether or not true CNS excitation occurs in the horse after methadone administration seems debatable at this time. Some references caution against the use of methadone in horses due to the potential for uncontrollable arousal. Just the opposite, some references state that an advantage of methadone in the horse is that it does not produce an excitatory phase. Differences of opinions may well relate to differences in dosages, rates of administrations and the condition of the horse at the time of injection. It has been recommended that methadone be administered in combination with atropine and promazine as a "lytic cocktail" in order to obtain preanesthetic sedation without excitation in the horse.

PRECAUTIONS

The morphine-like drugs are highly addictive not only in man but in other animals as well. That is, after repeated treatment with these drugs, the body in some way develops an actual dependence upon the drug. In addition, major side effects of narcotics are respiratory and cardiovascular depression.

Stimulants

Drugs that stimulate the CNS affect either the brain, the spinal cord, or both. Central nervous system stimulation results from the increased excitability of brain neurons (cells) produced by the stimulant drugs. The end result is a temporary increase in functional activity of the CNS. Stimulants of the CNS are used therapeutically to counteract anesthetic overdosage, to hasten recovery from anesthesia, to stimulate respiration, and to reverse the effects of certain toxic substances that depress the CNS. Amphetamine and amphetamine-like drugs are probably the most widely recognized CNS stimulants. They have been used as appetite depressants in humans and, in the past, as antidotes to overdosage of tranquilizers and other CNS depressants that are commonly abused by drug users.

Amphetamine: Amphetamine has been used in the past to counteract anesthetic overdosage in animals. Amphetamine temporarily stimulates the sensory cortex of the brain, resulting in greater mental responsiveness. Such psychic stimulation may momentarily override fatigue so that a horse seems to be in a state of arousal. However, pronounced CNS depression and even more pronounced fatigue occur as the effects of amphetamine rapidly diminish. Thus, amphetamine can produce a false sense of security, prompting attempts at physical activity that in reality may prove harmful rather than beneficial.

Severe and even fatal injuries have occurred to horses "doped" with CNS stimulants, such as amphetamine, in attempts to increase physical performance. Such examples of drug abuse should not be condoned by the horseman or his colleagues.

Another aspect of amphetamine that is frequently overlooked is that, in addition to CNS stimulation, this drug produces marked activation of the cardiovascular system. Intense stimulation of the heart and blood vessels occurs after amphetamine administration and damage to these tissues may result. For example, if a horse is suffering from an undiagnosed aneurysm (thin walled swelling) of a major blood vessel, administration of amphetamine could result in rupture of the blood vessel due to the pronounced increase in blood pressure that the drug produces.

Methylphenidate (Ritalin) is a nervous system stimulant that acts similarly to amphetamine, and has been abused in attempts to increase athletic performance of horses. Overdosage of methylphenidate results in severe convulsions.

Other CNS Stimulants: Other CNS stimulants include the xanthine compounds such as caffeine, theobromine, theophylline, and aminophylline. These compounds, of course, are found in certain beverage ingredients (i.e., coffee, tea, cocoa) and they act as mild CNS stimulants due to activation of the sensory and motor parts of the brain. They have been used in the past to produce respiratory and nervous system stimulation in horses and other animals.

Aminophylline has been used in attempts to assist breathing and reduce signs of abnormality in horses with chronic alveolar emphysema (broken wind or "heaves"); however, results are usually unsatisfactory. In fact, the xanthines are now infrequently used therapeutically. Strychnine is another example of a CNS stimulant used in the past but infrequently used at the present time.

Overdosage of any of the CNS stimulants can result in hyperthermia, severe agitation, excitability and convulsions. Self-inflicted wounds and death may occur.

Local Anesthetics

Local anesthetics are drugs that block the passage of nerve impulses when applied in effective concentration in the immediate vicinity of the nerve. Accordingly, these drugs provide relief from pain by preventing pain sensations from traveling up the sensory nerves to the brain.

Unlike the general anesthetics and hypnotics discussed in preceding sections, local anesthetics do not affect consciousness or other CNS functions in the horse. If administered in huge non-therapeutic dosages, however, local anesthetics produce incoordination and convulsions.

Local anesthesia is produced in the horse by several different methods including:

1. surface or topical anesthesia
2. infiltration anesthesia, in which the drug is injected directly in the surgical area
3. field block, in which the local anesthetic is injected around the surgical site so that sensory nerves supplying the site are blocked
4. nerve or regional block, in which the drug is injected into or near a major sensory nerve supplying a specific area
5. epidural block, in which the nerve roots in the vertebral canal are anesthetized

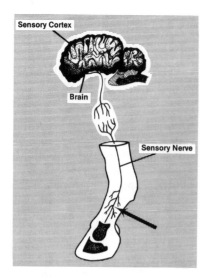

Fig. 22-1 A local anesthetic can be injected [arrow] to block nerve impulses traveling to the brain.

In the horse, commonly used methods of obtaining local anesthesia are surface, field, and infiltration anesthesia.

Drugs used to produce local anesthesia in the horse include: procaine (Novocaine), lidocaine (Xylocaine, Lignocaine), mepivacaine (Carbocaine), hexylcaine (Cyclaine), butacaine (Butyn Sulfate), tetracaine (Pontocaine), piperocaine (Metycaine) and proparacaine (Ophthaine). Most of the agents are used for particular types of local anesthesia, as outlined below.

SURFACE OR TOPICAL ANESTHESIA

This occurs when the local anesthetic is applied topically to mucous membranes or abraded skin. Unbroken skin prevents penetration of the drug; however, local anesthetics are usually effective in relieving pain from superficial wounds of the eye, mouth, nose or skin.

Butacaine (Butyn Sulfate) is often used to anesthetize the mucous membrane of the larynx when "roaring operations" are performed in conscious horses. Local anesthetics that are usually satisfactory for eye (ophthalmic) use include butacaine, tetracaine, piperocaine, and proparacaine in 0.5 to 5.0% solutions.

FIELD BLOCK ANESTHESIA

This method is accomplished by infiltrating the local anesthetic drug into the skin and deeper tissues surrounding, but not within, the site prepared for surgical incision. Another example of a field block is that type used when the forelimbs are "fired." In this case, the local anesthetic is injected into and underneath the skin around the circumference of a front leg in order to obtain local analgesia below the drug infiltration site. Drugs used to produce field block are also used to produce infiltration anesthesia.

INFILTRATION ANESTHESIA

This procedure is one of the most frequently used techniques to produce local anesthesia in horses. In infiltration anesthesia, small volumes of rather dilute solution of the local anesthetic drug are repeatedly injected subcutaneously and intradermally throughout the area to be anesthetized. This procedure is routinely used to prevent pain from minor surgical procedures (e.g., wound suturing, skin biopsy). If small amounts of the drug are first injected into the skin and more drug is injected as the needle is advanced, the horse should experience little pain.

Procaine is the most widely used local anesthetic in horses for both infiltration and field block. It is used in a 2.0% solution for these purposes. Mepivacaine is more potent than procaine, and is also administered as a 2.0% solution for both field and infiltration blocks. Lidocaine is more potent than procaine, and is injected as a 0.5 to 2.0% solution for infiltration anesthesia and a 1.0 to 2.0% solution for nerve blocks. Hexylcaine is 2 to 3 times as potent as procaine, and is used as a 5.0% solution for surface anesthesia and a 1.0 to 2.0% solution for infiltration or field block.

PRECAUTIONS

Sterile syringes and needles are always used when local anesthetics are injected, and aseptic precautions and preparation of the skin are followed in order to prevent bacterial infection. Small gauge needles are used in order to minimize trauma, and care is taken to ensure that the local anesthetic is not accidentally injected into an artery or vein. Local anesthetics are not injected into infected, inflamed areas since needle punctures may cause further spreading of the infection.

Muscle Relaxants

Relaxation of the voluntary (skeletal) muscles of the horse can be brought about by drugs that affect either the central nervous system or the spread of impulses from the peripheral nerves to the muscles. Centrally active muscle relaxants include certain tranquilizers such as meprobamate (Miltown, Equanil) and diazepam (Valium). The muscle relaxing effects of these drugs are believed to be mostly secondary to their tranquilizing actions.

CENTRALLY ACTING

Glyceryl guaiacolate (guaifenesin) is a centrally active muscle relaxant that has recently become somewhat popular for use in horses as a restraining agent or as a supplement to general anesthesia. A sterile 5% solution of this drug in 5% dextrose is administered intravenously at the usual dosage level of 1 ml of the solution per pound of body weight. Thus, a considerable volume of solution is usually required. The horse is usually recumbent for 15 to 30 minutes. When given in conjunction with thiamylal sodium, sedation and light anesthesia may last for 15 to 30 minutes.

Methocarbamol (Robaxin-V) is a centrally active muscle relaxant that is advocated by the manufacturer to be useful in reducing muscle spasms associated with acute inflammatory and traumatic conditions. This drug has little effect on normal muscle tone, but may be effective in reducing excessive skeletal muscle tone due to trauma, ligamentous strains, myositis (tying up), bursitis and synovitis. The dose in horses varies depending upon the severity of the condition, but 2 to 10 mg per pound administered intravenously is suggested by the manufacturer.

PERIPHERALLY ACTING

The peripherally acting muscle relaxants are called "neuromuscular blocking" drugs due to their site of action. They prevent the nerve impulse from reaching the skeletal muscles. They do this by blocking the specialized areas on the muscle cells that are normally activated by the chemical released from the nerve endings. Neuromuscular blocking agents are actually useful in horses only in select surgical procedures where profound muscle relaxation is needed in conjunction with general anesthesia. For example, peripherally acting muscle relaxants are sometimes used to facilitate surgical access to difficult body regions adjacent to large muscle masses. In some cases, muscle relaxants have been used to provide brief periods of restraint in horses to allow relatively minor surgical procedures such as simple castration.

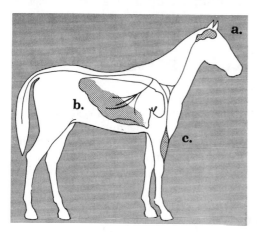

a. Brain. Site of action of general anesthetic.
b. Neuromuscular junction. Blocking site for respiratory muscle.
c. Neuromuscular junction. Blocking site for skeletal muscle.

Fig. 22-2   General anesthetics act on the brain, causing a loss of consciousness, while neuromuscular blocking agents act at the skeletal muscle level. Neuromuscular blocking agents have no effect on the central nervous system, do not cause loss of consciousness, and do not have an analgesic effect.

The neuromuscular blocking compounds were originally discovered by primitive tribes of South American Indians (although "discovery" by the modern world was centuries away). The local tribal medicine man concocted materials from particular plants in elaborate ceremonial procedures. The tips of the hunter's arrows, spears and blow-gun darts were dipped into the plant material concoction. When an animal was wounded by a poisoned weapon, it became paralyzed due to complete muscular relaxation, and died of suffocation. Early explorers brought back the plant materials which were called "curare." Drugs that produce neuromuscular paralysis are still called "curare-like" drugs.

It should be reemphasized that curare-like drugs are not anesthetics! They do not produce sedation, tranquilization, anesthesia or any loss of pain sensation. They "simply" block the nerve impulse at the points of nerve innervation to the muscle, causing paralysis so the horse can neither move nor breathe.

A synthetic curare-like drug relatively important to equine medicine is succinylcholine (Sucostrin). This drug was commonly used in the past and is still occasionally used in horses to provide restraint for brief surgical procedures, particularly simple castration. The rationale of this approach is based on the belief that surgical or "anesthetic" mortality (which is an important inherent risk in any surgery in the horse) is actually less when succinylcholine instead of a general anesthetic is used for support of castration. However, this is a highly controversial subject in equine medicine.

The horseman should be cognizant of the fact that when succinylcholine alone is used, the horse is completely conscious throughout the castration operation. The inhumaneness of submitting an animal to such an excruciatingly painful procedure should be considered.

In addition, respiration has to be carefully monitored and apparatus should be available for applying artificial respiration if needed. Furthermore, damage to the heart has been suspected in horses treated with succinylcholine, and aged or debilitated horses may respond excessively to this drug. Recent exposure to organophosphate insecticides or dewormers may cause severe potentiation and prolongation of the paralysis produced by succinylcholine. At the present time, succinylcholine is used most often in conjunction with CNS depressants and analgesics.

23

ANALGESIC AND ANTI-INFLAMMATORY DRUGS

This chapter deals with those drugs used in horses for relief from pain (analgesia), fever (antipyresis), and tissue inflammation (anti-inflammatory effect). These drugs are grouped together since several representative compounds exert all three of the effects mentioned in the preceding sentence. The drugs in this group include aspirin, phenylbutazone and several other agents with similar pharmacologic properties. Such drugs are usually referred to as nonnarcotic, or anti-inflammatory or mild analgesics, in order to distinguish them from the morphine-like narcotic drugs (discussed in another chapter). In relation to their anti-inflammatory effects, phenylbutazone and the aspirin-like compounds are referred to as non-steroidal anti-inflammatory drugs, in order to distinguish them from the cortisone-like steroid anti-inflammatory agents which are a different type of drug covered separately in the latter part of this chapter. In addition, a relatively new type of drug (Osteum: Schering) that is used in an effort to accelerate healing of certain types of inflammation is also included in this chapter as a drug alternative to "firing."

Narcotic and Nonnarcotic Drugs

As discussed in a previous chapter, the morphine-like narcotics produce profound analgesia and, depending upon the species and other factors, CNS sedation. This is accomplished by a marked depressant effect on brain centers resulting in an increase in the pain threshold of the sensory cortex. Narcotics are effective in reducing intense pain and pain of deep-seated visceral origin. However, these agents also affect various CNS functions not associated with pain sensation and, in the horse, may cause agitation and CNS arousal. The use of morphine and similar drugs is characterized by drug dependency, rigid legal control and the potential for variability of responsiveness of individual horses. With the occasional exception of meperidine (Demerol: Winthrop), narcotics are infrequently used in equine medicine.

On the other hand, phenylbutazone and the salicylate-like (aspirin) compounds do not cause drug dependency and, just as importantly, do not affect CNS behavioral patterns. They can indirectly enhance physical performance, but this is secondary to the relief from pain and inflammation that they provide. These drugs are effective only against pain of mild to moderate intensity. They are most useful against pain originating from inflammatory conditions of the muscles, bones or joints. The nonnarcotic analgesics decrease certain types of abnormally elevated fevers and decrease tissue inflammation. The latter effect, no doubt, contributes to the net pain-killing action of the phenylbutazone and aspirin-like drugs in horses.

General Aspects

Analgesic drugs are extensively used in humans. They are available in a multitude of over-the-counter preparations for relief from pain of headache, neuralgia, muscle ache, arthritis and other similar conditions. Such uses represent attempts to stop subjective symptoms in communicative patients. Indications for analgesic drugs are less common in horses, but include: laminitis, bone and joint disorders, muscle injury, and, in some cases, colic.

Certain of the analgesic agents have indeed proven to be exceptionally useful drugs in equines. However, it should be remembered that pain relief itself only masks the pain. It does not cure the horse of the ailment. In addition, anti-inflammatory drugs are contraindicated in infections unless an antibacterial drug is also administered, since spreading of the infection may result.

To reemphasize, the aspirin-like drugs are primarily effective against mild to moderate pain originating from the musculoskeletal system. The precise mechanism of analgesic and anti-inflammatory action is unknown. Since these drugs are most effective against pain associated with inflammation, it is believed that they interfere with the actions of pharmacologically active substances that are released from tissues in response to inflammation. For example, it is now known that prostaglandins (fatty acid substances) are synthesized in tissues in response to tissue injury and inflammation. Prostaglandins seem to sensitize local pain receptors to other tissue substances that are also increased in inflammation (e.g., bradykinin). Aspirin and phenylbutazone inhibit the synthesis of prostaglandin, thereby decreasing pain. Thus, a peripheral site of analgesic action is involved.

In addition, these drugs also exert part of their analgesic effect via a CNS action. However, this CNS effect is completely distinct from that of the narcotics! Aspirin-like drugs do not cause mental disturbances, hypnosis, or changes in CNS function other than changes in pain sensation (and temperature control). Furthermore, this effect is restricted to the more primitive brain centers and does not influence behavior. More specifically, these drugs do not produce CNS excitation or depression.

Precautions

Analgesia: As mentioned above, relief from pain by no means cures the pain-producing ailment, but simply provides relief to the horse. Pain is a natural sign indicating injury to the horse. If the primary condition is not corrected (either by other drugs or by allowing time for the body to heal), analgesia produced by a drug may, in the long run, prove to be a disadvantage. For example, the primary condition could become more complicated or, if the horse is forced to physically perform, the severity of the condition could worsen.

Anti-inflammation: Anti-inflammatory drugs have the capacity to prevent or reduce the local heat, redness, swelling and tenderness by which tissue inflammation is recognized by the observer. The signs of inflammation are reduced whether they are the result of injury caused by mechanical, thermal, radiation, infectious or allergic factors. In clinical use, the administration of anti-inflammatory agents is considered "palliative" therapy; that is, they can reduce the signs and discomfort but the underlying cause of the disease remains. The inflammatory manifestations are merely suppressed.

It should be remembered that inflammation (within limits) is an essential bodily process that represents the initial stages of the healing of damaged tissues. If inflammation and associated pain are prevented by drugs and the primary disorder is left untreated, harm rather than benefit may be the eventual result. Healing may be delayed and bacterial infection can spread due to the diminished inflammation. These factors are discussed further in relation to the individual drugs.

Adverse Side Effects: Although salicylate-like (aspirin) drugs have been used for at least a century, recent discoveries have provided critical information about both the beneficial and adverse effects of these and related drugs. For example, it is now known that aspirin, phenylbutazone and perhaps other similar-acting drugs affect blood clot formation. In man, aspirin can double the clotting time and this effect may persist for several days after administration. Phenylbutazone can also interfere with blood clot formation, and augment the activity of anticoagulant drugs. The clinical importance of increased bleeding tendency produced by these drugs is well established in human medicine, but is not clearly known in other animals.

It seems quite likely, however, that salicylates and phenylbutazone could increase the tendency for epistaxis (nosebleed) by slowing down blood clot formation. Perhaps the general increase in epistaxis that seems to be occurring in horses could be related to the increased use within recent years of anti-inflammatory, analgesic drugs. Although these aspects remain to be proven, the horseman should be well aware of the potential "anticoagulant" capabilities of the phenylbutazone and aspirin-like drugs.

In addition, many of the anti-inflammatory analgesic drugs can disrupt the functioning of those body tissues (e.g., bone marrow) that produce blood cells. These adverse side effects are infrequently produced in horses. However, serious and sometimes fatal blood disorders have occurred in humans who self-administered veterinary drugs intended for use only in horses. The horseman should be cognizant of the tendency for many drugs to be more toxic in man than in horses or other animals, particularly those drugs that can adversely affect blood-forming tissues.

Individual Drugs

Aspirin: Acetylsalicylic acid (commonly called aspirin) and its close relative, sodium salicylate, are common anti-inflammatory analgesics. They are used for relief of mild to moderate pain associated with inflammation of muscles, bones and joints. In horses, aspirin is now used more often for reducing fever than for relieving pain.

The antipyretic action of aspirin is achieved by "resetting" the "temperature thermostat" (thermo-regulatory center) of the brain. This causes sweating and dilation of peripheral blood vessels, allowing increased heat dissipation from the body surface. Aspirin drugs reduce fever if it is due to bacterial infection, but are ineffective against other types of fever, such as that due to heatstroke.

Aspirin and sodium salicylate are readily absorbed from the digestive tract, and tend to produce irritation of the stomach lining. This effect can be reduced by concurrent administration of an antacid such as sodium bicarbonate.

Dosages of aspirin in mature horses are 8 to 50 grams (depending on body weight) and the dose in foals is 0.5 to 6.0 grams. Aspirin is given orally, as is sodium salicylate, which is administered to mature horses in the dose of 20 to 100 grams. In foals, the dose of sodium salicylate is 0.5 to 6.0 grams.

Meclofenamic Acid: This drug is a new nonsteroidal anti-inflammatory agent that is distantly related to the salicylates. In the horse, it is indicated for the treatment of acute or chronic inflammatory conditions of the musculoskeletal system. Its mechanism of action is not known, but may be related to inhibition of prostaglandin synthesis.

The dose recommended by the manufacturer of meclofenamic acid (Arquel) is 1 mg per pound (1 gm per 1,000 lb body weight) administered orally once per day. The duration of treatment is for 5 to 7 days for both acute and chronic conditions. The commercial preparation is supplied in packets; the drug is mixed with the daily grain ration.

Meclofenamic acid should not be administered to horses with gastrointestinal, hepatic or renal disease. This drug can produce bleeding from the digestive tract, and may lower the hematocrit. The drug should be discontinued at the first signs of intolerance such as colic, diarrhea, appetite suppression, or blood in the feces.

Phenylbutazone: This drug (Butazolidin "Bute": Jensen-Salsbery) is an anti-inflammatory analgesic that is extensively used in horses. It has been advocated as treatment for various conditions involving the muscles, bones and joints. Examples include chronic arthritis, bursitis, lameness, rheumatism, chronic inflammation, myositis (tying up) and osteoarthritis.

Some medical sources consider that pain relief by phenylbutazone is secondary and due entirely to the reduction of inflammation and local edema produced by the anti-inflammatory action of the drug. Therefore, most recent medical references classify phenylbutazone as an anti-inflammatory agent rather than as an analgesic. In any case, the anti-inflammatory action of the drug and resulting relief from pain and lameness is well documented in horses.

Phenylbutazone is not believed to have either stimulatory or depressant effects on the CNS. That is, it does not produce a state of CNS arousal or a state of CNS depression. However, as with other drugs that decrease pain, phenylbutazone can indirectly affect physical performance as a result of diminished pain. It is advocated by many authorities that phenylbutazone does not increase the speed of a horse, but simply permits the animal to run (or perform) to his fullest potential. However, this aspect is still questioned by some.

Another important question involving phenylbutazone usage in the horse is whether or not the drug depresses a horse's natural survival instinct. This is an exceptionally difficult question to objectively answer. There is some evidence that phenylbutazone can, but does not necessarily have to, block the animal's instinct to protect himself from injury. Such a letdown in survival instinct could result in the horse failing to "let-off" or ease his physical effort if an injury should occur or seem imminent.

An extract from a statistical appendix to a California Horse Racing Board report was reprinted in the **Horseman's Journal** (November, 1976). It indicated that the incidence of "breakdowns" and "horses destroyed" on racetracks did not appreciably change during the first four years that controlled medication with phenylbutazone was allowed in that state. On the other hand, statements have been made that horses in Michigan and Pennsylvania's Keystone track were breaking down three or four times more often after controlled medication was allowed.

In Maryland, the state veterinarian has indicated that there seems to be no increase in the incidence of physical injuries to race horses since phenylbutazone was allowed as a controlled medication in that state. However, and very importantly, he believes the severity of injuries has increased since phenylbutazone was approved. This was based not on statistical surveys, but on his personal experience with racetrack horses. In particular, conditions that were mentioned included fractured knees and damage to the cannon bones and the extremities.

Whether or not the use of phenylbutazone and other comparable drugs encourages the racing and competing of unsound horses, thereby increasing the incidence and/or severity of physical breakdowns, remains to be definitively answered. In any case, the horseman should be well aware of the potential danger of masking pain alone, rather than trying to correct the primary ailment. Phenylbutazone is now allowed as a pre-race medication in some states.

In most cases that respond to phenylbutazone therapy, results are usually seen in one to four days. The oral dose of phenylbutazone in horses is 1 to 2 grams per 500 lbs of body weight (2 to 4 mg per lb). Intravenous doses are less, and accidental injection into an artery can produce severe toxic reactions. The prolonged daily administration of 2 grams of phenylbutazone for 32 days has caused necrotizing inflammation of the portal veins of the liver in horses. However, adverse side effects are infrequently seen in horses when phenylbutazone treatment is used for the recommended interval.

In man, phenylbutazone can produce exceptionally serious side effects. At this time, phenylbutazone is considered to be the most common cause of drug-induced blood (hematologic) disease in man. The most common hematologic side effect is thought to be "agranulocytosis," a condition in which the bone marrow cannot produce white blood cells. The more unusual hematologic side effect is "aplastic anemia"; in this condition, bone marrow is converted to fat and no blood cells are produced. Thus, the person affected suffers from anemia, infection and bleeding complications. An awareness of these disastrous complications is important to the horseman because it seems that some horsemen administer phenylbutazone to themselves! In 1975, a young jockey developed aplastic anemia and later died despite a bone marrow transplant from his brother. It was discovered that this jockey was self administering a veterinary preparation of phenylbutazone. There also seems to be some evidence that phenylbutazone may increase the vulnerability of some people to acute leukemia. All horsemen should be well aware of such examples of this form of "drug misuse" involving equine medications.

Specific points concerning the use of phenylbutazone in race horses have been compiled by the American Association of Equine Practitioners. These aspects are summarized and reprinted as follows:

1. Phenylbutazone (Butazolidin) is a very effective nonsteroidal anti-inflammatory agent in horses. Through its anti-inflammatory action, it is an analgesic (relieves pain) and is an antipyretic (reduces fever). **It is not an anesthetic.**
2. Phenylbutazone does not change a horse's innate ability to race, but by relieving inflammation may enable him to race nearer to his maximum capability.
3. Its mechanism of action is thought to be by inhibition of prostaglandins.
4. Onset of action occurs within a few hours and optimum effect lasts for less than 48 hours after the last dose.
5. In horses, phenylbutazone is safe; side effects and toxicity are rare at the usual doses.
6. Phenylbutazone can be detected in blood for 24 hours and occasionally up to 48 hours.

7. Although the quantity of phenylbutazone in the urine is not reliable for the determination of the time that the last dose of phenylbutazone was administered, reasonable estimates can be made by a comparison of the ratios of phenylbutazone to its major metabolites.
8. Trace amounts of phenylbutazone and its metabolites can be detected in urine for up to 96 hours by utilizing electron capture derivative formation and detection by gas chromatography.
9. The usual doses of phenylbutazone given on race day may interfere with the detection of other medications, depending upon analytical methods used.

Orgotein: This compound is a naturally occurring metalloprotein (metal containing protein) that is derived from beef liver. Orgotein (Palosein) is chemically distinct from the aspirin and phenylbutazone-like, anti-inflammatory drugs. It has no direct analgesic activity but provides relief from pain due to its anti-inflammatory effect and the resulting reduction of tissue inflammation.

Orgotein is a relatively new drug and probably will require additional research and clinical trial before its absolute benefits and toxicities are better defined. The long duration of therapy (several weeks) and associated rest period most likely contributes to beneficial results.

Orgotein (Palosein) is recommended by the manufacturer to be useful in reducing the signs of, and promoting healing from, soft tissue inflammation of the musculoskeletal system. Both acute and chronic conditions are reported by the manufacturer to respond to therapy with this drug. The usual dose in horses is 5 mg administered by deep intramuscular injection every other day for two weeks, and then twice a week for two to three additional weeks. This therapeutic regime represents a total of four to five weeks, a significant rest period that no doubt benefits the injured horse.

When therapy is started, transitory exacerbation (worsening) of the inflammatory condition and related lameness may occur prior to onset of improvement.

Naproxen: Naproxen (Equiproxen) is a new synthetic anti-inflammatory analgesic drug that also has antipyretic activities. It is chemically unrelated to phenylbutazone, the salicylates, or the steroid anti-inflammatory agents. It is classified chemically as an arylalkanoic acid.

Naproxen has been found to have good pain-killing effects in experimental studies. In the horse, it is used for treatment of inflammatory conditions and associated pain and lameness. It is particularly advocated by the manufacturer to be helpful in the treatment of myositis (tying up) and other soft tissue injuries of the musculoskeletal system. Since naproxen raises the pain threshold only in those states involving inflammation, the apparent analgesic properties are thought to be secondary to relief from inflammation.

For oral maintenance therapy, naproxen is administered twice daily at the dose of 4.5 mg per lb. An oral preparation of granules containing the drug is available for mixing with the feed.

The major side effect of naproxen in several animal species is gastrointestinal irritation; however, this does not seem to be a major problem in horses. This drug is reported by the manufacturer to be safe in pregnant mares, and to have no effect on breeding performance of stallions.

Dipyrone: This compound is an anti-inflammatory, antipyretic, analgesic frequently used in the horse. Dipyrone (Methampyrone, Novin) is not chemically related to aspirin or phenylbutazone, but is similar to aminopyrine, an aspirin substitute used in the past in humans.

This drug is most effective in equine colic and other conditions characterized by visceral smooth muscle spasms. Some controversy exists concerning the particular mechanism of colic relief produced by dipyrone. It has been reported to both produce analgesia and to directly relax intestinal smooth muscle. Therefore, it is considered by some authorities to be the drug of choice for spasmodic, non-obstructive colic. However, an experimental study of an intentionally induced form of colic in ponies indicated that the drug has essentially no analgesic effects. Perhaps this experimental type of colic is not truly representative of spontaneous spasmodic colic. Or, perhaps it is the spasmolytic effect rather than the analgesic effect that makes the drug popular in clinical incidences of spasmodic colic.

Dipyrone can be administered twice daily by the subcutaneous, intramuscular, or intravenous route. Dosage is 2.5 to 10.0 grams per mature horse, depending on body weight.

In man, dipyrone has been associated with hematologic (blood) disorders and, therefore, should not be used in horses with a history of blood disease. This drug should not be used in conjunction with phenylbutazone or barbiturates. In man, administration of dipyrone with chlorpromazine has been reported to produce serious hypothermia (lowering of body temperature), and such use is contraindicated. In horses, the concurrent use of dipyrone and phenothiazine tranquilizers probably should be avoided. Dipyrone can aggravate a bleeding tendency and should not be used in horses with epistaxis (nosebleed).

Pentazocine: This drug was chemically synthesized in a deliberate attempt to find drugs that would have the analgesic powers of narcotics without the undesirable side effects and potential for dependency. It is widely employed in horses for the control of abdominal pain associated with spasmodic colic. Pentazocine (Talwin: Winthrop) exerts its analgesic effects through a CNS depressant action. In addition, it has a direct relaxing effect on intestinal smooth muscle, thereby relieving pain caused by the abdominal cramping of spasmodic colic.

A major advantage of pentazocine is that, although it has some properties similar to morphine, it is not subjected to narcotic control laws. It is approximately one-quarter to one-third as potent as morphine on a mg to mg basis, but it can provide analgesia of about the same intensity as can morphine. The dose of pentazocine in horses is 0.25 to 2.0 mg per pound. This dose will usually provide analgesia for 15 to 90 minutes, depending upon the severity of the pain. If administered intravenously, the onset of analgesia usually occurs within three to eight minutes. After intramuscular or subcutaneous injection, the onset takes about 15 to 20 minutes.

Doses larger than 2.0 mg per lb may cause incoordination and muscle tremors. An advantage of pentazocine is the infrequent occurrence of CNS excitation and the low potential for addiction.

Dimethyl Sulfoxide (DMSO): DMSO has been used quite extensively in horses and other animals, including man. However differences in opinions of physicians (both human and veterinary) about the actual effectiveness of the chemical are widespread. For example, completely opposite responses were obtained from different veterinarians in a survey about DMSO that was published in the veterinary journal **Veterinary Medicine/Small Animal Clinician** (May, 1976). Favorable replies were in the majority and included "DMSO is a drug with such wide application and usefulness that it is a cornerstone of the practice." Disfavorable replies included "Products with DMSO in them have not been of any great value." These examples are given to point out to the horseman that the true therapeutic benefits of DMSO are not completely defined, some are still questionable, and much carefully controlled research needs to be done with this drug to verify or refute its many supposed benefits.

As is the usual case when a new drug is introduced, wide acclaim and flagrant claims have accompanied the use of DMSO in medicine. Some of the many actions that have been attributed to DMSO include:

1. increased membrane permeability to other drugs, thereby increasing their penetration into tissues
2. an anti-inflammatory effect
3. an antibacterial effect, and increased sensitivity of antibiotic-resistant bacteria to drugs
4. enhanced connective tissue repair of traumatized tissue
5. a local anesthetic effect
6. cholinesterase inhibition
7. a diuretic effect (increased urination)
8. interference with blood platelet aggregation

In horses, DMSO has been used in the treatment of acute lameness, lacerations, and other traumas to the musculoskeletal system. Administered intravenously, DMSO has even been used to treat pneumonia. For treatment of acute lamenesses, a solution of DMSO can be applied topically, often in conjunction with other topically applied agents. DMSO has also been administered intravenously to treat chronic or nonresponsive pneumonia in horses. A method used is 25 ml of a 90% solution combined with an antibiotic and administered intravenously once daily for three days. Horses with acute laminitis have been treated with 60 to 120 ml of DMSO (10% solution), plus 500 ml of electrolyte solution, but variable responsiveness occurred.

Administered without other drugs, DMSO has anti-inflammatory effects in horses, due in part to reduction of tissue edema. Arthritic conditions have been treated with topical applications of the agent. In addition, DMSO seems to increase the horse's response to certain other anti-inflammatory drugs. For example, the local antiarthritic effect of topically applied hydrocortisone was reported to be increased 10 fold when DMSO was used as the carrier. The ability of DMSO to increase the penetrability of other drugs depends on the chemical nature of the other drug, the route of administration and concentration of both DMSO and the other agent. Some drugs that may be affected are steroids, local anesthetics, antimicrobial agents and anticholinesterase agents.

The primary toxic effect of DMSO in animals seems to be alteration of the lens of the eye. In horses given 0.18 mg per lb cutaneously for 14 days, lens changes were not detected. However, when 0.27 mg per lb was applied similarly for two months, minor damage to the lens was found. It seems that DMSO is unlikely to cause ocular lens damage in horses unless used in relatively high doses over an extended period of time. When DMSO is applied topically, an applicator should be used. It can be absorbed from intact skin quite easily, and a "bitter almond" taste indicates that the person applying the medication has absorbed some of the drug into his circulation.

Steroid Anti-Inflammatory Agents

The adrenal glands are small endocrine glands located adjacent to the kidneys. There are two adrenal glands; each one is composed of an inner (medulla) and outer (cortex) portion. The medulla produces adrenalin (epinephrine) and noradrenalin (norepinephrine), as discussed in the chapter on Hormones.

The hormones produced by the adrenal cortex are the objects of this section. Included are several steroid hormones that are commonly referred to as the adrenal corticosteroids, and also several similar compounds that have been chemically synthesized. The more important naturally occurring corticosteroids are corticosterone and hydrocortisone (cortisol).

The corticosteroids are essential to life, and they affect various bodily functions including: electrolyte and water balance; metabolism of carbohydrates, proteins and fats; and functions of the cardiovascular system, the kidneys, the nervous system and various other tissues and organs.

The corticosteroids are further subdivided into the mineralocorticoids, which are primarily involved in water and electrolyte balance, and the glucocorticoids, which are primarily involved in carbohydrate metabolism. The glucocorticoids are the more important steroids in relation to clinical use in horses; these compounds exert a pronounced anti-inflammatory effect.

GENERAL ASPECTS

The adrenal cortex is stimulated by a hormone to produce the corticosteroids. This hormone is adrenocorticotropic hormone (ACTH), which is secreted by the pituitary gland of the brain. The pituitary and adrenal cortex interact through a complex "feed-back" system. That is, an increase in the release of ACTH from the pituitary into the circulation causes a stimulation of the adrenal cortex. The synthesis of steroid hormones by the adrenal glands is thereby increased. The resulting increase in the concentration of steroids in the blood then "informs" the pituitary to decrease production of ACTH. The decrease in ACTH, in turn, causes a decrease in synthesis of the adrenal corticosteroids. If the fall in steroid production becomes severe enough, the pituitary is again stimulated to increase ACTH formation, and the cycle repeats itself. This reciprocating feed-back (or "servo") system serves to maintain hormone production by the adrenal cortex in a closely controlled state.

Due to such complexities, it is obvious that the administration of exogenous (outside source) ACTH or corticosteroids can markedly disrupt endogenous (source from within the body) hormonal balance. For example, if corticosteroids are administered for a long period, the production of ACTH by the pituitary will decrease. In turn, the adrenal cortex will atrophy (decrease in size and function) due to the decrease in stimulation by ACTH. Corticosteroid production by the adrenals will decrease or stop. If therapy with the exogenous steroids is suddenly stopped under these circumstances, the horse will experience severe endocrine imbalance due to its inability to produce natural (endogenous) corticosteroids. Therefore, adrenocorticosteroid therapy should not be suddenly discontinued but should be gradually withdrawn, especially if therapy has been extended over a lengthy interval.

USE IN HORSES

Glucocorticoids have been used quite extensively in horses for the treatment of various lamenesses. In many cases, results are favorable, particularly if time is allowed to provide adequate rest in conjunction with steroid therapy. Administration can be by oral, intramuscular or local injection routes. In treatment of lamenesses associated with a swollen joint, muscle sheath or bursa, an ordinary procedure involves the sterile aspiration of excess fluid by hypodermic needle and syringe. The solution of corticosteroid is then injected through the same needle using another syringe. An antibiotic is often included in the injection if infection is present.

Intra-articular (into the joint) injection should be done only by the veterinarian, due to the need for precise anatomic location of the needle and the absolute requirement for aseptic techniques. Disastrous results can occur if the joint becomes infected!

Acute conditions such as carpitis (inflammation of the knee; "popped knee"), tarsitis (inflammation of the hock), gonitis (inflammation of the stifle) and inflammation of the cannon bones are usually responsive to corticosteroid and rest therapy. Other general conditions treated with corticosteroids include arthritis, tendonitis and bursitis. When applied locally to the skin or eyes, several of the corticosteroids are useful in reducing the inflammation associated with dermatitis or conjunctivitis.

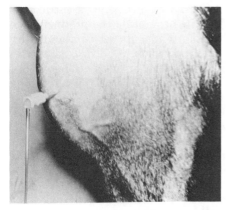

Fig. 23-1   Arthrocentesis. Excess synovial fluid is being drained from a joint capsule.

a.

b.

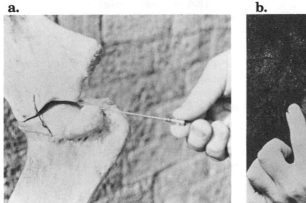 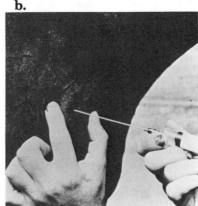

Fig. 23-2   Intra-articular injection.   a. Site of intended injection into the shoulder joint; note the length of needle required.   b. Actual injection.

PRECAUTIONS

As with other anti-inflammatory drugs, the corticosteroids do not cure any specific inflammation-producing disease. Their effects are palliative, and the underlying cause of the problem should be corrected. A sufficient rest period should be allowed in order to grant time for the horse's bodily mechanisms to correct the disorder. Particular caution is exercised if corticosteroids are used when an infectious condition is present. The anti-inflammatory action will promote dissemination of the infectious organism; a fulminating infection may result. In addition, the corticosteroids can delay normal wound healing processes.

CORTICOSTEROIDS

Adrenocorticotropic hormone (ACTH): ACTH is not a corticosteroid but exerts its anti-inflammatory effect by promoting the production by the adrenal glands of endogenous steroids. Thus, its anti-inflammatory effects are virtually identical to the corticosteroids. ACTH is not often used in horses, but has been reported to be useful in treating myositis if administered early in the condition. Dosage is from 50 to 150 international units (I.U.), administered intramuscularly (refer to Fig. 26-1).

Cortisone (Cortone, Cortogen): This was the first glucocorticoid available for clinical use; it is administered orally, intravenously or intramuscularly. It is converted within the body to hydrocortisone, which is actually the active principal. Dosage in horses is usually 1,000 to 1,500 mg, administered daily by intramuscular injection; or 50 to 250 mg if injected locally into bursa, tendon sheaths or joint capsules.

Prednisone (Deltra, Deltasone, Meticorten, Paracort): This steroid is about equally effective as cortisone, but is more potent on a mg to mg basis. Dosage in horses is from 100 to 300 mg, administered once daily by the intramuscular route. When injected locally into joints, tendon sheaths or bursa, the dose of prednisone is 50 to 250 mg.

Hydrocortisone (Cortef, Cortril, Hycortole, Hydrocortone): This drug can be given by the oral, intramuscular or intravenous routes. Some topical preparations are also available. The intramuscular dose is 1,000 to 1,500 mg; 50 to 250 mg is injected locally for treatment of arthritis, tendonitis or bursitis.

Prednisolone (Delta-Cortef, Hydeltra, Meticortelone): Prednisolone has about the same usefulness and effectiveness as prednisone. It can be administered orally or by injection. Dosage in horses is 100 to 300 mg, by the intramuscular route; 50 to 250 mg when injected for local effect. Prednisolone sodium succinate (Solu-Delta-Cortef) is a soluble form of prednisolone used for intravenous or intramuscular injection. Fluoroprednisolone (Predef) is a fluorinated prednisolone preparation used for oral or intramuscular administration.

Dexamethasone (Azium, Decadron, Deronil): This steroid is commonly used in the treatment of joint inflammation in horses. It is a potent steroid: dosage by intramuscular administration is only 2.5 to 5.0 mg, and 5 to 10 mg if given orally. Subsequent daily doses are usually reduced.

Triamcinolone (Aristocort, Kenacort, Vetalog): This agent has very little effect on water and electrolyte balance, and primarily exerts only glucocorticoid actions. It is about as effective as cortisone and other similar steroids. It sometimes causes weight loss and muscular weakness.

SODIUM OLEATE

"Firing" is a form of severe counterirritation used commonly in the past in attempts to increase recovery from conditions such as bucked shins or splints. Firing was performed (after local anesthesia and surgical scrubbing of the area) by burning numerous small holes through the skin over the cannon bones by use of a hot-iron cautery device. The severe inflammation that resulted, in conjunction with the necessarily long rest period, was believed to assist recovery from hair-line fractures of the cannon bones, splints, etc. However, the severe post-procedural pain associated with such techniques has prompted a search for more humane and more effective treatment procedures. Recently, a drug known as sodium oleate has shown promise as such a treatment.

Sodium oleate (Osteum) is a compound chemically related to the substance used in oleomargarine. Its mechanism of action is not clear; however, it is believed to accelerate the healing of bone and cartilage damage. This may either be due to primary stimulation of the healing process, or secondary to the rather pronounced counterirritation produced by the sodium oleate itself.

In any case, sodium oleate has been found in preliminary studies by several veterinarians to be useful in promoting healing and recovery from bucked shins and splints. In particular, a major reported advantage of the compound is the considerably accelerated healing time, thereby allowing physical training to recommence at an earlier than usual date. However, as is virtually always the case when a new drug therapy is introduced, perhaps the early wide and favorable comments on treatment with sodium oleate may prove to be somewhat overstated. No doubt, considerable further research and clinical trials will be necessary to establish the precise usefulness of sodium oleate in equine therapeutics.

Injection techniques for sodium oletate are shown in an accompanying illustration.

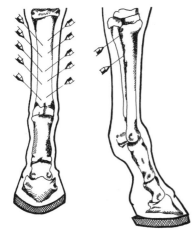

Fig. 23-3 Needle placement used in administering Osteum; bucked shins [left] and splint [right].

The manufacturer of Osteum makes the following recommendations: The amount of Osteum to be injected depends upon the area of response desired. An injection of 1 to 2 ml will produce a response of approximately 15 to 30 square centimeters. Larger areas require second injections. Total injected volumes should not exceed 10 ml. Immediate alcohol massage aids distribution of the injected solution, followed by bandaging. Local response to the compound includes swelling, pain and heat at the injection site. This is considered a normal response and will usually subside in 48 to 72 hours.

After treatment, the horse should be hand walked daily for one week. Controlled light work or training is encouraged beginning the second week after treatment. Normal work can be re-established as the animal improves. Osteum should not be administered within 30 days of the local injection of a corticosteroid. ♘

24

CARDIOVASCULAR DRUGS

The heart, arteries, veins, lymph vessels, blood, lymph and associated tissues comprise the cardiovascular system. These body constituents function to circulate nutrients and oxygen to all the cells of the body, and to transport metabolic wastes such as carbon dioxide and nitrogenous compounds from body tissues to excretory organs. Cardiovascular system dysfunction can result in immediate death or in prolonged debilitating illness. Accordingly, many drugs have been developed that affect the function of the heart, the blood vessels, or both. These drugs are referred to collectively as "cardiovascular drugs," the subject of this chapter.

It should be emphasized, however, that cardiovascular drugs are not extensively used in horses since primary diseases of the heart and blood vessels are recognized relatively infrequently in equines. Employment of cardiovascular drugs varies considerably in the different mammalian species depending upon the incidence of cardiovascular disease in the particular species.

General Aspects

In general, the occurrence of cardiovascular disease is considerably more frequent in man than in horses or other domesticated animals. Indeed, approximately 38 of every 100 human deaths are attributed to one form or another of cardiovascular disease. Such diseases include high blood pressure (hypertension), congestive heart failure, myocardial infarct (obstruction of blood flow to part of the heart muscle) or "heart attack," arteriosclerosis (hardening of the arteries), atherosclerosis (fatty deposits in the arteries) and various others. In the horse, such primary disorders as these rarely occur to any detectable extent. Circulatory problems seen in horses usually are secondary to:

1. systemic infection by bacteria or internal parasites
2. heartbeat irregularities
3. birth defects
4. shock

500

Infection

Bacterial infection of the heart muscle (myocarditis), the sack that encloses the heart (pericarditis) or the valves of the heart (valvular endocarditis) can occur as a sequela to pneumonia or other serious systemic infections. Arterial damage caused by migrating larvae of the internal parasitic worm, **Strongylus vulgaris**, is believed to occur in a large percentage of all horses. However, bacterial and larval infestations of cardiovascular tissues are not treated by cardiovascular drugs, but by appropriate antibacterial or anthelmintic therapy.

Heartbeat Irregularities

Heartbeat irregularities (cardiac arrhythmias) are fairly common in horses, but the clinical importance of such problems have not been determined. After exercise, some arrhythmias seem to be abolished and some seem less pronounced. Several drugs are available that tend to convert irregular heartbeat rhythm to a normal rhythm. These drugs are referred to as antiarrhythmic agents. Examples include quinidine, propranolol, and digitalis. The use of antiarrhythmic drugs is restricted to veterinarians because of the complexities in diagnosing cardiac arrhythmias and the need for hospital-like conditions where the electrocardiogram can be evaluated.

Birth Defects

Birth defects of the heart (congenital heart disease) is occasionally detected in horses but the prevalence of such problems has never been accurately determined. In some foals, the defect is so severe that death occurs shortly after birth. Most reports of cases of congenital heart disease in the horse are limited to a description of necropsy findings. Clinical signs associated with such problems are rarely known in detail. Since anatomical abnormalities are the basis for the condition, drugs cannot correct the problem.

Shock

Shock is a general term used to describe an acute and progressive failure of the cardiovascular system to provide adequate blood flow to body tissues. Characteristic signs include prostration or stupor and low blood pressure. Shock is considered predominately a cardiovascular disorder; however, it can be initiated by various factors. Hemorrhage, trauma, burns, allergic reactions and other important conditions that can precipitate a shock reaction are listed in an accompanying Table.

Any of the above listed conditions can initiate a sequence of circulatory (hemodynamic) events manifested initially by a fall in blood pressure. Hypotension seems to be the primary instigator that triggers the overall cardiovascular response that leads to the circulatory shock state. In response to hypotension, the nervous system of the horse attempts through neural reflexes to compensate for the low blood pressure. Peripheral vasoconstriction (constriction of the arteries of the skin and skeletal muscles) occurs, as does a shift of body water from tissues into the bloodstream. These responses are designed to increase the volume of blood in the circulation and to redistribute blood flow from the limbs to those organs that are vital for immediate survival (brain, heart, lungs). Thus, the signs of shock and the body's attempt to compensate for shock are characterized by hypotension, fast heart rate (tachycardia), blanching of the skin and mucous membranes, increased respiration and decreased urination.

If the corrective actions mediated by the horse's nervous system are not sufficient to compensate for and to overcome the shock state, then blood flow to vital organs and tissues become so depressed that tissue death occurs. An irreversible stage of shock is eventually reached and death results. The actual stage at which the irreversible form of shock is reached is not known. Neither is it known why some animals in shock respond to drug therapy and why others do not respond.

Depending upon the etiology (cause) of the shock condition, certain cardiovascular agents have proven useful in preventing development of the irreversible stage. However, drug therapy of shock is a highly controversial area in medicine, and many conflicting results have been reported by different scientists investigating shock therapy. Such differences in opinion no doubt reflect differences in experimental procedures, different animal species and different methods of producing experimental shock.

In any case, treatment of shock in horses must be administered by a veterinarian since therapy usually involves massive replacement of fluids to restore blood volume and blood pressure toward normal. Whole blood, plasma, plasma expanders, dextrose, or saline (salt) solution can be used depending upon the needs of the circulatory system. Drugs that increase the strength of the heartbeat and/or cause constriction of blood vessels are sometimes used in attempts to increase blood flow and blood pressure. Corticosteroids and antibiotics are often used as supportive therapy. Several types of agents that have been used to treat cardiovascular shock are given in an accompanying Table.

FIG. 24-1   TABLE 1
TYPES OF CARDIOVASCULAR SHOCK

Hemorrhagic	(Decreased Blood Volume)
Bacteremic	(Pathogenic Bacteria in Blood)
Septicemic	(Pathogenic Bacteria and Bacterial Toxins in Blood)
Burns	Thermal Injury)
Traumatic	(Severe Injury and Associated Pain)
Anaphylactic	(Immunologic-Allergic Reactions)
Cardiogenic	(Failure of Heart to Pump Blood)
Neurogenic	(Loss of Vasoconstrictor Nerve Impulses)
Combinations of Above Factors	

FIG. 24-2   TABLE 2
AGENTS THAT MAY BE USED IN TREATING
CIRCULATORY SHOCK CONDITIONS

Blood and Blood Substitutes
Whole Blood	Dextrose
Plasma	Lactated Ringers Solution
Dextran	

Alkalinizing Agents [decrease acidity of blood]
Sodium Bicarbonate

Vasoconstrictor Drugs
Epinephrine (Adrenalin)
Norepinephrine (Noradrenaline)
Methoxamine

Cardiac Stimulatory Agents
Epinephrine (Adrenalin)
Norepinephrine (Noradrenaline)
Isoproterenol
Digitalis
Calcium Ions

Corticosteroids

Antibiotics

25

DIURETICS

Diuretics are drugs that increase the volume of urine produced by the kidneys. Despite such a simple definition, a variety of different factors can be involved in the diuretic effects of drugs. The kidney is a complex organ, and the basic mechanisms whereby drugs can affect the volume of urine formation are beyond the scope of the present discussion. Actually, diuretics are used therapeutically in horses only in particular disease conditions, and their use must be carefully controlled by the veterinarian. However, diuretics are considered as a separate topic for two reasons that have importance to the horseman. First, diuretics are sometimes given to horses after races and some horse show events to facilitate urine collection for testing of drugs. Secondly, a commonly used diuretic, furosemide (Lasix: Hoechst-Roussel), is now being used fairly often in attempts to control nosebleed (epistaxis) in racehorses.

General Aspects

Diuresis, an increase in urine volume, can be produced in different manners. Water, for example, can have a diuretic effect if ingested in a large enough quantity. However, diuresis induced by increased water intake is of little therapeutic value since a net change in water balance does not occur. Diuretic drugs, on the other hand, can produce diuresis without necessitating an increase in water consumption. Thus, a net loss of body water is the result. Such an effect is often useful in the treatment of certain tissue disorders characterized by swelling and edema.

Edema, simply defined, is the abnormal collection of fluid in body tissues. Localized edema often occurs after trauma. Joint swelling, for example, is the result of an excess accumulation of joint fluid that is usually due to injury sustained by the joint and surrounding soft tissues. Fluid can also accumulate in body cavities such as the chest and abdomen. Excess fluid in body cavities usually occurs as a sequela (complication) to severe infection or circulatory problems. Edema of the lungs, known as pulmonary edema, can also occur leading to respiratory problems. If circulatory problems are severe enough to actually retard the normal flow of blood, edema can occur not only in the lungs and body cavities but also in the limbs. Generalized edema can also occur in association with certain serious systemic conditions such as purpura hemorrhagica.

Diuretic drugs are useful in treating such conditions since, by producing diuresis, these drugs cause a shift of body waters into the urine. This results in a net loss of body fluid. The initial effect occurring after administration of a diuretic is the movement of water from the blood into the urine. As the fluid portion of the blood is decreased, blood volume decreases proportionately, causing, in turn, a decrease in blood pressure. The decrease in blood volume and blood pressure causes an increased movement of tissue fluid from edematous tissues into the blood in an attempt by the body to restore blood volume and blood pressure toward normal. Thus, edema and related swelling are reduced, thereby providing relief from the pain associated with the increased pressure produced by the swelling. Also, due to the removal of excess tissue fluids and pressure, the healing process is assisted. In the case of pulmonary edema and related respiratory problems, breathing becomes less difficult due to the decrease in airway resistance that occurs after excess fluid and swelling are removed. However, diuretic therapy is usually only a supportive measure since edema may recur if the primary injury does not heal or if drugs or other therapeutic measures are not used to correct the primary problem.

Urine Collection

This aspect of the use of diuretics can be summarized in a few sentences. Briefly, diuretics are sometimes given to horses after a race in order to facilitate urine collection. The urine samples can then be analyzed for any traces of drugs. However, diuretics considerably alter the volume of post-race urine and can also affect the concentration of drugs in the urine.

The influence of furosemide on the concentration of phenylbutazone in both the blood and urine was tested in horses (abstracted in J.A.V.M.A. Volume 170, page 226, Jan. 15, 1977). Horses were first treated with 6.6 mg per kg (2.2 lb) of phenylbutazone, and then with 1 mg per kg of furosemide intravenously.

This diuretic had no important effects on the concentration of phenylbutazone in the blood. However, by increasing the volume of urine and thereby diluting the amount of phenylbutazone in the urine, furosemide reduced urinary concentrations of phenylbutazone 18-fold to concentrations which could affect drug detectability in routine screening tests. These studies show that it is probably not feasible to monitor compliance with phenylbutazone medication rules by means of urinalysis alone if the use of furosemide is permitted. However, furosemide treatment did not interfere with monitoring blood concentrations of phenylbutazone.

Epistaxis

In addition to the rational use of furosemide (Lasix) for reducing tissue edema, this agent is also used empirically in attempts to control epistaxis. As "empirical" indicates, the mechanism or reason why Lasix is useful in horses with nosebleed is not known. However, clinical experience by various racetrack veterinarians indicates that furosemide is of some benefit in preventing nosebleed in racehorses. Spontaneous nosebleed occurs in only a small number of horses; however, it is a serious problem in these animals since their running ability can be immediately affected, thus endangering other horses and jockeys.

Bleeding from the nose can obviously occur from a variety of factors, including: trauma, infection, tumors, lung damage, etc. The exact cause responsible for the spontaneous nosebleed seen in racehorses is not known, but infection, tumors and trauma are not thought to be primarily involved. Recently, it has been suggested that nosebleed seen in racehorses may actually be due to bleeding within the lungs. This bleeding may occur when small blood vessels of the microscopic air sacs (alveoli) of the lungs rupture in response to extreme exertion and/or forceful respiratory efforts. Blood leaking into the alveoli is then exhaled, coughed up, or sneezed and then drips from the nostrils (nares) as epistaxis.

Although the mechanism of action of furosemide in preventing nosebleed is not known, veterinarians indicated in a recent survey that an estimated 85% of the horses with epistaxis had the condition either reduced in severity or frequency or abolished completely by the drug. Perhaps as was recently suggested by a veterinary cardiologist (heart specialist), furosemide has, in addition to its diuretic effect on the kidney, a direct action on small blood vessels of the lung. This effect could render the vessels less prone to rupture. However, it is also possible that the decreased blood volume and blood pressure (produced as a result of the furosemide-induced diuresis) affect blood flow and pressure within the pulmonary (lung) circulation. For example, if blood volume and blood pressure are reduced due to diuresis, then pressure within small pulmonary blood vessels may be proportionately decreased. Thus, these vessels would be less likely to burst. Such an effect would represent a rational basis for the use of furosemide in preventing nosebleed.

It seems, however, that the use of furosemide in racehorses is not restricted to animals with nosebleed. Some racetracks require that each incidence of furosemide treatment be published in the daily record. The high incidence of use seems to indicate that furosemide is being used for purposes other than just the treatment of epistaxis. Perhaps furosemide is being used in racehorses because some people believe the drug facilitates physical performance.

Since such use represents a form of "drug misuse," several aspects of the use of furosemide should be considered. In some cases, furosemide has been given not only on the day of the race, but daily for several preceding days. Furosemide is usually given intramuscularly or intravenously in doses of 125 to 1,000 mg. In a survey, most responding veterinarians indicated the standard dose of furosemide was 200 mg given 3 to 4 hours prior to a race.

What are some of the potential consequences of such procedures in horses that do not actually have nosebleed? The most important questions are "Does the drug work?" and if so, "What does it work for?" If the first question relates to its effectiveness as a diuretic, furosemide very definitely "works," and is quite useful for collecting urine samples and for reducing edema.

Does furosemide work for epistaxis? If epistaxis is in fact caused by inflammation and disease of small airways in the lungs and if furosemide reduces edema and associated swelling of the small airway passages, then bleeding could be reduced.

Does furosemide increase performance of a racehorse? This question cannot be objectively answered at this time; however, it seems unlikely. In fact, strong argument can actually be made for adverse results of diuretics in performing horses. For example, in many cases it seems that trainers deny the horse feed and water from the time of furosemide injection until after the race. If this is true and if furosemide reduces blood volume and the amount of blood pumped by the heart per minute (cardiac output), then it seems likely that such horses are running in a mild state of dehydration and cardiovascular depression when compared to the pre-furosemide period. This means that there could be electrolyte disturbances and an increase in the viscosity of the blood. The results such serious and potentially adverse disturbances may actually exert on the performance of a horse remain to be determined.

Considerations concerning the use of furosemide in racehorses were summarized by members of the American Association of Equine Practitioners, and are reproduced herein as follows:

1. Injectable furosemide (Lasix) is an effective, safe diuretic (drug which causes increased urine production) which at the usual dose has its peak diuretic effect in about 20 minutes in horses, at which time it increases urine output up to 40-fold for a short time. Most of its diuretic effect is within the first two hours after injection.

2. During the first two hours, it decreases the pressure in the right side of the heart, decreases left atrial pressure, decreases cardiac output, and concurrently it increases peripheral (systemic) blood vessel resistance and heart rate.

3. It reduces edema (fluid) in the lungs and airway of horses with certain respiratory diseases by one or more mechanisms perhaps by lowering the pressure of the left atrium and/or increasing capacitance (ability to accept

blood) of the vessels of the lungs.

4. The mechanism by which Lasix helps prevent epistaxis (nosebleed) may result from the beneficial effect outlined in paragraph 3 above since most horses bleed from the lungs. Lasix also appears to affect the platelets which are important in the clotting mechanism.

5. The blood (plasma) level of Lasix declines rapidly. It can be detected in the urine by screening methods for the first 24 hours and by more sophisticated methods for up to 48 hours after injection.

6. Lasix does not affect the blood levels of other drugs.

7. During its peak diuretic effect, within two hours after injection, Lasix causes up to 40-fold dilution of certain drugs such as phenylbutazone (Butazolidin). However, Lasix administered more than four hours before race time does not significantly reduce the ability to detect those drugs studied to date.

8. There is no evidence that Lasix directly or indirectly affects the behavior of the horse.

9. Lasix cannot make horses race faster of perform better than their innate ability, but in many cases restores normal performance of horses which bleed.

26

HORMONES AND RELATED AGENTS

General Aspects

The endocrine system is an exceptionally complex organization of internal glands that participates to a major extent in the everyday regulation of bodily functions. This is carried out by the secretion from the endocrine glands of highly active substances, called hormones, into the blood stream. Hormones are circulated in the blood to their target organs, i.e., those particular tissues and body organs that the hormone affects. For example, the pituitary gland secretes several hormones, one of which is called follicle stimulating hormone or FSH. In the mare (and also in females of other mammalian species), FSH circulates in the blood from the brain to the ovaries where it stimulates the ovaries so that the development of ovarian follicles (which contain ova) is accelerated. In the stallion, FSH stimulates the testis to increase production of spermatozoa, i.e, spermatogenesis.

It should be remembered that hormones do not grant some "new power or function" to any particular tissue or organ, i.e., hormones (as is the case with any drug) can not make body parts perform any function that they do not normally perform. Rather, hormones act as regulators to increase, decrease, accelerate, decelerate, etc., normal activities of body tissues. Thus, a hormone can be defined as "a chemical substance produced in one part of the body that is transported in the blood to another area of the body, where it influences and regulates cellular functions."

From the above discussion, it can be appreciated that endocrine function is quite complex. Since normal "hormonal balance" can be easily disrupted by the administration of exogenous (outside-the-body source) hormones, hormone therapy in the horse is not administered indescriminately. Thus, hormone therapy in horses should only be administered by, or under close supervision of, the veterinarian.

Endocrine Glands

There are numerous endogenous (i.e., produced within the body) substances that have been discovered that comply with the definition of a hormone. However, there are only about a dozen major endocrine glands that are defined as producing the "classical" endocrine hormones. Although all of these glands are absolutely essential for normal bodily functions, a few are relatively more important than the others when the horse is considered. Major endocrine hormones, their target tissues and their major activities are summarized in the accompanying tables.

Hormone Therapy

In relation to the therapeutic use of hormones, two basic courses of action are recognized: replacement therapy and additive therapy.

Replacement therapy: This course of action involves the administration of small physiological amounts (i.e., amounts which correspond to the amounts normally present in the body) of a hormone, which acts to replace the hormone normally produced by a gland that is now failing in its hormone production capabilities. For example, if the thyroid gland has to be surgically removed, then it is necessary to administer exogenous thyroid hormone, thyroxine, to the horse in order to maintain body metabolism. Probably one of the most well recognized forms of replacement therapy involves the use of insulin in diabetes. Insulin is given only when the pancreas fails to produce adequate amounts of insulin, i.e., exogenous insulin is used to replace insulin normally provided by the pancreas.

Additive therapy: In contrast to replacement therapy, additive therapy involves the administration of relatively large amounts of a hormone in an attempt to achieve a specific effect not usually related to natural metabolic functions. For example, large doses of corticosteroids exert a rather pronounced anti-inflammatory effect, and are often used in horses for this purpose. In physiological situations, however, corticosteroids are regulators of protein, carbohydrate and other metabolic activities of various different tissue types.

A potential problem with additive therapy is that, due to the large amount of hormone usually required, serious side effects may result. In particular, the presence in the horse's body of large amounts of exogenous hormone can disrupt normal hormonal balance. These important factors are always considered when hormone therapy is required in horses.

In the remainder of this chapter, some of the major hormones and their uses are summarized. The reader should refer to the tables for hormonal source, target tissues and principal physiological actions of major hormones.

Metabolic Hormones

Thyroid Stimulating Hormone: This hormone is secreted by the pituitary gland, and it stimulates the thyroid gland to increase production of thyroxine, the thyroid hormone. TSH is rarely used therapeutically, but has occasionally been used to test for thyroid gland function.

Thyroxine: This hormone is secreted by the thyroid gland, and it affects all the cells of the body by increasing their metabolic rate. Thyroxine is used therapeutically in man and dogs when the thyroid gland fails to produce enough natural hormone. This condition is infrequently seen in horses. If therapy is not instituted in these cases, the patient becomes overweight, lethargic, and has a low metabolic rate. Goiter is a term used to describe enlargement of the thyroid, often seen in conjunction with iodine deficiency. If hypothyroidism is diagnosed in a horse, thyroid extracts have been used in the dosage of 2.5 to 5.0 grams per 100 pounds body weight.

Parathyroid Hormone (Parathormone): This hormone is produced by the parathyroid glands, and it is essential for regulation of the concentration of calcium dissolved in the blood (i.e., "ionized calcium"). Without the parathyroid glands and PTH, the horse will die from convulsions due to abnormally low serum concentrations of calcium. However, primary hypoparathyroidism (i.e., inadequate amounts) or hyperparathyroidism (i.e., too much PTH) is rarely seen in horses. On the other hand, secondary hyperparathyroidism can be induced in horses by improper, poorly balanced rations characterized by excess phosphorus in relation to calcium. Such diets are usually due to excess grain or grain by-products without appropriate calcium supplementation.

Bone formation problems, bone swelling and lamenesses are the principal clinical signs of nutritional hyperparathyroidism. Treatment involves correction of the improper ration.

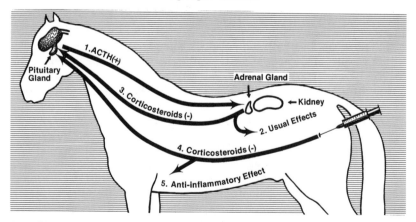

Fig. 26-1 Action of steriod anti-inflammatory drugs. 1. ACTH stimulates the adrenal gland to release corticosteriods into the bloodstream. 2. Corticosteroids affect body metabolsim, and 3. tell the pituitary gland to decrease ACTH production. 4. Large doses of exogenous corticosteroids decrease the ACTH released from the pituitary, and 5. produce an anti-inflammatory effect.

Insulin: This hormone is produced by the pancreas, and it serves to increase the movement of blood sugar (glucose) into cells for metabolic demands. When insulin secretion fails, glucose increases dramatically in the blood and in the urine, resulting in diabetes mellitus. Glucagon is another pancreatic hormone. It was recently discovered and acts to decrease movement of glucose into cells and works in a reciprocal manner with insulin. Diabetes is rarely encountered in horses.

Adrenal Corticosteroids: These hormones are produced by the outer (cortex) portion of the adrenal glands, in response to stimulation of the adrenal cortex by adrenocortical stimulating hormone (ACTH), a hormone released by the pituitary. Corticosteroids are used extensively in horses to reduce inflammation of the musculoskeletal system. The use of ACTH and corticosteroids is discussed in the chapter on "Analgesic and Anti-inflammatory Drugs."

Reproductive Hormones

Follicle Stimulating Hormone: This hormone is secreted by the pituitary gland. It stimulates the ovary, resulting in acceleration of ovarian follicle development. In males, FSH affects the testis by stimulating the production of sperm. FSH-like activity has been identified in pregnant mares' serum and in urine of pregnant women, as discussed in the following paragraphs.

Luteinizing Hormone: LH in the mare stimulates the ovarian follicle to maturation, estrogen production and finally ovulation. In stallions, Interstitial Cell Stimulating Hormone (ICSH), stimulates the testis to produce testosterone, the male sex hormone. LH, itself, is not used, but other products containing LH-like activity have been discovered, as discussed below.

Sheep's Anterior Pituitary Extract: An extract prepared from the pituitary glands of sheep contains both FSH and LH activity. Thus, it is useful both for stimulating development of follicles (by FSH activity) and for follicle maturation, induction of estrus through estrogen production and ovulation (by LH activity). It is used therapeutically in mares to stimulate ovulation, and to stimulate prepubertal, anestrous or sterile ovaries. The dose is usually 5 ml of the extract, equivalent to 5 mg FSH and 5 mg LH activity, by subcutaneous injection.

Pregnant Mare Serum Gonadotropin: "Gonadotropin" refers to stimulation of the gonads (i.e., ovaries and testes). The gonadotropins include FSH, LH, and ICSH. PMSG has primarily FSH-like activity with lesser amounts of LH-like activity. Thus, PMSG is referred to as a FSH-like hormone, and it is used widely in veterinary medicine to stimulate follicular growth in inactive ovaries of mature animals.

The ovaries of the noncycling mare are usually nonresponsive to PMSG in midwinter during the period of natural ovarian inactivity. However, PMSG will usually produce estrus in 5 to 8 days, followed by ovulation, if it is given in autumn or late winter. Dosage in horses is 1,000 to 2,000 units by subcutaneous, intramuscular or intravenous injection.

Human Chorionic Gonadotropin: This substance is found in the urine during the first 50 days of pregnancy in women. Its activity is primarily LH-like but also contains FSH-like activity. HCG is used in the mare to cause ovulation at time of breeding at the dose of 2,500 units by intravenous injection to 10,000 units by intramuscular injection. HCG is useful in stimulating the testicles of the stallion to increase production of the male sex hormone, testosterone.

Testosterone: This hormone is the male sex hormone, i.e., an androgen; it is produced by the testis and is responsible for development of genitalia, accessory sex organs and secondary sex characteristics of the male. Testosterone also exerts an anabolic effect, i.e., it increases tissue growth as will be discussed in a subsequent paragraph. Testosterone has been used in the stallion in attempts to treat infertility, hypogonadism, aspermia and decreased libido; however, useful results are not always obtained. Doses are usually 100-300 mg, 2 to 3 times weekly, by intramuscular injection of testosterone in oil.

Estrogen: This is the female sex hormone; it is secreted by the ovaries and is responsible for development of female sex characteristics, estrus, genitalia development etc. in the mare. Synthetic estrogens, such as diethylstilbesterol (DES), have largely replaced the more expensive natural estrogens. DES does not stimulate the ovaries, and will produce an artificial estrus with the usual external manifestations of heat but without ovulation unless ovulation would have occurred anyway. In mares that cycle, but show little outward evidence of estrus, DES has been used to induce a more receptive estrus when given in 5 to 25 mg doses intramuscularly. However, the proper timing of DES administration in the estrus cycle is essential if conception is to occur.

Progesterone: This hormone is produced by the corpus luteum of the ovary. The corpus luteum develops after ovulation, and its production of progesterone is important for maintenance of pregnancy. Progesterone has been used in attempts to prevent abortion, delay parturition, suppress estrus and synchronize estrus.

If pregnancy does not occur, the corpus luteum normally regresses and another estrus cycle is initiated. Sometimes, however, a corpus luteum persists, resulting in anestrus. Certain chemicals (e.g. prostaglandins) have been discovered that will cause regression of the corpus luteum, i.e., luteolysis. Such chemicals have been found to be useful in bringing non-breeding mares back into estrus cycle and for synchronizing estrus in broodmare operations. These aspects are considered below, under prostaglandins.

Synthetic Anabolic Hormones

In addition to its effect on male sexual characteristics, the male sex hormone (testosterone) also exerts an "anabolic" effect. "Anabolism" refers to the "building up" of tissues that occurs, for example, through increased protein synthesis in cells. Thus, male sex hormones (classified as a group by the term "androgens") increase the synthesis by the body of new tissues and therefore, enhance repair of damaged tissues. Such an anabolic effect has proven therapeutically useful.

Since the natural male hormone produces profound effects on sex characteristics, it would not be therapeutically useful as an anabolic agent since masculinization would also result. However, new synthetic hormone-like chemicals have been discovered that exert pronounced anabolic (i.e., tissue building) effects with minimal adrogenic (i.e., male sex hormone) activity. These compounds are receiving wide usage and evaluation in veterinary medicine at the present time. It will require considerably more research and clinical experience before all aspects of synthetic anabolic agents are defined, especially in horses; however, initial results appear promising. Stanozolol (Winstrol-V: Winthrop) and boldenone undecylenate (Equipoise: Squibb) are two anabolic steroids now available. These compounds have been recommended as an aid for treating debilitated horses when an improvement in weight, haircoat, and general physical condition is desired. Debilitation often occurs after major surgery, systemic disease, or prolonged anorexia. In clinical trials, it was reported by the manufacturer of Equipoise that at recommended doses this agent had a marked anabolic effect in debilitated horses: appetite improved, vigor increased, and improvement was noted in musculature and haircoat. Anabolic steroids may be particularly useful if there has been major tissue breakdown associated with the debilitating condition.

Although anabolic steroids may be useful in improving the general state of debilitated horses, thus aiding in correcting weight loss and improving appetite, they, of course, are not substitutes for well-balanced rations. As with any drug therapy, optimal results can be expected only when good management and feeding practices are observed. Anabolic steroids represent only a supportive or adjunctive therapy to the specific measures necessary to correct the primary disorder.

The dosage for Equipoise in horses is 0.5 mg per pound of body weight, intramuscularly. Treatment may be repeated at three week intervals. Response should be seen with one or two treatments. If masculinizing effects are seen, they are reported to be transitory; however, further injections should not be given. Caution: Possible side effects of anabolic steroids on breeding stallions and pregnant mares have not been determined at this time. These drugs should not be used in these animals.

Prostaglandins

These compounds occur to some extent in nearly all mammalian tissues. Their name was derived because they were first discovered in human semen, and it was thought they originated from the prostate glands.

Actually, prostaglandins are produced locally in a wide variety of tissues and do not depend upon any one organ for their source. In this respect, they do not strictly meet the definition of a hormone, but they are included in this chapter because of numerous similarities and their obvious connection with reproductive hormones.

Prostaglandins have a wide variety of different physiological actions, some of which are no doubt undiscovered at this time. It is likely, however, that prostaglandins are in some way involved in generation of local pain (refer to "Analgesics and Anti-inflammatory Drugs"), and there is considerable evidence that prostaglandins can affect different reproductive functions. In particular, these compounds can produce abortion through a luteolytic effect, i.e., by causing the regression of the corpus luteum (the small body on the ovary that produces the pregnancy-maintaining hormone, progesterone).

The ability of prostaglandins (particularly those chemically designated as "PGF_{2a}") and synthetically derived related chemicals to produce luteolysis in nonpregnant mares has proven therapeutically useful in regulating estrus, and therefore, breeding times, and also for increasing breeding success in difficult-to-breed mares, as follows:

1. Synchronization of estrus in estrus cycling mares: Mares treated with PGF_{2a} (dinoprost tromethamine, Prostin F_{2a}) or the synthetic analog prostalene (Synchrocept) during diestrus (4 or 5 days afer ovulation) have been reported to return to estrus within 2 to 4 days in most cases and to ovulate 8 to 12 days after injection.

2. Difficult-to-breed mares: In extended diestrus, there is failure to exhibit regular estrus cycles, which is different from true anestrus. Many mares described as anestrus during the breeding season may have a persistent corpus luteum (thereby inhibiting follicle development and estrus). Also, a proportion of maiden, lactating and "barren" mares that do not exhibit regular estrus cycles may be in extended diestrus due to the presence of a functional and persistent corpus luteum.

Treatment of such mares with PGF_{2a} or prostalene has been reported to usually result in regression of the corpus luteum followed by estrus and/or ovulation. In one study, mares that had been in clinical anestrus for an average of 58 days were treated with an injection of 5 mg PGF_{2a}, during the breeding season. Behavioral estrus was detected in 81 percent at an average time of 3.7 days after treatment, while ovulation occurred an average of 7 days after treatment. Of the mares bred, 59 percent were pregnant following an average of 1.4 services by the stallion during that estrus. Thus, prostaglandins may well prove to have clinically useful value in the treatment of certain breeding problems of mares.

However, several critical contraindications and precautions should be carefully considered when a prostaglandin is used:

1. Obviously, the reproductive status of any mare should be carefully evaluated before treatment with prostaglandin is attempted. For

example, this compound will not be useful if the mare is not properly cycling due to uterine infection rather than persistent corpus luteum!

2. Prostaglandin is ineffective if administered within 5 days of ovulation.
3. Prostaglandin should not be given to pregnant mares since abortion may result.
4. Prostaglandin should not be given to mares affected with reproductive, gastrointestinal, respiratory or cardiovascular disease.
5. The intravenous route of administration is contraindicated.
6. Nonsteroidal anti-inflammatory agents (e.g., phenylbutazone) should not be administered concurrently.

Prostalene (Synchrocept), as mentioned, is a synthetic analog of PGF_{2a} that is reported to have none of the adverse side effects of sweating, increased blood pressure and gastrointestinal function associated with PGF_{2a}. Indications for prostalene are basically the same as for Prostin F_{2a}.

Antihistamines

Antihistamines are not hormones; however, they are included in this chapter because they are used to counteract the effects of histamine, a substance sometimes described as a "local hormone." Histamine is not produced by any particular organ, but is released from several different tissues, particularly mast cells. Histamine is released from mast cells in response to burns, allergic reactions, and other types of trauma. In the horse, allergic reactions are probably the most important cause of histamine release.

After histamine is released from the mast cells, it produces many of the local signs associated with allergic injury, such as local swelling, redness, itching, and pain. In fact, the characteristic local signs that histamine produces are quite familiar to most people since such signs commonly occur with insect bites and stings. The local response to histamine has been described as the "triple response," since it is characterized by three signs, as follows:

1. a localized red spot at the immediate site of the insect bite; this red spot may later turn bluish
2. a brighter red flush or "flare" extended around the red center of the bite area
3. localized swelling (edema)

These signs are the result of histamine's actions on the permeability of local blood vessels, causing leakage of blood from the capillaries, along with other effects.

Histamine can also be released throughout the body in response to severe injury or, importantly, allergic reactions. The result is systemic changes that can include hypotension (low blood pressure), intense itching, wheals (localized swollen spots) such as urticaria, and respiratory problems. Drugs that prevent or reverse these effects of histamine are referred to as antihistamines, and they have found various usages in equine medicine.

Antihistamines are very useful in counteracting signs of allergic reactions to vaccinations, environmental allergies, urticaria, insect bites and stings, and other immunogenic-based responses. Purpura, lymphangitis, heaves, and laminitis have also been treated with antihistamines. Treatment may have to be repeated, since the effects of antihistamines may wear off before the condition has been resolved. Diphenhydramine (Benadryl: Parke-Davis) and promethazine (Phenergan: Wyeth) are commonly used antihistamines. Dosage varies with the individual drugs, and should be administered only by or under the supervision of a veterinarian. Antihistamines can cause depression and drowsiness or even hyperexcitability and convulsions, depending on dosage.

Fig. 26-2   TABLE 1
MAJOR ENDOCRINE HORMONES AFFECTING METABOLISM

Hormone	Source	Major Functions
Growth Hormone (GH) Somatotropin)	Pituitary	Accelerates body growth.
Thyroid Stimulating Hormone (TSH)	Pituitary	Stimulates thyroid gland to increase production of Thyroxine, the thyroid hormone.
Thyroxine	Thyroid	Increases metabolic rate of body tissues.
Adrenocorticotropic Hormone (ACTH)	Pituitary	Stimulates cortex of adrenal gland to increase production of corticosteroids.
Cortisol (major corticosteriod)	Adrenal Cortex	Affects various tissue metabolic processes.
Vasopressin (anti-diuretic hormone, ADH)	Pituitary	Increases water retention by the kidneys.
Insulin	Pancreas, beta cells	Increases entry of blood glucose into body cells, decreased blood glucose levels.
Glucagon	Pancreas, alpha cells	Raises blood glucose levels.
Parathyroid Hormone	Parathyroid	Calcium metabolism regulator.
Calcitonin	Thyroid	Calcium metabolism regulator.

Fig. 26-2 TABLE 2
MAJOR HORMONES AFFECTING REPRODUCTION

Hormone	Source	Major Functions
Follicle Stimulating Hormone (FSH)	Pituitary	(F) Stimulates growth of ovarian follicles. (M) Increases spermatogenesis.
Luteinizing Hormone (LH), or Interstitial Cell Stimulating Hormone (ICSH)	Pituitary	(F) Stimulates ovulation of ovarian follicles & production by ovaries of estrogen, the female sex hormone. (M) Stimulates secretion of male sex hormone, testosterone, by testis.
Prolactin (Luteotropic Hormone)	Pituitary	Stimulates milk production.
Oxytocin	Pituitary	Stimulates milk ejection.
Progesterone	Ovary (corpus luteum)	Maintains pregnancy.
Testosterone (Androgen)	Testis	Development and maintenance of male sex characteristics, and an anabolic effect (i.e., increased tissue growth).
Estrogen	Ovary	Development and maintenance of female sex characteristics, estrus inducing hormone.

(M) = male
(F) = female

27

VITAMINS AND MINERALS

Vitamins and minerals are essential for proper body growth and function. Because of the easy availability of most vitamins and minerals, these compounds have often been misrepresented, misunderstood, and misused. The indescriminate use of vitamins and mineral preparations is not only expensive, but may result in serious toxic effects and may even delay the diagnosis and treatment of an illness. When supplementation is required, care should be taken to maintain proper balances and levels since many vitamins and minerals interact with each other.

Vitamins

Vitamin supplementation may be necessary because of inadequate vitamin intake, a disturbance in absorption, or an increase in tissue requirement. An inadequate intake of vitamins may be caused by poor-quality feed, or a decrease in feed consumption. In some instances, a type of feed may destroy certain vitamins or cause an imbalance between vitamins (for example, bracken fern destroys vitamin B_1). A decrease in the absorption of vitamins may be caused by liver diseases, prolonged diarrhea, anemia, or digestive system disorders. An increase in tissue requirement, such as from pregnancy and lactation, growth, hard physical work, or diseases associated with increased metabolism, will automatically mean an increase in vitamin requirement. Since a deficiency of a single vitamin is rare, multiple vitamin therapy is usually recommended. For normal vitamin requirements, the recommended guidelines found in the text of FEEDING TO WIN should be satisfactory.

Vitamins are divided into two categories, depending on whether they are soluble in fat and oil, or in water. The fat-soluble vitamins are A, D, E, and K, while the water-soluble vitamins are the B complex vitamins and vitamin C.

FAT-SOLUBLE VITAMINS

Fat-soluble vitamins have several common characteristics in addition to their ability to dissolve in fats or fat solvents. These vitamins are stored mainly in the liver, although to a small extent they are also stored in other fatty tissue. An excess of any of the fat-soluble vitamins may cause toxic effects since large amounts can be stored, while utilization and excretion are slow. Fat-soluble vitamin deficiencies may occur during periods where there is interference with fat absorption, since absorption of these vitamins is similar to that of other fats.

VITAMIN A

Horses obtain vitamin A by ingesting carotene (the precursor to vitamin A) which is a yellow pigment occurring with chlorophyll in green plants. Carotene is then converted to vitamin A within the horse by an enzyme reaction in the intestine. Fresh green forages and high-quality hay, such as alfalfa, contain large amounts of carotene. The amount of carotene in old hay is questionable, however, since this substance is unstable and is affected by heat, light, and oxidation. A rich green colored hay is usually desirable, as the color may be some indication of its value. Pastured horses need to store enough vitamin A in the summer to meet their requirements during the winter months when the carotene content in grass is low.

Vitamin A is important in maintaining epithelial cell function, including the epithelial cells of the skin, eyes, and various mucosal membranes. An adequate amount of vitamin A will provide some resistance to parasites and infection, and will facilitate the healing of wounds that have been slow to repair due to the administration of anti-inflammatory agents. Vitamin A requirements increase during pregnancy, lactation, and growth, and may increase during periods of stress. Oral or injectable preparations can be used for supplementation in either a natural or synthetic form.

A deficiency in vitamin A is characterized by loss of appetite, night blindness, tearing (lacrimation), respiratory infections, and reproductive problems. Other signs may include convulsions, weakness, and keratinization of the cornea and skin (which lowers the body's natural defenses). Lameness resulting from hoof lesions may be another indication of vitamin A deficiency. Mineral oil interferes with the absorption of vitamin A, so a chronically colicky horse that is frequently dosed with the oil may develop a deficiency. Broodmares may also become deficient in vitamin A during the last months of pregnancy, due to depletion of winter stores of the vitamin. A severe vitamin A deficiency may even result in weak, blind, deformed, or dead offspring.

Vitamin A can be toxic if given in amounts greater than four times the storage capacity of the liver. Signs of vitamin A toxicity are similar to those of a deficiency, and may include brittle hoofs, lethargy, colic, hyperostosis (abnormal bone growth) and other bone disorders.

VITAMIN D

Vitamin D is stored in all the tissues of the body, but is concentrated primarily in the liver. The main functions of vitamin D are to assist calcium-phosphorus absorption, to maintain the necessary level of calcium in the blood, and to reabsorb calcium from bone. To some extent, vitamin

D acts as a hormone, since it is produced in the body, transported in the blood, and bodily functions are activated and influenced by it.

Horses almost always receive adequate amounts of vitamin D in sun-cured forages (legumes are the highest), or from direct sunlight. The ultraviolet rays of the sun activate skin sterols to produce vitamin D. Only about thirty to sixty minutes of daily exposure to sunlight is needed for an adequate amount of the vitamin to be synthesized.

Any drastic change in the levels of vitamin D, calcium or phosphorus, has an effect on body metabolism. Vitamin D plays an active part in the intestinal transportation of calcium and phosphorus, by increasing the absorption of the two minerals. If excessive amounts of calcium and phosphorus are introduced into the body, the available vitamin D is utilized in the absorption and distribution of the two minerals. If a vitamin D deficiency results, the absorption of calcium and phosphorus is limited and this in turn creates a deficiency in the two minerals. In young horses, a deficiency in vitamin D, resulting in decreased absorption of phosphorus and calcium, is the cause of rickets. In this disease, insufficient calcium and phosphorus in the blood prevent the normal conversion of cartilage into calcified bone. If the imbalance continues, calcium is eventually reabsorbed from the structural elements of bone, which may lead to osteomalacia.

The over-supplementation of vitamin D will cause an excessive amount of calcium and phosphorus to be absorbed into the blood. Instead of the normal process of bone formation or storage occurring, soft tissues are calcified. Calcium may even be deposited into the blood vessels and heart. Bone abnormalities, kidney damage, and calcification of the heart may result. Vitamin D toxicity is more often a problem than vitamin D deficiency, because of the tendency of horsemen to oversupplement with protein mixtures containing vitamins. Vitamins, A, D, and E are usually found in a high concentration in most protein supplements, so vitamin levels should be taken into account when feeding a protein supplement.

VITAMIN E

Vitamin E (alpha-tocopherol) is an essential compound and primarily functions to prevent oxidation (breakdown) of fats. As an antioxidant, alpha-tocopherol acts by inhibiting the oxidation of lipids (fats), thereby preventing them from deteriorating or becoming rancid. The most important function of vitamin E as an antioxidant is in the stabilization of cellular membranes. Cellular membranes are made up of lipoproteins, and the oxidation of these lipids could lead to massive ruptures of the cell walls. Vitamin E also functions as an antioxidant outside the body. It is often added to grains as a preservative, because it prevents the oils in the feed from becoming rancid. It should be remembered, however, that the vitamin E added to feed may be partially depleted in the antioxidating process, and the full amount of the vitamin may not be available to the horse as a supplement. There is still controversy over the other possible functions of vitamin E in horses. Some trainers and breeders believe (and some studies have indicated) that large doses of the vitamin improve performance and fertility, although this has not been conclusively proven.

There is a relationship between alpha-tocopherol and the mineral selenium, in that they both help to maintain cellular membranes. An adequate amount of vitamin E may lessen the body's requirements for selenium, and vice versa, but the two compounds are not interchangeable. A preparation of vitamin E and selenium is often administered by injection to treat or prevent azoturia and "tying up."

Alpha-tocopherol is found in cereal grains, high-quality hay, and wheat germ oil. Although there is usually sufficient vitamin E in the normal, well-balanced ration, some compounds (such as unsaturated fatty acids) destroy alpha-tocopherol, or prevent its utilization. If supplementation is necessary or desired, vitamin E can be found in commercial vitamin preparations, or in its natural form in wheat germ oil.

Vitamin E deficiency is uncommon in the horse, but may occur when some types of feed, such as weed seeds or cottonseed meal are ingested and destroy the vitamin. An alpha-tocopherol deficiency may result in muscle disorders, such as azoturia, and may have some effect on reproduction.

It appears that vitamin E is not toxic; however, it is a stored vitamin and is secreted slowly. There is a possibility that extremely large doses of the vitamin, over a prolonged period of time, could produce some toxic effects. Extreme caution should be used when using a vitamin E preparation containing selenium. Excessive amounts of selenium supplementation can be toxic.

VITAMIN K

The main function of vitamin K is in blood coagulation. The vitamin is synthesized in the horse's intestine from a precursor found in leafy green plants. It is then used in liver cells for the synthesis of prothrombin, which is one of the ten factors needed for the clotting of blood. Vitamin K may also be involved with several other compounds necessary for blood clotting.

Supplementation may be indicated when there is bleeding, or when other compounds inhibit or destroy vitamin K. An adequate level of the vitamin is especially important in pregnant mares because there is danger of hemorrhaging after foaling if the blood does not properly clot. Race horses suffering from epistaxis (nosebleed), can be treated with vitamin K in conjunction with vitamin C (refer to "Epistaxis"). Supplementation may be needed when a horse receives high doses of antibiotics, since prolonged oral medication with these agents can destroy the bacteria that synthesize vitamin K in the intestine. Even when a horse does synthesize enough vitamin K, a deficiency may develop if moldy hay or sweet clover is ingested. Dicoumarol, a compound found in spoiled sweet clover and some moldy hays, counteracts the action of prothrombin and inhibits blood clotting. Since vitamin K is synthesized in the distal portions of the intestines, much of it may be passed out in the feces. Coprophagy (eating of feces) is common in horses deficient in this vitamin. If supplementation is necessary, the veterinarian will recommend either oral doses or injections of vitamin K.

A delayed clotting time of the blood is the most common sign of vitamin K deficiency, and an injury such as a contusion may cause considerable bleeding and the formation of a hematoma. When there is a severe vitamin K deficiency, the horse may even hemorrhage spontaneously at body openings.

WATER-SOLUBLE VITAMINS

Water-soluble vitamins are distributed more uniformly in the tissue than the fat-soluble vitamins, so there are no large deposits, such as that of vitamin A in the liver. The stores that do exist are used up fairly quickly or excreted, so toxicity is usually not a problem if kidney function is normal.

The water-soluble vitamins are available from plant and animal sources. Mature horses are usually able to derive adequate amounts from feed or by synthesization in the cecum. Supplementation may be necessary if there is an insufficient amount of feed, if absorption is disrupted, or if a horse is suffering from a chronic disease. Additional vitamins may also be indicated when the tissue requirements are greater, such as in young foals and hard-working older horses. Interference with absorption may be a problem when there is prolonged diarrhea, when some types of plants are ingested, or when large doses of antibiotics are given.

The water-soluble vitamin category is comprised mainly of vitamin C, and the B complex vitamins, which include:

B_1 (thiamin)	biotin
B_2 (riboflavin)	pantothenic acid
B_6 (pyridoxine)	choline
niacin (nicotinic acid)	inositol
B_{12} (cyanocobalamin)	folic acid

B COMPLEX VITAMINS

Many of the B vitamins are components of coenzymes and function in basically similar manners. Only B_1, B_2, B_6, niacin, and B_{12} will be discussed, since their functions and requirements are the best understood in the horse. There is no evidence available that indicates supplementation with other B vitamins is beneficial; however, all the B complex vitamins can be easily given by the addition of brewer's yeast in the grain ration. Many of the B vitamins are available either separately or combined in injectable solutions.

Vitamin B_1

Vitamin B_1 (thiamin) functions in metabolism by acting as an enzyme which helps break down carbohydrates into a usable energy form (sugars). B_1 is found in green leafy plants, well-cured hay, and whole cereal grains.

Thiamin is not normally deficient in horses; however, a steady diet of bracken fern destroys the vitamin and can cause deficiency signs. It is also believed that laryngeal hemiplegia (roaring) may be related to a thiamin deficiency. Signs of a deficiency may include weight loss, diarrhea, weakness, and muscular incoordination. If a severe B_1 deficiency is not corrected, the horse may go into convulsions and eventually die from cardiac failure.

Vitamin B_2

Vitamin B_2 (riboflavin) is important in cellular function, and is a component in some enzymes which affect the metabolism of carbohydrates and protein. It is found to some extent in green leafy forages and in a higher concentration in brewer's yeast.

Signs of a B_2 deficiency may include slow growth, dermatitis and infertility. Riboflavin deficiency has also been implicated as a possible cause of periodic ophthalmia or "moon blindness." This disease is characterized by lacrimation (discharge of tears) and photophobia, and in severe cases, blindness. Although an insufficient amount of riboflavin may precipitate "moon blindness," the vitamin is usually ineffective in the treatment of this condition.

Vitamin B_6

Vitamin B_6 (pyridoxine) forms an enzyme that is important in amino acid and protein metabolism. Yeast, bran, and wheat germ oil all contain considerable amounts of B_6. Pyridoxine is not a dietary essential of the horse since it is normally synthesized in the cecum. A B_6 deficiency is extremely rare, but may include signs such as dermatitis and weak muscle action.

Niacin

Niacin is a component of several enzymes which are essential in metabolism. Except for corn, cereal grains consumed by horses tend to be high in tryptophan (an amino acid), which can be converted by the horse into niacin. Therefore, this vitamin rarely needs to be supplemented in a horse's ration.

Vitamin B_{12}

Vitamin B_{12} (cyanocobalamin) promotes the formation of blood cells (hematopoiesis). It also functions in protein metabolism as it forms several coenzymes, and is a growth promoter. The exact dietary requirements of the horse for cyanocobalamin are not known, although it is sometimes given intramusclarly in the treatment of myositis, weakness, anemia, and anorexia (loss of appetite). Some horsemen and veterinarians believe that B_{12} also produces a sense of well-being.

VITAMIN C

Vitamin C (ascorbic acid) is required for the production of some amino acids, as well as collagen (connective tissue). Vitamin C is active in the formation of cartilage, aids ossification, and encourages the healing of wounds, burns and fractures. For this reason, ascorbic acid is believed to be beneficial when given to a stressed horse. For example, it sometimes helps in healing when given after surgery. Ascorbic acid is not needed in the mature horse's diet, since it is synthesized in the horse.

Minerals

Minerals are inorganic compounds, which are essential for sound skeletal development and normal metabolism. The minerals vital to the horse include:

sodium	zinc
chloride	iron
calcium	copper
phosphorus	manganese
potassium	fluorine
magnesium	selenium
iodine	cobalt

Although these minerals are vital, many are only required in minute amounts and excesses can prove highly toxic. Most minerals have an interrelationship, and an abnormally high level of one mineral may affect the requirements of other minerals. Therefore, to maintain a mineral balance, proper proportions are as important as adequate levels.

Minerals are typically consumed by a horse through feed and water supplies which contain minerals derived from the soil. Therefore, a soil lacking in an important mineral will produce forage which is also low in that mineral. Ideally, an analysis of water and soil should be done to determine what mineral deficiencies are present, and what type of dietary supplementation is needed. Hay and feed analysis can be very beneficial in balancing the diet of a stalled horse.

Minerals are supplied to horses in a variety of ways. In the free-choice method, minerals are supplied in either block or loose form. Blocks were originally intended for cattle, which prehend with their tongue. Since horses prehend (pick up food) with their lips, it is difficult for them to consume enough minerals from a block to meet their requirements. Therefore, a loose salt form is the preferred method of providing free-choice minerals. Minerals can also be force-fed by mixing a supplement in the horse's ration, by using mineralized water, or by using grains and forages high in mineral content. The force-feed method is unsatisfactory in most instances, since it is difficult to supply the necessary minerals at just the right levels and proportions. It is usually better to provide salt and trace mineral salt free-choice so that the horse can self-feed at his own rate.

SODIUM CHLORIDE

The mineral needed in a horse's diet in the greatest amount is sodium chloride salt. Sodium chloride is a salt, meaning a combination of an acid and a base, but it is not the only one. However, sodium chloride is commonly referred to simply as salt. As well as being a nutrient, the addition of salt in the diet makes feed and minerals more palatable. Sodium chloride is vital in maintaining the proper fluid and electrolyte balance in the body. Since salt is regularly excreted in the urine, as well as being used in bodily functions, at least 60 grams a day should be supplied to adult horses. Lactating mares will need more salt, since some is lost in supplying milk to the foal. Supplemental salt is also required by horses under conditions of hot weather and hard exercise, since sodium chloride helps regulate the cooling mechanism in the body and is excreted through sweat (perspiration is 0.7% salt).

Salt is easily supplied by mixing it in the feed and by providing it in loose form. Since the salt needs of individual horses will vary, only the minimum requirement should be added to the horse's ration. Additional salt can be provided with a free-choice supply. However, horses may consume too much salt, if they have been salt-deprived and are suddenly allowed access to salt, or if they are confined in stalls for long periods of time and become bored. In this circumstance, the free-choice salt may be supplied in a block, in order to limit the horse's salt intake. Whichever way salt is supplied, it should be constantly available and ample water should always be supplied .

A sodium chloride deficiency will decrease the horse's appetite and water intake. The horse may show signs of fatigue and heat exhaustion. In addition, a salt deficiency retards growth, reduces lactation and causes a rough haircoat. A horse suffering from a deficiency of this or any other mineral, may begin chewing wood, or eating dirt and other non-food objects.

Sodium chloride toxicity is not common, but when it occurs, will cause a severe fluid imbalance and may prove fatal. Excessive sodium chloride intake is a danger if the animal is fed a ration overly supplemented with salt. In addition, toxicity may occur if a horse is supplied salt without access to sufficient water, or if the only water available is high in saline content.

CALCIUM AND PHOSPHORUS

One of the oldest mineral interrelationships known is that of calcium and phosphorus. Calcium and phosphorus are especially crucial in the growth process of young horses where the proper amounts of both minerals are required in order for cartilage to be converted into calcified bone (ossification). The bones also serve as storage for the calcium-phosphate complex until it is needed. This reserve will be utilized during periods of insufficient intake, periods of stress, and during pregnancy and lactation.

Calcium and phosphorus have other functions in addition to their roles in bone structure. Calcium is vital in many bodily functions, and phosphorus is important in metabolic reactions involving enzymes and vitamins.

Calcium and phosphorus must be in the correct ratio or the two minerals will combine into compounds which cannot be absorbed in the intestine. A severe and long-term imbalance can cause serious diseases. A horse on a well-balanced diet should receive the proper ratio of the two minerals, since a good quality hay is high in calcium, and grains are normally high in phosphorus. (Refer to "Nutrition" or to the text FEEDING TO WIN for information on the proper calcium to phosphorus ratio).

Calcium and phosphorus not only affect each other, but are also affected by other elements, vitamins and hormones. Supplementation of calcium and/or phosphorus may be needed when there is an interference in absorption, when there is an imbalance of the two minerals in the diet, or when there is an increase in requirement. The primary vitamin which affects calcium and phosphorus is vitamin D. This vitamin is now thought to be a major factor influencing the metabolism of the two minerals. Some organic acids (such as phytic acid and oxalic acid) found in feeds interfere with mineral absorption by combining with calcium and phosphorus to form unabsorbable compounds. The same is true when metals, such as magnesium, iron, and aluminum, are ingested in great quantities. The metals combine with phosphorus to form unabsorbable phosphate compounds. There may be an imbalance of calcium and phosphorus in the feeds of certain geographical regions where there are deficiencies, or heavy deposits, of one mineral or the other.

The calcium-phosphorus ratio should also be thought of in terms of bodily requirements. There is an increased need for the two minerals (especially calcium) in very old horses, broodmares, young horses, and horses subjected to periods of stress. Horses suffering from a severe deficiency may even chew on rocks, dirt, wood, etc. If supplementation is indicated, ground limestone is a good source of calcium, sodium phosphate is a good source of phosphorus, and bone meal and dicalcium phosphate are convenient sources of both minerals.

To understand how excesses or deficiencies of calcium or phosphorus affect the body, it is necessary to examine the relationship of calcium in blood to calcium in bone. While a much greater quantity of calcium is needed in the formation of bone, the most important role of calcium in the body is to participate in functions such as muscle contraction, blood coagulation, and transmission of nerve impulses. Calcium is also needed for the activation of some enzyme systems, and the transference of particles through cell membranes. In short, the calcium level in the blood must be kept within narrow limits for life to continue. To maintain this important calcium level in the blood, the body involuntarily initiates a series of reactions when the level drops. When the calcium intake or absorption is low, the level of calcium in the blood is lowered. The parathyroid gland releases parathormone, which in turn signals the activation of vitamin D from the liver. Parathormone and vitamin D work together to reabsorb calcium stored in bone thereby re-elevating the calcium level in the blood back toward normal. If the low calcium imbalance continues, the stored calcium will eventually be depleted and calcium will be taken from the structural elements of bone. Bone structure is ultimately sacrificed so the rest of the body (nerves, muscles, etc.) can continue functioning. This is the reason that a calcium deficiency shows up as bone disorders rather than nerve or muscle disorders. The phosphorus ratio is very important because it works with or against calcium in absorption and bone formation.

A calcium-phosphorus deficiency interferes with the normal metabolism of the entire body. Chronic imbalances in the calcium-phosphorus ratio will cause diseases such as nutritional secondary hyperparathyroidism. In this disease, parathormone is continually released to rebalance the low calcium-high phosphorus ratio in the blood. The hormone raises the calcium level in the blood by constantly reabsorbing calcium from bone. As this process continues, calcium is taken from the structural portion of the bones and is replaced by fibrous tissue. Since calcium is one of the main structural elements in bone, the density and strength of the bones is greatly reduced. The horse is usually stiff in the joints, and lameness and fractures are not uncommon.

Osteomalacia or "big head" disease may result from nutritional secondary hyperparathyroidism. It is also caused by low intake or absorption of calcium, and may be complicated by a high phosphorus intake. The bone demineralization process continues, and fractures may result even under conditions where stress is minimal. Another characteristic of the disease is a shifting lameness accompanied by soreness and swelling in the joints and around the bones. In severe cases, the swelling around the softened facial bones is very noticeable and creates the appearance of a "big head." Osteomalacia occurs most frequently in broodmares, where the disease may result in abortion and infertility. A broodmare's requirement for calcium is greatly increased during pregnancy when the mineral stores are used up in the development of the fetus, and during lactation when an abundant supply of calcium is needed for the production of milk. Epiphysitis, sometimes referred to as "open knees," is another disease sometimes caused by an imbalance in the calcium-phosphorus ratio. It is commonly found in well-fed young horses where there is an over-feeding of phosphorus accompanied by a calcium deficiency. It may even occur in foals where the ingestion of phosphorus is excessive and the intake of calcium is normal (refer to "Epiphysitis").

In horses, the interrelationship of calcium and phosphorus is complex and imbalance may create serious problems. Consultation with a veterinarian, along with a soil and feed analysis, is recommended before supplementation of either mineral is begun. (For more information on the calcium-phosphorus ratio, refer to the text FEEDING TO WIN.)

POTASSIUM

Potassium is an essential mineral in horses, and is the third most abundant mineral in the body. It is active in helping to maintain proper muscle and nerve function and may function in other less understood biological processes as well. Potassium is abundant in plants and a diet that is at least half fiber should provide an adequate amount of the mineral. A diet low in fiber, molasses, or oil meals may also be low in potassium. When supplementation is needed, it is usually provided in the form of oral doses of potassium chloride (Lite salt is a good source of potassium).

It is possible for a horse to become slightly deficient in potassium when suffering from prolonged diarrhea or starvation, or when given a diuretic drug, such as furosemide. The signs of a deficiency may include lack of appetite, poor growth, and, in extremely severe cases, muscular weakness and paralysis.

Toxicity is rare since a horse will not voluntarily consume excessive amounts of potassium. However, large amounts of the mineral may interact with magnesium and cause grass tetany.

MAGNESIUM

Magnesium is found in all cells and is necessary for protein synthesis and muscle function. It is another mineral usually found in sufficient amounts in forages. Unless a horse is severely deficient in magnesium, a mineralized salt supply should be an adequate source.

Magnesium deficiency may cause hyperirritability and incoordination, and in rare instances, seizures and death may follow.

Toxicity due to ingestion is uncommon, since magnesium is not easily absorbed and it is efficiently excreted by the kidneys. Toxicity can occur, however, if an excessive amount of magnesium salts is given too quickly intravenously. The usual effect of this toxicity is paralysis, which can result in death by respiratory failure and cardiac arrest.

IODINE

Iodine is essential in nutrition, since iodine deficiency will automatically result in thyroid dysfunction. The main role of iodine in the thyroid gland is in the production of the hormone thyroxin. Thyroxin is essential for the normal function of the central nervous system and is critically important in regulating the metabolic rate of all body cells. Most of the iodine contained in the body is concentrated in the thyroid glands, and any new iodine absorbed is immediately stored there.

Iodine is found in soil and water, and there is generally more iodine in roughage than in grains. There are areas where iodine is deficient in soil and water. Goiter is so prevalent in these areas that they are known as "goiter belts." Iodized salt is usually all the supplementation that is needed; however, kelp or potassium iodine can be added to feed if necessary.

Broodmares that are deficient in iodine will often give birth to weak or dead foals. Signs of iodine deficiency include loss of haircoat color, unthriftyness, sterility, and enlarged thyroid glands or goiter (the most common sign).

An excessive amount of iodine can also cause goiter, as well as loss of weight, restlessness, and an increased and irregular heartbeat. Any therapy involving iodine should be watched carefully to make sure the dosage is correct.

ZINC

The most important function of zinc is its role in the synthesis of RNA (ribonucleic acid). Zinc is essential for good skin and haircoat, as well as proper growth and healing. There are no known wide geographical areas deficient in zinc, and most forages contain more than adequate levels of the mineral. The zinc in a mineralized salt supply is usually adequate, but if a horse is on a high calcium or high protein diet, especially when the protein is derived from soybeans, additional dietary zinc may be needed. In such cases, zinc oxalate or zinc carbonate can be added directly to the salt supply.

Signs of zinc deficiency are slow growth rate, deformed hoofs, bad skin and haircoat, incomplete wound healing, anemia, and weight loss. Zinc toxicity is rarely a problem due to the unpleasant taste of zinc compounds.

IRON

Iron is found mainly in the hemoglobin in blood, where small amounts are necessary for blood formation and oxygen transport (refer to "Hematology"). Supplementation is usually not needed since iron is found in sufficient quantities in plants and water. Also, little iron is excreted from the body since the iron from dead cells is salvaged and reused. Supplementation other than a mineralized salt supply is usually in the form of iron salts or iron concentrates.

Supplemental iron is not recommended except as a treatment for iron deficiency. An iron deficiency will result in anemia, poor growth, listlessness, and a rough haircoat.

Supplemental iron is commonly given to race horses, but care should be taken when it is given to any healthy animal, since the body is not very efficient at excreting excess iron. Signs of iron toxicity include lethargy, diarrhea, and shock.

COPPER

Copper is only needed in trace amounts in the horse. It is necessary for iron absorption, and is also involved in tissue metabolism and in blood and bone formation. It is usually found in satisfactory supply in most feedstuffs. However, supplementation may be needed in areas deficient in copper, or where other minerals interact with copper and reduce its absorption in the body (for example, areas high in molybdenum may be deficient in copper). If additional copper is necessary, besides what is contained in a mineralized salt supply, an organic form of copper can be injected.

Insufficient copper may limit the absorption and utilization of iron and therefore cause anemia. A copper deficiency also interferes with connective tissue metabolism and may result in abnormal bone development and decreased hair pigmentation.

Toxicity depends not only on how much copper is ingested, but also on what the concentration is of molybdenum, sulfur, iron, and zinc in the diet, since these minerals limit copper absorption. Copper is accumulated largely in the liver and excessive amounts may cause renal dysfunction and central nervous system damage.

FLUORINE

It is not known whether fluorine is an essential trace element, and no deficiencies have been recognized. An excess of fluorine, from mineralized water, high-fluorine feed, or force-fed mineral supplements, can cause defective teeth, loss of appetite, and a poor haircoat. The only treatment for fluorine toxicity is to reduce intake. A change of food or water may be necessary to eliminate the source.

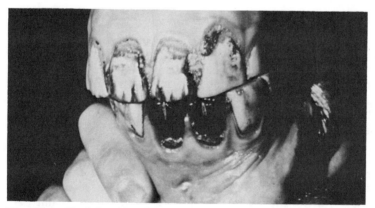

Fig. 27-1   Toxic levels of flourine can result in defective teeth.

SELENIUM

Selenium is essential in the diet in trace amounts, but extreme care should be taken because it is toxic when given in excess. Selenium is necessary for growth and fertility and is also used in the treatment of some cell degenerating diseases. Selenium's most important known function is to protect cellular membranes. Selenium may be an essential component in an enzyme that breaks down highly oxygenated compounds which might otherwise damage the delicate cell membranes.

This mineral is found in plants in varying amounts depending upon the plant. There are areas where toxic amounts are contained in the plants, but there are also areas where selenium is almost completely absent. The bodily requirement of the mineral depends on such variables as what kind is ingested and how much vitamin E is present. Selenium in a vitamin E preparation is the most common form of supplementation, but should not be used without the advice of a veterinarian. Linseed meal is also a source of selenium.

A lack of this mineral may cause "white muscle disease" in foals and may be a cause of "tying up" in older horses. Selenium, in conjunction with vitamin E, is often administered in the prevention and treatment of azoturia. Signs of a deficiency may include loss of hair, liver lesions, muscle degeneration, and decreased fertility.

Horses will not ingest plants containing large amounts of selenium, because of the taste, unless no other forage is available. Selenium toxicity interferes with the metabolism of vitamins A and C and decreases oxygen utilization. Signs of selenium poisoning are colic, diarrhea, fever, weak pulse, blindness, and hoof sloughing. Because of the severe toxic effects of selenium, a horse's diet (especially in high-selenium areas) should be carefully regulated to ensure an excessive amount of the mineral is not ingested.

COBALT

The amount of cobalt required in a horse's system is very minute, but is necessary for the synthesis of vitamin B_{12}. Although the amount of cobalt needed is usually found in plants, there are some cobalt deficient areas. If supplementation is required, cobalt salt can be added to the horse's salt supply.

Signs of cobalt deficiency may include weakness, decrease in appetite, and anemia. Cobalt is relatively non-toxic, but if absorbed in great quantities, the effects are the same as those of a deficiency.

28

FLUIDS AND ELECTROLYTES

The following factors are considered by the veterinarian when fluid therapy is required in horses:

1. When should fluid therapy be used?
2. What solution should be used?
3. How much fluid should be used?
4. How fast should the solution be given?
5. What route of administration should be used?
6. How is the success of the therapy evaluated?

The answers to these questions depend upon the history of the horse involved plus a knowledge of how the particular disease affects the water and electrolyte (ion) balance of the body.

Some of the more important ions are; sodium, chloride, potassium, bicarbonate, and calcium. The usual purpose of fluid and electrolyte therapy is to correct dehydration and/or electrolyte imbalances. These problems may occur as a result of intestinal, kidney, heart, and liver diseases, as well as from trauma and a number of other diseases. Fluids are used to correct acidosis or alkalosis, to treat shock, to provide nourishment, and to stimulate organ function (e.g., kidney function). Examples of situations that may require fluid therapy are:

colic
surgical procedures
diarrhea
jaw fractures

The rate of fluid and/or electrolyte replacement should parallel the extent of the dehydration. The initial rate of administration may be very rapid and then be decreased as improvement in the condition becomes evident. As much as 40 to 60 liters of fluid may be given rapidly under pressure to a horse in shock. This rapid administration may continue until urination occurs or until the first hour has elapsed, whichever happens first. After that time, the rate is reduced each hour and continued until the maintenance and replacement fluid requirements of the horse are met. The normal maintenance requirement of a 1000 pound horse is approximately four and one-half gallons per day. This is the fluid loss due to loss via feces, sweat, the respiratory tract, and the formation of urine. Fluid loss is generally increased during illness due to conditions such as fever, diarrhea, or blood loss. Replacement requirements are computed from the percent of dehydration and by the weight of the horse.

Route Of Administration

The most commonly used route of fluid administration in the horse is the intravenous route. If fluids, antibiotics and drugs are to be administered over an extended period (several days), an indwelling catheter may be placed in the jugular vein. Because of the large volume of fluid sometimes required in horses for initial therapy, five - one gallon containers of distilled water, to which the appropriate amount of powdered electrolytes (e.g., Eltradd IV-4000 Powder: Haver-Lockhart) has been added, are frequently used to supply electrolytes.

Surgical patients are very often given fluids during the course of a surgical procedure. This is because postoperative kidney function is often decreased by as much as 30%. In addition, metabolic and respiratory acidosis may develop due to the incomplete lung ventilation which results when a large animal is on its side or back during surgery. A commonly used solution is lactated Ringer's solution which contains the following:

6.0 gm NaCl
0.3 gm KCl
0.22 gm $CaCl_2$
5.0 ml 60% sodium lactate
sufficient water to make 1 liter of solution

The degree of acidosis may be monitored by the following tests: plasma bicarbonate, blood pH, and blood pCO_2 (blood gases). Sodium bicarbonate is sometimes added to the fluid to help combat acidosis.

The hematocrit or packed cell volume (PCV) is monitored to determine the extent of hemoconcentration. The normal PCV is 32 to 44%. In colic, the PCV may be as high as 65%, indicating the need for rapid administration of large volumes of fluid. Conversely, the PCV could be as low as 5% (the blood is very diluted at this volume) in the case of blood loss anemia in postparturient hemorrhage in the mare, or in neonatal isoerythrolysis in the foal. In the case of the foal, because of its small size, a blood transfusion would be feasible.

The nasogastric route of fluid administration (i.e., the stomach tube) will be used in some cases to provide fluid and nourishment. Depending on the size of the horse, up to 2 gallons of solution may be administered at one time using a stomach pump and stomach tube.

Endurance and competitive trail riders frequently carry powdered electrolytes or electrolyte boluses, such as Electrofin Tabsules (Haver-Lockhart), which are added to the horses' water at rest stops. The use of these products is an attempt to maintain normal electrolyte balance during competition and to keep up fluid intake. A horse must be accustomed beforehand to the taste of the added electrolytes since some horses are sensitive to any alterations in the taste of their water supply.

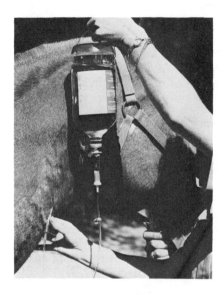

Fig. 28-1 Fluids and electrolytes are usually administered intravenously.

Points To Remember

1. Dehydration will affect a foal much faster than an adult.
2. Old horses with chronic diseases (e.g., kidney problems) require more water than other horses.
3. Horses require more water if they are very active or if the weather is hot and/or humid.
4. Some drugs, e.g., corticosteroids and diuretics, change fluid and electrolyte needs.
5. Horses that have been anesthetized may require additional fluids while in surgery and have increased water requirements for a few days post-surgically.
6. Large volumes of fluids may be lifesaving in the treatment of shock. It is only recently that the total volume of fluid required to supply maintenance as well as replacement requirements has been fully appreciated. 🐎

29

TOXIC SUBSTANCES

General Aspects

A "poison," also called a "toxicant," can be defined as any substance that causes deleterious effects in a living organism. From this rather broad definition, it can be inferred that any substance could prove to be poisonous (and, thus, a "poison") if its dosage and route of entry into the bodily systems are not restricted. This indeed is the case, and substances that are normally considered perfectly safe (and even essential for life) can, under certain conditions, prove to be toxic. Oxygen, for example, as imperative as it is for life, can produce harmful effects if artificially administered in excessive amounts for too long a period. Obviously, however, oxygen intoxication is of little importance to the horseman; whereas, toxicosis produced by insecticides or other chemicals routinely used around livestock is quite relevant to equine husbandry. Therefore, this chapter contains a summation of several selected "environmental poisons" that the horse may come in contact with by ingestion or other means. "Drug toxicities" are covered in other chapters in conjunction with the individual drug categories.

As a general rule, toxic effects of chemicals can be divided into two major groups:

1. toxic effects associated with therapeutic drugs; that is, adverse side effects of drugs
2. toxic effects of environmental substances; "environmental" in this instance referring to virtually any poisonous substance within the environment (either natural or manmade) that the horse may accidentally encounter.

Cautions

Although treatments for certain poisons, when known, are summarized in the following pages, these are included only to familiarize the horseman with procedures that may be used by the veterinarian. Diagnosis of poisonings is certainly one of the most difficult tasks encountered by the veterinarian. In many cases, absolute diagnosis is not possible until post-mortem tissue samples are analyzed by a diagnostic laboratory. Thus, treatment of poisonings should not be attempted by the horseman except in cases of extreme emergencies. This is particularly true since, in some cases, antidotes for one type of poisoning may actually compound the toxicosis associated with a different type of poisoning.

If poisoning is suspected, the veterinarian should be immediately contacted, and the horseman should then:

1. try to provide comfort for the horse until the veterinarian arrives
2. attempt by examination of the premises to determine what chemicals or environmental substances could have been in contact with the horse

Several poisons are listed in Tables 1-7 according to the primary clinical signs or lesions that they produce, as follows:

1. poisons causing physical disfigurement or lameness (Table 1)
2. poisons causing respiratory difficulties (Table 2)
3. poisons causing stimulation or depression of the nervous system (Tables 3 & 4)
4. poisons causing gastrointestinal distress (Table 5)
5. toxicity of chlorinated hydrocarbons (Table 6)

A method of characterizing poisons according to degree of toxicity is given in Table 7, and a listing of several treatments for certain poisonings is given in Table 8.

Nervous System Poisons

Chlorinated Hydrocarbons: These compounds are often included in insecticide dips and sprays and in tree and field pesticides. Some are quite safe, whereas some are too toxic to be safely used in horses and other mammals. Toxic levels can be as low as 10 mg per lb of body weight with the highly toxic compounds, and as high as 2,800 mg per lb of body weight with less toxic chlorinated hydrocarbons. Care should always be exercised when these chemicals are used in horses other than healthy adults, and some are contraindicated in very young, very old, debilitated, or ill horses. Some of the individual chlorinated hydrocarbons and their characteristic effects in horses are summarized in Table 6.

Organophosphates: These chemicals are cholinesterase inhibitors (refer to "Gastrointestinal Drugs"). In addition to signs of severe colic (Table 5), organophosphates can produce convulsions, profuse salivation tremors, muscle weakness and, finally, exhaustion and death (Tables 3 & 4). Organophosphates are now widely used in equine medicine as insecticides and dewormers, and the horseman should become thoroughly familiar with the toxic signs produced by these chemicals. Further, accurate records should always be maintained of organophosphate usage in horses since these agents can interact with other drugs, thereby greatly increasing the incidence of toxic reactions. Atropine is a specific and usually effective antidote for organophosphate poisonings.

Thallium: Some rodenticides contain this chemical; it is quite toxic to horses and produces muscle tremors, depression, paralysis and inability to swallow (dysphagia) (Tables 3 & 4).

1-(Naphthyl)-2-Thiourea (ANTU): Sometimes used as a rodenticide, ANTU is toxic to the horse since it cannot vomit the chemical, as do other species like the dog. Severe depression of the nervous system terminates in death without convulsions (Tables 3 & 4).

Gastrointestinal Poisons

Organophosphates: These compounds are often used as insecticides in fields and orchards and as equine dewormers as mentioned previously. Toxicity varies from compound to compound and may be induced by quantities as low as 1 mg per lb to as much as 1,000 mg per lb of body weight. Signs seen in horses include: colic, severe diarrhea, abdominal cramping, kicking at the abdomen, biting at the flanks, profuse salivation, constricted pupils, general muscular weakness, tremors, and eventual death due to convulsions and respiraatory arrest. Atropine is the primary antidote for organophosphate poisoning, repeated when necessary at two hour intervals (Table 5). Trichlorfon and dichlorvos are two organophosphates used in equine dewormers.

Phenol (Creosote): This compound is commonly used as a wood preservative, and horses that crib wood in the stable or corral are, of course, prone to phenol intoxication. Toxic signs include abdominal distress, depression, ataxia, muscle tremors, convulsions and eventually, paralysis and death. Specific treatments are not available.

Selenium: Selenium toxicosis is often referred to as "alkali disease." It can occur when horses are fed forage or grain grown on soils high in selenium content. In addition to intestinal disorders, selenium toxicity can produce loss of hair from mane and tail, abnormal hoof growth, hoof loss, restlessness and emaciation. No specific treatments are available (Table 5).

Heavy Metal Poisons

Arsenic: This chemical is sometimes included in insecticides, herbicides, wood preservatives, and rodenticides (Table 5). Therefore, arsenic intoxication in horses is usually accidental and the result of improper management. However, the possibility of malicious use should be considered if a thorough examination of the premises fails to identify inadvertent availability to the horse of arsenic-containing compounds.

Arsenic is a tissue toxin and, thus, adversely affects different body organs. Acute intoxication is usually characterized by profuse hemorrhagic diarrhea with shreds of intestinal mucous membrane in the fecal material. Signs of colic and straining while defecating (tenesmus) are also frequently seen. In late stages of acute intoxication, dehydration and shock usually occur in association with muscular weakness. Chronic toxicity in horses and mules is usually characterized by emaciation and attacks of colic.

Once the signs of arsenic poisoning occur, treatment is of little value. A laxative may prove helpful to increase elimination of any arsenic remaining in the gut. Sulfur-containing drugs have been used as antidotes since they combine with arsenic and render it chemically inert. Sodium thiosulfate and British Anti-Lewisite (BAL, 1 mg per lb every 3-4 hours) have been used for this purpose. As is always the case, prevention is much more effective than treatment.

Lead: Lead poisoning (plumbism) in horses is usually a chronic condition associated with prolonged ingestion of lead-containing substances such as paint, boiled linseed oil, lead shot, and automobile batteries (Table 5). The major toxic effects of lead poisoning are gastrointestinal disorders due to hemorrhagic gastroenteritis, central nervous system damage, and degeneration of peripheral nerves. Signs of lead toxicity in horses include diarrhea, colic, emaciation, nerve damage (paralysis of lips, muscle atrophy), stiffness of joints, and incoordination. Importantly, roaring with dyspnea (difficulty in breathing) is also seen in plumbism in horses, and a dark demarcation line (lead line) may be present on the gums.

Treatment involves attempts to chelate (chemically bind) the lead with other chemicals so it can be eliminated from the body. Given orally, magnesium sulfate (epsom salt) forms an insoluble non-toxic precipitate with lead that is not absorbed from the digestive tract. Calcium versenate, a chelating agent, can be administered parenterally for the same basic reason: to "tie up" lead into a non-toxic form.

Mercury: This compound is sometimes used as a fungicide and preservative on seed grains, and treated grains are one of the most common sources of mercury intoxication in horses. Mercury has also been included in some antiseptic and counterirritant preparations. Signs of mercury toxicity are sudden in onset, and characterized by gastroenteritis, colic, depression, and shock. If the animal survives the acute toxic stage, then the severe kidney damage that subsequently develops may prove fatal.

If substances high in protein (e.g., eggs, milk, serum) can be administered orally, some of the mercury within the gut may be rendered unavailable for absorption into the horse's system. Fluid therapy, to assist the kidneys, and BAL have also been used as treatments of mercury poisoning.

Plant Poisons

As a general rule, most poisonous plants are not palatable; therefore, horses will rarely eat them except under certain conditions such as:

1. when there is insufficient forage
2. when poisonous plants or their seeds are mixed with hay or grain
3. when poisonous plant material (clippings, etc.) are placed where a
   horse is accustomed to eating

Therefore, plant poisoning can usually be avoided if the horseman is vigilant and continues looking for and eliminating undesirable plants. Several poisonous plants are included in Tables 1-3.

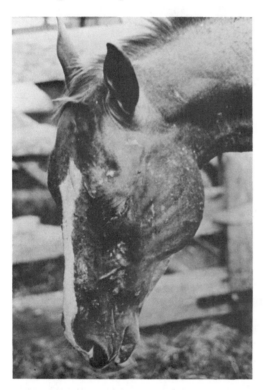

Fig. 29-1 **Toxic plants can cause severe reactions, as in this case of sneezeweed.**

A few of the poisonous plants that have been associated with toxicosis in horses are as follows:

Castor Beans: Although the leaves and stalks of this plant **(Ricinus communis)** are relatively nontoxic, the bean is exceptionally poisonous. The horse seems to be particularly susceptible to ricin (the toxic principal in the bean), much more so than sheep or cattle. Death has been reported in horses ingesting as little as 7 grams (about 20 beans) of castor beans, but it usually takes about 150 beans to kill a 1,000 lb horse. Castor bean toxicosis is characterized by severe, profuse watery diarrhea due to enteritis. It may be produced within hours or 2-3 days after ingestion. Signs of severe colic accompany the diarrhea and death occurs with convulsions. Supportive treatment is given and the veterinarian may administer fluids intravenously.

Oleander: Nerium oleander is an ornamental shrub that is exceptionally toxic due to its severe disrupting effects on the heart beat rhythm. A total of 50 to 60 dried leaves (about 40-50 grams) can kill a 1,000 lb horse. Diarrhea and straining may also be seen. Treatment usually involves supportive measures.

Bracken Fern: This plant produces central nervous system disorders in horses. Ingestion must occur for 30-60 days before toxicosis is seen. Signs include weight loss and staggering. The vitamin thiamine hydrochloride is given for 7-14 days as treatment.

Yellow Star Thistle: This plant, (**Centaurea solstitalis**), is a member of the sunflower family; it produces a disease of the nervous system called Nigropallidal Encephalomalacia or "chewing disease." Mortality is quite high once signs are evident. Chewing difficulties, persistent chewing movements, and inability to drink and eat are produced. No effective treatment has been found, and death is usually the result of starvation.

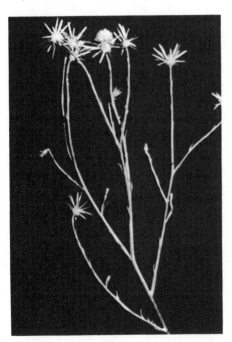

Fig. 29-2 Yellow star thistle affects the nervous system, causing a characteristic difficulty in chewing.

Yellow Bristle Grass: This grass (**Setaria glauca, S. lutescens**) produces a mechanical stomatitis due to the awns becoming embedded in the gingiva. Local erosion and ulceration result. Healing is rapid once the grass awns are removed.

Lupines: These plants belong to the pea family. They produce diarrhea and an unusual high-lifting of the feet. Depression also occurs, and no specific treatment is available.

Senecio spp.: This group of plants is one of the largest in the plant kingdom, and is considerably widespread. These plants are usually not eaten by horses if good forage is available, however, an increased incidence of ingestion seems to be associated with unusual pasture conditions such as drought or after excessive rain. Toxicity in the horse is characterized by liver damage and/or central nervous system disturbances. Intoxicated horses exhibit a staggering gait and aimless wandering, and may develop jaundice (yellow discoloration of tissues) due to liver damage. Prognosis is usually poor and, other than removal of the plant, treatment is symptomatic.

Chinaberry: This group of rapidly growing shade trees **(Melia spp.)** contain an unidentified toxic substance in all above-ground parts of the plant, particularly the berries. Within a few hours, the affected animal will show a general weakness and lack of coordination, loss of appetite, and constipation. Treatment consists of the administration of mineral oil through a stomach tube. The horse may recover within 1-2 days.

Locoism: A variety of leguminous plants commonly called milk vetches **(Astragalus spp** and **Oxytropis spp)** can produce signs of "locoism" or locoweed poisoning in horses when ingested in sufficient quantity. Horses will usually not graze such plants if other forage is available; however, in some strange cases, certain horses seem to become "addicted" and may actually search out locoweeds. Locoism is a problem only at certain times, usually during the summer.

Signs of locoweed intoxication, as its name implies, are characterized by behavioral disturbances, such as abnormal gait, aimless wandering, "head-pressing" against stationary objects, severe reaction to restraint and, terminally, convulsions. Prognosis is poor and treatment is supportive.

Sudan Hybrid Pasture: A syndrome characterized by inflammation of the bladder (cystitis) and posterior ataxia has been associated with hybrid-sudan pasture. This syndrome has been seen primarily in the northwest part of Texas in horses fed only the sudan grass. Lesions of the spinal cord are seen, and no specific treatment is available. Prevention is obtained by feeding other feeds when horses are placed on sudan pasture.

Moldy Corn: Leukoencephalomalacia, a type of brain damage, has been associated with ingestion of moldy corn or corn stalk pasture. This condition more commonly occurs during the fall months when wet conditions favor fungal growth. Horses usually graze contaminated forage for 2-3 weeks before signs appear. Signs include muscle tremors, weakness, lack of coordination, swallowing difficulties, and jaundice if the horse lives for several days. Treatment consists of supportive care since no specific antidote has been identified.

Grass Tetany: This condition is associated with lush pastures and is due to lowered magnesium concentration in the blood. Muscle spasms, tremors, and ataxia are produced, but they respond well to intravenous therapy with magnesium and calcium solutions.

Deadly Nightshade: This plant **(Atropa belladonna)** is a member of the Solanaceae (potato family), or belladonna plants. Related plants include jimson weed and henbane. The toxic principle is atropine and atropine-like compounds. Signs produced include constipation and central nervous system disorders. Treatment involves the careful use of cholinergic drugs (refer to "Gastrointestinal Drugs.")

Spoiled Sweet Clover: The critical clinical signs of spoiled sweet clover intoxication are related to the toxic principle, dicoumarol, contained in such plants. This chemical has a pronounced anticoagulant effect in the blood. Thus, it prolongs clotting time, resulting in hemorrhage, bloody discharge from body openings, hematomas under the skin and around joints, and hemorrhagic shock. Treatment includes injections of vitamin K (0.5 to 1.0 mg/lb), but a sudden cure is not seen. Rather, recovery will gradually occur if the poisoning was identified early enough.

Botulism: This condition is caused by a toxin produced by the bacterium **Clostridium botulinum**. It is included in the section on poisonous plants since plant feeds sometimes become contaminated with Clostridium, especially spoiled and decaying ensilage. Also, although rarely a problem in horse management, decaying carcasses often become contaminated with this bacterium. If a horse suffers from dietary deficiency resulting in abnormal appetite (pica), then it may ingest dead animals contaminated with **Cl. botulinum**. Botulinum toxin attacks those nerves that supply the voluntary muscles. Thus, botulism (sometimes called "limber neck") produces a disorder characterized by muscular paralysis of the throat, jaw and neck regions. Other muscles may also be affected, causing the horse to stagger and stumble, finally terminating in a flacid paralysis, usually within 3-6 days after ingestion of the toxin. Treatment is of little value once signs have developed, and the prognosis is poor.

Cyanide Poisoning: Johnson grass, sudan grass, cherry laurel, and sorghum are cyanogenic plants that yield hydrocyanic (prussic) acid after digestion by gastrointestinal enzymes. This acid is a tissue poison that can produce death within a brief interval. Poisoning is usually a result of ingestion of the involved plants after they were wilted, stunted, trampled, frost damaged or treated with 2,4-D. Signs of toxicity include severe convulsions and respiratory distress. Treatment consists of carefully controlled intravenous injection of sodium nitrate and sodium thiosulfate solution. Large doses of vitamin B_{12a} (hydroxocobalamin) may also be helpful. If a horse survives for two hours after the signs develop, recovery usually occurs.

Cantharidin (Blister Beetle) Poisoning: Alfalfa hay may be contaminated with blister beetles **(Epicauta vitatta)** that contain cantharidin, which is an intense irritant and nephrotoxic. Signs of cantharidin poisoning include uneasiness, diarrhea, sweating, high fever (106°F), rapid respiration, and a rapid, thready pulse. Death may occur within 4-6 hours to several days.

The veterinarian may give the horse supportive treatment to minimize shock, including fluid therapy and corticosteroids. The horse should not be dosed with mineral oil since it will increase the absorption of cantharidin, although it can be given protectants by stomach tube to decrease absorption. Regardless of treatment, however, the prognosis is very poor.

FIG. 29-3 TABLE 1
POISONS CAUSING PHYSICAL DISFIGUREMENT OR LAMENESS

Poisons Causing Bone, Tooth, Hoof and Hair Abnormalities	Poisons Causing Skin Lesions	Plant Poisons Causing Fetal Deformities
Fluoride (chronic poisoning)	Chlorinated Naphthalene	Tobacco
Selenium (chronic poisoning)	Corrosives	Seleniferous plants
Cadmium, Lead, Thallium	Organomercurials	Jimsonweed, Wild Cherry
Plants: Sweet Peas, Sorghums	Thallium	Poison Hemlock, Lupines
Day-Blooming Jessamine	Polybrominated Biphenyls	Locoweeds, Sweet Peas
	Mold toxins: Ergots	

FIG. 29-4 TABLE 2
POISONS CAUSING RESPIRATORY DIFFICULTIES

Poisons Depressing the Respiratory Centers of the Brain

Methaldehyde
Alcohols

Poisons Decreasing Oxygen Uptake from the Lungs

ANTU (Alpha Naphthyl Thiourea)
Hydrogen Sulfide
Ammonia Gas & Compounds
Nitrogen Oxide Gasses
Sulfur Oxide Gases
Petroleum Products

Poisons Decreasing Oxygen Transport to Tissues

Nitrate
Methylene Blue
Carbon Monoxide
Chlorate
Copper
Iron
Plant Poisons:
  Oleander, Staggergrass,
  Indian Tobacco, Bracken Fern,
  Sweet Clover, Wild onion, Cottonseed
Snake Venoms

Unknown Mechanisms

Lupines, Locoweeds
Cocklebur Sprouts
Poison Hemlock
Tobacco
Dutchman's-breeches
Squirrel Corn

Poisons Decreasing Oxygen Utilization by Tissues

Hydrogen Sulfide Gas
Cyanide

Poisons Increasing Tissue Oxygen Demands

Nitrophenols
Chlorophenols

FIG. 29-5   TABLE 3
POISONS CAUSING STIMULATION OR DEPRESSION
OF THE CENTRAL NERVOUS SYSTEM

Poisons Directly Damaging the Brain or Spinal Cord

Salt (water deprivation)
Hexachlorophene
Mold Toxin
Organomercurials
Plants: Locoweeds, Sweet Peas
  Sensitive Fern

Unknown Mechanisms

Chlorinated Hydrocarbons
Lead
Mold Toxins: Ergot
Plants: Bitterweed, Ground Lichen,
  Bracken Fern, Horsetails, Milkweeds,
  Ohio Buckeye, Horse Chestnut,
  Indian Tobacco, Carolina Jessamine,
  Lupines, Squirrel Corn, Dutchman's-
  breeches, Fitweed, Water Hemlock,
  Poison Hemlock

Poisons Acting on Specific Nervous Functions

Organophosphates
Carbamate Insecticides
Strychnine
Fluoroacetate
Nicotine
Plants: Tobacco, Jimson Weed,
  Henbane, Deadly Nightshade

FIG. 29-6 TABLE 4
PESTICIDES CAUSING STIMULATION
OR DEPRESSION OF THE NERVOUS SYSTEM

Chemical	Use	Toxic Level	Major Signs	Treatment
Chlorinated Hydrocarbons	Insecticides Field and Tree Pesticides	Variable and may be acute or chronic from 10 mg/lb to 2800 mg/lb.	Convulsions and colic, intermittent in type.	Sedate to effect with chloral hydrate-magnesium sulfate or barbiturates to control the CNS disturbance.
Fluoroacetate	Rodenticides	5 mg/lb kills in a few hours.	Intermittent Convulsions, colic, possibly diarrhea.	There is no effective antidote for horses.
Organophosphates	Pesticides Dewormers	From less than 1 mg/lb to more than 1000 mg/lb.	Terminal-type convulsions, colic, muscular weakness, salivation.	Atropine and 2-PAM to effect.
Strychnine	Pesticides	1 to 2 mg/lb	Convulsions.	Control convulsions with chloral hydrate or barbiturates, complete quiet.
Thallium	Rodenticides	14 mg/lb	Tremors, depression, paralysis.	Diphenylthiocarbazone is not very practical for horses.
ANTU	Rodenticides	14 mg/lb	Severe depression, death without convulsion, pulmonary edema.	No effective antidote.

FIG. 29-7 TABLE 5
POISONS CAUSING GASTROINTESTINAL DISTRESS

Poison	Use	Toxic Level		
Arsenic	Insecticides Herbicides Rodenticides	Oral, acute - 12-220 mg/lb; Chronic - 1-3 gm per day for 14 wks to kill	Acute: possibly diarrhea; Chronic: emaciation in horses and mules.	Remove the source and give both symptomatic and supportive treatment. BAL has limited use in the horse.
Lead	Paints Insecticides	Oral, acute - 5-20 gm/1000 lbs	Dyspnea with roaring, weakness, central nervous system disturbance, stiffness of joints, lead line on gums.	Chronic: 2% saline-sugar sol. of Ca-EDTA. Acute poisoning may kill before diagnosis or treatment can be made.
Selenium (Alkali disease)	Forage or grain on seleniferous soils	1.5 mg/lb	Loss of hair from mane and tail, softened and abnormal hoof, listlessness and emaciation.	Remove from exposure; give supportive and symptomatic treatment.
Organo-phosphates	Insecticides Dewormers	From less than 1 mg/lb to 1000 mg/lb	Horses have colic, general muscular weakness, perspiration, salivation, may develop convulsions.	Atropine and 2-PAM.
Phenol (Creosote)	Wood preservatives	Acute: 30 gm is lethal; Chronic: as little as 0.1 mg/lb	Acute: depression, ataxia, convulsions, paralysis and terminal muscular tremors. Chronic: contact burns, and slower changes with encephalitis.	Remove from exposure and give both symptomatic and supportive treatment.

BAL = British Anti-Lewisite

FIG. 29-8   TABLE 6
TOXICITY OF CHLORINATED HYDROCARBON PARASITICIDES

Compound	Common Use	LD 50 Oral	Comments
DDT and Chlordane	Sprays Dusts Dips	Acute: 250 mg/kg	Poisoning in horses is rare if properly used. Dangerous if a contaminant of feed or water. Most susceptible are very young, very old, debilitated and malnourished horses and gestating mares. Use calcium gluconate and supportive agents as necessary. DDT is secreted in the milk in large amounts.
Lindane	Dusts Dips Sprays	Acute: 250 mg/kg Chronic low	Unapproved for milking females and all meat animals, as it is eliminated in the milk and stored in the fat. Avoid use on the very young or very old animals, and avoid contamination of feed or water. Control convulsions with chloral-hydrate barbiturate-type sedatives and use supportive treatment including calcium gluconate.
Heptachlor	Field Spray and Dust	Acute: 90 mg/kg Chronic low	Too toxic for use on mammals. Use sedation as for Lindane and the same supportive treatments.
Methoxychlor	Dusts Sprays Dips	Acute: 2800 mg/kg or more	Virtually nontoxic for horses under practical conditions. It is the least toxic of the chlorinated insecticides in common use. Not eliminated in the milk.
Aldrin Dieldrin Isodrin Endrin	Field or Seed Spray	Acute: less than 75 mg/kg Chronic low	Aldrin, Dieldrin, Isodrin, Endrin and others of this immediate group are too dangerous for use on mammals. In accidental poisoning, use sedation and liberal amounts of calcium gluconate and supportives as necessary.
Toxaphene (Camphene)	Dips or Sprays	Acute: 60 mg/kg Chronic: 330 mg/kg	Toxaphene is one of the most effective agents against ticks and mites and is safe if properly used except for young colts, aged or debilitated animals.

LD50 = Lethal dose 50% = the average amount that will kill 50% of the horses it is administered to

FIG. 29-9 TABLE 7
CLASSIFICATION OF POISONS
ACCORDING TO DEGREE OF TOXICITY

Classification	A Likely Single Lethal Dose [mg per lb body weight]	Equivalent for a 1,000 lb horse
1. Practically Nontoxic	More than 7,500 mg	More than 16.5 lbs
2. Slightly Toxic	2,500 mg to 7,500 mg	From 5.5 lbs to 16.5 lbs
3. Moderately Toxic	250 mg to 2,500 mg	From 0.5 lbs to 5.5 lbs
4. Very Toxic	25 mg to 250 mg	From 5/6 oz to 0.5 lbs
5. Extremely Toxic	2.5 mg to 25 mg	From 1/14 oz to 5/6 oz
6. Supertoxic	2.5 mg or less	About 1/14 oz or less

FIG. 29-10 TABLE 8
COMMONLY USED ANTIDOTES FOR CERTAIN POISONINGS

Poisoning	Antidote	Comments
Arsenic	BAL or British Anti-Lewisite	1st day: .625 mg/kg, 4 I.M. doses 2nd day: .625 mg/kg, 4 I.M. doses 3rd day: .6 mg/kg, 2 I.M. doses 4th day: 1.2 mg/kg, 1 I.M. dose
Lead	NaCa EDTA	I.V., 50 ml/100 lbs liveweight, divided in 3 or 4 doses per day, for 2 or 3 days at a time.
Organophosphate Insecticides	Atropine, 2-PAM	Repeated in 2 or 3 hours, if necessary.
HCN or Prussic Acid	Thiodex (Ft. Dodge) Trypan Blue and Sodium thiosulfate	100 to 200 ml, I.V., or to effect; can be repeated if necessary.
Insect stings and drug shock emergencies	Epinephrine Corticosteroids Antihistamines	Calcium gluconate with dextrose and magnesium solutions given slowly, I.V. to effect. Epinephrine injectable, 1/1000, is given S.C., 4 to 8 ml.

30

IMMUNOLOGY

Animals are in constant contact with many pathogenic organisms. Immunity is the successful resistance of a host to disease-producing organisms, and immunology is the study of the mechanisms of protection against the organism. Immunization as a protection from disease is based on the ability of the body's immune system to combat the antigens of the infectious organism (virus, bacteria, etc.).

Definitions

The following definitions are given to assist in understanding the principles of immunity.

Antigen: Immunogen; various substances (usually foreign proteins) that, as a result of contacting the appropriate tissues of an animal's body, produce a state of sensitivity and/or resistance to infection or toxic substances. This response requires 7-14 days after initial contact.

Antibody: Substance which reacts with a particular antigen; its production may be stimulated by exposure to the antigen through natural infection or vaccination.

Antitoxin: An antibody formed in response to antigenic poisonous substances of biologic origin, such as bacterial exotoxin, e.g., those elaborated by **Clostridium tetani** (the causative agent of tetanus). The term generally refers to the whole or globulin fraction of serum from animals (usually horses) immunized by injections of a specific toxoid. Produces a transient passive immunity, e.g., tetanus antitoxin.

Toxin: A poisonous substance that is an integral part of a cell, an extracellular product (exotoxin), or both. Toxins are formed during metabolism and growth, especially of certain microorganisms.

Toxoid: A toxin that has been treated (commonly with formaldehyde) so as to destroy its toxic property, but that still retains its antigenicity, i.e., is capable of stimulating the immune response and producing active immunity, e.g., tetanus toxoid.

Vaccine: Any preparation intended for stimulating the active immunologic response: a biological, e.g., equine influenza vaccine, rhinopneumonitis vaccine, encephalomyelitis vaccines. Administration is usually by

552

injection, but ingestion is preferred in some instances, and nasal sprays are occasionally used.

Bacterin: A bacterial vaccine made from a suspension of bacteria, killed generally by heat or chemical means, and used to enhance immunity, e.g., **Streptococcus equi** (strangles) bacterin.

Autogenous: Refers to vaccines prepared from bacteria or viral particles obtained from the infected animal, e.g., autogenous wart vaccine (viral), or autogenous bacterin from **Streptococcus zooepidemicus** (bacterial).

Booster: A dose of vaccine given at some time after the initial dose to enhance the effect and protection; the response of the immune system will be more rapid and protection will be sooner than the 7-14 days required with the initial dose.

Primary Defense Mechanisms

A horse is protected by primary defenses and/or by secondary defense mechanisms which are either natural or acquired. Primary defense mechanisms hinder or prevent the passage of disease-producing agents into the tissues. The epithelial coverings (such as skin and mucous membranes), act as physical barriers and aid in the destruction of many pathogens. The skin may destroy some pathogenic organisms on contact due to the presence of normal skin flora (bacteria), or due to the active enzymes in sweat. The inner surfaces of the body are protected to some extent by the enzymes and local antibodies found in mucous. Normal bodily discharge, such as tears, vaginal secretions, and urine, help defend the animal by effectively sweeping foreign materials out of the body. Respiratory secretions are coughed up or swallowed, and organisms which are swallowed quickly contact the highly acidic gastric juice of the stomach and are destroyed.

Secondary Defense Mechanisms

Secondary defenses deal with agents that manage to enter the tissues in spite of the primary defenses. Secondary defenses are either provided by natural resistance or acquired immunity. Natural resistance is classified as individual, genetic, or species resistance. It is an inherited immunity which exists in an individual, a breed, or a species from birth and is unrelated to any acquired immunity. An example of inherited immunity is the lack of susceptibility of man, horses, dogs, and cats to foot-and-mouth disease and rinderpest (cattle plague).

ACQUIRED IMMUNITY

Acquired immunity may be either active or passive, and this type of immunity is the basis for the use of biologicals in a vaccination program. Active acquired immunity is produced by the animal in his own body after vaccination, or after recovering from the disease.

Vaccines can be toxoids, antitoxins, bacterins, killed viral vaccines, or modified or live viral vaccines. Toxoids cause the best immunogenetic response. Bacterins produce some immunity, but are not as effective as are live virus vaccines. The live vaccines will cause a mild case of the disease to stimulate the immunogenetic system. Some inflammation is necessary to initiate the development of antibodies, and causes either a swelling at the site of the injection or a mild case of the disease. The degree of inflammation present will depend on the horse's individual response and on the type of vaccine given; killed virus vaccines cause less reaction.

The inflammation caused by infection (or by vaccination with live vaccine) precipitates the manufacture of antibodies, which are proteins that neutralize specific antigens. It takes approximately five days for these antibodies to become present in the blood stream, and 7-14 days for them to attain an effective level. Subsequent to the control of the original infection, the level of antibodies in the blood will decrease. However, the body will remember that specific antigen, and when exposed later to that same antigen, will very rapidly produce the appropriate antibodies. This is the reason behind the administration of periodic "booster" shots.

A non-immune animal can obtain passive acquired immunity by the transference of antibodies from an immune animal which has been vaccinated or has previously recovered from the disease. However, the immediate temporary resistance the non-immune animal receives is of short duration and lasts only 20-30 days. In the horse, passive acquired immunity is accomplished several ways:

1. transfusion of whole blood, plasma, or serum (for example, tetanus antitoxin)
2. gamma globulin fractions from the blood of an immune animal injected into a non-immune animal
3. the ingestion of colostrum (first milk of the mare)

Antibody levels in the colostrum are ten times that of serum levels and must be ingested by the foal in the first day of life to be utilized. This is especially important since the placental transfer of antibody from dam to fetus does not occur in the equine species. Vaccinating the mare with tetanus toxoid a month prior to foaling will assure a high antibody content in the mare's colostrum at foaling. Colostrum may be frozen and saved for those rare instances when the mare has none, the mare dies, or when neonatal isoerythrolysis is suspected.

IMMUNODEFICIENCY

Occasionally, the immune system may fail to adequately function, resulting in immunodeficiency. This condition is most commonly seen in newborn foals which, for some reason, either do not receive colostrum or are unable to absorb the antibodies in colostrum. The foal will have little disease resistance, but if his immune system is competent, he will respond to vaccination. Primary immunodeficiency occurs when the immune system fails to develop in the fetus. The foal will be partially or totally unprotected against pathogenic organisms when the passive antibody levels acquired from the mare's colostrum fall off. Adult horses may develop secondary immunodeficiency. This type of deficiency may result when the horse's system is overly stressed, such as by malnutrition or disease. The degree to which the immune system is inhibited varies with each type of immunodeficiency, but in all cases there is an increase in susceptibility to pathogens. (Refer to "Immunodeficiency" under "Foal Diseases and Disorders.")

BIBLIOGRAPHY

Adams, O.R. **Lameness in Horses**. 2nd ed.   Philadelphia: Lea and Febiger, 1972.

Adams, O.R. **Lameness in Horses**. 3rd ed.   Philadelphia: Lea and Febiger, 1974.

Beeman, G.M.   **Know First Aid for your Horse**. Omaha: Farnam Horse Library, 1972.

Blood, D.C. and J.A. Henderson. **Veterinary Medicine**.   Baltimore: William and Wilkins Co., 1974.

Brander, G.C. and D.M. Pugh. **Veterinary Applied Pharmacology and Therapeutics**.   Baltimore: William and Wilkins Co., 1971.

Burns, S.J. and W.C. McMullan. **Junior Clinics Equine Section**.   Texas A&M Univ., College of Vet. Medicine.

Clarke, E.G.C. and M.L. Clarke.   **Veterinary Toxicology**.   Baltimore: William and Wilkins Co., 1975.

Codrington, W.S. **Know your Horses**. London: J.A. Allen and Co., 1972.

Davidson, J.B. **Horseman's Veterinary Advisor**. Arco, N.Y.:   1975.

Dukes' Physiology of Domestic Animals. Ed. M.J. Swenson. Ithaca, N.Y.: Comstock Publishing Associates, 1970.

Dunn, A.M. **Veterinary Helminthology**. Philadelphia: Lea and Febiger, 1969.

Ensminger, M.E. **Horses and Horsemanship**. Danville, Ill.: The Interstate Printers and Publishers, Inc., 1969.

Equine Medicine and Surgery. 2nd ed. Ed. E.J. Catcott and J.F. Smithcors. Wheaton, Ill.: American Veterinary Publications, Inc., 1972.

Evans, J.W., A. Borton, H.F. Hintz, and L.D. Van Vleck. **The Horse**. San Francisco: W.H. Freeman and Co., 1977.

Feeding to Win. Ed. D.M. Wagoner. Grapevine, Tx.: Equine Research Publications. 1973.

Frandson, R.D. **Anatomy and Physiology of Farm Animals**. Philadelphia: Lea and Febiger, 1972.

Frank, E.P. **Veterinary Surgery**. 7th ed. Minneapolis: Burgess Publishing Co., 1964.

Gelatt, K.N., R.L. Peiffer, Jr., and L.W. Williams. "The Status of Equine Ophthalmology."**The Journal of Equine Medicine and Surgery**, 1 Jan. 1977, pp.13-19.

Goth, A. **Medical Pharmacology**. 8th ed. St. Louis: C.V. Mosby Co., 1976.

Greeley, R.G. **The Art and Science of Horseshoeing**. Philadelphia: J.B. Lippincott, 1970.

Hayes, M.H. **Veterinary Notes for Horseowners**. 16th ed. N.Y.: Arco, 1974.

The Illustrated Veterinary Encyclopedia for Horsemen. Ed. D.M. Wagoner. Grapevine, Tx.: Equine Research Publications, 1977.

Jones, L.M. **Veterinary Pharmacology and Therapeutics**. 4th ed. Ames, Iowa: Iowa State University Press, 1977.

Journal of Equine Medicine and Surgery. Vol.I January 1977
Davis, L.E. and A.P. Knight.   "Review of the Clinical Pharmacology of the Equine Digestive System." pp.27-35.

Scott, E.A. and D.J. Kunze. "Ovariectomy in the Mare: Presurgical, Surgical and Postsurgical Considerations." pp. 5-12.

Journal of Equine Medicine and Surgery. Vol.I   February 1977
Naylor, J.M. "The Nutrition of the Sick Horse." pp. 64-70.

Journal of Equine Medicine and Surgery.   Vol. I   March 1972.
Houpt, K.A.   "Horse Behavior: Its Relevancy to the Equine Practitioner." pp. 87-94.

Journal of Equine Medicine and Surgery.   Vol. I   April 1977.
Bello, T.R., S. D. Gaunt and B.J. Torbert. "Critical Evaluation of Environmental Control of Bots (Gasterophilus Intestinalis) in Horses." pp. 126-130.
Huston, R., G. Saperstein, and H.W. Leipold. "Congenital Defects in Foals." pp. 146-161.

Leahy, J.R. and P. Barrow. **Restraint of Animals**. 2nd ed. Ithaca, N.Y.: Cornell Campus Store, 1953.

Le Clair, R.A. **Veterinary Pharmaceuticals and Biologicals. 76/77**   Philadelphia: F.A. Davis Co., 1976.

Lindholm, A., H.E. Johansson and P. Kjaersgaard. "Acute Rhabdomyolysis ("Tying-Up") in Standardbred Horses." **Acta Vet. Scand.**, 15 (1974), 1-15.

Marlin, H, and S. Savitt. **How to Take Care of your Horse until the Vet Comes**. N.Y.: Dodd, Mead, and Co., 1975.

Merchant, I.A. and R.A. Packer. **Veterinary Bacteriology and Virology**. 7th ed. Ames, Iowa: Iowa State University Press., 1971.

The Merck Index. 8th ed. Ed. P.G. Stecher. Rahway, N.J.: Merck & Co., Inc., 1968.

557

The Merck Veterinary Manual. 4th ed. Ed. O.H. Siegmund. Rahway, N.J.: Merck and Co.,Inc., 1973.

Meyers, F.H., E. Jawetz and A. Goldfien. **Review of Medical Pharmacology.** 4th ed. Los Altos, Ca.: Lanhe Medical Publications, 1974.

Myers, V.S. and J. McClure. "Equine Dental Care and Aging." **Stud Manager's Handbook.** Vol.II Agriservices Foundation, pp. 211-215.

McKibbin, L.S. and A. Sugerman. **Horse Owner's Handbook.** Philadelphia: W.B. Saunders, 1977.

McMullan, W.C. **Equine Dermatology.** Texas A&M Univ., College of Veterinary Medicine

Naviaux, J.L. **Horses in Health and Disease.** N.Y.: Arco., 1976.

Nutrient Requirements of Horses. 3rd ed. Washington, D.C.: National Academy of Sciences., 1973.

Oehme, F.W. and J.E. Prier. **Textbook of Large Animal Surgery.** 3rd ed. Baltimore: William and Wilkins, 1975.

The Pharmalogical Basis of Therapeutics. Ed. L.S. Goodman and A. Gilman. N.Y.: Macmillan, 1975.

Proceedings of the 1st National Horsemen's Seminar. Fredericksburg, Virginia. 1976 Program.

Proceedings of the 17th Annual Convention of the American Association of Equine Practitioners. Ed. F.J. Milne. 1972
Fries, J.H. "Freeze-Branding the Foal." pp.147-149.
Gelatt, K.N. "Equine Ophthalmology." pp. 323;336.
Mansman, R.A., J.D. Wheat and S.S. Jang. "Diagnostic Usefulness of Transtracheal Aspiration in the Horse." pp. 143-146.
Metcalf, J.W. "Improved Technique in Sarcoid Removal." pp. 45;47.
Owen, D. "Arthrocentesis Techniques in Treating Equine Joint Disease." pp. 263-267.
Proctor, D.L. and H.S. Conboy "A practical Approach to Shock Therapy." pp. 313-320.
Walker, E.R. "The Treatment of Acute and Chronic Wounds Below the Carpal and Tarsal Areas." pp. 49-52.

Proceedings of the 18th Annual Convention of the American Association of Equine Practitioners. Ed. F. J. Milne. 1973
Beeman, G.M. "A Surgical Approach to the Repair of Equine Wounds." pp. 163-172.
Herthel, D.G. "Technique of Intestinal Anastomosis Utilizing the Crushing Type Suture." pp. 303-306.
Keeran, R.J. "Equine Ovariectomy: Anesthesia and Positioning." pp. 41-42.
McDonald, D.R. "Diagnosis and Therapy of Common Eye Conditions." pp. 381-384.
Page, E.H. "Common Skin Diseases of the Horse." pp. 385-399.
Scott, B. "Equine Insurance: Its Relationship to the Practicing Veterinarian." pp. 11-15.

Proceedings of the 19th Annual Convention of the American Association of Equine Practitioners. Ed. F.J. Milne. 1974
DeGroot, A. and D.E. Bresler. "Acupuncture - A Pilot Program in the Horse." pp. 213-218.
Johnson, J.H., H.E. Garner, D.P. Hutcheson and J.G. Merriam. "Epistaxis." pp. 115-121.
Owen, D. "Local Nerve Blocks." pp. 153-156.
Swanson, T.D. "Restraint in Treatment." pp. 147-151.
Swanstrom, O.G. and M. Lindy. "Therapeutic Swimming." pp. 315-322.
Wheat, J.D. "Sinus Drainage and Tooth Repulsion in the Horse." pp. 171-176.

Proceedings of the 20th Annual Convention of the American Association of Equine Practitioners. Ed. F.J. Milne. 1975
Adams, O.R. "A Review of Treatments for Navicular Disease." pp. 47-59.
Aubrey, F.B. "Equine Insurance Problems." pp. 31-35.
Bello, T.R., G. F. Ambrorski and B.J. Torbert. "Practical Equine Parasitology, Based on Recent Research." pp. 97-118.
Johnson, J.E. "Ringbone: Treatment by Ankylosis." pp. 67-80.
Kemen, M.J. "Clinical Aspects of Equine Influenza." pp. 119-126.

Proceedings of the 21st Annual Convention of the American Association of Equine Practitioners. Ed. F.J. Milne. 1976.
Boles, C.L. "Epiglottic Entrapment and Pharyngeal Paralysis: Diagnosis and Treatment." pp. 29-34.
Fackelman, G.E., C.F. Reid, M. Leitch and R Cimprich. "Angular Limb Deformities in Foals." pp. 161-176.
Farris, H.E., F.T. Fraunfelder, and C.T. Mason. "Cryosurgery of Equine Cutaneous Neoplastic and Non-Neoplastic Lesions." pp. 177-190.
Hackathorn, T.A. "A Practical Approach to the Chronic Pharyngitis/Gutteral Pouch Problem." pp. 35-41.
Loomis, W.K. "The Practioner's Approach to the Handling of the Acute Abdominal Crisis." pp. 123-126.
Norrie, R.E. "The Treatment of Joint Disease by Saline Lavage." pp. 91-94.
Raker, C.W. "Endoscopy of the Upper Respiratory Tract of the Horse." pp. 23-28.
Shideler, R.K. and D.G. Bennet. "Diagnosis in Equine Colic." pp. 197-201.

Wheat, J.D. "Fractures of the Head and Mandible of the Horse." pp. 223-228.

Proceedings of the 22nd Annual Convention of the American Association of Equine Practitioners. Ed. F. J. Milne. 1977.
Currie, A.K. and S.W.J. Seager. "Anhidrosis." pp. 249-251.
Knowles, R.C. "Equine Infectious Anemia (EIA)--1976 Update in the United States." pp. 121-126.
McMullan, W.C. "Equine Dermatology." pp. 293-326.
Stannard, A.A. "Equine Dermatology." pp. 273-292.
Swanson, T.D. "Treatment of Rattlesnake Bites." pp. 267-268.

Progress in Equine Practice. Vol.I Ed. E.J. Catcott and J.F. Smithcors. Santa Barbara, Ca.: American Veterinary Publications, Inc., 1966.

Progress in Equine Practice. Vol.II Ed. E.J.Catcott, and J.F. Smithcors. Wheaton, Ill.: American Veterinary Publication, Inc., 1970.

Radeloff, R.D. **Veterinary Toxicology.** Philadelphia: Lea and Febiger, 1970.

Rapidan River Farm Digest. Ed. J. C. Hagan. Spring, 1975.
Allen, W.R. "Prostaglandin: Breeding Breakthrough " pp. 50-55.
Conner, J. "Weaning the Foal" pp. 167-169.

Rapidan River Farm Digest. Ed. J.C. Hagan, Summer, 1975.
Kenney, R.M. "Prostaglandins in Horse Breeding " pp. 43-49.
McCollum, W.H., J.T. Bryans and W.E. Wise. "Equine Viral Arteritis " pp. 225-226.
Swerczek, T.W. "Diseases of Foals " pp. 68-76.
Wise, W.E., J.H. Drudge and E.T. Lyons. "Controlling Internal Parasites of the Horse " pp. 33-39.
Wise, W.E. and T.W. Swerczek. "Equine Tetanus " pp. 213-214.
Wise, W.E. and T.W. Swerczek. "Taxus (Yew) Poisoning" pp. 152-153.

Rapidan River Farm Digest. Ed. J. C. Hagan, Winter, 1976.
Ensminger, M.E. "The Newborn Foal" pp. 161-163.
Finocchio, E.J. "Kidney Disease in the Horse--Fact or Fiction " pp. 204-205.
Jefferson, D.A. "Blood Loss in the Horse " pp. 233-236.
Lowe, J.E. and H.F. Hintz. "Founder" pp. 135-141.
Ricketts, S.W. "Foaling and the Newborn Foal " pp. 86-93.

Roberts, S.J. **Veterinary Obstetrics and Genital Diseases.** 2nd ed. Ann Arbor, Michigan: Edwards Brothers, Inc., 1971.

Rooney, J.R. **The Lame Horse--Causes, Symptoms, and Treatment.** No.Hollywood, Ca.: Wilshire Book Co., 1976.

Rossdale, P.D. **The Horse.** Arcadia, Ca.: California Breeders Association, 1972.

Rossdale, P.D. and S.W. Wreford. **The Horse's Health from A to Z.** N.Y.: Arco, 1974.

Rossdale, P.D. and S.W. Ricketts. **The Practice of Equine Stud Medicine.** Baltimore: Williams and Wilkins, 1974.

Rossdale, P.D. **Seeing Equine Practice.** London: Heinemann Veterinary Books, 1976.

Rossoff, I.S. **Handbook of Veterinary Drugs.** N.Y.: Springer Publishing Co., 1974.

Schalm, O.W., N.C. Jain,and E.J. Carroll. **Veterinary Hematology.** Philadelphia: Lea and Febiger, 1975.

Serth, G.W. **The Horseowner's Guide to Common Equine Ailments.** No. Hollywood, Ca.: Wilshire Book Co., 1974.

Smith, H.A., T.C. Jones and R.D. Hunt. **Veterinary Pathology.** 4th ed. Philadelphia: Lea and Febiger, 1972.

Straiton, E.C. **The Horseowner's Vet Book.** Philadelphia: J.B. Lippincott Co., 1973.

Strong, C.L. **Horses' Injuries.** London: Faber and Faber Ltd., 1967.

Textbook of Veterinary Physiology. Ed. J.E. Breazile. Philadelphia: Lea & Febiger, 1971.

Veterinarians' Product and Therapeutic Reference. Ed. R.M. Grey. Edward Nottage, 1972.

Veterinary Reference Service Update 1976 Large Animal Edition AVP. Ed. J.T. Smithcors.

Way, R.F. and D.A. Lee. **The Anatomy of the Horse.** Philadelphia: J.B. Lippincott Co.

Way, R.F. **Horse Anatomy--Illustrated.** N.Y.: Dreenan Press Ltd., 1973.

Willis, L.C. **The Horse Breeding Farm.** N.Y.: A.S. Barnes, 1976.

APPENDIX

1. Normal Vital Functions
2. Calculating Dosages
3. Diluting Solutions
4. Physiological Saline Solution
5. Conversion Factors and Measurements
6. Diagnostic Laboratory Services
7. Mare Foaling Calendar
8. Sites of Lameness
9. Skeleton of the Horse
10. Points of the Horse
11. Planes of Reference

APPENDIX 1
NORMAL VITAL FUNCTION VALUES OF THE HORSE

RESPIRATION (resting)
Normal Range   8 - 16
Normal Average   12

PULSE RATE (resting)

Mature Horses	30 - 40 pulses/minute
Foals (birth - 2 weeks)	100
Foals (4 weeks - 6 months)	70
Colts and Fillies (6 - 12 months)	45 - 60
Young Horses (1 - 2 years)	40 - 50

TEMPERATURE (rectal)

Normal Range	99.5 - 101.5°F	(37.5 - 38.6°C)
Normal Average	100.5°F	(38°C)
Fever		
mild	100.5 - 102.5°F	(38.0 - 89.2°C)
moderate	102.5 - 104.0°F	(39.2 - 40°C)
high	104.0 - 106.5°F	(40.0 - 41.2°C)
very high	above 106.5°F	(above 41.2°C)

HEMATOLOGY VALUES

Erythrocytes

Red Blood Cell Count (RBC)
range   6.9 - 11.6 millions/cu. mm
average 8.8
Packed Cell Volume (PCV or Hematocrit)
range   29-49.5%
average 39.1%
Hemoglobin (Hbg)
range   9.5-16.4 gm/100 ml
average 12.9
Mean Corpuscular Volume (MCV)
range   39-52 10^{-12}/ml
average 45.5
Mean Corpuscular Hemoglobin Concentration (MCHC)
range   31-35%
average 32.5%

Leukocytes

White Blood Cell Count (WBC)
range   6-13 thousands/cu. mm
average 9.1
Neutrophils
range   35-75
average 55
Lymphocytes
range   15-50
average 35
Eosinophils
range   1-10
average 4
Basophils
range   0-3
average 1

BLOOD CHEMISTRY VALUES

Glucose
range   60 - 100 (mg/100 ml, mg%)
average 73
Urea Nitrogen
range   10 - 20
average 15
Uric Acid
range   0.5 - 1.1
average .8
Creatinine
range   1.2 - 1.9
average 1.5
Calcium
range   11.2 - 13.4 (mg%)
average 12
Magnesium
range   2.2 - 2.8 (mg%)
average 2.5
Phosphorus
range   2.4 - 4.0 (mg%)
average 3

Sodium
range   146 - 152 (mEg/L)
average 149
Chloride
range   98 - 106
average 102
Potassium
range   2.7 - 3.5
average 3.3

Serum Protein   (gm/100 ml)   6.5 gm/100 ml
pH   7.4
Coagulation Time   (minutes)   3 - 15
Volume as a % of Body Weight   9%

560

URINE VALUES
     Specific Gravity
               range   1.025 - 1.060
               average   1.040
     pH range   7.5 - 8
     Quantity
               range   5 - 8 (liters/day)
     Appearance   (yellow, cloudy)

NORMAL RANGES OF REPRODUCTIVE ACTIVITY
     Puberty
               range   10 - 24 months
               average   18 months
     Estrous Cycle Length
               range   19 - 23 days
               average   21 days
     Estrus Period Length
               range   4.5 - 7.5 days
               average   5.5 days
     Ovulation   1-2 days before end of estrus
     Optimum Breeding Time   3 - 4 days before end of estrus
     Gestation Length
               range   330 - 345 days
               average   336 days

APPENDIX   2

CALCULATING DOSAGES

As part of the treatment for a horse suffering from an infectious ailment,the veterinarian may prescribe antibiotic injections. Since these may have to be given frequently, the veterinarian might simply instruct the horseowner to administer the drug so that the veterinarian himself will not have to make frequent calls just to give an injection. In such a case, the horseowner will have to adjust the recommended dosage for horses to fit the particular horse involved.

EXAMPLE:

A 1,000 lb. horse suffering from a respiratory disease is to be given an injection of penicillin at the rate of 10,000 units/kg. The type of penicillin provided by the veterinarian contains 400,000 units/ml. How many ml of the drug should the horseowner administer?

Step 1.
Check the table of approximate conversion factors to change 10,000 units/kg into units/lb.:

$$10,000 \text{ units/kg} = X \text{ units/lb}$$
$$10,000 \text{ units/kg} \times .454 = 4,540 \text{ units/lb}$$

Step 2.
Determine how many units of the drug a 1,000 lb. horse will require:

$$1,000 \text{ lb} \times 4540 \text{ units/lb} = 4,540,000 \text{ units.}$$

Step 3.
Figure out how many ml of 400,000 units/ml drug are needed to provide 4,540,000 units:

$$4,540,000 \text{ units} = X (400,000 \text{ units/ml})$$
$$4,540,000 \text{ units} \div 400,000 \text{ units} = x \text{ ml}$$
$$11.35 = \text{the number of ml necessary.}$$

Step 4.
Since ml are approximately equivalent to cubic centimeters (cc), the horseowner can use a large syringe (a 20cc one, for example) and fill it with penicillin up to the 11 or 12cc mark. It would be almost impossible to accurately measure exactly 11.35cc of penicillin, so the figure can be rounded off. In this instance, rounding off can be safely employed but it should not be commonly done without the knowledge and consent of the veterinarian.

It is vital that the horseowner realize that drugs are not administered in "cc's" or "ml's", but rather in units (I.U., mg) per volume (ml). Different brands and formulations of the same drug vary considerably in strength and potency, so dosage of any medication must be calculated for each individual horse, taking into account the concentration of the product used.

APPENDIX 3

DILUTING SOLUTIONS

It is occasionally necessary to dilute a solution according to its expected use. For example, a 70% solution of ethyl alcohol (for use as a topical antiseptic) must be diluted to a 5% solution for intravenous use (as a poison antidote).

The criss-cross method can be employed to determine how many parts of the original solution and dilutent are required to make a solution of a certain strength. With this method, the percentage of the solution desired is subtracted from the percentage of the original solution; this gives the parts of dilutent that are necessary. Next, the percentage strength of the dilutent (in the case of water, this is always 0%) is subtracted from the percentage of the solution desired; this gives the parts of the original solution that are required.

> **EXAMPLE:**
> 70% alcohol (original solution %) -5% alcohol (desired solution %) = 65 (parts of the dilutent needed).
>
> 5% alcohol (desired solution %) --0% (diluting with water) = 5 (parts of the original solution required).

APPENDIX 4

PHYSIOLOGICAL [NORMAL] SALINE SOLUTION

Physiological saline solution is isotonic with the body's fluid. This means that it contains the same ion concentration as blood and tears. It is used for many veterinary procedures, for example, in tracheal washing, or to rinse a wound, because it is non-irritating and will not cause edema. Because of these properties it is considered preferable to water for wound lavage.

To make this solution, mix warm water with sodium chloride (table salt; use the non-iodized type) in the following proportions:

> **1 teaspoonful sodium chloride/473.2 ml [1 pint] warm water.**

This formula will result in an approximately 0.9% sodium chloride solution.

APPENDIX 5

COMMON MEASUREMENTS AND CONVERSION FACTORS

The two major systems of weights and measurements in use in the United States are the Metric and U.S. systems. For your convenience and to enable you to fully utilize VETERINARY TREATMENTS AND MEDICATIONS FOR HORSEMEN, the following tables are provided. They will enable you to easily convert from one system of measurement to another.

When dealing with the metric system, remember the relationship between each unit of measure:

> 10 millimeter = 1 centimeter
> 100 centimeter = 1 meter
> 1,000 meter = 1 kilometer
> 1,000 milliliter = 1 liter
> 1,000 milligram = 1 gram
> 1,000 gram = 1 kilogram

LENGTH

U.S. System	Metric System
1 inch [in] = 2.54 cm	1 millimeter [mm] = 0.03937 in
1 foot [ft] = 30.48 cm	1 centimeter [cm] = 0.3937 in
1 yard [yd] = 91.44 cm	1 meter [m] = 39.37 in
	or 3.2808 ft
	1 kilometer = 0.6214 mile

To convert from the U.S. system to the Metric system of length, multiply the number of U.S. units by the number of Metrics units per U.S. unit.

Example:
To change 12 inches to centimeters, multiply the number of inches by the number of centimeters per inch.

12 in x 2.54 cm per in = 30.48 cm

To convert from the Metric system of length to the U.S. system, multiply the number of metric units by the number of U.S. units per metric unit.

Example
To change 2 meters to inches, multiply the number of meters by the number of inches per meter.

2m x 39.37 in/m = 78.74 in

VOLUME

U.S. System	Metric System
1 ounce [oz] = 29.573 ml	1 milliliter [ml] = 0.0338 oz
1 pint [pt] = 473.166 ml	1 liter [l] = 33.8148 oz
1 quart [qt] = 946.332 ml	or 2.1134 pt
	or 1.0567 qt
	or .2642 gal

For practical purposes, 1 quart is usually considered approximately equivalent to 1 liter.

To convert from the U.S. System of volume to the Metric system, multiply the number of U.S. units by the number of Metric units per U.S. unit.

Example:
To change 8 fluid oz to ml, multiply the number of fluid oz by the number of ml per fluid oz.

8 fluid oz x 29.573 ml/fluid oz = 236.584 ml

To convert from the Metric system of volume to the U.S. system, multiply the number of Metric units by the number of U.S. units per Metric unit.

Example:
to change 350 ml to oz multiply the number of oz per ml.

350 ml x .0338 oz/ml = 11.834 oz

WEIGHT

U.S. System	Metric System
1 oz = 28.3 gm	1 gram [gm] = 0.03527 oz
1 lb = 453.6 gm	1 kilogram [kg] = 2.2046 lb
1 ton = 907.18 kg	1,000 milligram [mg] = 1 gm

To convert from the U.S. system of weight to the Metric system, multiply the number of U.S. units by the number of Metric units per U.S. unit.

Example:
To change 12 oz to grams, multiply the number of oz by the number of grams per oz.

12 oz x 28.3 gm/oz = 339.6 gm

To convert from the Metric system of weight to the U.S. system, multiply the number of Metric units by the number of U.S. units per Metric unit.

Example:
To change 2.5 kg to lbs multiply the number of kg by the number of lb per kg

2.5 kg x 2.2046 lb/kg = 5.5115 kg

APPROXIMATE HOUSEHOLD MEASURES

It may sometimes be necessary to use a household item to measure a medication or solution. The following table will enable you to make approximately equivalent measures.

1 teaspoonful = 5 ml [or 5 cc]
3 teaspoonsful = 1 tablespoonful
1 tablespoonful = ½ fluid oz = 15 ml
1 jigger = 1½ fluid oz = 45 ml
1 cup = 8 fluid oz = 240 ml

APPROXIMATE CONVERSION FACTORS

This table can be used to convert dosages to the appropriate form for the system of body weight used.

To Convert	To	Multiply by
grains/lb	mg/lb	64.8
grains/lb	mg/kg	143
mg/lb	grains/lb	0.015
mg/lb	mg/kg	2.2
mg/kg	grains/lb	0.007
mg/kg	mg/lb	0.454

TEMPERATURE

There are two major systems of temperature measurement that are commonly used today, Fahrenheit and Centigrade (there are other temperature systems used mainly by the scientific community). The Fahrenheit system is set up so that water freezes at 32°F and boils at 212°F, while in the Centigrade system, water freezes at 0°C and boils at 100°C.

To convert Fahrenheit degrees to Centigrade degrees, subtract 32 from the number of Fahrenheit degrees, multiply the remainder by 5, and divide the result by 9.

Example: 72°F -32 = 40
40 x 5 = 200
200 ÷ 9 = 22.2°C

To convert Centigrade degrees to Fahrenheit degrees, multiply the number of Centigrade degrees by 9, divide the result by 5, and then add 32.

Example: 38°C x 9 = 342
342 ÷ 5 = 68.4
68.4 + 32 = 100.4°F

TEMPERATURE CONVERSION TABLE

Fahrenheit	Centigrade	Fahrenheit	Centigrade
230°	110°	100.4°	38°
212	100	99.5	37.5
203	95	98.6	37
195	90	97.7	36.5
185	85	96.8	36
176	80	95.9	35.5
167	75	95	35
158	70	93.2	34
149	65	91.4	33
140	60	89.6	32
131	55	87.8	31
122	50	86	30
113	45	77	25
111.2	44	68	20
109.4	43	59	15
107.6	42	50	10
105.8	41	41	+5
104.5	40.5	32	0
104	40	23	-5

APPENDIX 6

STATE DIAGNOSTIC LABORATORY SERVICES

Virology and Serology Procedures	Sample Required
Mare Immune Pregnancy test (MIP)	mare serum
Equine Infectious Anemia (AGID)	equine serum
Influenza A1 (HI)	acute† and convalescent† serum
Influenza A2 (HI)	acute and convalescent serum
Venezuelan Equine Encephalomyelitis (HI)	acute and convalescent serum
Western Equine Encephalomyelitis (HI)	acute and convalescent serum
Eastern Equine Encephalomyelitis (HI)	acute and convalescent serum
Equine Rhinopneumonitis (SN) (Serum Neutralization)	acute and convalescent serum; single sample of little diagnostic value, as it only indicates exposure or vaccine response.
Toxoplasma (IFA)	Titers 1:64 or higher indicate exposure
Neonatal Isoerythrolysis (Coombs test)	Foal EDTA (unclotted) blood
Crossmatch of Blood Types	Mare serum vs. stallion EDTA
Brucella (Card or Plate)	Titers 1:50 or higher: positive
Leptospirosis (Plate Agglutination)	Titers 1:160 or higher: positive

Toxicology Procedures
Various toxic chemicals and plants can be identified.

Hematology Procedures
Complete Blood Chemistry (CBC) is available.

Parasitology Procedures
Fecal samples, skin biopsy samples, affected tissues can be examined for parasites.

Pathology Procedures
The following tissues may be sent in for examination:

urine specimen: live animal	intestine
blood specimen: live animal	heart
stomach contents	brain
liver‡	spleen
kidney‡	fetal fluids
lung‡	

† Acute sample is taken at the time of illness, while a convalescent sample is taken 2-3 weeks later.

‡ Always sent for examination

APPENDIX 7
MARE FOALING CALENDAR

This mare foaling calendar, based on an average gestation period of 336 days, can be used to determine the approximate foaling date of the mare, if the breeding date is known. Use the columns marked "Date Bred" to locate the day on which the mare was bred; across from that date will be a date from a column headed "Date Due to Foal" which is the day, a little over eleven months later, on which the mare can be expected to foal. Of course, 336 days is an average, and many mares may foal within about ten days either before or after the date given in this table.

During leap year, the foaling dates opposite February 29 through December 31 should be moved back one day because of the extra day added to February.

DATE BRED	DATE DUE TO FOAL	DATE BRED	DATE DUE TO FOAL	DATE BRED	DATE DUE TO FOAL
Jan. 1	Dec. 3	Mar. 1	Jan. 31	May 1	Apr. 2
2	4	2	Feb. 1	2	3
3	5	3	2	3	4
4	6	4	3	4	5
5	7	5	4	5	6
6	8	6	5	6	7
7	9	7	6	7	8
8	10	8	7	8	9
9	11	9	8	9	10
10	12	10	9	10	11
11	13	11	10	11	12
12	14	12	11	12	13
13	15	13	12	13	14
14	16	14	13	14	15
15	17	15	14	15	16
16	18	16	15	16	17
17	19	17	16	17	18
18	20	18	17	18	19
19	21	19	18	19	20
20	22	20	19	20	21
21	23	21	20	21	22
22	24	22	21	22	23
23	25	23	22	23	24
24	26	24	23	24	25
25	27	25	24	25	26
26	28	26	25	26	27
27	29	27	26	27	28
28	30	28	27	28	29
29	31	29	28	29	30
30	Jan. 1	30	Mar. 1	30	May 1
31	2	31	2	31	2
Feb. 1	3	Apr. 1	3	Jun. 1	3
2	4	2	4	2	4
3	5	3	5	3	5
4	6	4	6	4	6
5	7	5	7	5	7
6	8	6	8	6	8
7	9	7	9	7	9
8	10	8	10	8	10
9	11	9	11	9	11
10	12	10	12	10	12
11	13	11	13	11	13
12	14	12	14	12	14
13	15	13	15	13	15
14	16	14	16	14	16
15	17	15	17	15	17
16	18	16	18	16	18
17	19	17	19	17	19
18	20	18	20	18	20
19	21	19	21	19	21
20	22	20	22	20	22
21	23	21	23	21	23
22	24	22	24	22	24
23	25	23	25	23	25
24	26	24	26	24	26
25	27	25	27	25	27
26	28	26	28	26	28
27	29	27	29	27	29
28	30	28	30	28	30
		29	31	29	31
		30	Apr. 1	30	Jun. 1

DATE BRED	DATE DUE TO FOAL	DATE BRED	DATE DUE TO FOAL	DATE BRED	DATE DUE TO FOAL
Jul. 1	Jun. 2	Sep. 1	Aug. 3	Nov. 1	Oct. 3
2	3	2	4	2	4
3	4	3	5	3	5
4	5	4	6	4	6
5	6	5	7	5	7
6	7	6	8	6	8
7	8	7	9	7	9
8	9	8	10	8	10
9	10	9	11	9	11
10	11	10	12	10	12
11	12	11	13	11	13
12	13	12	14	12	14
13	14	13	15	13	15
14	15	14	16	14	16
15	16	15	17	15	17
16	17	16	18	16	18
17	18	17	19	17	19
18	19	18	20	18	20
19	20	19	21	19	21
20	21	20	22	20	22
21	22	21	23	21	23
22	23	22	24	22	24
23	24	23	25	23	25
24	25	24	26	24	26
25	26	25	27	25	27
26	27	26	28	26	28
27	28	27	29	27	29
28	29	28	30	28	30
29	30	29	31	29	31
30	Jul. 1	30	Sep. 1	30	Nov. 1
31	2	Oct. 1	2	Dec. 1	2
Aug. 1	3	2	3	2	3
2	4	3	4	3	4
3	5	4	5	4	5
4	6	5	6	5	6
5	7	6	7	6	7
6	8	7	8	7	8
7	9	8	9	8	9
8	10	9	10	9	10
9	11	10	11	10	11
10	12	11	12	11	12
11	13	12	13	12	13
12	14	13	14	13	14
13	15	14	15	14	15
14	16	15	16	15	16
15	17	16	17	16	17
16	18	17	18	17	18
17	19	18	19	18	19
18	20	19	20	19	20
19	21	20	21	20	21
20	22	21	22	21	22
21	23	22	23	22	23
22	24	23	24	23	24
23	25	24	25	24	25
24	26	25	26	25	26
25	27	26	27	26	27
26	28	27	28	27	28
27	29	28	29	28	29
28	30	29	30	29	30
29	31	30	Oct. 1	30	Dec. 1
30	Aug. 1	31	2	31	2
31	2				

APPENDIX 8   SITES OF LAMENESS

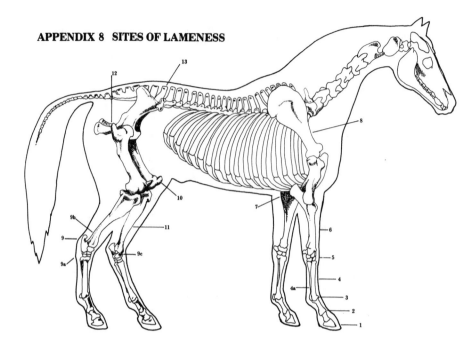

1: contracted heels
    sand cracks
    keratoma
    laminitis
    sidebones
    quittor
    navicular disease
    P3 fractures
    pedal osteitis
    pyramidal disease

2: contracted flexor tendons
    ringbone

3: windpuffs
    osselets
    sesamoiditis
    suspensory ligament sprain
    weak flexor tendons
    constriction of the annular ligament
    stocking up

4: bucked shins
    splints

4a: bowed tendon

5: epiphysitis
    hygroma of the carpus
    carpitis
    ruptured extensor carpi radialis

6: strain of the superior carpal check ligament
    radial nerve paralysis

7: capped elbow

8: sweeny

9: capped hock
    luxated superficial flexor tendon

9a: curb

9b: thoroughpin

9c: occult spavin
    bog spavin
    bone spavin

10: gonitis
    upward fixation of the patella

11: stringhalt
    ruptured peroneus tertius

12: coxitis
    dislocation of the hip joint
    crural paralysis
    pelvic fracture

13: sacroiliac joint subluxation
    over-riding dorsal spinous processes

APPENDIX 9 SKELETON OF THE HORSE

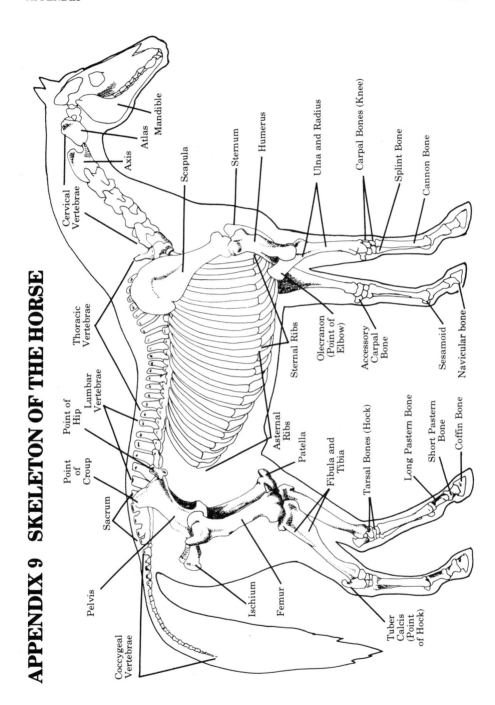

Mandible
Atlas
Axis
Cervical Vertebrae
Scapula
Sternum
Humerus
Ulna and Radius
Carpal Bones (Knee)
Splint Bone
Cannon Bone
Olecranon (Point of Elbow)
Accessory Carpal Bone
Sesamoid
Navicular bone
Sternal Ribs
Thoracic Vertebrae
Point of Hip
Lumbar Vertebrae
Point of Croup
Sacrum
Pelvis
Coccygeal Vertebrae
Ischium
Femur
Patella
Asternal Ribs
Fibula and Tibia
Tarsal Bones (Hock)
Long Pastern Bone
Short Pastern Bone
Coffin Bone
Tuber Calcis (Point of Hock)

APPENDIX 10   POINTS OF THE HORSE

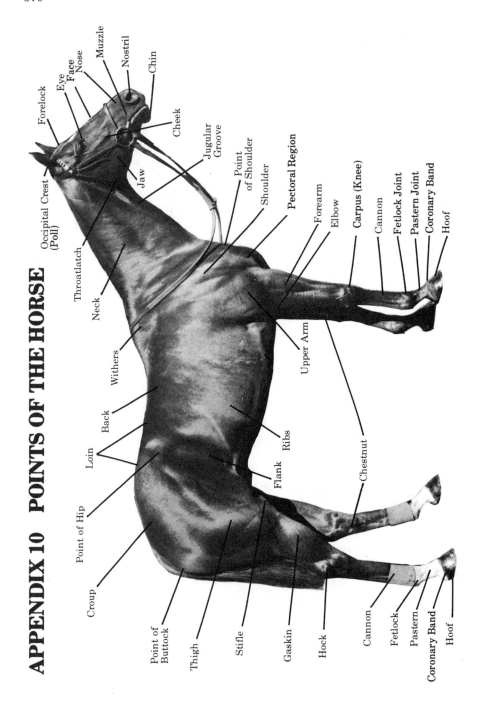

Forelock
Eye
Face
Nose
Muzzle
Nostril
Chin
Cheek
Jugular Groove
Point of Shoulder
Shoulder
Pectoral Region
Forearm
Elbow
Carpus (Knee)
Cannon
Fetlock Joint
Pastern Joint
Coronary Band
Hoof
Occipital Crest (Poll)
Jaw
Throatlatch
Neck
Withers
Back
Loin
Upper Arm
Point of Hip
Croup
Point of Buttock
Thigh
Stifle
Gaskin
Flank
Ribs
Hock
Chestnut
Cannon
Fetlock
Pastern
Coronary Band
Hoof

APPENDIX 11   PLANES OF REFERENCE

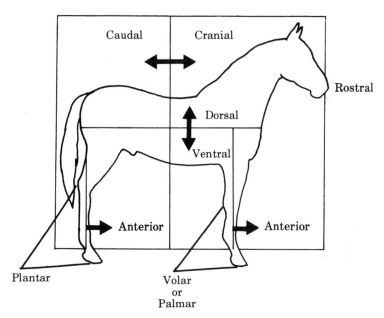

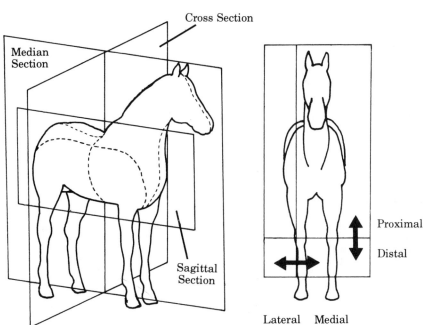

PREFIXES AND SUFFIXES

ab-: From, away.
ad-: Toward.
arthr-, arthro-: Denotes a joint.
auto-: Pertaining to self.
blepharo-: Pertaining to the eyelid.
brachy-: Short.
brady-: Slow.
cardio-: Relating to the heart.
-centesis: Aspiration.
cephalo-: Head.
chondro-: Pertaining to cartilage.
chorio-: Relating to a membrane.
costo-: Relating to the ribs.
cysto-: Relating to the bladder.
-cyte: Denotes a cell.
derm-, derma-, dermat-, dermato-, dermo-: Signifies skin.
dys-: Signifies painful, bad, abnormal, or difficult.
ecto-: On, without, on the outside.
-ectomy: Operative removal of a given part.
-emia: Blood.
endo-: Within.
enter-, entero-: Relating to intestines.
exo-: Outside.
gnath-, gnatho-: Denotes relationship to the jaw.
hepat-: Denoting the liver.
hemo-: Signifies blood.
hydro-: Denotes relationship to water.
hyper-: Signifies above, beyond, excessive.
intra-: Within.
iso-: Equal, alike, or the same.
-itis: Denotes inflammation of a given part.
leuko-: White.
lyso-: Splitting, destruction.
mal-: Ill or bad.
meta-: After, subsequent to, behind.
myco-: Relating to fungus.
-oma: Denotes a tumor or neoplasm.
-osis: Denotes a process, particularly a disease or morbid process.
-osteo: Denotes relationship to bone or bones.
para-: Beside, beyond, apart from.
peri-: Around.
-phage, phago-: Eating or devouring.
pneumo-: Relating to the lungs.
pyo-: Relating to pus.
rhino-: Denotes relationship to the nose.
-rrhage: Denotes excessive flow.
-rrhea: Denotes flow or discharge.
septic-: Pertaining to pus forming or pathogenic organisms.
supra- Above or over.
syn-: Associated with.
epi-: Denotes on, upon, following, or subsequent to.
tachy-: Fast.
toco-: Relating to birth.
-tomy: Cutting or incising.
trans-: Denotes across or through.
-uria: Pertaining to the urine.
vaso-: Related to a vessel or a duct.

GLOSSARY

A

ABDOMINOCENTESIS: Withdrawal of fluid through a needle into the abdominal cavity.

ABDUCTION: A drawing away from the median plane of the body.

ABORT: To expel a fetus before it is viable.

ABORTIFACIENT: Substance which causes abortion.

ABRASION: A wound caused by the wearing away of the top layer of skin aand hair by friction.

ABSCESS: A localized collection of purulent material in a cavity formed by disintegration of tissues.

ACETABULUM: Pelvic structure which receives the head of the femur to make the hip joint.

ACIDOSIS: A condition of acid accumulation in the body due to disruption of the normal acid base balance.

ACTH: Adrenocorticotropic hormone; a hormone secreted by the anterior pituitary gland that acts primarily on the adrenal cortex, stimulating its growth and secretion of corticosteroids. The production of this hormone is increased in times of stress.

ACTIVE IMMUNIZATION: Acquired immunity due to the presence of antibodies formed in response to an antigen.

ACUTE: Having a short and relatively severe course.

ADDUCTION: A drawing toward the median plane of the body.

ADHESION: Abnormal firm fibrous attachment between two structures.

ADJUVANT: A substance added to a prescription to increase the action of the main ingredient; in immunology, a vehicle used.

ADRENOCORTICAL: Pertaining to the cortex of the adrenal gland.

AEROBE: A microorganism that lives and grows in the presence of oxygen.

AEROPHAGIA: Spasmodic swallowing of air followed by the belching of air from the stomach.

AGGLUTINATION TITER: The highest dilution of a serum that causes clumping of bacteria or other particulate antigens.

ALIMENTARY CANAL: The tract extending the length of the body from lips to anus in which digestion occurs.

ALKALOID: A bitter organic basic substance found in plants, such as atropine, morphine, nicotine.

ALKALOSIS: Disturbance of acid base balance resulting in excess base or a deficit of acid or carbon dioxide.

ALLERGEN: A protein or non-protein substance capable of inducing allergy or hypersensitivity.

ALLERGY: A hypersensitive state acquired through exposure to a particular allergen, reexposure resulting in an alteration of the normal reaction to the substance.

ALOPECIA: Loss of hair.

ALVEOLAR PERIOSTITIS: An inflammation of the outer bone of the tooth socket due to infection, and marked by suppuration and pain.

ALVEOLI: Tooth sockets.

ANABOLIC: Pertaining to any constructive process, particularly the process in which simple substances are converted into living tissue; building of muscle and condition.

ANAEROBE: An organism capable of growing in the complete, or almost complete, absence of oxygen.

ANALGESIC: A drug that relieves pain without the loss of conciousness.

ANAPHYLAXIS: An unusual allergic reaction to a foreign protein or drug which results in a state of shock.

ANASTOMOSE: To create a connection between two hollow or tubular structures, as divided ends of intestine or blood vessels.

ANDROGENS: Hormones which produce masculine characteristics.

ANEMIA: A blood disorder characterized by abnormally low red blood cell count, hemoglobin concentration, or packed cell volume.

ANESTHETIC: A drug or agent that is used to abolish the sensation of pain.

ANESTRUS: A period of sexual inactivity between two estrous cycles.

ANEURYSM: A blood-filled sac formed by an abnormal dilation of the wall of an artery, a vein, or the heart.

ANHIDROSIS: An abnormal deficiency of sweat.

ANHYDROUS: Containing no water.

ANKYLOSIS: Fusion of joint surfaces due to disease, injury, or surgical procedure.

ANNULAR: Shaped like a ring.

ANOREXIA: Loss of appetite.

ANOXIA: Lack of oxygen.

ANTAGONISTIC: In opposition, as when referring to two drugs that nullify each other's actions.

ANTERIOR: Situated in front of or in the forward part of an organ, or toward the head end of the body.

ANTERIOR SYNECHIA: Adhesion of iris to cornea.

ANTERIOR UVEAL TRACT: The iris and ciliary body.

ANTHELMINTICS: Agents (drugs) that are destructive to worms; the drugs that are active in commercial dewormers.

ANTIBIOTIC: A chemical substance produced by a microorganism which has the capacity, in dilute solutions, to inhibit the growth of or to kill other microorganisms.

ANTIBODY: A protein in the blood or other body fluid that interacts with a specific antigen to neutralize it.

ANTICOAGULANT: Substance which prevents clotting of blood; used in collecting blood samples, e.g., sodium acid citrate.

ANTIDOTE: A substance used to combat the effect of a poison.

ANTIGEN: Any substance, such as a toxin, foreign protein, bacterium or tissue cell, which enters the body and causes the formation of an antibody.

ANTIHISTAMINE: A drug which counteracts the effects of histamine, especially useful in allergic reactions.

ANTI-INFLAMMATORY: An agent that counteracts or suppresses the inflammatory response.

ANTIMYCOTICS: Fungistatic and fungicidal agents.

ANTIOXIDANT: A substance which prevents destruction through oxidative processes.

ANTIPHLOGISTIC: An agent that counteracts inflammation.

ANTIPRURITIC: An agent that prevents or relieves itching.

ANTIPYOGENIC: An agent that prevents suppuration or the formation of pus.

ANTIPYRETIC: An agent that reduces fever.

ANTISEPTIC: An agent that prevents the decay or decomposition of tissue by inhibiting the growth and development of microorganisms.

ANTISERUM: A serum that contains antibodies.

ANTISPASMODIC: An agent that relieves muscle spasms, usually referring to smooth muscle spasms, as of the digestive system.

ANTITOXIN: An antibody to the toxin of a microorganism, to a zootoxin, or to a phytotoxin, that combines with the toxin, causing its neutralization.

ANTITUSSIVE: An agent that prevents or relieves coughing.

ANTIVENIN: A proteinaceous material used in the treatment of poisoning by animal venom.

ANURIA: Little or no excretion of urine.

APICAL: Pertaining to the top or tip of a structure.

APLASTIC: Pertaining to a lack of development of an organ or tissue.

APOCRINE: A type of glandular secretion that contains part of the secreting cell.

APONEUROSIS: A flattened tendinous expansion which runs from a muscle attachment to the muscle body.

APPOSITION: The placing of things in proximity, as when bringing together the edges of a wound for suturing.

AQUEOUS HUMOR: The fluid produced in the eye, occupying the anterior and posterior chambers of the eye, and diffusing out of the eye into the blood.

ARCADE: An anatomical structure resembling a series of arches, usually referring to the surface of the jaws that holds the teeth.

ARRHYTHMIA: Any variation from the normal heartbeat.

ARTERIES: Vessels through which oxygen-enriched blood passes away from the heart toward the various parts of the body.

ARTERIOLES: The arteries of capillary beds.

ARTHRITIS: Inflammation of joints.

ARTHROCENTESIS: Puncture and aspiration of joint fluid.

ARTHROCHONDRITIS: Inflamed joint cartilage.

ARTHRODESIS: Surgically induced fusion of a joint.

ARTICULAR: Pertaining to a joint.

ARTICULATION: Junction between two or more bones.

ARTIFICIAL INSEMINATION: Depositing semen into the vagina or cervix by artificial means.

ASCITES: Collection of fluid in the abdomen, as in congestive heart failure.

ASEPTIC: Sterile.

ASPECT: The part of a surface facing in any designated direction.

ASPERMIA: Failure of formation or emission of sperm.

ASPHYXIATION: Suffocation.

ASPIRATE: The act of inhaling, or the withdrawal of fluids or gases from a cavity by suction.

ASPIRATION BIOPSY: A biopsy in which the tissue is obtained by the application of suction through a needle attached to a syringe.

ASSIMILATION: The transformation of food into living tissue.

ASTRINGENT: An agent, usually applied topically, which causes local contraction of blood vessels and stops discharge.

ASYMMETRY: Lack of symmetry.

ATARACTIC: A tranquilizer.

ATAXIA: An inability to coordinate voluntary muscular movements; incoordination.

ATONY: Lack of normal tone or strength.

ATRESIA: Congenital absence or closure of a normal body opening, as in atresia ani.

ATROPHY: A decrease in size or wasting away of a body part or tissue.

ATTENTUATE: To render thin or less virulent by passage of a microorganism through host species or by repeated growth on laboratory media.

AUSCULTATION: The act of listening for sounds within the body, chiefly for determining the condition of the lungs, heart, pleura, abdomen, and intestines.

AUTOCLAVE: An apparatus that sterilizes by using steam under pressure.

AUTONOMIC NERVOUS SYSTEM: The part of the nervous system that regulates the internal environment of the body that is not under conscious (voluntary) control; composed of sympathetic and parasymphathetic systems.

AUTOPSY: The postmortem examination of a body.

AVASCULAR: Not supplied with blood vessels.

AVULSION: The tearing away of part of a structure, e.g., avulsion fracture.

AZOTURIA: A disease of horses marked by a sudden attack of perspiration and paralysis of the hindquarters and by the passing of light red to dark brown urine. It occurs in horses that, after being engaged in continuous work, are rested with no decrease in feed and then returned to work.

B

BACTERIA: Any microorganism of the class Schizomycetes.

BACTERICIDAL: Destructive to bacteria.

BACTERIN: A suspension of killed bacteria used as a vaccine to stimulate the production of antibodies.

BACTERIOSTATIC: An agent that inhibits the growth or multiplication of bacteria.

BARREN MARE: One that is not pregnant.

BAR SHOE: A corrective shoe that uses either a half-bar or a full-bar across the frog from heel to heel; creates extra pressure on the frog.

BARKER FOAL: Convulsive syndrome; neonatal maladjustment syndrome.

BASE-NARROW: The distance between the center lines of the limbs at their origin is greater than the center lines of the feet on the ground; will be broad-chested.

BASE-WIDE: Opposite of base-narrow.

BEAN: A hard mass of smegma that collects around the urethral process at the end of the penis.

BENIGN: Not malignant or recurrable, with a favorable outlook for recovery.

BIFURCATION: The site where a single structure divides into two branches.

BIG KNEES: Abnormal growth caused by epiphysitis or resulting from concussion.

BILATERAL: Having two sides or pertaining to both sides.

BILIRUBIN: A bile pigment formed from the breakdown of hemoglobin when red blood cells are destroyed.

BIOLOGICAL: A medicinal preparation made from living organisms or their products, including vaccines, antitoxins, serums, etc.

BIOPSY: The removal and microscopic examination of a minute portion or tissue from a living body to aid in diagnosis.

BLEMISH: A minor conformation fault, caused by either an injury of occurring congenitally, that is considered unattractive but does not interfere with the horse's soundness.

BLEPHAROSPASM: Spasm of the eyelids that causes partial or complete closure of the eye.

BLIND SPAVIN: See Occult Spavin.

BLISTER: A counterirritant applied to the skin to cause blistering and inflammation, used to treat chronic or subacute inflammations of joints, tendons or bones.

BLOOD POISONING: Septicemia.

BLOOD PRESSURE: The pressure of the blood on the walls of the arteries, dependent on the energy of the heart action, the elasticity of the walls of the arteries, and the volume and viscosity of the blood; systolic and diastolic pressure.

BOG SPAVIN: A chronic distension of the tibiotarsal joint capsule of the hock with synovial fluid.

BOLUS: A rounded mass of food or medicine which is given orally.

BONE CUTTER: A forceps-like instrument, originally designed to cut bones, that can also be used successfully to remove the sharp points on a horse's teeth.

BONE SPAVIN: A lameness originating in the hock which is characterized by either exostosis or bone destruction on the inner surface of the hock.

BOOSTER: Second or subsequent dose of vaccine.

BORBORYGMI: Sounds caused by the passage of food, fluid, and gas through the digestive system. These sounds are increased in spasmodic colic and diarrhea, and decreased in impaction.

BOT: The larvae of botflies, which are parasitic in the stomach; Gastrophilus species.

BOTULISM: A type of food poisoning caused by the neurotoxin of Clostridium botulinum; characterized by abdominal pain, nervous system signs, secretion disturbances, mydriasis, etc.

BOWED TENDON: Damage to the flexor tendons or tendon sheaths below the carpus that results in inflammation; syn. tendosynovitis.

BOWLINE KNOT: A particular knot that will not slip or jam.

BRACE: An alcohol-based substance applied to horses' legs after exercise.

BRACHYGNATHISM: An abnormally short lower jaw; syn. parrot mouth.

BRADYCARDIA: An abnormally slow heart rate.

BREAKOVER: The act of rolling the hoof forward, lifting the foot from the ground heel first, as the horse moves forward.

BROAD SPECTRUM ANTIBIOTIC: An agent that is effective against a variety of organisms; describes the range of certain antibiotics, such as ampicillin.

BRONCHIAL DILATOR: A drug that will dilate (enlarge) the bronchi and other air passages of the respiratory system.

BRUISE: A contusion caused by impact without laceration.

BUCCAL: Pertaining to the cheek.

BUCK KNEES: Syn. over at the knees; anterior deviation of the carpus.

BUCKED SHINS: A periostitis of the anterior surface of the cannon bone, usually occurring on the forelegs of young horses that are strenuously exercised.

BUN: Blood urea nitrogen.

BURSA: A sac or sac-like cavity filled with fluid and situated at places in the tissue at which friction would otherwise develop, e.g., navicular bursa.

BURSITIS: An inflammation of a bursa, occasionally accompanied by the formation of a calcified deposit in the underlying tendon.

BUTTRESS FOOT: A form of low ringbone in which the horse's hoof and coronary region become pyramidal in shape due to bony enlargement at the front of the coffin bone.

C

CACHEXIA: Wasting and malnutrition.

CAESAREAN SECTION: Incision through the abdominal and uterine walls for the delivery of a fetus.

CALLUS: Localized hyperplasia of the epidermis of the skin due to friction or pressure; an unorganized meshwork which forms around the site of a fracture and is eventually replaced by bone during healing.

CANCELLOUS: Spongy tissue of bone.

CANKER: Chronic hypertrophy of the horn-producing tissues of the foot, especially the frog and the sole.

CANNULA: A tube inserted into a body cavity to transfuse or draw off fluid.

CAPILLARIES: Minute vessels that connect the arterioles and venules, forming a network in nearly all parts of the body. Their walls act as semipermeable membranes for the interchange of various substances between the blood and tissue fluid.

CAPILLARY ACTION: The action by which a liquid is elevated in a tube through the attraction of its surface molecules to those of the tube.

CAPILLARY REFILL TIME: The time required for normal blood flow and color to return to an area of the gingiva to which pressure has been applied.

CAPPED ELBOW: A soft flabby swelling over the point of the elbow due to trauma.

CAPPED HOCK: An inflammation of the bursa over the point of the hock caused by trauma.

CAPS: Deciduous premolar teeth.

CARBOHYDRATES: Sugars and starches.

CARCINOMA: A malignant neoplasm derived from epithelial cells that tends to metastasize.

CARDIAC CYCLE: The actions of the heart during one complete heartbeat.

CARDIAC OUTPUT: The amount of blood pumped from the heart during each beat.

CARDIOVASCULAR: Pertaining to the heart and blood vessels.

CARPAL: Pertaining to the knee.

CARPITIS: Acute or chronic inflammation of the carpus, causing swelling, pain, and lameness; may involve the joint, bone, and associated ligaments.

CARTILAGE: A specialized type of fibrous connective tissue, often associated with joint surfaces.

CASLICK'S OPERATION: An operation to correct pneumovagina that involves suturing the upper vulvar lips together.

CATABOLISM: Breaking down of protein and loss of muscle.

CATALYST: A substance that brings about increased rate of a chemical reaction without being itself consumed by that reaction.

CATAPLASM: See Poultice.

CATARACT: An opacity of the lens of the eye.

CATHARTIC: An agent that causes evacuation of the bowels.

CATHETER: A flexible tubular instrument for withdrawing fluids from, or introducing fluids to a body cavity, e.g., urinary catheter, indwelling intravenous catheter, etc.

CAUDAD: Toward the tail; opposite of cephalad.

CAUDAL: Referring to a position near the tail.

CAUSTIC: Burning, corrosive, and destructive to living tissue.

CAUTERIZE: To destroy or coagulate tissue with a hot iron, electric current, or caustic substance.

CAUTERY: The application of a caustic substance, a hot iron, or an electric current to destroy living tissue.

CELLULITIS: Purulent inflammation of subcutaneous tissues.

CELLULOSE: A carbohydrate that appears only in plants and cannot be digested by horses; also referred to as fiber.

CEPHALAD: Toward the head; opposite of caudad.

CEREBROSPINAL FLUID: Fluid containing salts, proteins, and sugar which bathes the spinal cord and brain stem.

CERVICAL: Pertaining to the neck, or to the neck of any organ or structure, such as the cervix of the uterus.

CHEMOTHERAPY: The treatment of disease by chemical agents.

CHOKE: A partial or complete esophageal obstruction that may cause death through perforation of the esophagus or degeneration and death of the tissues due to pressure.

CHOLINERGIC: Refers to the parasympathetic nerve endings which release acetylcholine.

CHONDRITIS: Inflamed cartilage.

CHONDROIDS: Relating to or resembling cartilage.

CHONDROMALACIA: Softening of the articular cartilage, especially in the patella.

CHORIOALLANTOIC SAC: Placenta.

CHORIORETINITIS: An inflammation of the choroid and the retina of the eye.

CHRONIC: Long-term, continued, not acute.

CILIA: Minute hair-like processes that move in a swaying motion.

CIRCUMDUCTION: The circular movement of an eye or leg.

CLOT: A semi-solidified mass of red blood cells and fibrin.

COAGULATE: To form a blood clot or insoluble fibrin clot.

COFFIN BONE: Third phalanx, P3.

COGGINS TEST: An agar gel immunodiffusion test used to determine the presence of EIA antibodies in a blood sample.

COLIC: Acute abdominal pain.

COLLAGEN: The main fibrous protein of skin, bone, tendon, cartilage and connective tissue.

COLLATERAL: Secondary or accessory; a small side branch, as of a blood vessel or nerve.

COLLODION: A clear, viscous liquid that dries to a transparent film when applied over wounds as a protective covering.

COLOSTRUM: The first milky secretion from the mammary glands of the mare, with high protein and protective antibody content, secreted shortly before and for a few days after delivery of a foal.

COMA: A state of unconsciousness from which the animal cannot be aroused.

COMMINUTE: To break or crush into small pieces.

COMPOUND FRACTURE: A fracture that has broken the skin.

COMPRESSION BANDAGE: A bandage that is applied tightly over the site of inflammation to provide pressure to the area and reduce swelling.

COMPRESSION SCREW: A special kind of screw used to fix bone fragments together.

CONCUSSION: A violent jar or shock; in head injury, consciousness is impaired or lost.

CONDYLE: A rounded projection on a bone.

CONFORMATION: The shape or contour of the body or body structures.

CONGENITAL: Existing at and usually before birth; referring to conditions that may or may not be inherited.

CONGESTION: Excessive abnormal accumulation of blood in a part of the body.

CONJUNCTIVITIS: Inflammation of the membrane that lines the eyelid and covers part of the eyeball.

CONNECTIVE TISSUE: The tissue which binds together and is the support of the various structures of the body, made up of fibroblasts, collagen fibrils, and elastin fibrils.

CONSOLIDATION: The process of becoming solid, as when, in pneumonia, the lung becomes firm as the air spaces fill up with exudate.

CONSTIPATION: Infrequent or difficult evacuation of the feces.

CONTAGIOUS: Able to spread from one animal to another.

CONTAMINANT: Foreign material such as microorganisms in a wound or bacteria introduced accidentally to a bacterial culture.

CONTRACTED HEELS: A condition in which the foot is contracted and narrowed at the heel, caused by a lack of frog pressure and moisture.

CONTRAINDICATE: To render any particular method of treatment as undesirable or improper.

CONSTRICTION: An area of compression and of drawing together; a stricture.

CONTUSION: A bruise; an injury that does not break the skin.

CONVALESCENCE: Period of recovery from surgery or injury.

COPROPHAGY: The eating of feces.

CORIUM: Modified vascular tissue inside the horn of the hoof which produces the horn: perioplic corium, coronary corium, laminar corium, sole corium, and frog corium.

CORONARY: Pertaining to the heart; encircling in the manner of a crown, as applied to blood vessels, ligaments, or nerves; the coronary band encircles the hoof.

CORPORA NIGRA: Pigmented nodules on the upper and lower edge of the pupil which break up light to protect the inner eye structures.

CORTICOSTEROIDS: A term applied to hormones of the adrenal cortex or to any other natural or synthetic compound having a similar activity. They have systemic and metabolic effects and inhibit the inflammatory process.

CORTISONE: A hormone from the adrenal cortex with anti-inflammatory properties that affects carbohydrate, water, and mineral metabolism; changes fibrous tissue growth, and reduces resistance to infection.

COUNTERIRRITANTS: An agent that produces a superficial irritation and increased blood flow to a part.

COXITIS: Inflammation of the hip joint.

CRANIAL: Pertaining to the cranium (skull), or to the anterior end of the body.

CREPITATION: The noise made by rubbing together the ends of a fractured bone. A sound like that made by rubbing the hair between the fingers.

CROSS-FIRING: Condition in which the inside toe or wall of a hindfoot strikes the inner quarter or undersurface of the opposite forefoot.

CROSS-MATCHING: Process of testing blood of one individual against that of another prior to transfusion or foal nursing first colostrum.

CRYOSURGERY: The destruction of tissue by the application of extreme cold, used in the treatment of sarcoids, etc.

CRYPTORCHIDISM: A developmental defect marked by the failure of the testes to descend into the scrotum.

CULTURE: A growth of microorganisms of living tissue cells.

CURB: A thickening of the plantar tarsal ligament, resulting in an enlargement below the point of the hock, and marked by inflammation and lameness.

CURETTAGE: The removal of growths or other material from the wall of a cavity, usually by scraping.

CURETTE: A spoon-shaped instrument used to remove material, e.g., from the uterus, from a bony surface, etc.

CYCLOPLEGICS: Agents that paralyze the ciliary muscles of the eye, causes mydriasis, e.g., atropine.

CYST: Any normal or abnormal closed cavity or sac, lined by epithelium, particularly one that contains a liquid or semi-solid material.

CYSTITIS: Inflamed urinary bladder.

D

DEBILITATE: To weaken.

DEBRIDE: To remove foreign material and contaminated or dead tissue, usually by sharp dissection.

DECIDUOUS TEETH: The first teeth which are shed at maturity.

DECUBITUS: Ulcers or sores formed from prolonged lying down, especially on the hip, stifle, elbow, and bony prominences of the head.

DEHISCE: To split open.

DEMINERALIZE: To excessively eliminate mineral or inorganic salts from individual tissues, especially bone, e.g., osteomalacia.

DENTIGEROUS CYST: A tumor containing different kinds of material such as hair or tooth tissue. Also known as an ear fistula or conchal sinus.

DERMAL: Pertaining to the skin.

DERMATITIS: Inflammation of the skin.

DERMATOMYCOTIC: Referring to a superficial fungal infection of the skin.

DESICCATION: The act of drying up.

DESMITIS: Inflammation of a ligament.

DESMOTOMY: The cutting or division of ligaments.

DESQUAMATING: The peeling of the epithelial layer.

DEWORMER: Any of a number of commercial products containing anthelmintics; administered by stomach tube, syringe, or through feed to control parasites.

DEXTROSE: Glucose; a monosaccharide that is widely distributed in nature, is the carbohydrate found in the blood of animals where it is an immediate source of energy.

DIARRHEA: Abnormal frequency and liquidity of fecal discharges.

DIASTOLE: The period of dilatation of the heart, coinciding with the interval between the first and second heart sounds.

DIATHERMY: Heating of the body tissues by high-frequency electromagnetic radiation.

DIESTRUS: A short period of sexual quiescence occuring between metestrus and proestrus.

DIFFUSED: Not localized; widely spread.

DIGITAL: Pertaining to the long and short pastern bones and the coffin bone, i.e., Pl, P2, P3.

DILATATION: The condition of being dilated or stretched beyond normal dimensions.

DISINFECTANT: A chemical or physical agent used to kill bacteria on inanimate objects; generally considered too toxic for use on animals.

DISLOCATION: The displacement of any part, usually referring to a bone or joint.

DISSEMINATE: Scatter or spread over a considerable area.

DISTAL: Remote; more removed from the point of attachment or any point of reference; opposite of proximal.

DISTEMPER: Strangles, an infectious bacterial disease characterized by mucopurulent inflammation of the respiratory mucous membrane.

DISTENSION: The act of being swollen or enlarged from internal pressure.

DIURETIC: An agent that increases the production of urine.

DORSAL: Pertaining to the back or denoting a position more toward the back surface; opposite of ventral.

DRENCHING: The pouring of liquid medication down an animal's throat.

DROPPED ELBOW: Loss of control of the forelimb because of radial nerve paralysis.

DRY-COAT: Anhidrosis, the lack of the ability to sweat.

DUCT: A passage with definite walls.

DUMMY FOAL: A foal suffering from the convulsive syndrome caused by a lack of oxygen at birth; also called barker foal.

DURATION: The length of time that an illness or condition lasts.

DYSENTERY: A disorder characterized by inflammation of the intestines and abdominal pain. There will be blood and mucus in the frequent stools, and it can be caused by chemical irritants, bacteria, protozoa, or parasitic worms.

DYSFUNCTION: Disturbance or impaired function of an organ.
DYSPHAGIA: Difficulty in swallowing.
DYSPNEA: Difficult or labored breathing.
DYSTOCIA: Abnormal labor or childbirth.
DYSURIA: Difficulty in passing urine.

E

ECBOLIC: Pertaining to rapid labor.
ECTROPION: The outward turning of the edge of the eyelid.
ECZEMA: Any non-specific inflammation of the outermost layer of skin.
EDEMA: An accumulation of abnormally large amounts of fluid between cells in the tissues.
EFFICACY: Effectiveness or the ability to produce a desired effect.
ELECTROCARDIOGRAM: A graphic tracing of the electrical impulses produced by the heart muscle.
ELECTROLYTE: A substance present in body fluids which is capable of conducting electricity in various body functions such as nerve impulses, oxygen and carbon dioxide transport, and muscle contraction.
ELECTRORETINOGRAPH: An instrument for measuring the electrical response of the retina of the eye to light stimulation.
ELECTUARY: A medicinal preparation consisting of a powdered drug made into a paste with honey or syrup; a confection.
EMACIATED: The condition of being excessively thin, in a wasted condition.
EMBOLISM: The sudden blocking of an artery by a clot or foreign material carried by the bloodstream.
EMBRYOTOMY: The dismemberment of a fetus in the uterus to facilitate delivery.
EMOLLIENT: Drug which softens or soothes irritation.
EMPHYSEMA: See Heaves.
EMPIRICAL: Based on experience.
EMULSIFIER: An agent used to produce an emulsion.
EMULSION: A preparation of one liquid distributed in small globules throughout another liquid.
ENAMEL: The white, compact, and very hard substance that covers and protects the dentine of the crown of a tooth.
ENCEPHALITIS: Inflammation of the brain.
ENCEPHALOMYELITIS: Inflammation of the brain and spinal cord.
ENDEMIC: A disease constantly present, at a low level, in the animal population.
ENDOCRINE: Secreting internally; applied to organs and structures which secrete hormones into the blood or lymph that have an effect on other parts of the body, the target organs.
ENDOCRINOLOGY: Study of endocrine glands and their hormones.
ENDOGENOUS: Originating within the body.
ENDOSCOPE: An instrument for the examination of the interior of a hollow organ such as the bladder.
ENDOTOXIN: A heat-stable toxin present in the bacterial cell.
ENGORGEMENT: Hyperemia; local congestion; excessive fullness of any organ or vessel.
ENTERIC: Pertaining to the intestines.
ENTERITIS: Inflammation of the intestine, particularly the small intestine.
ENTERECTOMY: Resection of the intestine.
ENTEROTOMY: Incision into the intestine, used in such conditions as colic.
ENTEROTOXEMIA: A condition characterized by the presence in the blood of toxins produced in the intestines.
ENTROPION: The inward turning of the eyelid.
ENZYME: A protein which acts as a catalyst (helps cause or accelerate) a chemical reaction, as in digestion of feed, without being consumed in the process.
EPIDEMIC: A disease that is not normally present that attacks many animals in a community simultaneously.

EPIDERMIS: The outer epithelial portion of the skin.

EPIDURAL: On or outside of the fibrous covering of the brain and spinal cord.

EPILATION: The removal of hair by the roots.

EPIPHORA: Tearing.

EPIPHYSIS: The cartilaginous growth plates at the ends of long bones.

EPISIOTOMY: A surgical incision of the vulva.

EPISTAXIS: Nosebleed.

EPITHELIAL: Pertaining to the epithelium, which is the covering of the internal and external surfaces of the body, including the lining of vessels and other small cavities.

EPSOM SALT: Magnesium sulfate.

ERYTHROCYTES: Red blood cells; transport inspired oxygen from the lungs to body tissues.

ERYTHROPOIESIS: The formation of red blood cells.

ESCHAROTIC: A corrosive or caustic agent, such as those used to remove granulation tissue.

ESR: Erythrocyte sedimentation rate; the rate of settling and separation of red blood cells in a volume of drawn blood.

ESTROUS: Pertaining to estrus.

ESTRUS: A period of sexual receptivity in the female during which she ovulates and is able to conceive; the heat period.

ETIOLOGY: The cause of a disease.

EUTHANASIA: An easy or painless death; mercy killing.

EVACUATION: An emptying, as of the bowels.

EXCISION: Removal of an organ or part of a structure by cutting.

EXCRETION: The act of eliminating the body's waste materials.

EXOCRINE: A glandular secretion that is delivered to the body surface, e.g., sweat gland.

EXOGENOUS: Originating from outside the body.

EXOSTOSIS: A benign bony growth projecting outward from the surface of a bone; may cause mechanical interference.

EXOTOXIN: Extracellular toxin.

EXPECTORANT: Promoting the ejection of mucus or other fluids from the lungs and trachea.

EXPIRATION: The act of breathing out.

EXTENSOR: Any muscle that extends a joint; opposite of flexor.

EXTRAVASATION: A discharge or escape of blood or other substance from a vessel into the tissues.

EXUDATE: Fluid or cells which have escaped from blood vessels into tissues or onto tissue surfaces, usually as a result of inflammation.

F

FASCIA: White fibrous tissue sheets beneath skin or between muscles.

FEBRILE: Characterized by fever.

FERMENTATION: Enzymatic decomposition of a complex organic compound into simpler compounds.

FETID: Having a disagreeable odor.

FEVER: Elevation of body temperature above the normal.

FIBRIN: An elastic filamentous protein active in coagulation of the blood.

FIBROCARTILAGINOUS: Cartilage which contains a large amount of fibrous connective tissue.

FIBROMA: Benign tumor of fibrous tissue.

FIBROSIS: The formation of fibrous tissue during the reparative process.

FIBROUS ADHESION: A fibrous band or structure by which organs or other structures abnormally adhere to one another.

FIBROUS CONNECTIVE TISSUE: Tissue consisting of elongated cells, fibroblasts, and collagen.

FIRST INTENTION HEALING: The preferred method of healing in which the opposing edges of a wound are perfectly aligned and no granulation tissue fills the defect.

FISTULA: An abnormal passage between two organs or from an internal organ to the surface of the body.

FLACCID: Flabby and without tone.

FLATULENCE: Pertaining to excessive amounts of air or gases in the stomach or intestine which may be expelled through the anus.

FLEXION: The act of bending.

FLEXOR: Any muscle that flexes a joint; opposite of extensor.

FLOAT: The rasp used to file a horse's teeth.

FLOATING: The act of filing a horse's teeth to remove the sharp edges.

FOAL HEAT: The first heat period which occurs approximately nine days after a mare has foaled; also called nine-day heat.

FOMENTATION: Warm and moist applications applied for treatment; a poultice.

FORCEPS: An instrument used for compressing or grasping tissues in surgery, or for handling sterile dressings and surgical supplies.

FORGING: A type of limb contact during movement, in which the toe of the hind foot hits the bottom of the forefoot on the same side as it leaves the ground.

FOSSA: A hollow or depressed area.

FOUNDER: The crippling condition caused by laminitis.

FOUNDER RING: A ring in the hoof wall that results from improper keratin synthesis following an attack of laminitis.

FRACTIONATION: In radiology, division of the total dose of radiation into small doses given at intervals; given in this manner, radiation usually causes less biological damage than the same total dose administered at one time.

FRESHEN: To trim the edges of a wound before suturing.

FUNDUS: The interior part of the eye exposed to view through the ophthalmoscope.

FUNGICIDES: Agents that destroy fungi.

FUNGISTATIC: Pertaining to agents that retard the growth and development of fungi.

FUNGUS: A general term used to denote a group of organisms responsible for the mycotic diseases, e.g., ringworm, phycomycosis.

FUSION: The abnormal coherence of adjacent parts of bodies, e.g., arthrodesis.

G

GAMMA RAYS: Photons released spontaneously by a radioactive substance.

GAMMA RAY THERAPY: A type of radiation therapy using gamma rays to treat conditions such as neoplasms.

GANGRENE: Death of tissue, usually due to loss of blood supply; may be wet or dry.

GASTRIC: Pertaining to the stomach.

GASTRIC DILATATION: Excessive distension of the stomach, as in grain overload toxicity.

GENERAL ANESTHETIC: Drug used for surgery to produce complete unconsciousness and to abolish pain sensation.

GINGIVA: The gums of the mouth.

GLAUCOMA: Eye disease marked by an increase in the intraocular pressure which causes changes in the optic disk and results in blindness.

GLUCOSE: A sugar which is a principal source of body energy.

GONAD: An organ that produces sex cells; ovaries or testes.

GONITIS: Inflammation of the stifle joint.

GRANULATION TISSUE: The formation in wounds of small rounded masses of tissue, composed of capillaries and connective tissue cells which grow outward to fill the wound defect. See Second Intention Healing.

GRAVITATIONAL EFFECTS: Effects caused by gravity, such as abdominal edema in which the force of gravity pulls the excess fluids down to the lowest point on the midline.

GRUEL: A semi-liquid food made from cereal grain.

GUT STASIS: A condition in which normal passage of the intestinal contents is impaired by lack of peristaltic movement.

H

Hb: Hemoglobin.

HEALTH CERTIFICATE: A certificate from a veterinarian stating that a horse was sound and free from any contagious disease at the time of examination.

HEAT: See Estrus.

HEAT EXHAUSTION: Hyperthermia; circulatory collapse and shock caused by high environmental temperature, high humidity, and poor ventilation.

HEATSTROKE: Hyperthermia; caused by the same situations as heat exhaustion, but is more serious. Sweating usually stops, and heatstroke can often end in death.

HEAVES: A respiratory ailment, characterized by forced expiration and dyspnea, resulting from the rupture of alveoli in the lungs, and caused by such things as allergies, dust, etc.

HEEL CALKS: Short protrusions from the underside of each heel of a horseshoe; used on racing shoes to provide better traction.

HELMINTH: Worm.

HEMATINIC: An agent which improves the quality of the blood, increasing the hemoglobin level and the number of erythrocytes.

HEMATOCRIT: Syn. packed cell volume (PCV). The fraction of the total blood volume, expressed as a percentage, that is occupied by the erythrocytes; abbreviated HCT.

HEMATOLOGY: The study of blood and blood-forming organs.

HEMATOMA: A localized collection of blood, usually clotted, in an organ, space, or tissue due to a break in the wall of a blood vessel.

HEMATOPOIETIC: Affecting the formation of red blood cells.

HEMATURIA: Blood in the urine.

HEMOCONCENTRATION: Increase in blood concentration due to a decrease in fluid volume.

HEMODYNAMIC: Pertaining to blood circulation.

HEMOGLOBIN: The oxygen-carrying protein pigment of the red blood cells.

HEMOGLOBINURIA: The presence of free hemoglobin in the urine.

HEMOLYSIN: Naturally occurring substance which destroys erythrocytes.

HEMOLYSIS: The release of hemoglobin by the destruction of red blood cells.

HEMOPHILIA: A hereditary deficiency of a clotting factor in the blood.

HEMORRHAGE: The escape of blood from the vessels; bleeding.

HEMOSTATIC AGENT: A substance which checks or stops the flow of blood.

HEPATIC: Pertaining to the liver.

HERNIA: The protrusion of a portion of an organ or tissue through an abnormal opening in another structure, e.g., muscle wall, mesentery, etc.

HISTAMINE: A chemical compound which dilates capillaries, constricts the smooth muscle of the lungs, and increases secretions of the stomach; substance released in anaphylactic reations and shock.

HIVES: See Urticaria.

HOLOCRINE: Type of gland in which the entire secreting cell forms secreted matter of gland, e.g., sebaceous gland.

HOOF TESTER: A pincer-type instrument used to gently pinch hoofs to find any sore areas. The hoof is compressed between the prongs of the tester; when this is done to an area of inflammation, the horse will flinch.

HORMONE: A chemical substance produced in the body by a gland or body organ which travels in the blood or lymphatic system to a distant specific organ, the target organ, to regulate the activity of that organ.

HYALOID VESSEL: An artery present in the eye of the fetus which is commonly present at birth and usually degenerates during the first two weeks of life.

HYDROKINETIC: Pertaining to moving water, as in a whirlpool bath.

HYDROPHILIC: Readily absorbing water.

HYDROTHERAPY: The application of water in any form, internally or externally, in treating disease or illness.

HYDROTHERMAL: Relating to the temperature effects of water.

HYGROMA: A sac distended with a serous fluid.

HYPERCALCEMIA: Excess calcium in blood.

HYPERCAPNIA: Excess of carbon dioxide in blood.

HYPEREMIA: An excess of blood in a part causing redness and congestion.

HYPEREXCITABILITY: Abnormal excitation of the nervous system.

HYPEREXTENSION: Extreme or excessive extension of a limb beyond its normal limit.

HYPERFLEXION: Overflexion of a limb or part beyond its normal limit.

HYPERKALEMIA: Excess potassium in blood.

HYPEROSTOSIS: Syn. exostosis; abnormal enlargement of bone.

HYPERPLASIA: Overdevelopment of tissue or an organ due to an increase in the number of cells.

HYPERTENSION: High blood pressure.

HYPERTHERMIA: Temperature above normal.

HYPERTONIC: Pertaining to a solution which, when bathing cells, causes a flow of water out of the cell across the cell membranes.

HYPERTROPHY: The enlargement or overgrowth of an organ or part due to an increase in size of its constituent cells.

HYPHEMA: Bleeding (hemorrhage) into the anterior chamber of the eye.

HYPNOTICS: Drugs that induce sleep.

HYPOCALCEMIA: Abnormally low levels of blood calcium.

HYPOFLEXION: Decreased flexion in muscles and tendons of the legs.

HYPOGONADISM: Abnormally decreased activity of the gonads, with retarded growth and sexual development.

HYPOPLASIA: Underdevelopment of tissue or an organ due to a decrease in the number of cells.

HYPOPYON: Pus in the anterior chamber of the eye.

HYPOTENSION: Low blood pressure.

HYPOTONIC: Pertaining to a solution which, when bathing cells, causes a flow of water into the cell across the cell membranes.

HYPOTHERMIA: Temperature below normal.

HYPOVOLEMIA: Abnormally decreased circulating blood volume.

HYPOXIA: Low oxygen content in inspired air, blood or tissues.

I

ICTERUS: See Jaundice.

IMMUNIZATION: The process of rendering a subject immune, e.g., through vaccination.

IMMUNODEFICIENCY: A deficiency in antibody response, leaving the animal susceptible to infection.

INANITION: A starved condition, with marked weight loss, weakness, and a decreased metabolism caused by severe malnutrition.

INCISION: A cut produced by a surgeon's scalpel.

INCUBATION PERIOD: The period of development of an infectious disease from the time the disease-producing organism enters the body until signs of the disease appear.

INDWELLING CATHETER: A piece of tubing seated in a structure to allow continuous drainage or repeated application of medication, e.g., intravenous catheter, urinary catheter.

INFARCTION: The formation of an area of dead tissue resulting from obstruction of circulation to the area by a clot.

INFLAMMATION: A condition of tissues characterized by pain, heat, redness, swelling and various exudations as a reaction to injury. It serves to eliminate harmful substances and damaged tissue.

INFLUENZA: An acute viral infection involving the respiratory tract, occurring in isolated cases, in epidemics, or in pandemics striking many continents simultaneously or in sequence. It is marked by inflammation of the nasal mucosa, the pharynx, and conjunctiva.

INFUSION: The therapeutic introduction of a fluid, such as saline solution, into the body by the force of gravity.

INGESTA: Consumed feed and fluids.

INGESTION: The act of taking food, medicines, etc., into the body by mouth.

INNERVATION: The distribution or supply of nerves to a part. The supply of nervous energy or of nerve stimulus sent to a part.

INOCULATE: Syn. vaccinate. The introduction of a vaccine or disease-producing organism into the body.

INTERCOSTAL: Between ribs.

INTERFERENCE: The striking of the inside of one leg with the inside of the hoof or shoe of the opposite leg. Impact point may be from the coronary band up to the carpus or hock.

INTEROSSEOUS: Between bones.

INTESTINAL FLORA: The bacteria normally present within the intestine.

INTRA-ARTICULAR: Within a joint.

INTRADERMAL: Within the skin.

INTRAMUSCULAR: Within a muscle.

INTRATHECAL: Within a sheath.

INTRAUTERINE: Within the uterus.

INTRAVENOUS: Within a vein.

INTRAVENOUS OUTFIT: The needle, syringe, plastic tubing, and fluid vial used to make a large volume intravenous injection; if an indwelling catheter is used, plastic tubing is temporarily placed into the vein and the fluid injected through it.

INTUSSUSCEPTION: Telescoping of one section of the intestine into the lumen of an adjoining part of the intestine causing blockage.

INVOLUNTARY: Performed independently of the will; contravolitional.

IRIDENCLEISIS: A surgical procedure to reduce intraocular pressure.

IRIDOCYCLITIS: Inflamed iris and ciliary body, e.g., periodic ophthalmia.

IRRIGATION: See Lavage.

ISCHEMIA: Deficiency of blood supply to a part.

ISOERYTHROLYSIS: Destruction of erythrocytes by isoantibodies.

ISOIMMUNIZATION: Development of antibodies against an antigen derived from a genetically dissimilar individual of the same species.

ISOTONIC: A fluid exerting the same osmotic pressure as another; e.g., isotonic saline solution is compatible with body cells and will not cause shrinking or swelling of cells.

ISOTONIC SALINE SOLUTION: A 0.9% sodium chloride (salt) solution.

ISOTOPE: A chemical element having the same atomic number as another, but possessing a different atomic mass.

I.U.: International unit.

J

JACK SPAVIN: An exceptionally large bone spavin.

JAUNDICE: A syndrome characterized by hyperbilirubinemia and deposition of bile pigment in the skin and mucous membranes with resulting yellow appearance of the patient.

JOINT: An articulation; the place of union or junction between two or more bones of the skeleton.

JOINT MOUSE: A small chip of bone enclosed in the joint space.

K

KELOID: A sharply elevated, irregularly shaped, enlarging scar.

KERATIN: An insoluble protein which is the principal constituent of epidermis, hair, nails, and horn.

KERATOMA: A horny tumor on the inner surface of the wall of a horse's hoof.

KETONE BODIES: Normal metabolic products: acetone, acetoacetic acid, beta-hydroxybutyric acid.

KNOCK-KNEE: Epiphysitis occurring in foals (sometimes because of diet deficiency).

L

LABIAL: Pertaining to a lip.

LACERATION: A torn, ragged wound.

LACRIMATION: The secretion and discharge of tears.

LACTATION: The secretion of milk.

LACTIC ACID: An organic acid normally present in muscle tissue, produced by anaerobic muscle metabolism. It may also be produced in carbohydrate material by bacterial fermentation.

LAMINAE: Thin, flat plates or layers. The insensitive laminae lining the hoof wall interlocks with the sensitive laminae of the foot.

LAMINITIS: Inflammation of the laminae of a horse's foot.

LAPAROTOMY: A surgical incision through the abdominal wall.

LARVA: An early developmental stage, usually the feeding form of insects or worms.

LARYNGEAL HEMIPLEGIA: Paralysis of one side of the larynx.

LARYNGEAL VENTRICULOTOMY: Surgical stripping of the laryngeal ventricles to correct roaring.

LARYNGOSCOPIC EXAMINATION: A direct visual examination of the larynx through the use of an instrument such as an endoscope.

LATERAL: Pertaining to a side or outer surface; a portion further from the midline of the body or of a structure.

LAVAGE: The washing out of a cavity or wound with a stream of fluid.

LAXATIVE: An agent that acts to promote evacuation of the bowel; a cathartic or purgative.

LEG BRACE: A soothing liniment or lotion used on the legs to cool and tone up the legs before or after exercise; usually contains water, alcohol, menthol, etc.

LEPTOSPIROSIS: Acute bacterial disease characterized by increasing hemolytic anemia.

LESION: An abnormal change in the structure of a part due to injury or disease.

LETHARGY: Condition of drowsiness or indifference.

LEUKOCYTES: White blood cells or white blood corpuscles.

LEUKOCYTOSIS: A temporary increase in the number of leukocytes in the blood due to infection, inflammation, etc.

LEUKOPENIA: Abnormally low level of white blood cells.

LIBIDO: Sexual drive.

LIGAMENT: A band of fibrous tissue that connects bones and/or cartilage.

LIGATE: To tie off a vessel or part with a suture of catgut, steel, silk, etc.

LIME: Calcium oxide, used as a disinfectant.

LIME WATER: A mixture of calcium hydroxide and water in the proportions of 1:700, used as an antacid.

LINEA ALBA: The tendinous median line of the ventral abdominal wall between the pairs of abdominal muscles.

LINGUAL: Pertaining to the tongue.

LINIMENT: An oily, soapy, or alcoholic liquid preparation used on the skin and applied with friction.

LIPOMA: A benign fatty tumor.

LOCKJAW: See Tetanus.

LONG PASTERN: First phalanx, P1.

LUMBAR: Pertaining to the loins, the part of the back between the thorax and the pelvis.

LUXATION: Dislocation.

LYMPH: A transparent yellowish liquid containing mostly white blood cells and derived from tissue fluids; the fluid content of the lymphatic system.

M

MALIGNANT: Tending to become progressively worse and result in death; in the case of neoplasms, refers to uncontrollable growths which tend to disseminate and recur after removal.

MALABSORPTION: Impaired intestinal absorption of nutrients.

MALNUTRITION: A nutrition disorder caused by either an imbalanced or insufficient diet, or due to poor absorption and utilization of nutrients.

MANGE: A contagious skin disease caused by various types of mites.

MASSAGE: The therapeutic rubbing and kneading of the body tissues to loosen adhesions, relax tense muscles, etc.

MASTICATION: The process of chewing food.

MASTITIS: Inflammation of the mammary gland.

MECONIUM: A dark green, adhesive material in the intestine of the full-term fetus, being a mixture of the secretions of the intestinal glands and some amniotic fluid.

MEDIAL: Pertaining to the middle or inner surface; a position closer to the midline of the body or of a structure.

MEDIUM: Any preparation or substance, when referring to a culture, that is used to support the growth of microorganisms.

MEMBRANE: A thin layer of tissue which covers a surface, lines a cavity, or divides a space or organ.

METABOLISM: The sum of physical and chemical activities whereby the function of nutrition is effected. See Anabolism and Catabolism.

METASTASIS: The spread of neoplasms from the primary site to other parts of the body.

METESTRUS: The period of sexual rest following estrus in female mammals.

METRITIS: Inflammation of the uterus.

MICROORGANISMS: Minute, microscopic organisms such as bacteria, viruses, molds, yeasts, and protozoa.

MINERAL DEPOSITS: Extraneous inorganic matter collected in the tissues or in a cavity.

MINERALIZATION: The process of being impregnated with minerals.

MIOSIS: Contraction of the pupil; opposite of mydriasis.

MIOTIC: Any drug that causes the pupil to constrict.

MITRAL VALVE: Referring to the mitral bicuspid, or left A-V valve of the heart.

MODIFIED LIVE VIRUS: A virus that has been taken from the natural state and raised in a laboratory under somewhat unnatural conditions. Because of the unnatural conditions in which it was raised, the virus does not have the disease-causing abilities of a virus in the natural state, but it still has the properties of stimulating the production of antibodies when injected into an animal. The stimulation of antibody production makes it valuable as a vaccine.

MOIST RALES: An abnormal respiratory sound, occurring with fluid in the air passages, heard through auscultation.

MONORCHID: Individual with only one testis descended.

MOTILITY: The ability to move; peristalsis when referring to the intestines.

MUCOID: Resembling mucus.

MUCOPURULENT: Containing both mucus and pus.

MUCOSA: A mucous membrane, e.g., lining of eyelid, mouth, gums, vagina.

MUCOUS MEMBRANES: The mucosa which secrete mucus, a slimy secretion of the glands. Usually refers to the mucosa of the eyelid, vagina, mouth, and gums.

MUCUS: The free slime of the mucous membranes, composed of secretion of the glands.

MURMUR: An abnormal periodic sound of short duration of cardiac or vascular origin.

MUSCLE: An organ which, by contraction and relaxation, produces the movements of an animal organism.

MUSCLE RELAXANT: An agent that specifically aids in reducing muscle tension.

MUSCLE TREMOR: An involuntary trembling or quivering of a muscle.

MUTATION: Change in position of the fetus in the uterus.

MYCOTIC: Fungal.

MYDRIATIC: Any drug that dilates the pupil; opposite of miosis.

MYOGLOBIN: A ferrous complex pigment which gives muscle its characteristic color and acts as a store of oxygen.

MYOPATHY: Any disease of a muscle.

MYOSITIS: Inflammation of a voluntary muscle.

N

NARCOSIS: A reversible state of stupor.

NARCOTICS: Drugs that induce sleep and relieve pain at the same time.

NARROW SPECTRUM ANTIBIOTIC: A term used to describe an agent that is effective against only a limited number of organisms or a specific organism; describes the range of certain antibiotics.

NASOLACRIMAL: Pertaining to the nasal opening of the tear-producing apparatus.

NECROPSY: Examination of a body after death; autopsy.

NECROSIS: Death of a cell or group of cells which is in contact with living tissue.

NEMATODE: Internal parasitic worms.

NEONATAL: Pertaining to newborn animal.

NEONATAL ISOERYTHROLYSIS: A severe red blood cell destroying disease of newborn foals; hemolytic jaundice in foals.

NEOPLASM: A new and abnormal growth of tissue; such as a tumor.

NEPHRITIS: Inflammation of the kidney.

NERVES: Cordlike structures, visible to the naked eye, comprising a collection of nerve fibers which convey impulses between a part of the central nervous system and some other region of the body.

NEURAL: Pertaining to a nerve or to the nerves.

NEURECTOMY: The excision of a part of a nerve.

NEUROMA: A tumor or new growth largely made up of nerve cells and nerve fibers; a tumor growing from a nerve.

NEUROTOXIC: Poisonous or destructive to nerve tissue.

NEUTRALIZE: To make a substance neither acid nor base.

NEUTROPHILIA: Increase in number of neutrophil white cells in blood; sign of infection.

NF: National Formulary (United States).

NICTITATING MEMBRANE: Third eyelid.

NINE-DAY HEAT: Also called foal-heat; the period (usually 9-11 days after foaling) during which mares show signs of heat.

O

OCCLUSION: Bite; the relationship between the biting surfaces of the maxillary and mandibular teeth when they are in contact.

OCCULT SPAVIN: A term for typical spavin lameness without external signs.

OMENTUM: A fold of peritoneum extending from the stomach to adjacent organs in the abdominal cavity.

OPEN KNEES: A condition, usually the result of a mineral imbalance, wherein the profile of the knee is irregular due to the enlarged epiphysis of the lower end of the radius and carpal bone deviation toward the back.

OPHTHALMIA: Severe inflammation of the eye or conjunctiva.

OPHTHALMOLOGY: That branch of medicine dealing with the eye, its anatomy and physiology, etc.

OPHTHALMOSCOPE: An instrument containing a perforated mirror and lenses used to examine the interior of the eye.

OPTIC: Pertaining to the eye.

ORBIT: Eye socket.

ORIFICE: The entrance or outlet of any cavity in the body.

ORTHOPEDIC: Pertaining to the correction of bone disorders.

OSMOTIC PRESSURE: The pressure, dependent on molar concentration and absolute temperature, that is associated with osmosis.

OSSIFY: To change or develop into bone.

OSTEITIS: Inflammation of a bone.

OSTEOMALACIA: Condition characterized by softening of the bones; usually due to a calcium-phosphorus deficiency.

OSTEOMYELITIS: Inflammation of bone caused by a pyogenic (pus producing) organism.

OSTEOPOROSIS: Abnormal rarefaction of bone; seen in big head.

OTOSCOPE: An instrument for inspecting the ears.

OVER-REACHING: A faulty gait in which the toe of the hind hoof strikes the heel of the forefoot.

OXYGENATED: Saturated with oxygen.

P

P1: First phalanx; long pastern.

P2: Second phalanx; short pastern.

P3: Third phalanx; coffin bone.

PALLIATIVE: Medical treatment that provides relief without a cure.

PALLOR: Paleness, absence of skin coloration.

PALMAR: Pertaining to the flexor surface of the foreleg.

PALPABLE: Perceptible by touch.

PALPATION: The act of feeling with the hand.

PALPEBRAL: Refers to eyelid.

PAPILLOMA: A growth of epithelial tissue (warts).

PARACENTESIS: The surgical puncture of a cavity for aspiration of a fluid.

PARALYSIS: Loss or impairment of motor function in a part due to nerve damage.

PARASITE: A plant or animal which lives upon or within another living organism at whose expense it obtains some advantage.

PARASYMPATHETIC: A subsystem of the autonomic nervous system.

PARATHORMONE: Hormone secreted by the parathyroid glands, instrumental in maintaining proper calcium levels in the body.

PARENTERAL: Administration of medication through some other route than the alimentary canal, such as subcutaneous, intramuscular, etc.

PARIETAL: Pertaining to the walls of a cavity.

PARROT MOUTH: A congenital defect of imperfectly meshed teeth, similar to buck teeth.

PARTURITION: The act or process of giving birth.

PASSIVE IMMUNITY: Acquired immunity produced by administration of preformed antibody.

PATENT: Open.

PATHOGEN: Any disease-producing microorganism or material.

PATHOLOGICAL: A diseased condition.

PCV: Packed Cell Volume; the number of packed red cells in milliliters per 100 ml of centrifuged blood; hematocrit.

PECTORAL: Pertaining to the chest.

PEDUNCULATED: On a stalk.

PERACUTE: Excessively acute; pertains to disease.

PERCUSSION: The act of striking a part with short, sharp blows as an aid in diagnosing the condition of the parts beneath by the sound obtained.

PERIARTICULAR: Situated around a joint.

PERINEAL: Pertaining to the area between the anus and the scrotum or vulva.

PERIODIC OPHTHALMIA: Recurrent uveitis; often referred to as "moon blindness," this inflammatory disease of the eye is the most common cause of blindness in the horse.

PERIOPLE: The layer of soft, light-colored horn covering the outer aspect of the hoof.

PERIOSTEAL: Pertaining to the connective tissue covering of the bones.

PERIOSTEITIS or PERIOSTITIS: Inflammation of the periosteum (bone covering).

PERIOSTEUM: A specialized connective tissue covering all bones of the body which is capable of forming bone.

PERIPHERAL CIRCULATORY SYSTEM: The part of the circulatory system that carries blood to and from the outer parts of the body.

PERISTALSIS: Waves of contraction along the muscular walls of the intestine and other hollow organs which propel the contents.

PERITONEUM: The serous membrane lining the abdominopelvic cavity and enveloping the viscera.

PERITONITIS: Inflammation of the peritoneum; a condition marked by exudations in the peritoneum of serum, fibrin, cells, and pus.

PERIVASCULAR: Situated around a vessel.

PERMEABILITY: The state of being pervious or penetrable.

PETRISSAGE: Massage in which the muscles are kneaded and pressed.

pH: Symbol for the measurement of alkalinity and acidity; pH 7 is neutral, greater than 7 is alkaline, less than 7 is acid.

PHAGOCYTE: Any cell that ingests microorganisms or other cells and foreign particles.

PHARMACOLOGY: The science that deals with drugs, their sources, appearance, chemistry, action and use.

PHARYNGITIS: Inflammation of the pharynx.

PHOTODYNAMIC AGENT: An agent that reacts in the sunlight.

PHOTOPHOBIA: An abnormal aversion to light.

PHOTOSENSITIZATION: An excessive reaction of the skin to sunlight, resulting in swelling and inflammation.

PLANTAR: Pertaining to the sole of the foot; syn. palmar.

PLASMA: The liquid portion of the blood, contains fibrinogen.

PLASMA EXTENDERS: A substance which can be transfused to maintain plasma volume of the blood.

PLATELETS: Disk-shaped structures found in the blood of all mammals and chiefly known for their role in blood coagulation. Also called blood platelets and thrombocytes.

PLEXIMETER: A veterinary instrument used to perform percussion.

PNEUMOVAGINA: Air in the vagina, the single most common cause of female infertility due to infection.

POLYCYTHEMIA: An increase in the total red blood cell mass of the body.

POLYDIPSIA: Persistent, excessive thirst.

POLYURIA: Passage of an abnormally large volume of urine in a given period; frequent urination.

POSTERIOR: Situated in back of; toward the rear end of the body.

POSTERIOR SYNECHIA: Adhesion of iris to lens.

POSTERIOR UVEAL TRACT: The choroid.

POSTMORTEM: After death.

POSTPARTUM: Occurring after delivery, with reference to the mother.

POSTPARTURIENT: Occurring after delivery.

POULTICE: A soft, moist mass about the consistency of cooked cereal, spread between layers of muslin, linen, gauze, or towels and applied hot to a given area in order to create moist local heat or counterirritation.

PRECIPITATE: To cause a substance in a solution to settle and form solid particles.

PREHENSION: The act of seizing or grasping, as when the horse grasps food with the lips.

PROGNATHISM: Marked protrusion of the lower jaw.

PROGNOSIS: The prospect of recovery from a disease or injury.

PROLAPSE: The passing outwards of part of an organ or the organ itself through a natural body opening or tear.

PROLIFERATE: To multiply; to grow by reproducing similar cells.

PROPHYLACTIC: An agent that tends to prevent disease.

PROSTHESIS: An artificial substitute for a missing part of the body.

PROTEIN: Any group of complex compounds which contain nitrogen and are composed of amino acids.

PROTHROMBIN: Precursor of the coagulating protein present in plasma.

PROUD FLESH: Excessive granulation tissue.

PROXIMAL: Nearest, closer to the point of attachment or any point of reference.

PRURITIS: Intense itching.

PULP: The soft substance at the center of the horse's teeth.

PULSE: Rhythmic throbbing of an artery which may be felt with the finger, caused by blood forced through the vessel by contractions of the heart.

PUNCTURE: A wound that is deeper than it is wide.

PURGATIVE: An agent that causes cleansing or evacuation of the bowels.

PURULENT: Consisting of or containing pus; the formation of or caused by pus.

PUS: A liquid inflammation product containing leukocytes.

PUSTULES: Visible collection of pus within or beneath the epidermis.

PYOMETRA: An accumulation of pus within the uterus.

PYRAMIDAL DISEASE: Also called buttress foot, a form of low ringbone, a new abnormal bone growth which may be due to fracture or periostitis or osteitis of extensor process of the coffin bone.

Q R

QUARANTINE: Restriction placed on the entrance to and exit from the place or premises where a case of communicable disease exists.

QUIDDING: A condition in which the horse takes food into his mouth, chews it, and then drops the bolus of chewed food out of his mouth; can be caused by dental disease, facial paralysis, or other disorders affecting the horse's ability to swallow.

QUITTOR: A chronic, deep-seated inflammation of the lateral cartilages, characterized by necrosis of the inflamed part.

RADIATION: Particulate rays, such as alpha, beta, and gamma rays.

RADIATION THERAPY: Treatment using x-rays, beta rays, and gamma rays to destroy or retard the growth of tumors, and treat certain areas with artificial inflammation.

RADIOGRAPH: A film of internal structures of the body produced by the action of x-rays or gamma rays on a specially sensitized film.

RADIOLOGY: The medical science that uses radiant energy in the treatment of disease.

RADIOLUCENT: Transparent to x-rays; shows as a dark area on radiograph.

RADIOPAQUE: Opaque to x-rays; shows as a white area on radiograph.

RALES: Any abnormal respiratory sound.

RBC: Red blood cells, erythrocytes.

RECURRENT UVEITIS: Periodic ophthalmia or moon blindness.

RECUMBENCY: A lying down position.

RECURRENT: Returning after intermissions.

RED BLOOD CELLS: Hemoglobin-carying corpuscles in the blood that transport oxygen; also called erythrocytes.

REHABILITATION: The restoration of normal form and function after injury or illness.

RELAPSE: The return of a disease after it has apparently ceased.

REMITTENT: Abating for awhile, at intervals, and then returning.

RENAL: Pertaining to the kidney.

REPULSION: The pushing back of the fetus into the uterus, usually done before any correction of dystocia is attempted.

RESECTION: Surgical removal of part of a structure and reconstruction of the remaining structure.

RESPIRATION: The exchange of oxygen and carbon dioxide between the atmosphere and the cells of the body.

RETINAL DETACHMENT: A condition associated with periodic ophthalmia or injuries that may affect the eye. Often causes blindness in the eye affected.

ROSTRAL: Toward the nose.

ROUGHAGE: The indigestible fiber in the diet needed to give bulk and to keep the digestive system functioning properly.

RUBEFACIENT: An agent that reddens the skin. First stage of irritation characterized by mild redness.

RUPTURE: A breaking or tearing of tissue.

S

SALINE SOLUTION: A salt-containing solution.

SALVE: A thick ointment.

SARCOIDS: A tumor composed mainly of connective tissue which appears on the skin as the most common tumor of horses.

SARCOMA: An often highly malignant tumor made up of a substance like the embryonic connective tissue.

SCALE: A thin layer of cornified epithelial cells on the skin.

SCALPEL: A small surgical knife, usually with a convex blade edge.

SCOUR: Severe diarrhea, especially in foals.

SCURFING: The process of forming thin, dry scales on the skin.

SEBORRHEA: A skin disease, probably the result of an abnormal production of keratin. Usually a secondary disease in horses following dermatitis or eczema.

SECOND INTENTION HEALING: Healing by granulation ; scar tissue will form.

SECONDARY CONDITION: A condition derived from or consequent to a primary condition.

SECRETE: To produce and give off cell products.

SEDATIVE: An agent that reduces and controls excitement.

SEDIMENT: Particles that settle out of a fluid left standing, such as blood or urine sediment.

SELENIFEROUS: Selenium containing.

SEMILUNAR VALVES: Resembling a crescent, or half-moon, found in the heart.

SEMICOMATOSE: The condition of a stupor from which the subject can be aroused.

SENSITIVITY TEST: Test for susceptibility of an infectious organism for an antibiotic.

SEPSIS: The presence of pathogenic organisms.

SEPTICEMIA: Disease associated with disease-producing microorganisms or their poisons in the blood; blood poisoning.

SEQUELA: Any complication following or caused by a disease or ailment.

SERIAL BLOOD SAMPLES: Blood chemistries done at intervals during the course of the disease to aid in diagnosis, prognosis and therapy.

SERUM: The clear liquid which results from the clotting of blood; whole blood without the corpuscles and fibrinogen.

SEROUS: The clear liquid portion of the blood or any body fluid that separates after complete clotting; blood plasma with the fibrinogen removed.

SESAMOIDITIS: An inflammation of the proximal sesamoid bones, usually involving both osteitis and periostitis.

SHEATH: A tubular structure enclosing or surrounding an organ or part, e.g., tendon sheath.

SHOCK: A condition of acute peripheral circulatory failure due to derangement of circulatory control or loss of circulating fluid.

SHORT PASTERN: Second phalanx, P2.

SIDEBONES: Ossification of the two lateral cartilages of the wings of the coffin bone.

SIGN: Evidence of a disease, as observed by someone other than the patient.

SLAKED LIME: Calcium hydroxide.

SLOUGH: Dead tissue in the process of separating from the body.

SMEGMA: The secretion of sebaceous glands, especially the cheesy secretion found in the sheath of the stallion or gelding.

SOLUTION: The homogeneous mixture of one or more substances dispersed in a sufficient quantity of dissolving medium.

SPASM: A sudden, involuntary contraction of a muscle or constriction of a passage.

SPASMODIC: Pertaining to periodic sudden, involuntary contractions of one or more muscles, accompanied by pain.

SPASMOLYTIC: Checking spasms, antispasmodic.

SPAVIN: An exostosis, usually medial, of the hock joint.

SPECIFIC GRAVITY: The ratio of the weight or mass of a given volume of a substance to that of an equal volume of another substance used as the standard (water is the standard for liquids and solids).

SPECULUM: An instrument for showing the interior of a passageway or cavity of the body.

SPECULUM, MARE: A hollow tube, usually about sixteen inches long and one and one-half inches in diameter, used to examine the vagina and cervix.

SPERMATOZOA: Mature male sex cells, the specific output of the testes; sperm.

SPHINCTER: A ringlike band of muscle fibers that constricts a passage or closes an opening, e.g., anal sphincter.

SPONDYLITIS: Inflamed vertebrae.

SPONGY BONE: See Cancellous Bone.

SPRAIN: A joint injury in which some of the fibers of a ligament are ruptured.

STERILE ABSCESS: One which contains no microorganisms.

STIMULANTS: Any agent or remedy that produces stimulation.

STOCK UP: Swelling of the horse's lower legs due to restricted exercise.

STRAIN: An overstretching or overexertion of some part of the musculature.

STRANGULATED HERNIA: One in which the hernial ring has narrowed, trapping a piece of the intestine. This affects the circulation and may cause death of the tissue.

STRANGURY: Slow and painful urination, caused by urethra and bladder spasm.

STRESS: Forcibly exerted influence or pressure.

STRIATION: Stripe, e.g., skeletal muscle is striated.

SUBACUTE: Somewhat acute, between acute and chronic.

SUBCUTANEOUS: Beneath the skin.

SUBCUTICULAR: Situated beneath the epidermis.

SUBLUXATION: An incomplete or partial dislocation.

SUBPALPEBRAL: Under the eyelid.

SUPERFICIAL: Pertaining to or situated near the surface.

SUPER-SATURATED SOLUTION: A solution containing more of the ingredient than can be held in solution permanently; the ingredient will fall to the bottom of the solution if allowed to stand.

SUPPORTIVE TREATMENT: That which is mainly directed at sustaining the strength of the patient.

SUPPURATIVE: Producing pus.

SUSPENSION: A preparation of a finely divided drug intended to be incorporated (suspended) in some suitable liquid before it is used.

SUTURE: A stitch used to close a wound.

SYMPTOM: Evidence of a disease, as perceived and described by the handler.

SYMPTOMATIC: Pertaining to or of the nature of a symptom.

SYNDROME: A set of signs which occur together usually indicating a particular type of disease process.

SYNERGISM: The total effects of combined agents which is greater than the simple sum of their individual effects.

SYNOVECTOMY: Excision of a synovial membrane.

SYNOVIAL FLUID: A transparent fluid, resembling the white of an egg, secreted by the synovial membrane and contained in joint cavities, bursae and tendon sheaths for lubrication.

SYSTEMIC: Pertaining to or affecting the body as a whole.

SYSTOLE: The contraction or period of contraction of the heart.

T

TACHYCARDIA: Unusually fast heart rate.

TEASER: A stallion used to find mares in estrus by observing the mares' behavior.

TENDINITIS: Inflammation of tendons and tendon-muscle attachments.

TENDON: A fibrous cord of connective tissue which attaches muscle to bone or other structures.

TENDOSYNOVITIS: Inflammation of a tendon sheath.

TENECTOMY: The cutting out of a lesion of a tendon or of a tendon sheath.

TENOTOMY: The cutting of a tendon.

THERAPEUTIC: Curative.

THERAPEUTIC INDEX: In drug use, the margin between the safe dose of a drug that will effect a cure, and the toxic dose that will kill the patient.

THERAPY: The treatment of disease.

THROMBIN: Enzyme causing blood to clot.

THROMBOSIS: The formation of a blood clot which remains attached at the point of formation in the blood vessel causing an obstruction.

TISSUE: An aggregation of similarly specialized cells united in the performance of a particular function.

TOPICAL: Pertaining to a particular surface area.

TORSION: Twisting, as in torsion of the intestines in colic.

TORTICOLLIS: A contraction of the cervical muscles, causing a twisted neck and an abnormal position of the head.

TOURNIQUET: An instrument for the compression of a blood vessel by application around an extremity to control the circulation and prevent the flow of blood to or from the distal area.

TOXEMIA: A general intoxication or poisoning sometimes due to the absorption of bacterial products (toxins) formed at a local source of infection.

TOXIC: Pertaining to, or of the nature of poison.

TOXIN: An organic poison, usually a protein produced by a living organism.

TOXOID: A modified bacterial exotoxin that has lost its toxicity but retains the properties of stimulating the formation of antitoxin.

TRACHEOSTOMY: The formation of an artificial opening into the trachea.

TRANQUILIZER: An agent that produces a quietening or calming effect, without changing the level of consciousness.

TRANSFUSION: The introduction of whole blood or blood component directly into the bloodstream.

TREPHINE: A crown saw for removing a circular area of bone, chiefly from the skull.

TRICUSPID VALVE: Having three cusps; referring to the left A-V valve of the heart.

TROCAR: A sharp-pointed, hollow instrument for piercing the wall of a cavity.

TUMOR: A mass of new tissue which persists and grows independently of its surrounding structures and which has no useful function.

UV

ULCER: A hollowed-out space on the surface of an organ or tissue due to the sloughing of dead tissue.

ULCERATED: Affected with or of the condition of an ulcer.

ULTRAVIOLET LIGHT: Light waves with powerful actinic and chemical properties with wavelengths between 1800 and 3900 angstroms.

UNILATERAL: Affecting one side only.

URACHUS: Tube connecting the fetal bladder with the placenta.

URINALYSIS: A physical, chemical, or microscopic analysis or examination of urine.

URINE: The fluid excreted by the kidneys, passed through the ureters, stored in the bladder, and discharged through the urethra.

URTICARIA: An allergic condition characterized by the appearance of wheals on the skin surface. Also known as hives.

USP: United States Pharmacopeia.

UVEAL TRACT: The iris, ciliary body and choroid.

VACCINATION: The injection of vaccine for the purposes of inducing immunity.

VACCINE: A suspension of attenuated or killed microorganisms administered for the prevention or treatment of infectious diseases.

VASCULAR TISSUE: Tissue with a good supply of blood vessels.

VASOCONSTRICTOR: Causing constriction of the blood vessels.

VASODILATION: Dilation or enlargement of a vessel; causes increased blood flow to the area.

VECTOR: An animal (insect or mammal) that transmits a disease-producing organism.

VEIN: A vessel through which the deoxygenated blood passes from various organs or parts back to the heart.

VENOM: A poison, specifically, a toxic substance normally secreted by a snake, insect, or other animal.

VENOUS: Pertaining to the veins.

VENTRAL: Denoting a position more toward the lower surface of the body.

VENULES: Small veins in capillary beds.

VERMINOUS: Pertaining or due to worms.

VERSION: Change of the polarity of the fetus in the uterus in relation to the mare.

VESICANTS: A counterirritant agent which produces blistering and scurfing of the skin.

VESSEL: Any channel for carrying a fluid.

VIABLE: Alive or capable of living.

VIRULENT: Characterized by being exceedingly pathogenic or noxious.

VIRUS: One of a group of minute infectious agents, usually not seen in a light microscope, and characterized by a lack of independent metabolism and by the ability to replicate only within living host cells.

VISCERA: The internal organs.

VISCERAL: Pertaining to the large internal organs in the thoracic, abdominal, and pelvic cavities, especially in the abdomen.

VISCOUS: The state of a fluid that has a high degree of friction between its molecules; gluey, sticky.

VITREOUS HUMOR: The clear, gelatinous substance filling the area behind the lens in the eye.

VOLAR: Indicating the back or bottom surface of the forearm, knee, fetlock, pastern, or hoof.

VOLATILE: Tending to evaporate quickly.

VOLUNTARY: Accomplished in accordance with the will.

VOLVULUS: A knotting and twisting of the intestines that causes an obstruction and colic.

WXYZ

WARTS: An epidermal tumor caused by a papilloma virus.

WAXING: The collection of a drop of dry collostrum at the end of each teat which occurs 18-48 hours before foaling.

WBC: White blood cell count; number of white blood cells in a specific volume of blood.

WEB: The width of the horseshoe from the inner to the outer edges of the metal.

WHEALS: Smooth, slightly raised areas of the skin surface which are redder or paler than the surrounding areas.

WINDGALLS: Also called windpuffs; a distension (overfilling) of the synovial sheath between the suspensory ligament and the cannon bone, or of the synovial sheath between the long pastern and the middle inferior sesamoidean ligament.

WINDSUCKING: An undesirable habit of some horses in which the animal grasps the manger or other object with the incisor teeth, arches the neck, makes peculiar movements with the head, and swallows quantities of air; also called cribbing.

X-RAYS: Roentgen rays, electromagnetic vibrations of short wavelength that penetrate most substances to some degree, used to take radiographs of the body, thus locating fractures, etc.; are used in the treatment of some conditions because of their tissue ionizing ability.

INDEX

G

K

Kanamycin, 467
Kaolin, 446, 457
Keloids, 307
Kenacort, 496
Keratitis
  ectropion, 317
Keratolytic Agents, 449
Keratoma, 224
Kicking, 88
Kidney, 323
Knee, 248 - 251
  carpitis (popped knees), 251
  epiphysitis, 248 - 249
  hygroma of the carpus, 249 - 251
  ruptured extensor carpi radialis, 249
Knock-Knees, 208 - 209
Knocked Down, 265
Knots, 98 - 102
  bowline knot, 98
  cotton neck-rope, 98
  foreleg tie, 101 - 102
  quick-release knot, 98
  tail tie, 98 - 101
  tying a hindleg/use of a sideline, 102
Knuckling Over
  traumatic division of the digital extensor
  tendon, 241 - 242
Kopertox, 468

L

Laboratory Techniques, 359 - 375
  abdominal paracentesis, 374 - 375
  biopsy, 371 - 373
  culture and sensitivity testing, 373 - 374
  hair analysis, 370 - 371
  hematology, 359 - 369
  tracheal aspiration, 375
  urinalysis, 369 - 370
Lacerations, 124
  corneal, 315
Lameness
  examination, 14 - 15
  foot, 223
  general conditions affecting the musculoskeletal system, 214
Laminitis, 225 - 229
  acute laminitis, 225
  chronic laminitis, 226
  corrective shoeing, 353
  general treatment, 226 - 228
  grain founder, 228
  grass founder, 229
  mechanism of laminitis, 225
  postparturient founder, 228 - 229
  road founder 229
  water founder, 229
Lanolin
  emollient, 445
Laparotomy, 404 - 405
  lateral laparotomy, 405
  midline laparotomy, 405
Lard

  emollient, 445
Laryngeal Hemiplegia
  surgical correction, 400
Laryngeal Ventriculotomy, 400
Laughing Gas, 473
Laxatives, 453
Lead Poisoning, 541
Leg and Foot Examination, 29 - 36
  basic checks for lameness, 30 - 31
  specific tests and use of diagnostic aids, 31 -
  36
Leg Bandages, 134
  leg injuries, 134
  leg protection, 134
Leg Injuries, 134
  bandaging the knee, hock, & fetlock, 135
  cold water bandage, 141 - 142
  hot water bandage, 142
  ice bandage, 142
  poultice bandage, 139 - 140
  pressure bandages, 138 - 139
  sweat bandage, 141
  temporary cast bandage, 137
  "Thomas Jones" emergency splint for a
  fracture, 138
Leg Protection, 143
  exercise bandage, 144
  rundown bandages and speed patches, 145
  running bandages, 144 - 145
  standing and shipping bandages, 143
  support bandage, 143 - 144
Leptospirosis
  vaccine, 54
Leukoencephalomalacia, 544
Librium, 474
Lidocaine, 480
Lignocaine, 480
Lime, 463
Liniments and Braces, 148
Linseed Oil
  emollient, 445
  irritant cathartic, 454
Lip Tattooing, 44
Lipomas
  colic, 268
Liver, 322 - 323
Liver & Kidney Conditions, 322 - 323
Local Anesthetics, 479 - 481
  field block anesthesia, 480
  infiltration anesthesia, 481
  precautions, 481
  restraint, 114
  surface or topical anesthesia, 480
Locally Acting Enzymes, 449 - 450
Locoism, 544
Lone Star Tick, 68
Long Bone Fracture Repair
  considerations in, 219 - 220
Louse
  horsebiting, 66
  horsesucking, 66
Lubricants
  intestinal, 453
Lugol's Iodine, 463
Lupines, 543
Luteinizing Hormone [LH], 513
Luxated Superficial Digital Flexor Tendon, 257
Luxations & Subluxations, 220
Lye, 463